Pharmacology in Veterinary Anesthesia and Analgesia

Pharmacology in Veterinary Anesthesia and Analgesia

Edited by

Turi Aarnes
The Ohio State University
College of Veterinary Medicine
Columbus, OH, USA

Phillip Lerche
The Ohio State University
College of Veterinary Medicine
Columbus, OH, USA

WILEY Blackwell

Library of Congress Cataloging-in-Publication Data
Names: Aarnes, Turi K. (Turi Kenna), editor. | Lerche, Phillip, editor.
Title: Pharmacology in veterinary anesthesia and analgesia / edited by Turi
  Aarnes, Phillip Lerche.
Description: Hoboken, NJ : Wiley-Blackwell, [2024] | Includes
  bibliographical references and index.
Identifiers: LCCN 2024000508 (print) | LCCN 2024000509 (ebook) | ISBN
  9781118975138 (cloth) | ISBN 9781118975145 (adobe pdf) | ISBN
  9781118975152 (epub)
Subjects: MESH: Anesthesia–veterinary | Analgesia–veterinary |
  Anesthetics–pharmacology | Anesthetics–adverse effects
Classification: LCC SF914 (print) | LCC SF914 (ebook) | NLM SF 914 | DDC
  636.089/796–dc23/eng/20240124
LC record available at https://lccn.loc.gov/2024000508
LC ebook record available at https://lccn.loc.gov/2024000509

Cover Design: Wiley
Cover Image: Dr. Phillip Lerche; Dr. Turi Aarnes

Set in 9.5/12.5pt STIXTwoText by Straive, Pondicherry, India

SKY10068204_022624

Dedication

I would like to thank my colleague, Turi Aarnes, on two fronts. First, Turi's dedication to improving animal care and comfort is exemplary, as demonstrated by her clinical expertise as well as her research focus on the pharmacology of anesthetic and analgesic drugs. Second, for her work on this book; it would not have been published without her unparalleled organizational skills and attention to detail.
I would also like to thank my family for their constant support.
-Phillip Lerche

I would like to thank my family and friends for their support. I would also to like to thank my co-editor Phillip Lerche for his commitment to completing this project. He was my teacher and colleague for many years and I appreciate all he taught me.
-Turi Aarnes

Contents

List of Contributors

Turi K. Aarnes DVM, MS, DACVAA
Associate Professor
Dept. of Veterinary Clinical Sciences
The Ohio State University
Columbus, OH
USA

Anusha Balakrishnan BVSc, DACVECC
Director of Emergency Certificate Education
Veterinary Emergency Group
Chapel Hill, NC
USA

Linda Barter BVSc, MVSc, PhD, DACVAA
Professor
Dept. of Surgical and Radiological Sciences
University of California, Davis
Davis, CA
USA

Sébastien Hyacinthe Bauquier DVM, PhD, DACVAA
Associate Professor
Dept. Of Veterinary Clinical Sciences
University of Melbourne
Melbourne
Australia

Gianluca Bini DVM, DACVAA
Assistant Professor
Dept. of Veterinary Clinical Sciences
Oklahoma State University
Stillwater, OK
USA

Teresa A. Burns DVM, MS, PhD, DACVIM (LAIM)
Associate Professor
Dept. of Veterinary Clinical Sciences
The Ohio State University
Columbus, OH
USA

Jennifer E. Carter DVM, MANZCVS, DACVAA, MClinEd
Professor
Dept. of Veterinary Clinical Sciences
University of Melbourne
Melbourne
Australia

Andrew Claude DVM, DACVAA
Associate Professor
Dept. of Clinical Sciences
Oregon State University
Corvallis, OR
USA

Laurie Cook DVM, DACVIM (Neurology)
Clinical Associate Professor
Dept. of Veterinary Clinical Sciences
The Ohio State University
Columbus, OH
USA

S. Bryce Dooley DVM, MS, DACVAA
Veterinary Anesthesiologist
Allied Veterinary Anesthesia Associates
Chadds Ford, PA
USA

Julien Guillamin Doct Vet, DACVECC, DECVECC
Associate Professor
Dept. of Clinical Sciences
Colorado State University
Fort Collins, CO
USA

Bonnie L. Hay Kraus DVM, DACVS, DACVAA
Associate Professor
Dept. of Veterinary Clinical Sciences
Iowa State University
Ames, IA
USA

Ashley C. Hechler DVM, MS, DACVIM (Neurology)
Neurologist and Neurosurgeon
Bark City Veterinary Specialists
Park City, UT
USA

John A.E. Hubbell DVM, MS, DACVAA
Chief of Anesthesia
Rood and Riddle Equine Hospital
Paris, KY
USA

Martin Kennedy DVM, DACVAA
Veterinary Anesthesiologist
Dept. of Dental Care & Oral Surgery
The Veterinary Dental Group
Nashville, TN
USA

Jeffrey Lakritz DVM, PhD, DACVIM, DACVCP
Professor
Dept. of Veterinary Clinical Sciences
The Ohio State University
Columbus, OH
USA

Phillip Lerche BVSc, PhD, DACVAA
Professor – Clinical
Dept. of Veterinary Clinical Sciences
The Ohio State University
Columbus, OH
USA

Lydia Love DVM, DACVAA
Clinical Assistant Professor
Dept. of Molecular Biomedical Sciences
North Carolina State University
Raleigh, NC
USA

Manuel Martin-Flores MV, DACVAA
Associate Professor
Dept. of Clinical Sciences
Cornell University
Ithaca, NY
USA

Daniel M. Sakai MV, DACVAA
Assistant Professor
Dept. of Small Animal Medicine & Surgery
University of Georgia
Athens, GA
USA

Reza Seddighi DVM, MS, PhD, DACVAA
Professor
Dept. of Large Animal Clinical Sciences
University of Tennessee
Knoxville, TN
USA

Caitlin Tearney DVM, DACVAA
Assistant Professor
Dept. of Veterinary Clinical Sciences
University of Minnesota
St. Paul, MN
USA

Lance C. Visser DVM, MS, DACVIM (Cardiology)
Associate Professor
Dept. of Clinical Sciences
Colorado State University
Fort Collins, CO
USA

Erin Wendt-Hornickle DVM, DACVAA
Associate Professor
Dept. of Veterinary Clinical Sciences
University of Minnesota
St. Paul, MN
USA

Craig Willette DVM, MS, DACVAA
Clinical Assistant Professor
Dept. of Veterinary Clinical Sciences
Iowa State University
Ames, IA
USA

Preface

The practice of veterinary anesthesia is continually evolving as the understanding and treatment of animal diseases expands. Our patients are living longer than ever before, often with one or more co-morbidities that require ongoing treatment with pharmaceuticals, many of which can have an impact on anesthetic management. Newer drugs, and different formulations of drugs, are also being added to the veterinarian's armamentarium in the various veterinary specialties, for example, behavior medicine and cardiology. It is not always easy to collate relevant information about the impact of anesthesia on a specific drug, or the impact of a drug on anesthesia, as information is often scattered throughout the academic literature.

Our aim with compiling this volume is to create a single reference dedicated to anesthetic drug pharmacology, and anesthetic interactions with drugs commonly used to treat health problems in animals. We hope that this textbook will be a useful reference for anyone performing veterinary anesthesia, whether they are a specialist veterinarian, a private practitioner, a veterinary technician, or a student.

We would like to thank all of the contributing authors without whom this book would not have been possible. We also want to thank Tim Vojt of the Biomedical Media department of The Ohio State University College of Veterinary Medicine.

1

Pharmacokinetics and Pharmacodynamics

Phillip Lerche and Jeffrey Lakritz

Introduction

Pharmacokinetic studies describe the time course of drugs from administration to removal from the body, and pharmacodynamics evaluates the effects drugs have on the various body systems. The basic concepts of pharmacokinetics and pharmacodynamics with reference to drugs commonly used in the peri-anesthetic period will be reviewed in this chapter. The unique aspects of inhalant anesthetic pharmacokinetics are discussed in Chapter 10.

Pharmacokinetics

Drug disposition refers to the processes of absorption, distribution, metabolism and excretion within the body after the drug is administered. In order for drugs to exert their effects when given by routes other than intravenous administration (IV), they must first be absorbed into the central compartment (i.e. the systemic circulation), from where they are distributed to the site of action. Distribution is followed by metabolism (biotransformation) and, finally, the drug and/or its metabolites are eliminated from the body (Caldwell et al. 1995).

Absorption and Bioavailability

Absorption refers to the movement of a drug from its site of administration into the central compartment. Most anesthetic and other drugs given in the peri-anesthetic period are given IV, thus bypassing the absorption phase. Advantages to this include the ability to have an almost immediate effect, (e.g. IV induction of anesthesia with propofol allows for rapid tracheal intubation, thus protecting the airway), to titrate the dosage to effect, to administer large volumes, and for emergency treatment. A disadvantage is that an overdose can rapidly lead to serious side effects.

In order to be absorbed, drugs must cross cell membranes. Drugs that are weak acids or weak bases are typically ionizable. That is, in solution, they exist in two forms: the non-ionized form which is lipid soluble and readily diffusible, and the ionized form which has lower lipid solubility and is poorly diffusible. Distribution of ionizable drugs across cell membranes is related to the drug's pK_a, which is the pH at which 50% of the drug is ionized, and 50% is non-ionized. In the presence of a pH higher than a weak acidic drug's pK_a, dissociation will be favored, and in the presence of a pH lower than that drug's pK_a, non-ionization will be favored. The opposite is true for weak bases – at a pH below the pK_a, the drug will be more ionized, while a pH above the pK_a will result in more non-ionized drug (see Table 1.1). As an example, a weakly acidic drug will be readily absorbed in the highly acidic environment of the stomach as the pH favors non-ionization, whereas a weakly basic drug will be more non-ionized and readily absorbed in the alkaline environment of the small intestine.

Absorption can be a passive process (e.g. diffusion), or an active process (via active transporters). Most anesthetic drugs move across cell membranes by passive diffusion along a concentration gradient. The family of ABC transporters actively removes some drugs from cells and includes the P-glycoprotein (P-gp) transporter that is coded by the *ABCB1* (*MDR1*) gene. In dogs that have homozygous mutations of this gene, P-gp transporters are nonfunctional. This can result in toxicity with some drugs (e.g. ivermectin in Collies), as well as prolonged activity of acepromazine and opioids (Deshpande et al. 2016; Martinez et al. 2008).

Bioavailability is the fraction (*F*) of a drug that reaches the central compartment after administration, and can be expressed as follows:

$$F = \text{amount of drug entering the systemic circulation} / \text{amount of drug administered}$$

Table 1.1 Impact of pH on ionization of weak acids and weak bases as it relates to a drug's pK_a, and the impact on absorption.

	$pH = pK_a$	$pH < pK_a$	$pH > pK_a$
Weak acid	Non-ionized = ionized $$HA \rightleftharpoons A^- + H^+$$	Non-ionized > ionized Absorption ↑	Non-ionized < ionized Absorption ↓
Weak base	Non-ionized = ionized $$BA \rightleftharpoons B + H^+$$	Non-ionized < ionized Absorption ↓	Non-ionized > ionized Absorption ↑

pK_a is the pH at which the drug is in equilibrium between the non-ionized and ionized form. The non-ionized form of the drug is more lipophilic and therefore more readily absorbed.
$\rightleftharpoons$ indicates that non-ionized and ionized forms are in equilibrium.

Bioavailability therefore ranges from 0 to 1, depending on route of administration. $F = 1$ after IV administration of drugs. Drugs given by the subcutaneous (SC) and intramuscular (IM) routes typically result in bioavailability above 0.75. Bioavailability after oral administration is highly variable, and dependent on multiple factors (e.g. impact of gastric enzymes on the drug, incomplete absorption in the presence of food, rate of gastric emptying, presence of enteric coating). Drugs absorbed in the gastrointestinal tract (GI) enter the hepatic portal circulation and can undergo first-pass biotransformation and elimination in the liver prior to entering the central compartment.

Drugs that can be absorbed via the oral mucosal surface (oral trans-mucosal, OTM), e.g. dexmedetomidine, buprenorphine, enter the central compartment via venous drainage from the head and neck to the cranial vena cava (Dent et al. 2019; Enomoto et al. 2022). Giving medication by this route has the advantage of being technically less challenging than giving injections, and therefore useful in minimizing stress in patients who are uncooperative for IM, IV, or SC administration. Absorption via the OTM route is determined by the Fick principle of diffusion, where the amount absorbed is directly proportional to drug concentration, drug lipophilicity, the surface area of and duration of contact with the tissue and is indirectly proportional to thickness of the tissue. The presence in the oral mucosa of enzymes that break down peptides can also limit drug absorption via this route (Zhang et al. 2002). Drugs delivered by this route can also be lost to the GI tract due to swallowing, which is likely to result in decreased bioavailability.

Intranasal (IN) administration offers similar advantages to the OTM route in that a large surface area with good blood supply is available for absorption. Naloxone given IN to dogs, for example, was rapidly absorbed with F = 0.32, and buprenorphine administered using a nasal atomization device had F = 0.57 (Wahler et al. 2019; Enomoto et al. 2022). Drawbacks to this route of administration include the drug being lost due to sneezing, head shaking or swallowing. Some animals actively resist placement of nasal drugs, making administration difficult. The presence of excess mucus in the nasal cavity may also decrease absorption.

Absorption of topical and transdermal formulations of drugs (e.g. the topical formulation of buprenorphine Zorbium®, fentanyl patches) occurs via the skin and, as a general rule, is determined by the lipid solubility of the drug and the surface area available (Kukanich and Clark 2012). In the case of fentanyl patches, other factors also play a role (location, body fat composition at the site of placement, body temperature). Damage to the skin surface can enhance absorption of drugs.

The formulation of a drug can impact its absorption. Several drugs with analgesic properties are available in sustained-release formulations that extend the period of absorption over time (e.g. fentanyl patch, liposome encapsulated bupivacaine) (Bartholomew and Smith 2023).

Distribution

After a drug is absorbed into the central compartment, it is distributed to the tissues. Distribution is impacted by regional blood flow and the tissue groups with high blood flow (the vessel rich group) such as the brain, heart, liver, and kidneys initially receive most of the drug. Delivery to the other tissues of the body (muscle, other viscera, skin, fat) takes longer.

Many drugs bind to plasma proteins. Acidic drugs typically bind to albumin, and basic drugs to α_1-acid glycoprotein. Plasma protein binding decreases free drug available for absorption. Decreases in plasma protein binding due to decreased number of binding sites, e.g. with hypoproteinemia, will result in increased drug being unbound in plasma. Many anesthetic drugs are given to effect, e.g. propofol which is highly protein bound (97%), thus, decreased protein binding has limited relevance clinically. The impact of decreased protein binding resulting in an increase in unbound drug may have relevance when the therapeutic index is narrow, e.g. IV lidocaine.

Drugs can accumulate in tissues through tissue binding. The tissue will then act as a reservoir for the drug. Commonly, lipophilic drugs accumulate in adipose tissue.

The endothelial cells of the brain have tight endothelial junctions, thus forming part of the blood-brain barrier. The more lipid soluble a drug is in its unbound, non-ionized form, the more likely it is to cross the blood-brain barrier. Similarly, highly lipid soluble drugs can cross the placenta. Ion trapping of basic drugs may occur in the fetus as the pH is slightly lower than 7.4.

Cessation of drug effect(s) usually occurs when the drug is cleared from the body via metabolism and excretion. In some cases, redistribution of a drug from its site of action to another tissue group can occur. For example, thiopental is cleared slowly, while anesthetic effects wear off relatively rapidly. Return to consciousness cannot be explained by metabolism alone, and is due in part to redistribution (Russo and Bressolle 1998).

Metabolism (Biotransformation)

Lipophilic drugs must be biologically transformed into hydrophilic metabolites in order to be excreted in urine. Metabolism of most drugs occurs via first-order kinetics, i.e. a fraction (or percentage) of the drug is metabolized per unit time. Some drugs, e.g. ethanol (alcohol), are metabolized via zero-order kinetics, i.e. a fixed amount of drug is metabolized per unit time.

The main site of metabolism is the liver, and biotransformation occurs in two steps via microsomal enzyme activity. Firstly, phase 1 reactions change the parent drug via oxidation, reduction, or hydrolysis. Phase 1 enzymes include cytochrome P450 (CYP) enzymes, non-CYP enzymes, and flavin-containing monooxygenase (FMO) enzymes. Metabolism via these enzymes results in exposure of, or addition of, a functional group, e.g. -OH, $-COOH$, $-SH$, -O-, or NH_2 to the drug molecule. Functional group addition usually makes the drug inactive, but does not make the drug less lipophilic. Some inactive drugs (called prodrugs) can be activated by phase 1 reactions. Metabolites of active drugs are usually inactive; however, some may have biological effects. Additionally, some drugs can induce activity in phase 1 enzymes, resulting in increased clearance of other drugs biotransformed in the same pathway, e.g. pentobarbital increases the clearance of propranolol (Branch and Herman 1984). Secondly, enzymes involved in phase 2 reactions conjugate the products of phase 1 with another molecule (e.g. an acetyl group, glucuronic acid, glutathione, sulfate), resulting in metabolites that are more hydrophilic, which makes them pass more easily into the aqueous environment of urine or bile. Phase 2 enzymes include glucuronosyltransferases, glutathione-S-transferases (GST), methyltransferases, N-acetyl-transferases (NAT), and sulfotransferases (SULT).

The lung is a site for drug metabolism, with the most important enzymes being CYP, FMO, carboxyl esterase, GST, NAT, and SULT (Enlo-Scott et al. 2021). Drugs can also be metabolized in the kidneys and the GI tract (e.g. biotransformation by transferases) (Rowland et al. 2013). In plasma, drugs can undergo Hoffman elimination, e.g. atracurium, and ester hydrolysis, e.g. remifentanil (Neill et al. 1983; Egan et al. 1993).

Elimination

The kidney is the main organ of drug elimination, and both unchanged drug and drug metabolites can be excreted into the urine. Compounds that are highly lipophilic are less readily eliminated compared to water soluble (polar) molecules, which move into the aqueous urine more easily. The process of renal elimination involves glomerular filtration, active tubular secretion, and passive tubular reabsorption. Glomerular filtration rate (GFR) and whether or not a drug is protein bound determines how much drug enters the proximal renal tubular lumen. Only compounds that are not bound to proteins are available for filtration. Non-ionized forms of drug (i.e. more lipophilic) can be reabsorbed from the distal renal tubular lumen via passive diffusion. The pH of the urine will influence reabsorption in the same way that pH influences absorption. Acidic urine will favor reabsorption of weak acids and excretion of weak bases, whereas alkaline urine will favor reabsorption of weak bases and excretion of weak acids.

Drugs can also be excreted by the liver into bile, which then enters the intestinal tract. Parent compounds and metabolites can be reabsorbed from the intestines. This is referred to as enterohepatic recycling, and can lead to extended drug activity.

Pharmacokinetic Models

Mathematical modeling of pharmacokinetics is used to describe the time course of a drug's disposition in the various body compartments. Drug disposition is comprised of drug distribution and elimination. Key parameters affecting drug disposition include bioavailability (defined above), apparent volume of distribution (often abbreviated to volume of distribution), elimination half-life and clearance.

Apparent Volume of Distribution

Apparent volume of distribution (V) is the theoretical fluid volume that would be required to produce a given plasma (or blood) concentration (C) for the amount of drug in the body (A).

$$V = A/C \qquad (1.1)$$

If a drug is administered IV, then A is equal to the dose administered

$$V = Dose/C \qquad (1.2)$$

The apparent volume of distribution can vastly exceed the body's total fluid volume for highly lipophilic drugs. For example, V for propofol is reported as 6.5 l/kg in dogs (Nolan and Reid 1993). In other words, V does not usually correspond to a physiologic volume of the body like blood volume. If V is known for a drug, Eq. (1.2) can be used to calculate the dose needed to achieve a specific C.

$$\text{Dose} = V \cdot C \tag{1.3}$$

Elimination Half-Life

The concentration immediately after a dose is administered IV, C(0), can be extrapolated from a C versus time (t) plot. Anesthetic and analgesic drugs are commonly eliminated by first-order kinetics. When a semilogarithmic plot of C is graphed against time (Figure 1.1a), the straight line obtained is described by the following equation, where k is the slope of the line:

$$\ln C = \ln C(0) - kt \tag{1.4}$$

Equation (1.4) can be transformed by taking the antilogarithm of both sides.

$$C = C(0) \cdot e^{-kt} \tag{1.5}$$

Both sides can be multiplied by V, giving:

$$V \cdot C = V \cdot C(0) \cdot e^{-kt} \tag{1.6}$$

Since $V \cdot C$ represents the amount of drug in the body (A), and $V \cdot C(0)$ is the dose, then:

$$A = \text{Dose} \cdot e^{-kt} \tag{1.7}$$

Equations (1.5) and (1.7) can be used to estimate C and A at any point in time. Elimination half-life ($t_{1/2}$) is defined as the time it takes for C to decrease by half (Figure 1.1a, b). It follows that one half-life would be the time taken for C(0) to decrease to ½ of C(0). Equation (1.5) can therefore be expressed as:

$$\tfrac{1}{2} \cdot C(0) = C(0) \cdot e^{-kt_{1/2}} \tag{1.8}$$

This can be simplified to:

$$\tfrac{1}{2} = e^{-kt_{1/2}} \tag{1.9}$$

Inverting yields:

$$2 = e^{kt_{1/2}} \tag{1.10}$$

The natural logarithm of both sides gives:

$$0.693 = kt_{1/2} \tag{1.11}$$

This can be rearranged as follows to give $t_{1/2}$:

$$t_{1/2} = 0.693/k \tag{1.12}$$

The constant, k, represents the slope of the line from Eq. (1.4) and can also be calculated using Eq. (1.12) if the

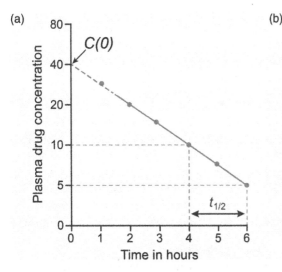

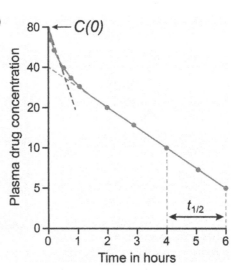

Figure 1.1 Semilogarithmic plots of plasma concentration of drug vs time. (a) Plasma concentrations plotted over time yield a straight line. The first plasma sample is taken at one hour after IV administration. Extrapolation of the line (the dashed portion of the line) yields the plasma concentration at time 0: C(0). Elimination half-life ($t_{1/2}$) is the time required for plasma concentration to decrease by 50%. If the extrapolated C(0) matched the measured C(0), this plot would represent a one-compartment pharmacokinetic model, where the drug does not distribute outside of the central compartment. The log of plasma concentration vs time relationship can be described by the equation for a single straight line. (b) Increased frequency of plasma sampling between 0 and 1 hour results in the line obtained becoming curved between those time points. In this theoretical example, the latter part of the curve is identical to 1.1a, however C(0) is not accurately predicted by extrapolation of this terminal part of the curve. This shows that the drug distributes into more than one compartment, i.e. the central compartment and a tissue compartment. In a two-compartment model, the equation describing the curve is comprised of two lines, one for each compartment.

value for $t_{1/2}$ is known. It can also be related to the amount of drug in the body (A) as it changes over time by differentiating Eq. (1.7):

$$dA/dt = -k \cdot dose \cdot e^{-kt_{1/2}} \qquad (1.13)$$

Since $A = Dose \cdot e^{-kt}$,

$$dA/dt = -k \cdot A \qquad (1.14)$$

dA/dt is the rate of change of a drug in the body and is equal to the rate of elimination. Rearranging Eq. (1.14) yields:

$$k = \text{rate of drug elimination / amount of}$$
$$\text{drug in the body} \qquad (1.15)$$

The rate constant k in Eq. (1.15) describes elimination and is known as the elimination rate constant. Equation (1.7) can be arranged to show that the fraction of drug remaining in the body (A/dose) equals e^{-kt}.

$$A/dose = e^{-kt} \qquad (1.16)$$

From Eq. (1.11), $k = 0.693/t_{1/2}$, therefore:

$$A/dose = e^{-0.693/t_{1/2}} \qquad (1.17)$$

The right side of Eq. (1.17) can also be expressed in general terms of the number of half-lives, n, that have passed since the drug was given, where $n = t/t_{1/2}$.

$$A/dose = e^{-0.693n} \qquad (1.18)$$

The value of $e^{-0.693}$ is ½, giving:

$$A/dose = \left(\tfrac{1}{2}\right)^{n} \qquad (1.19)$$

The fraction of drug remaining in the body for different values of n can be determined (Table 1.2). After five half-lives approximately 3% of the original dose is left, i.e. 97% has been eliminated. While a drug will continue to be in the body in evermore declining fractions of the original

Table 1.2 Fraction of the drug as a percentage remaining in the body as it relates to the number of elapsed half-lives.

Number of half-lives (n in Eq. (1.20))	Fraction of drug remaining (%)	Fraction of drug eliminated (%)
0	100	0
1	0.5 × 100 = 50	50
2	0.5 × 50 = 25	75
3	0.5 × 25 = 12.5	87.5
4	0.5 × 12.5 = 6.25	93.75
5	0.5 × 6.25 = 3.125	96.875
6	0.5 × 3.125 = 1.5625	98.4375

A drug is considered to have been effectively eliminated after five half-lives.

dose, in practical terms, it can be considered to have been effectively eliminated after five half-lives.

Clearance

Total body, i.e. systemic, clearance (CL) relates the concentration of a drug to its rate of elimination. When clearance is at a constant rate:

$$\text{Rate of elimination} = CL \cdot C \qquad (1.20)$$

Since the rate of elimination = $k \cdot A$ (Eq. (1.15)), and $A = V \cdot C$ (Eq. (1.3)),

$$\text{Rate of elimination} = k \cdot V \cdot C \qquad (1.21)$$

Rearranging Eq. (1.20) gives:

$$CL = \text{rate of elimination}/C \qquad (1.22)$$

Substituting rate of elimination = $k \cdot V \cdot C$ from Eq. (1.21) yields:

$$CL = k \cdot V \qquad (1.23)$$

From Eq. (1.12), $t_{1/2} = 0.693/k$, and from Eq. (1.23), $k = CL/V$. Half-life can therefore be related to the independent variable's clearance and volume of distribution as follows:

$$t_{1/2} = 0.693 \cdot V/CL \qquad (1.24)$$

Clearance can be determined independently of the elimination half-life. Equation (1.22) can be used to express the amount of drug eliminated in a period of time (dt) as follows:

$$\text{Amount eliminated during dt} = CL \cdot C \cdot dt \qquad (1.25)$$

If dt represents a short interval of time, e.g. one minute, $C \cdot dt$ is equal to the area under the drug concentration versus time curve (AUC) for that short period of time. The AUC for the entire time course of elimination is given by mathematical integration of the whole drug concentration vs time curve such that:

$$AUC = \text{amount of drug eliminated}/CL \qquad (1.26)$$

When a drug is administered IV, the amount of drug eliminated is equal to the dose. Rearranging Eq. (1.26) yields:

$$Dose = CL \cdot AUC \qquad (1.27)$$

Clearance can therefore be determined independently of volume of distribution and $t_{1/2}$. Equations (1.23) and (1.27) can be used to determine volume of distribution. Rearranging Eq. (1.23) gives $V = CL/k$. Substituting for clearance gives:

$$V = Dose/\left(AUC \cdot k\right) \qquad (1.28)$$

Equation (1.28) shows that volume of distribution can be calculated without extrapolating to time zero from the concentration versus time curve that was described earlier.

The most important organs involved in eliminating drugs are the liver and kidneys. Other organs can also contribute to clearance e.g. the lungs. Total body clearance is therefore given by:

$$CL = CL_{hepatic} + CL_{renal} + CL_{other} \qquad (1.29)$$

Hepatic Clearance The amount of drug that enters the liver via the arterial blood supply equals hepatic blood (Q_H) × the drug concentration in arterial blood (C_A). Similarly, the amount of drug exiting the organ is Q_H × the drug concentration in venous blood (C_V). Rate of elimination is therefore:

$$\begin{aligned} \text{Rate of elimination} &= Q_H \cdot C_A - Q_H \cdot C_V \\ &= Q_H \cdot (C_A - C_V) \end{aligned} \qquad (1.30)$$

Since clearance equals rate of elimination/drug concentration, Eq. (1.30) can be related to clearance by dividing both sides by C_A.

$$CL_H = Q_H \cdot (C_A - C_V)/C_A \qquad (1.31)$$

In Eq. (1.31), $(C_A - C_V)/C_A$ is termed the extraction ratio (ER), giving:

$$CL_H = Q_H \cdot ER \qquad (1.32)$$

The processes responsible for drug elimination that occur in the liver, indeed, in any organ, do not have infinite capacity, and can become saturated. This occurs when the rate at which a drug is presented to the liver exceeds the liver's capacity to clear the drug. The maximum capacity of an organ to clear a drug is referred to as the intrinsic clearance (CL_i) of that organ. ER and CL_i are related as follows:

$$ER = CL_i/(Q + CL_i) \qquad (1.33)$$

Combining Equations (1.33) and (1.31) gives the relationship between hepatic clearance and intrinsic clearance:

$$CL_H = Q_H \cdot CL_i/(Q_H + CL_i) \qquad (1.34)$$

When intrinsic clearance is very small compared to hepatic blood flow, CL_i in the denominator of Eq. (1.34) can be ignored, giving:

$$CL_H = Q_H \cdot CL_i/Q_H \qquad (1.35)$$

Equation (1.35) can then be expressed as:

$$CL_H = CL_i \qquad (1.36)$$

In this case, clearance depends on the intrinsic clearance of the liver and not hepatic blood flow.

When the amount of drug presented to the liver is much less than the intrinsic clearance for that drug, clearance is a function of hepatic blood flow. CL_i in the denominator of Eq. (1.34) can be ignored, giving:

$$CL_H = Q_H \cdot CL_i/CL_i \qquad (1.37)$$

This can then be written as:

$$CL_H = Q_H \qquad (1.38)$$

As an example, lidocaine is cleared very efficiently by the liver, and therefore clearance is determined by hepatic blood flow. This is demonstrated in a study by Feary et al. (2005) which showed that clearance of lidocaine administered as an infusion to awaken horses was 29 ml/min/kg, whereas in sevoflurane anesthetized horses clearance was 15 ml/min/kg, a reduction of approximately 50% (Feary et al. 2005). The decrease in clearance is attributed to decreased liver blood flow as a result of the significant decrease in cardiac output that occurs under inhalant anesthesia in horses.

Renal Clearance Renal clearance (CL_R) is defined as the rate of change of drug in the urine compared to the plasma concentration of drug.

$$CL_R = \text{excretion rate}/C \qquad (1.39)$$

Renal clearance is determined by renal filtration, renal tubular secretion and renal tubular reabsorption.

$$\begin{aligned} CL_R = (&\text{filtration rate} + \text{secretion rate} \\ &- \text{reabsorption rate})/C \end{aligned} \qquad (1.40)$$

If secretion and reabsorption rates are low, renal clearance is then a function of GFR.

$$CL_R = GFR/C \qquad (1.41)$$

Additionally, only a drug that is free (i.e. not protein bound) is available for renal clearance. The unbound fraction of drug (fu) is given by the following, where C_u is the concentration of unbound drug:

$$fu = C_u/C \qquad (1.42)$$

Renal filtration rate is then:

$$\text{Filtration rate} = GFR \cdot fu \cdot C \qquad (1.43)$$

If there is no renal secretion or reabsorption, the filtration rate in Eq. (1.41) can be replaced using Eq. (1.43), giving:

$$CL_R = GFR \cdot fu \cdot C/C \qquad (1.44)$$

Renal clearance is therefore:

$$CL_R = GFR \cdot fu \qquad (1.45)$$

In cases were fu = 1, i.e. when a drug does not bind to proteins, renal clearance is equal to the GFR. When renal clearance exceeds or is less than the GFR, this indicates that the drug is being actively secreted by, or is being reabsorbed from, the renal tubules.

Compartmental Models

Compartmental models of drug disposition are used to obtain pharmacokinetic variables that help to predict drug concentration, and therefore drug effect(s). Statistical pharmacokinetic software uses drug plasma concentrations over time to predict the model that fits best. Most drugs can be modeled as one-, two- or three-compartment models. The first compartment is referred to as the central compartment, and the others are peripheral compartments.

A one-compartment model is shown in Figure 1.2a. A dose of drug given directly into, or absorbed into, the compartment (I represents input) distributes into the volume (V) of the compartment, and is eliminated over time (k is the elimination constant). In the case of a one-compartment model, the change in plasma concentration over time [C(t)] is described by the following exponential equation:

$$C(t) = e^{-kt} \qquad (1.46)$$

The semilogarithmic plot of plasma concentration vs time yields a single straight line, like the one shown in Figure 1.1a. The dose required to reach a target plasma concentration for a one-compartment model can be calculated using Eq. (1.3), clearance can be determined from Eq. (1.23), and $t_{1/2}$ from Eq. (1.24).

In the case of a two-compartment model, the drug is eliminated from the central compartment and distributed to (and can return from) a peripheral compartment (Figure 1.2b). The semilogarithmic plasma concentration vs time plot will yield a curve comprised of two overlapping straight lines (Figure 1.1b). The initial phase has a steeper slope compared to the second phase. Change of plasma drug concentration over time in a two-compartment model is given by:

$$C(t) = Ae^{-\alpha t} + Be^{-\beta t} \qquad (1.47)$$

A three-compartment model has two peripheral compartments connected to the central compartment with different equilibration rates (rapid and slow) (Figure 1.2c). This model's semilogarithmic plasma concentration vs time plot will be comprised of three overlapping straight lines. The equation for change of plasma concentration over time contains three exponential terms:

$$C(t) = Ae^{-\alpha t} + Be^{-\beta t} + Ce^{-\gamma t} \qquad (1.48)$$

Compartmental pharmacokinetic analysis is a simplification of how drugs are distributed within the body, as each organ has its own specific blood flow. Physiologic-based models can be used to give a clearer picture of a drug's pharmacokinetics. Pharmacokinetic parameters can also be determined using non-compartmental analysis. A discussion of pharmacokinetics of these models is outside the scope of this chapter.

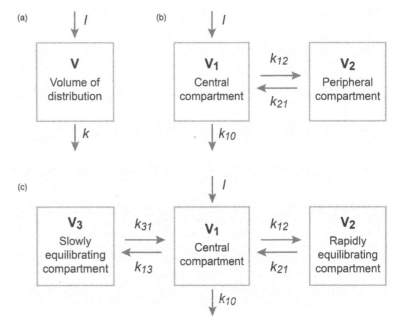

Figure 1.2 Compartmental pharmacokinetic models. (a) A one-compartmental model, where the compartment is the central compartment, i.e. the drug does not move out of the blood into the tissues. *I* represents input, i.e. IV drug dose or a drug that enters the compartment via absorption. V represents volume of distribution, and k is the elimination constant. (b) A two-compartment model showing a central compartment and a peripheral tissue compartment with their own volumes of distribution, V_1 and V_2. k_{12} and k_{21} are the equilibrium constants between the compartments, and k_{10} is the elimination constant. (c) A three-compartment model showing two peripheral compartments connected to the central compartments. The two peripheral tissue compartments are a more rapidly equilibrating one and a more slowly equilibrating one. Each compartment will have its own volume of distribution, with multiple constants describing drug equilibration between compartments.

Infusion Pharmacokinetics

Up to this point, the pharmacokinetics of a single dose have been discussed. For a continuous drug effect, repeated boluses can be given, with peaks and troughs of drug plasma concentration stabilizing after about 5 half-lives (Figure 1.3). A true steady state plasma concentration (C_{ss}) can be achieved by administering a drug by infusion. This is useful for drugs with a narrow therapeutic range, and for those with very short half-lives, e.g. catecholamines like norepinephrine where $t_{1/2}$ is measured in minutes. Use of infusions is commonplace in veterinary anesthesia, e.g. to provide analgesia and/or reduce inhalant requirements (opioids, lidocaine, ketamine), for cardiovascular support (inotropes) or as total IV anesthesia (propofol).

Since it takes about 5 half-lives to reach steady state, a bolus or loading dose can be given for drugs that have relatively long half-lives (Figure 1.4). This can be determined using Eq. (1.3). If V_{SS} equals volume of distribution at steady state, then:

$$\text{Loading dose} = C \cdot V_{SS} \qquad (1.49)$$

Loading doses are useful when the half-life of a drug is relatively long, so that the desired plasma concentration at steady state can be reached sooner. In a one-compartment model, once steady state has been reached, the rate at

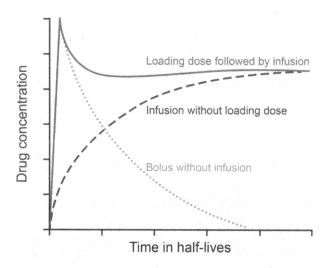

Figure 1.4 Semilogarithmic plot of drug concentration vs time for a constant rate infusion with and without a loading dose. The blue line (dotted) represents the plasma concentration vs time course of a loading dose. The red line (dashed) represents the time taken to reach steady state after starting a constant rate infusion. To reach steady state earlier, a loading dose can be given (purple solid line).

which a drug needs to be added is equal to the desired plasma concentration × clearance.

$$\text{Maintenance infusion rate} = C \cdot CL \qquad (1.50)$$

Note that once a true plasma concentration steady state has been reached, kinetics can be characterized as a zero-order process, i.e. a fixed amount of drug is added and removed per unit time. This concept also applies to the pharmacokinetics of fentanyl patches, where a specific dose per unit time is delivered (Lötsch et al. 2013). Equation (1.50) is also valid for two- and three-compartment models once all compartments have reached equilibrium. This may not occur for some time, particularly with slowly equilibrating tissue compartments. Under circumstances where it takes hours to reach equilibration, using this equation will underestimate the plasma concentration, since the drug will still be moving into the third compartment. The following equation is used for an infusion where the drug distributes in a three-compartment model, where C_T is the target plasma concentration:

$$\begin{aligned}&\text{Maintenance infusion rate}\\&= C_T \cdot V_1 \cdot \left(k_{10} + k_{12}e^{-k_{21}t} + k_{13}e^{-k_{31}t} \right)\end{aligned} \qquad (1.51)$$

For example, in dogs, after an IV bolus of propofol (4 mg/kg), use of a constant rate infusion of propofol (0.4 mg/kg/min) for maintenance of anesthesia for

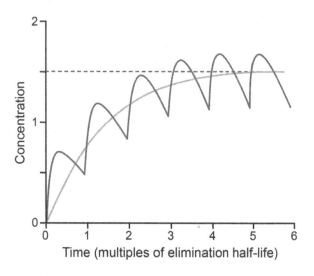

Figure 1.3 Semilogarithmic plot of drug concentration vs time comparing intermittent dosing to constant rate infusion. Time is given in multiples of elimination half-life, the time it takes drug concentration to increase (or decrease) by 50% from a previous value. It takes approximately 5 half-lives to reach steady state. The blue curve demonstrates peaks and troughs of drug concentration observed with intermittent dosing. Administration of a drug by constant rate infusion (orange curve) smooths out the peaks and valleys, allowing a drug to reach a steady state (dashed line).

60 minutes resulted in a steady rise in plasma concentration (Nolan and Reid 1993). This rise in plasma concentration can be ameliorated by decreasing the rate of infusion in a stepwise fashion over time. This is most commonly achieved in veterinary anesthetic practice by manually changing the rate of delivery of an infusion (or syringe) pump. Pharmacokinetic data can be used in conjunction with computer programing to create devices that can deliver a drug to target a specific plasma concentration, i.e. target-controlled infusion systems. The operator chooses the target plasma concentration, and the device alters the infusion rate in accordance with pharmacokinetic data to achieve that concentration. Target-controlled infusion systems have been evaluated for propofol in dogs and cats, and for ketamine in ponies, however, this anesthetic delivery technique remains a research tool in veterinary anesthesia (Beths et al. 2001; Cattai et al. 2016; Levionnois et al. 2010).

The concept of elimination half-life was previously discussed in the context of administering a single bolus with minimal distribution to peripheral compartments. When a drug is given by infusion over a period of time long enough to allow significant distribution to peripheral compartments, the concept of context-sensitive half time is useful. Context-sensitive half-time is the time for drug plasma concentration to decrease by 50% when the drug is being administered by infusion such that plasma concentration is at steady state. Context-sensitive half-time is not a fixed value, instead, it increases as the duration of infusion administration increases until equilibrium among compartments is reached.

Pharmacodynamics

Pharmacodynamics is the study of the effect of drugs on the body, with the vast majority of drugs acting via interaction with receptors. Molecules, both endogenous (e.g. natural hormones) and exogenous (e.g. drugs), that bind to receptors (R) are referred to as ligands (L).

Receptors

Receptors can be grouped into families based on shared structure and similarity of function. Major receptor families relevant to drugs used in the peri-anesthetic period include ion channels, transmembrane enzymes and G protein-coupled receptors (GPCR). Ion channels include voltage-gated channels, e.g. sodium channels which are a target for local anesthetics, and ligand-gated channels, e.g. neurotransmitter receptors like gamma-aminobutyric acid (GABA), a target for some injectable anesthetics such as propofol. Transmembrane receptors that are linked to intracellular enzymes include receptor tyrosine kinases like the insulin receptor. The family of GCPRs is large, and includes opioid, adrenergic and muscarinic receptors. In the basal state, GPCR consist of seven membrane-spanning helixes coupled with an intracellular G protein consisting of three subunits (Gα, Gβ, and Gγ) that forms a complex connected to the intracellular helix loops, with GDP connected to the Gα subunit (Figure 1.5). Binding of a ligand to the receptor results in a conformational change that stimulates GDP release and binding of GTP to the Gα subunit. The activated Gα unit and Gβγ complex are now able to bind to effectors, resulting in actions, or signals, via second

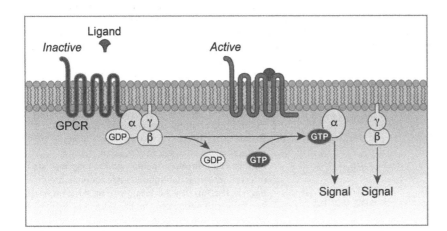

Figure 1.5 G protein-coupled receptor. In the basal state, G protein-coupled receptors consist of seven membrane-spanning helixes coupled with an intracellular G protein. The G protein consists of three subunits (Gα, Gβ, and Gγ) that forms a trimeric complex connected to the intracellular helix loops, with GDP connected to the Gα subunit. Binding of a ligand to the receptor results in a conformational change that stimulates GDP release and binding of GTP to the Gα subunit. The activated Gα unit and Gβγ dimer are now able to bind to effectors, resulting in actions, or signals, via second messengers. Ligands can be endogenous (e.g. hormones, neurotransmitters, opioids) or exogenous (e.g. drugs, toxins).

messengers like cyclic AMP. Traditionally, GPCRs were thought to be inactive in the basal state, only becoming active through ligand binding. More recently, it has been shown that these receptors can exist in two states in the absence of ligand binding: they can be inactive (R) or have some basal level of activity (R*). This two state model can be expressed as follows:

$$R \rightleftharpoons R^*$$

When a ligand is present, the ligand-receptor relationship is:

$$L + R \rightleftharpoons LR \rightleftharpoons LR^*$$

Drug-receptor Interactions

Drug action at a receptor is influenced by the degree to which it binds to the receptor (affinity) as well as the drug's ability to cause a response once bound to the receptor (efficacy).

A drug with high affinity for a receptor will bind more readily to a receptor than a drug with low affinity. Therefore at equilibrium, a greater fraction (or percent) of a high affinity drug will be bound to receptors compared to a low affinity drug.

Ligands (drugs) that produce an increased response when they bind to receptors are called agonists (Figure 1.6). The ability of a drug to produce an effect is known as its efficacy. A full agonist is a ligand that can activate a receptor to a maximal extent (e.g. morphine). Agonists that produce a submaximal response are referred to as partial agonists (e.g. buprenorphine). Morphine is therefore more efficacious than buprenorphine. Ligands are said to be antagonists when they effectively occupy the receptor and do not change its level of activity (e.g. naloxone). Antagonism can be competitive or non-competitive. Antagonism from a competitive antagonist can be overcome by increasing the concentration (i.e. dose) of an agonist. In contrast, non-competitive antagonism cannot be overcome by increasing the concentration of an agonist. Some drugs can have agonist activity at one receptor, and antagonist activity at another (e.g. butorphanol, which is a kappa opioid receptor agonist and a mu opioid receptor antagonist). Such drugs are referred to as agonist-antagonists. Ligands can also decrease the level of activity when binding to a receptor that has a basal level of activity, i.e. receptors in the R* state, in which they are referred to as inverse agonists (Sato et al. 2016).

Potency refers to the amount of drug required to exert an effect. If less drug (lower plasma concentration) is required to produce an effect compared to another drug, the first drug is more potent, i.e. as potency increases, the more a dose/effect curve moves to the left (Figure 1.7). Note that in Figure 1.7, all three drugs are able to reach maximum

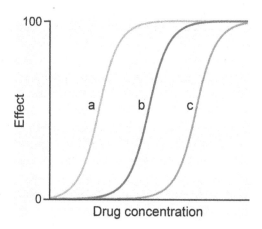

Figure 1.7 Potency. Potency is the amount of a drug required to exert an effect. Drug *a* is more potent than drugs *b* and *c* because a lower plasma concentration is required to exert the same effect as either *a* or *b*. Note that all three drugs shown here have the same efficacy.

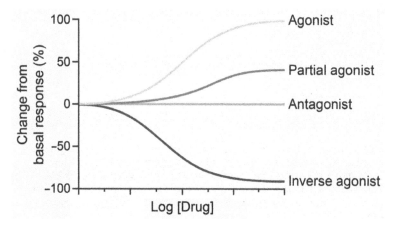

Figure 1.6 Efficacy. The ability of a ligand (drug) to bind to a receptor and produce an effect is known as its efficacy. A full agonist is a ligand that can activate a receptor to a maximal extent. Agonists that produce a submaximal response are referred to as partial agonists. Antagonists are ligands that occupy a binding site on a receptor and prevent changes to the basal level of activity of that receptor. Ligands that decrease basal receptor activity are termed inverse agonists, which can have partial or full activity. Note that all four of the ligands shown in this figure have the same potency and different efficacies.

effect, and therefore have equal efficacy. Compare this to Figure 1.6 where the full agonist, partial agonist, antagonist and inverse agonist have equal potency, but different efficacy.

Receptor populations, and therefore response to drugs, is not always uniform within a species, often as a result of genetic mutation. The study of inherited variability in response to drugs is termed pharmacogenomics and is discussed in Chapter 2.

Pharmacokinetic/Pharmacodynamic Modeling

Studies that relate pharmacokinetics to pharmacodynamics (PK/PD) studies are used to provide information relating plasma concentration to drug effect. In an ideal world, the veterinary anesthetist would have access to PK/PD models for all drugs used in the perioperative period, in both awake and anesthetized animals, that also take important disease states (e.g. hepatopathy, renal insufficiency, hypovolemia) into account. This would inform decision making when selecting drug dosages and rates of administration in healthy and ill animals, as well as expectations for drug effects, both wanted and unwanted. In reality this is not the case, particularly when it comes to disease states. When this information is unavailable, it is prudent to give drugs to effect where possible, and to monitor patients closely for side effects.

References

Bartholomew, K. and Smith, L.J. (2023). The effectiveness of liposome-encapsulated bupivacaine compared to standard bupivacaine for anesthesia of the maxilla in dogs. *J. Vet. Dent.* 12: 8987564231179885 https://doi.org/10.1177/08987564231179885.

Beths, T., Glen, J.B. et al. (2001). Evaluation and optimisation of a target-controlled infusion system for administering propofol to dogs as part of a total intravenous anaesthetic technique during dental surgery. *Vet. Rec.* 148: 198–203.

Branch, R.A. and Herman, R.J. (1984). Enzyme induction and beta-adrenergic receptor blocking drugs. *Br. J. Clin. Pharmacol.* 17 (Suppl 1): 77S–84S.

Caldwell, J., Gardner, I. et al. (1995). An introduction to drug disposition: the basic principles of absorption, distribution, metabolism, and excretion. *Toxicol. Pathol.* 23: 102–114.

Cattai, A., Pilla, T. et al. (2016). Evaluation and optimisation of propofol pharmacokinetic parameters in cats for target-controlled infusion. *Vet. Rec.* 178: 503.

Dent, B.T., Aarnes, T.K. et al. (2019). Pharmacokinetics and pharmacodynamic effects of oral transmucosal and intravenous administration of dexmedetomidine in dogs. *Am. J. Vet. Res.* 80: 969–975.

Deshpande, D., Hill, K.E. et al. (2016). The effect of the canine ABCB1-1Δ mutation on sedation after intravenous administration of acepromazine. *J. Vet. Intern. Med.* 30: 636–641.

Egan, T.D., Lemmens, H.J. et al. (1993). The pharmacokinetics of the new short-acting opioid remifentanil (GI87084B) in healthy adult male volunteers. *Anesthesiology* 79: 881–892.

Enlo-Scott, Z., Bäckström, E. et al. (2021). Drug metabolism in the lungs: opportunities for optimising inhaled medicines. *Expert Opin. Drug Metab. Toxicol.* 7: 611–625.

Enomoto, H., Love, L. et al. (2022). Pharmacokinetics of intravenous, oral transmucosal, and intranasal buprenorphine in healthy male dogs. *J. Vet. Pharmacol. Ther.* 45: 358–365.

Feary, D.J., Mama, K.R. et al. (2005). Influence of general anesthesia on pharmacokinetics of intravenous lidocaine infusion in horses. *Am. J. Vet. Res.* 66: 574–580.

Kukanich, B. and Clark, T.P. (2012). The history and pharmacology of fentanyl: relevance to a novel, long-acting transdermal fentanyl solution newly approved for use in dogs. *J. Vet. Pharmacol. Ther.* 35 (Suppl 2): 3–19.

Levionnois, O.L., Mevissen, M. et al. (2010). Assessing the efficiency of a pharmacokinetic-based algorithm for target-controlled infusion of ketamine in ponies. *Res. Vet. Sci.* 88: 512–518.

Lötsch, J., Walter, C. et al. (2013). Pharmacokinetics of non-intravenous formulations of fentanyl. *Clin. Pharmacokinet.* 52: 23–36.

Martinez, M., Modric, S. et al. (2008). The pharmacogenomics of P-glycoprotein and its role in veterinary medicine. *J. Vet. Pharmacol. Ther.* 31: 285–300.

Neill, E.A., Chapple, D.J. et al. (1983). Metabolism and kinetics of atracurium: an overview. *Br. J. Anaesth.* 55 (Suppl 1): 23S–25S.

Nolan, A. and Reid, J. (1993). Pharmacokinetics of propofol administered by infusion in dogs undergoing surgery. *Br. J. Anaesth.* 70: 546–551.

Rowland, A., Miners, J.O. et al. (2013). The UDP-glucuronosyltransferases: their role in drug metabolism and detoxification. *Int. J. Biochem. Cell Biol.* 45: 1121–1132.

Russo, H. and Bressolle, F. (1998). Pharmacodynamics and pharmacokinetics of thiopental. *Clin. Pharmacokinet.* 35: 95–134.

Sato, J., Makita, N. et al. (2016). Inverse agonism: the classic concept of GPCRs revisited. *Endocr. J.* 63: 507–514.

Wahler, B.M., Lerche, P. et al. (2019). Pharmacokinetics and pharmacodynamics of intranasal and intravenous naloxone hydrochloride administration in healthy dogs. *Am. J. Vet. Res.* 80: 696–701.

Zhang, H., Zhang, J., and Streisand, J.B. (2002). Oral mucosal drug delivery: clinical pharmacokinetics and therapeutic applications. *Clin. Pharmacokinet.* 41: 661–680.

Further Reading

Basic pharmacodynamic and pharmacokinetic concepts have been discussed in this chapter. An expanded discussion of these and more advanced pharmacologic concepts can be found in the following texts.

Brunton, L.L., Hilal-Dandan, R., and Knollman, B.C. (ed.) (2018). *Goodman & Gilman's The Pharmacological Basis of Therapeutics, 13*e. Wolters Kluwer.

Derendorf, H. and Schmidt, S. (ed.) (2020). *Rowland and Tozer's Clinical Pharmacokinetics and Pharmacodynamics: Concepts and Applications, 5*e. McGraw-Hill Education.

2

Pharmacogenetics in Veterinary Anesthesia and Analgesia

Jeffrey Lakritz

Introduction

Veterinary Pharmacogenomics, is the study of inherited variability in response to drugs in veterinary species and has been extensively reviewed (Mosher and Court 2010; Court 2013a; Garcia 2014; Mealey 2006; Martinez et al. 2013). Initially known as pharmacogenetics, early studies of single-gene defects were useful in defining the effects of drugs administered on specific enzymatic functions (or lack of effects). (Kalow 1971; Vesell 1969; Mahgoup et al. 1977; Smith 2001;).

Newer studies utilize whole genome sequencing to study genomic variation (single nucleotide polymorphism [SNP], CNV, mutations, etc.) to evaluate the impact of changes in the sequences of DNA and correlates these to reactions associated with unexpected effects on the individual or population levels to determine the cause. This field of discovery combines pharmacology and genomics to identify genetic determinants of drug efficacy, failure or toxicity. Ultimately, pharmacogenomic testing could provide the clinician information allowing selection of safe and effective medications used in a dosing regimen tailored to an individual's genetic makeup. In horses, a genetic mutation of the skeletal muscle sodium channel gene is associated with muscle fasciculations, spasm, and hyperkalemia (Spier et al. 1989). Currently, tests addressing genetic variation of cell-membrane drug transporters are available for dogs to determine the presence of polymorphisms of the *ABCB1* gene (P-glycoprotein transporters). Prior knowledge of the patient's genotype can allow individualization of therapy to reduce the incidence of toxicity associated with common pharmacologic agents that are substrates of this important protein (Mealey 2008). For the anesthesiologist, knowledge of species and breed-specific drug disposition, drug response and their association with genetic polymorphisms is currently in its infancy. Perhaps at some point, this information could provide critical input when deciding on patient-specific anesthetic and pain management protocols.

Pharmacogenetics – Historical Perspectives

The relationships between inherited traits and individual responses to food, natural products, and disease have been described and their potential association with inheritance attributed to a number of individuals (Nebert 1999; Kalow 1971; Vesell 1969; Mahgoup et al. 1977; Smith 2001). Studies describing human population diversity related to the effects of drugs were published as early as the mid-1950s (Motulsky 1957; Remmer and Merker 1963, Kalow 1971). However, it was not until 1988 when the genetic basis for polymorphisms leading to altered metabolism of debrisoquine and many other drugs were reported (Gonzalez et al. 1988). The completion of the human genome project in 2003 provided the framework on which the study of genetic polymorphisms of drug-metabolizing enzymes and drug receptors in humans could be conducted. These, and more recent methods, have led to pre-therapy genetic screening for patients requiring drugs previously associated with serious adverse events (McLeod and Yu 2003) and to optimize longstanding drug therapies, effectively minimizing adverse effects (Burns et al. 2013). Through collaboration, the impetus to develop high-density SNP and haplotype maps have proven useful in the study of genetic markers, predictive of serious adverse events associated with drug therapy (Columbia Systems Biology 2022).

The early human studies of genetic polymorphisms were focused on drug metabolizing enzymes. As newer technologies become available (genome-wide association studies)

Pharmacology in Veterinary Anesthesia and Analgesia, First Edition. Edited by Turi Aarnes and Phillip Lerche.
© 2024 John Wiley & Sons, Inc. Published 2024 by John Wiley & Sons, Inc.

it has been possible to differentiate contributions of the immune system and other host responses from genetic causes of adverse reactions associated with polymorphisms in the CYP450 enzymes and other cellular pathways (Daly 2012). These studies quantify changes in the genetic code producing loss of / altered function mutations which could be useful in characterizing a disease as well as developing new treatments.

Understanding how the genetic make-up of an individual alters their responses to administered drugs is a goal of human medicine. Knowledge of whether a given drug, when dosed appropriately, would provide the anticipated response, exaggerated responses or no response at all, would prevent adverse drug reactions. Adverse events associated with therapeutic drugs do occur and, many in humans, are associated with genetic polymorphisms that alter the drugs' disposition. These polymorphisms may manifest as dose related when drug dose is inappropriate or could occur even at low doses.

In humans, well-characterized variations in response to administration of a particular drug have been associated with variation in the genetic code (Gonzalez et al. 1988; Steward et al. 1997; Rieder et al. 2005). The debrisoquine/sparteine and warfarin polymorphisms were discovered based upon clinical observations of the effects of drugs on patients and followed by pharmacogenetic studies to identify gene variations. Clinical observations leading to discovery of the nature of relevant variability in response to drugs remain important to anesthesia.

At present, there are few examples where variant gene coding results in clinical differences in drug disposition in veterinary medicine (Paulson et al. 1999; Mise et al. 2004; Tenmizu et al. 2006; Mealey et al. 2001; Blaisdell et al. 1998).

Polymorphisms, such as the well-described clinical sensitivity to avermectin drugs in herding dogs has been shown to be associated with a sequence variation in the canine *ABCB1* gene resulting in the expression of a truncated and inactive membrane transport protein (Mealey et al. 2001). From studies of this polymorphism in dogs, it has become apparent that this defect is widespread across a number of breeds (Mealey and Meurs 2008). A number of other studies document expression of genes or of drug sensitivity or drug interactions in several important veterinary species. For example, it is widely known that some drugs are less rapidly eliminated by cats due to limited formation of glucuronide conjugates (Court 2013b). Thus, the use of acetaminophen in cats is contraindicated due to toxicity associated with the combined failure of expression of the appropriate uridine diphosphate glucuronosyltransferase isoform in this species and the inability to acetylate toxic intermediates (Court and Greenblatt 2000). Many of these known peculiarities across species were observed as clinically apparent sensitivity or adverse reactions in patients before the elucidation of the molecular genetic cause (Paul, et al. 1987; Mealey et al. 2001; Court and Greenblatt 2000), while others are strongly suggestive of a genetic polymorphism (Robertson et al. 1992; Sams and Muir 1988; Mandsager, et al. 1995; Zoran et al. 1993). Many other polymorphisms of drug metabolism and drug receptors have recently been documented, but additional effort will be required to both characterize the function or expression of the gene product(s) and link these variations with clinical effects. Once the precise mechanism(s) are defined, markers may be developed to test individual or groups of animals to identify animals with potential for drug sensitivity (as is done for *ABCB1* Δ dogs).

The goals of anesthesia are to immobilize, render unconscious and alleviate pain to facilitate procedures performed on animals varying from a few grams to hundreds of kilograms body weight. Veterinary anesthesia commonly utilizes multi-modal techniques that rely on drug–drug interactions to promote anesthesia and analgesia (Papich 2007). While commonplace, the use of sedative, anesthetic and analgesic combinations could be associated with risks in some animals.

The use of multiple drugs in combination may provide substantial clinical benefit; however, the use of combinations of anesthetic, analgesic and other drugs could also result in unwanted effects (toxicity if drug interactions produce adversity; no benefit if antagonism occurs). This is especially true in geriatric, diseased or injured patients where concurrent medications and physiologic changes are of concern. While still unknown in most cases, an animal's genetic make-up can alter pharmacokinetics or pharmacodynamics of a drug(s) (one usually does not observe the consequences of altered PK/PD until after the drug is administered). Defining clinically important observations with genetically altered metabolizing enzymes, drug receptors or other proteins should reduce these adversities through selection of the most appropriate medication for the patient. Conversely, drugs may be designed to limit or prevent adversities once the therapeutic target is identified. There are likely to be numerous other breed, species and gender-related variations in animal responses to drugs. Some differences may be related to nutrition, environment or concurrent medications and may result from drug–drug interactions (Krein et al. 2014). Others may be the result of variations in the genetic code within individual animals that alter drug disposition and lead to appropriate responses, exaggerated responses or no response at all.

While there are a number of excellent reviews evaluating pharmacogenetics in small animals, there are still significant gaps in knowledge of whether these variations are associated with altered disposition and potentially adverse reactions (Mosher and Court 2010; Court et al. 2013; Mealey 2006; Martinez et al. 2013). For now, knowledge of species- and breed-specific responses to administered drug(s) should be considered with every patient. As one encounters patients who consistently respond outside of the norm during anesthetic procedures, consideration of potential genetic variations responsible for functional alterations in important genes, gene expression and metabolism should be considered. As newer drugs are tested and approved for use in veterinary species, this information may become more available. Until then, acknowledging that clinical observations foster the study of differences in drug disposition will promote greater recognition of these concerns (Paulson, et al. 1999; Mise et al. 2004; Tenmizu et al. 2006; Mealey et al. 2001).

Pharmacogenetics – Current Situation

Compared with the human field, veterinary pharmacogenetics is a relatively new area of research. Like human medicine, the discovery of genetic variation in terms of drugs has been led by pharmacologists in academia and industry as well as veterinarians making observations of clinical patients. Currently, there are several enzyme transporter or receptor polymorphisms identified based upon responses to drugs, drug disposition and, in some cases, therapeutic effects or toxicities. While most of the variations have been described in companion animals and most involve drug-metabolizing enzymes, newer studies have focused on other variations (drug receptors) and some large animal species (horses). After reading this chapter, it will become evident that we still have a long journey to complete. With newer technologies emerging daily, pharmacogenetic studies of animals will continue to progress.

Completion of the canine (Lindblad-Toh et al. 2005), feline (Pontius et al. 2007), bovine (Elsik et al. 2009), equine (Wade et al. 2009), ovine and caprine (Jiang et al. 2014; Du et al. 2014) genomes, has led to substantial progress toward an understanding of the genetic basis for animal disease susceptibility, productivity and, more recently, studies evaluating the variation in responses to drugs in individual animals. Adapting the technologies developed through the human genome project are important to completion of similar studies in veterinary species (Alpay et al. 2014; Tonomura et al. 2015; Mucha et al. 2015; Forsberg et al. 2015; Hendrickson 2013). Like human medicine, the study of genetic polymorphisms in veterinary species could demonstrate the genetic basis for the wide variations in therapeutic response between individual animals (Kennerly et al. 2009). More recent studies confirm prior suggestions that genetic polymorphisms of drug metabolism are also present in large animals. Knowledge of these variations should provide information about why some animals respond the way they do to anesthetics and analgesics (Krein et al. 2014).

Pharmacogenetics – Cytochrome P450 Function

Cytochrome P450 monoxygenases are membrane bound, heme-containing enzymes that play important roles in the disposition of many drugs, endogenous and exogenous substances (Hrycay and Bandiera 2015; Klassen 2013).

Cytochrome P450 are named based upon the gene sequence similarity into families (CYP1, CYP2, CYP3, etc.), subfamilies (CYP1A, CYP2B, etc.) and when they were sequenced (number: CYP1A2, CYP2B11, etc.) (Court 2013a). It has become apparent that functional characteristics (specificity, substrate, and inhibitor selectivity) produce differing clinical phenotypes. Multiple isoforms of CYP450 are co-expressed in the same tissue and substrate specificity of each cytochrome P450 form may demonstrate significant overlap. As two unique enzymes expressed by the same tissue metabolize the same drug, identifying a polymorphic enzyme is difficult without monitoring specific metabolites produced, sequencing the gene or protein and characterizing the biological function of each expressed enzyme.

The cytochromes are present in virtually all organisms and appear to function very similarly (Fink-Gremmels 2008). While traditionally thought to have conserved functions, and mainly expressed by the liver, enzyme expression and substrate and inhibitor specificity demonstrates significant phenotypic variability across the wide variety of veterinary species and breeds. It is now known that intestine, lung, kidney, adrenal and other organs express substantial amounts of cytochrome P450 whose profile differs significantly from that of the liver (Mealey et al. 2008a; Trepanier 2006; Sivapathasundaram et al. 2001; Tyden et al. 2014).

These enzymes function in concert to catalyze hydrolysis, reduction, oxidation and conjugation reactions (Parkinson et al. 2013). Drug metabolism processes create metabolites. For some drugs (pro-drugs), metabolism is required for a drug's function. Without the appropriate enzymatic processes, drugs would not be eliminated and could accumulate over time and may produce toxicity (Riviere 2009). These initial processes usually decrease, sometimes enhance and, in some cases, modify the physiologic effects of a particular drug.

After a drug is oxidized, hydrolyzed or reduced, a second system of enzymes (phase II, conjugation) adds functional groups to promote elimination. Drug metabolism is a key factor in the disposition of drugs administered to animals. Without these key proteins, drug activity may be prolonged due to accumulation and toxicity could be observed (Riviere 2009). Despite conserved functions of many drug-metabolizing enzymes, variation in substrate specificity of these enzyme systems is common (Fink-Gremmels 2008). With significant differences in substrate specificity, as well as enzyme expression level and location within and across species, extrapolation between species is not reasonable with currently available methods (Fink-Gremmels 2008). It is also recognized that multiple enzymes may metabolize the same drug which, in the case of a genetic polymorphism of one enzyme (rendered non-functional), the animal may not demonstrate clinically relevant differences in drug disposition or effect except at supra-therapeutic levels. Substrates known to be metabolized by human CYP450 enzymes are metabolized by dog, horse or other species' CYP450 enzymes, but do so with much different rates, substrate and inhibitor concentrations (Martinez et al. 2013). Together, these limit the usefulness of cross-species or breed comparisons due to lack of complete characterization of individual enzymes or lack of knowledge of specific substrates for each animal's enzyme (Fink-Gremmels 2008). Differential expression of CYP450 isozymes within the gut, lung, kidney and liver having wide-substrate selectivity add to the aforementioned complexities.

Expression of recombinant CYP450 enzymes has allowed for more precise assessment of substrate specificity (Miskimins Mills et al. 2010; Aidasani et al. 2008; Shou et al. 2003). In studies comparing recombinant, expressed enzymes with whole-liver microsomal preparations, differences in the activity of a specific P450 between these two preparations suggests multiple CYP450s participate in the metabolism of a particular substrate. This may sometimes be discernable by evaluation of the specific metabolites produced.

At present, at least seven different canine cytochrome P450 enzymes have been cloned and expressed and their activities characterized *in vitro* (Miskimins Mills et al. 2010; Aidasani et al. 2008; Shou et al. 2003). Several classes of CYP450 enzymes have also been cloned and expressed in cats, horses, swine, and ruminants.

Recent studies, recognizing the importance of the dog in the assessment of metabolism, pharmacokinetics, safety and efficacy of drugs in human drug discovery have produced data addressing substrate specificity of dog CYP450 as a means of developing isoenzyme-selective markers (Shou et al. 2003). Similarly, recombinant canine CYP450 enzymes have been used to evaluate substrates and inhibitors of specific CYP450 isozymes with the goal of predicting drug–drug interactions (Miskimins Mills et al. 2010). These studies have demonstrated *in vivo* drug interactions with

substrate-inhibitor combinations: caffeine-fluvoxamine, midazolam-ketoconazole, and temazepam-ketoconazole. This knowledge could shed light onto whether a drug is a substrate or inhibitor of specific CYP450's allowing further study aimed at analyzing the potential of drug–drug interactions through targeted screening prior to widespread use (Miskimins Mills et al. 2010). Together with the development of high throughput study technologies, evaluation of their function may be conducted in a more precise and rapid manner (Aidasani et al. 2008). Although some inconsistencies remain, these studies will be valuable in evaluation of variant enzymes in animals with known polymorphisms (Martinez et al. 2013; Paulson et al. 1999).

Genetic Variations in Drug Disposition

Genetic variation in drug Absorption, Distribution, Metabolism and Excretion (ADME) is based upon changes within the sequence of DNA an animal inherits. Sequence variation is commonly associated with SNPs where a single base is changed, from one of the four nucleotide bases to another, and alteration of the protein encoded for may occur. The genetic code is arranged such that there are 61 codons (three letter words) defining the 20 different amino acids (leucine and arginine are represented by six codons, valine, serine, proline, threonine, alanine, and glycine by four codons, etc.). There is one start codon (ATG; representing methionine) and three stop codons (TAA, TAG, TGA). If the DNA sequence (codon = three sequential bases comprising a specific amino acid) changes such that the amino acid remains the same, there is often no or little change in protein function (TTT → TTC; A synonymous SNP). These changes are often clinically silent (single-base change, which does not change the amino acid sequence of protein) unless the DNA polymorphism results in alterations in DNA binding sites. If the codon changes such that the reference sequence changes to another amino acid (CTT → CCT; A non-synonymous SNP), the protein sequence changes, and altered protein folding can occur that modifies the active site and/or activity of the enzyme. For example, a change from leucine (CTT) → proline (CCT) could produce steric limitations on formation of the active site of the enzyme or reduce the stability of the protein leading to premature degradation. In rare instances, the change in protein sequence may augment protein function (Otero et al. 2015). Conversely, if a frameshift occurs (deletion, insertion) and the codon changes to a premature stop codon, protein synthesis stops and either a truncated protein is expressed (ABCB1 Δ) or the abnormal protein is degraded (CYP2B11). One well-described, non-synonymous polymorphism leads to deletion of the nascent CYP4501A2 protein and loss of function in laboratory beagle colonies (Mise et al. 2004; Tenmizu et al. 2006). Many other genetic polymorphisms have been described in animals; at present, their clinical relevance has yet to be elucidated.

Genetic polymorphisms of drug metabolism enzymes and transporters are generally silent, at least until the animal is exposed to a drug or xenobiotic substrate metabolized or handled by a deficient enzyme or transporter. Without analysis of drug disposition and metabolite production, clinical adversity may not be observed. Early observations in humans administered an adrenergic antagonist drug "debrisoquine," suggested marked variation in responses to this drug for hypotension. Some individuals had clinically relevant problems when taking this medication (individuals possessing two mutant alleles – poor metabolizer phenotype), while others demonstrated improved clinical signs (two functional alleles – extensive metabolizers; one functional, one mutant allele – intermediate phenotype) or exhibited no response to therapy (more than two functional alleles – ultra-rapid metabolizers). Individuals were segregated based upon clinical manifestations of drug sensitivity (severe hypotension) or normal (normal blood pressure). For debrisoquine, poor metabolizers (excrete mainly unchanged parent drug in urine) demonstrated marked responses to administration of this drug (hypotension) in comparison to extensive metabolizers (excrete greater proportion of metabolite in urine). Analytic characterization of drug and metabolite(s) in blood or urine is currently a valuable tool.

After demonstrating these polymorphic phenotypes (Idle and Smith 1979), the genetic basis for this defect was later shown to be a polymorphism in CYP450 2D6 (Gonzalez et al. 1988). Subsequent studies demonstrating this deletion polymorphism results in altered drug ADME for over 20 additional, commonly used medications (Eichelbaum and Gross 1990).

Unlike polymorphic CYP450 2D6 mutations in humans, many described in animals became apparent due to adverse reactions, or simply differing drug disposition (Mise et al. 2004; Tenmizu et al. 2006; Paulson et al. 1999). These dogs were administered the drug in pre-clinical studies to define the drug disposition in humans; the effect of the drug was silent and the polymorphism became apparent only after plasma drug analysis. Likewise, genetic polymorphisms of drug transporters leading to altered drug disposition or effect result in homozygous normal dogs, heterozygous normal/mutant ABCB1Δ and homozygous mutant/mutant ABCB1 Δ (Mealey et al. 2001; Mealey 2006).

Currently, the most completely characterized veterinary drug metabolizing enzyme polymorphisms where DNA changes are associated with altered drug disposition are those observed in canine CYP2D15, CYP1A2, and ABCB1Δ

(Mise et al. 2004; Tenmizu et al. 2006; Mealey et al. 2001; Mealey 2006). The reported changes have been documented in humans, lab animals, and companion animals. Recent studies have documented a number of polymorphisms in horses and ruminants. While a young science in veterinary medicine, it would be prudent to consider drug-interactions as well as genetic variation in cases which do not produce the appropriate response to anesthetics and analgesics. Clinical observations will be critical in the identification of these responses and eventually elucidation of the mechanisms associated with them.

Pharmacogenomics of Drug Metabolism in Veterinary Patients – Polymorphisms of CYP450

Cytochrome P450 1A2

Cytochrome P450 1A gene expression is transcriptionally regulated by the aryl-hydrocarbon receptor complex (AhR) which binds to DNA response elements increasing transcription of CYP4501A proteins in response to the presence of a variety of aromatic hydrocarbons and some proton pump inhibitors (Parkinson et al. 2013). Induction of CYP450 1A may be modulated by the expression and activity of other CYP450 enzymes (Parkinson et al. 2013).

A series of pharmacokinetic studies in dogs described a common CYP450 1A2 polymorphism in populations of laboratory beagles (Mise et al. 2004; Tenmizu et al. 2006). This genetic polymorphism (CYP450 1A2 1117 C>T) results in the formation of a premature stop codon resulting in the expression of an inactive protein. For at least for two experimental drugs, (AC-3933 or YM-64227), the dogs were phenotyped by observing dramatically altered drug disposition (Mise et al. 2004; Tenmizu et al. 2006). At present, it is unclear whether or not significant changes in the disposition of these drugs can be predicted to occur due to polymorphism. However, one study demonstrated the inhibition of CYP450 1A2 by fluoroquinolone antibiotics (inhibitor of CYP4501A2) significantly altered the pharmacokinetics of theophylline (substrate of CYP4501A2) by reducing clearance and augmenting the area under the curve with accumulation of theophylline in beagle dogs (Intorre et al. 1995). Others have demonstrated noncompetitive inhibition of CYP4501A2 by fluoroquinolones that vary between individual members of this class of antibiotics (Regmi et al. 2005). These studies support the idea that animals expressing this polymorphism may be at risk when administered drugs which are primarily metabolized by CYP1A2. Further study of drugs suspected of causing adverse reactions in genotyped animals would be extremely valuable. At present, only one study has evaluated the metabolism of a drug in CYP4501A2 genotyped dogs (Whiterock et al. 2012). However, while this polymorphism was originally described in laboratory beagles, several additional studies demonstrated this polymorphism in a large number of pure- and mixed-breed dogs (Aretz and Geyer 2010; Scherr et al. 2010). A recent review of this subject precisely collated the expression of this common polymorphism in mixed and pure-bred dogs (Court 2013a,b). At least 24 mixed and pure-breed dog breeds possess at least one mutant allele. The percentage of each breed population expressing the TT allele varies greatly, as does the frequency of this mutant in different populations of studied dogs (by country or region) (Aretz and Geyer 2010; Scherr et al. 2010). Like the polymorphism in ABCB1-Δ, monitoring the responses to drugs administered (plasma drug concentrations) in genotyped dogs, would be useful to define both the reason for potential polymorphic phenotypes and the clinical impact of this polymorphism.

The CYP4501A1/2 genes have been cloned and sequenced in cats, with two different forms of CYP4501A2 being characterized (Tanaka et al. 2006). No studies have evaluated CYP4501A polymorphisms in the cat at present. Expression of CYP1A enzymes in large animals has demonstrated the presence of the gene and activity of CYP4501A enzymes in the horse and cow (Tyden et al. 2014; Sivapathasundaram et al. 2001).

Cytochrome P450 2B

Cytochrome P450 2B enzymes are important in drug metabolism of many drugs used in veterinary species (Martinez et al. 2013). Cyclophosphamide is activated by CYP2B enzymes producing active, cytotoxic metabolites (phosphoramide and acrolein) (Chong-Sheng et al. 2004). In fact, canine CYP2B11 is seven-to-eight-fold more active in hydroxylating cyclophosphamide and ifosfamide than rat CYP2B1. Cytochrome P450 2B11 metabolizes a number of other drugs of importance to a wide variety of diseases (Michalowska et al. 2014). Cytochrome P450 2B11 metabolizes and is inhibited by drugs co-administered in balanced anesthetic protocols (ketamine and midazolam) (Baratta et al. 2009). Cytochrome P450 is inducible with phenobarbital being a very potent inducer of this enzyme. For most dogs and other species, barbiturates were generally used as anesthetic agents and in a wide variety of clinical situations. In greyhound dogs, metabolism of drugs differs significantly from mixed-breed or other breeds of dogs. As demonstrated by Sams et al. (1985) administration of thiobarbiturates to greyhounds resulted in prolonged anesthetic recovery times and was thought to be associated with lower expression or a less functional CYP450 in

greyhounds (Sams et al. 1985; Sams and Muir 1988). Plasma drug concentrations of thiobarbiturates after dosing did not decline exponentially after dosing, like those observed in mixed-breed dogs suggesting a saturable enzymatic process. These authors later induced CYP450 by administration of phenobarbital for 16 days. Afterward, it was apparent that metabolism of thiobarbiturates was greatly improved in greyhounds and similar to the kinetics of mixed-breed dogs. After phenobarbital induction, cytochrome P450 metabolism was pharmacokinetically a linear process (Sams and Muir 1988). Later, Mandsager et al. (1995) demonstrated that greyhounds treated with chloramphenicol (inhibitor of CYP450 2B11) and then administered propofol intravenously (IV) by infusion increased the half-life of elimination, reduced clearance by half and prolonged recovery from propofol-induced anesthesia (Mandsager et al. 1995).

Propofol is also metabolized by cytochrome P450 2B11 based upon chemical and antibody inhibitors as well as substrate specificity studies in dogs (Hay Kraus et al. 2000). Propofol is popular because of rapid onset and recovery from anesthesia. However, greyhounds demonstrated slower drug clearance and longer recoveries after administration (Robertson et al. 1992; Zoran et al. 1993; Mandsager et al. 1995). Greyhound microsomal metabolism of propofol was consistently >3 fold lower than beagle or mixed-breed dogs. Further, propofol metabolism was inhibited by chloramphenicol and an antisera to CYP2B suggesting that this isoform plays a significant role in propofol metabolism and may be deficient compared with mixed-breed and beagle dogs (Court et al. 1999). More recently, a number of polymorphisms have been described in dog cytochrome P4502B11; however, the association between these polymorphisms and altered drug metabolism has yet to be demonstrated (Gagliardi et al. 2015;). Martinez et al. (2020), demonstrated hepatic microsomes of greyhound livers metabolized CYP2B11 substrates slower in part due to reduced expression of this protein in spite of equivalent or higher mRNA for this cytochrome. (Martinez et al. 2020). Re-sequencing of the genome revealed three haplotypes of CYP2B11 that were differentiated based upon sequence variation in the 3′-untranslated region of the mRNA. Greyhounds demonstrated the highest expression of the three-haplotypes that led to truncation of the transcripts and ultimately lower expression of CYP2B11. (Martinez et al. 2020. Pharmacogenomics of poor drug metabolism in greyhounds: Cytochrome P450 (CYP)2B11 genetic variation, breed distribution, and functional characterization. Nature/Scientific Reports. https://doi.org/10.1038/s41598-019-56660-z.)

Cytochrome P450 2B6 has been shown to be expressed in the small intestine and lung, but not in the liver of cats

(Okamatsu et al. 2016). The recombinant protein metabolized substrates of human 2B6 and was inhibited by medetomidine and atipamezole, ticlopidine and sertraline (Okamatsu et al. 2016).

Cytochrome P450 27B1 (1α-hydroxylase) catalyzes the conversion of calcidiol into calcitriol (1,25-dihydroxyvitamin D3). There was a single case report of a unique mutation of the DNA encoding *CYP45027B1*, in a three-month old Siamese cat demonstrating lethargy, gait abnormalities and pain (Grahn et al. 2012). Elevated serum PTH, low iCa, but normal 25-hydroxyvitamin D3 and low serum 1,25-dihydroxyvitamin D3 suggested low 1α-hydroxylase activity as a cause as previously reported (Geisen et al. 2009). Complete analysis of this gene demonstrated six SNPs, one of which resulted in truncation of the protein (loss of 297 amino acids) (Grahn et al. 2012). The affected kitten's normal littermate was heterozygous at all of these SNPs (Grahn et al. 2012).

Ketamine is metabolized by the equine liver (Mossner et al. 2011). The ortholog of human CYP4502B6 in horses has been cloned, expressed and functional characterizations performed. In addition, several polymorphisms were identified and characterized (Peters et al. 2013). The cloning and expression of this enzyme revealed three polymorphisms, one of which altered an amino acid from valine to isoleucine (exon 2; c.226G>A) and two others in exon 3, one of which was associated with an amino acid shift from glycine to glutamic acid (c.356G>A). This enzyme metabolized racemic ketamine to norketamine, hydroxynorketamine, and dehydronorketamine *in vitro*. Since *CYP450 2B6* metabolizes ketamine as well as other co-administered drugs in horses and it can be induced by phenobarbital (humans, dogs, ruminants), studies of drug interactions and polymorphisms resulting in altered metabolism should expand our capabilities to predict potential drug interactions and perhaps responses (Peters et al. 2013). Fluconazole administration to treat ocular disease in horses was associated with prolonged recovery time when ketamine and midazolam were used as induction agents. This is likely a DDI, however further study may be prudent.

Cytochrome P450 2C

While there appears to be greater hepatic expression of the CYP4502C isoforms in canine liver than other enzymes, little is known about substrate selectivity and inhibition of this enzyme. Further, most studies evaluating veterinary drug metabolism or inhibition also demonstrate other CYP450 isoforms can metabolize the same substrates making observations of the drugs which are specific for 2C subfamily less informative. To date, several members of the cytochrome P450 2C subfamily has been identified in dogs.

Canine *CYP4502C21* is expressed in the dog liver and was present within all dogs tested (Blaisdell et al. 1998). A second gene (*CYP4502C41*) was also cloned but had only 70% identity to *CYP4502C21*. Cytochrome P450 2C is induced by phenobarbital and mildly inhibited by ketoconazole and vincristine (Aidasani et al. 2008). More effort to define substrate and inhibitors for these enzymes is needed as there has been little characterization to date.

Equine cytochrome P450 2C92 was cloned, expressed, and functionally analyzed *in vitro*. It appears to metabolize diclofenac slower than human *CYP4502C9*, metabolizes tolbutamide and S-warfarin comparably to the human orthologs, but metabolized S-mephenytoin poorly compared to human enzymes (DiMaio Knych et al. 2009). CYP450 2C (bovine, porcine) have also been studied with some predictable findings (Zimin et al. 2009). While no conclusions can be made regarding substrate selectivity or genetic polymorphisms, enzymatic activity and protein expression are documented for both phase I (CYP450) and phase II (GSTx) processes. Further, for some enzymes, rates of substrate metabolism and protein expression in duodenal microsomes did not vary between veal calves and adults (similar activity for CYP2C and 3A substrates; no to little activity or expression for CYP1A) (Virkel et al. 2009). Other studies have demonstrated that maintaining plasma insulin concentrations at normal or elevated levels in dairy cows and sheep down regulated expression of CYP 2C and CYP 3A while feeding glucogenic substrates (propionic acid, propylene glycol, corn starch) modifies expression of hepatic enzymes (Lemley et al. 2008; Lemley et al. 2010). These data suggest cytochrome P450 2C enzymes perform species-specific functions in horses and ruminants. It is also interesting that breed and dietary components may have a measurable effect on drug metabolism in ruminants. However, to date, little is known about drug interactions or polymorphisms leading to altered metabolism in these species.

Cytochrome P450 2D

The first descriptions of the genetic basis of polymorphic drug metabolism in humans and dogs were those observed in cytochrome P450 2D (Gonzalez et al. 1988; Paulson et al. 1999). Over 100 different polymorphisms of human CYP450 2D6 have been demonstrated; many of which demonstrate altered metabolism of drugs (Martignoni et al. 2006). Cytochrome P450 2D is expressed by the liver, albeit at lower levels than other CYP450 isoforms and has been shown to oxidize a wide variety of anti-arrhythmics, beta-blockers, dextromethorphan and methadone in several species (Martignoni et al. 2006). It is suggested that CYP4502D metabolizes nearly 25% of the drugs labeled for use in humans (Martignoni et al. 2006; Corado et al. 2016).

In dogs, evaluation of celecoxib disposition demonstrated distinct differences in plasma concentrations, half-life of the terminal phase, clearance, distribution volumes, and area under the curve in dogs given IV (5 mg/kg body weight) and oral doses (7.5–25 mg/kg body weight) of celecoxib (Paulson et al. 1999). In this study, *in vitro* metabolism of celecoxib by recombinant canine *CYP2B11*, *CYP2C21*, *CYP2D15*, and *CYP3A12* demonstrated that the highest oxidative activity for celecoxib and bufuralol (a substrate for human CYP4502D6) was observed with *CYP2D15*. However, when dog-liver microsomal preparations from extensive and poor metabolizer dogs were evaluated *in vitro*, there was poor concordance between celecoxib and bufuralol metabolism, suggesting the contributions of other enzyme(s). This study was the first to suggest that the involvement of genetic variants of cytochrome P450 identified in dogs utilized in their study population was associated with altered metabolism of celecoxib.

There is also evidence that inhibition of CYP450 2D is similar in humans and dogs, suggesting the well-characterized variation in humans may also occur in canines. As such, one could imagine that the propensity for drug interactions would be similar depending upon the use of selected drugs in dogs. *In vitro* evidence supports the possibility of drug interactions as demonstrated inhibition of dog CYP450 2D by ondansetron (42% inhibition), ketoconazole (82% inhibition), clomipramine (84% inhibition), and fluoxetine (54% inhibition) (Aidasani et al. 2008). Whether or not inhibition of co-administered drugs is relevant clinically has not been well characterized. However, ketoconazole is useful as a CYP450 inhibitor to reduce the dose of other drugs while augmenting their plasma concentrations (Myre et al. 1991; Archer et al. 2014). Similarly, with evidence for three differing clones of the wild-type gene, of which two render the animals phenotypically different from the wild type CYP450 2D15 animal, suggests variability in metabolism (inactive or active) of a drug(s) could result in unpredictable consequences (Roussel et al. 1998).

Recently, the ortholog of human CYP450 2D6 in horses (CYP450 2D50) was cloned and expressed and evaluated in 150 horses (Corado et al. 2016). Sequence evaluations of these horses demonstrated 126 exonic SNPs were present; 31 of which were present in more than one horse. Of these polymorphisms, seven were predicted to cause alteration in the function of this enzyme (Corado et al. 2016). These investigators then administered a probe substrate drug (tramadol) to genotyped horses to determine the metabolic ratio (tramadol:O-desmethyltramadol). In this subset of genotyped horses, the tramadol:O-desmethyltramadol ratios segregated into poor, extensive and ultra-rapid metabolizers. Considering the importance of CYP450 2D to the metabolism of human drugs, many of which are also used "off-label" in horses, there appears to be significant information to further investigate whether this key enzyme (or other subfamilies) could promote adverse drug events in horses. Further, considering the stringent regulation of the use of pharmaceuticals in athletic performance horses, genotypic information could be very important in the estimation of withdrawal times to ensure compliance with drug-use guidelines (Corado et al. 2016; Knych et al. 2012).

Polymorphisms of cytochrome P450 2D subfamily enzymes of animals, like humans, appear to be relatively common. While the clinically demonstrable effects of these SNPs have not been described, they contribute to the metabolism of a large number of drugs. As such, further study would be appropriate to define potential adverse reactions associated with clinical signs and altered disposition.

Cytochrome P450 2E

CYP450 2E1 is a major, constitutively expressed P450 in the human liver having a significant role in metabolism and toxicity of small molecules. One of the major concerns with metabolites of this enzyme is the production of reactive metabolites capable of producing injury or promoting carcinogenesis. Ketone bodies, ethanol, isoniazid, acetaminophen, methoxyflurane, and sevoflurane are substrates of CYP450 2E (Court et al. 1997; Tanaka et al. 2005). This enzyme appears to play protective roles in under-nutrition by conversion of fatty acids and ketones to useable substrates in the body (Lieber 2004). Some of these substrates are also inducers of enzyme activity. Cytochrome DNA and protein sequences are well conserved across those species examined, with the exception of ruminants (Lankford et al. 2000; Court et al. 1997; Nebbia et al. 2003). The substrate, chlorzoxazone, used in human studies, is efficiently metabolized to 6-hydroxychloroxazone and the enzyme is inhibited by diethyldithiocarbonate in some but not all species (Court et al. 1997). This system has been studied in humans, mice, rats, rabbits, ferrets, monkeys, cats, dogs, horses, and cattle liver microsomes and demonstrated all species metabolize this substrate and it is inhibited by diethyldithiocarbonate. Two studies demonstrated one SNP (T1453C) resulting in an amino acid change from tyrosine to histidine (Lankford et al. 2000) and 12 amino-acid differences in 2 CYP 2E enzymes in the cat (Tanaka et al. 2005). Interestingly, while there were 12 amino-acid residue differences between the two feline proteins, only one of these differences resulted in an altered amino-acid sequence (representing a change from aspartic acid to glutamic acid). Further work is necessary to determine the presence of polymorphisms in other species and whether there are functional differences in this enzyme with drugs relevant to anesthesia.

Cytochrome P450 3A

In humans, cytochrome P450 3A enzymes consist of CYP 3A4, 3A5, and 3A7 (Ingelman-Sundberg et al. 2007). This subfamily of enzymes has wide substrate specificity and metabolizes the majority of drugs used clinically as well as functions to metabolize key endogenous substrates (Ingelman-Sundberg et al. 2007). These enzymes are mainly expressed by the liver, but expression is considerable in the gastrointestinal (GI) tract as well as other locations (Mealey et al. 2008a; Tyden et al. 2012; Nebbia et al. 2003). Cytochrome P450 3A enzymes are very inducible with some drugs (rifampicin) in human and dog liver whereas dexamethasone does not induce CYP3A enzyme in dogs (unlike humans) (Nishibe et al. 1998; Zhang et al. 2006). CYP 3A isoforms are also inhibited by a variety of other drugs. Ketoconazole and several other drugs are potent inhibitors of CYP3A in dogs and humans. Currently, ketoconazole's inhibition of CYP3A isoforms is utilized as a drug-interaction with cyclosporine to allow lower doses of cyclosporine, maintaining therapeutic blood levels of this immunomodulatory agent (Archer et al. 2014; Myre et al. 1991; Lu et al. 2005). Some macrolide antibiotics are also potent suicide inhibitors of CYP3A subfamily enzymes (Ludden 1985; Martignoni et al. 2006).

In humans, the three enzymes differ in their expression, with *CYP3A7* expressed in the fetus, *CYP3A5* expression throughout life and *CYP3A4* is the major adult form of *CYP3A* (Ingelman-Sundberg et al. 2007). It is not known whether there are differences in *CYP3A12* and *CYP3A26* expression during the lives of dogs or other animals. However, in the dog *CYP3A12* and *CYP3A26* are expressed in the liver, however, the 3A26 isoform hydroxylates steroids poorly in comparison to 3A12, and hepatic expression of *CYP3A26* is greater than that of *CYP3A12* (Fraser et al. 1997). It is also interesting that duodenal expression of *CYP3A12* over 3A26 was predominant in the dog (Mealey et al. 2008a). The *CYP3A26* migrates at a slightly higher molecular mass in SDS-PAGE gels and key polymorphisms between 3A12 and *CYP3A26* reside in the substrate recognition sites of the enzymes (Fraser et al. 1997; Martinez et al. 2013). Paulson et al. (1999), described another variant enzyme (*CYP3A12*2*) with five amino-acid differences from the reference *CYP3A12*. The variant *CYP3A12*2* enzyme demonstrated lower enzymatic activity toward testosterone substrate than the reference allele.

The cytochrome P450 3A subfamily of enzymes has also been extensively studied in ruminants, swine, and horses. Bovine nasal and olfactory mucosa was evaluated by Dhamankar et al. (2013) showing by RT-PCR, cDNA microarray and immunofluorescence that *CYP3A4*, and a 3A4-like enzyme was expressed in these regions of the respiratory tract. Tyden et al. (2012), demonstrated *7-CYP3A* genes expressed in the lung parenchyma and airways of horses. Further, DiMaio Knych et al. (2010), demonstrated three separate hepatic forms, which were distinct from those evaluated in earlier reports (Schmitz et al. 2010). The results of these studies underscore the variability in substrate selectivity, expression and enzymatic activity across species. As with other subfamily members, polymorphisms likely exist but remain to be characterized.

Other Polymorphisms of Relevance Based upon Clinically Recognized Phenomena – Drug Transporters

As noted above, drug-transporter polymorphisms have been demonstrated to result in severe adverse reactions in dogs and potentially other species. The seminal work by Mealey et al. (2001) proved that clinically observed signs of apparent dose-dependent toxicosis (100–2500 μg/kg body weight) in some collies, but not others (at doses up to 2500 μg/kg body weight) were associated with a four base-pair deletion in the *ABCB1* gene (Mealey et al. 2001; Paul et al. 1987). This gene encodes the ATP-binding cassette protein (Mealey 2008). Membrane-bound transporters are expressed in many cell types including intestinal epithelial cells, capillary endothelial cells of the brain, biliary canalicular cells and epithelial cells of the renal tubules, placenta, and testicle (Mealey et al. 2001). The functions of these transporters are to actively (ATP dependent) pump xenobiotics out of the cell. Gut luminal drug or other xenobiotic are absorbed into cells based upon lipophilicity and are actively pumped back into the lumen of bowel. This function is suggested to be protective of the organism and is conserved across organisms from bacteria, protozoa and nematodes (Mealey et al. 2001). P-glycoprotein functions normally with a wide variety of compounds including chemotherapeutics, immunomodulators, anti-parasitic agents, steroids, and many other compounds.

As with other genetic polymorphisms or mutations, animals possessing these variant genetics appear outwardly normal, until they are exposed to a substrate for the protein. Once exposed to a substrate, the poorly functional or absent P-glycoprotein does not remove the drug from the cell and toxicity develops. Ivermectin sensitivity in collies results from the accumulation of high levels of drug within the central nervous systems (CNS) of these dogs. Mealey and colleagues demonstrated that the four base-pair mutation in the *ABCB1* gene creates a nonsense codon leading to the premature stop codon for synthesis of this protein (Mealey et al. 2001). Homozygous mutant dogs display toxicity (salivation, vomiting, confusion, ataxia, tremors) with doses greater than 120 μg/kg, while homozygous wild-type dogs do not. Heterozygous normal/mutant dogs may show toxicity at higher doses of ivermectin or after multiple daily doses (Mealey et al. 2001). Other macrocyclic lactones have also been reported to result in neurologic sequelae in these dogs (Barbet et al. 2009). Of similar importance, the ABCB1Δ genotype in dogs is associated with a wide variety of adverse reactions to other drugs used in this species. Dogs homozygous for the ABCB1Δ mutation are at much greater risk for adverse drug reactions when administered a wide variety of drugs from other classes. Mealey and coworkers have demonstrated that loperamide, vincristine, vinblastine, doxorubicin, digoxin, and cyclosporine, among others, are substrate molecules of P-gp (Coelho et al. 2009; Kaiser et al. 2007; Henik et al. 2006; Lind et al. 2013; Sartor et al. 2004). It is presently accepted that dogs possessing at least one copy of the ABCB1Δ mutation receiving standard dosages of vincristine for chemotherapy of neoplasia demonstrate hematologic toxicity due to the prolonged residence of the drug (Mealey et al. 2008b). For the anesthesiologist, other drugs such as acepromazine and loperamide as substrates of P-gp in dogs and other species suggest that dogs with the ABCB1-1Δ mutation may respond differently to sedatives, analgesics or anesthetics than wild-type P-gp expressing dogs (Deshpande et al. 2016; Sartor et al. 2004). Deshpande and coworkers demonstrated that standard doses of acepromazine in homozygous mut/mut collies resulted in prolonged sedation when compared to normal dogs and suggested dosage reductions or selection of differing pre-anesthetic/sedation drugs would be prudent (Deshpande et al. 2016). Considering that humans who carry similar polymorphisms in their drug metabolizing or efflux transporter pumps demonstrate adverse reactions to the administration of opiates and other drugs categorizing clinical responses of patients to administered drugs could lead to further understanding of how these polymorphisms in veterinary patients result in abnormal clinical reactions (Madadi et al. 2013).

Similar nonsense mutations of *ABCB1* were reported in cats (Mealey and Burke 2015). Of the eight animals evaluated in one study, one was homozygous for a double mutation of the *ABCB1* (1930_1931 deletion TC) (Mealey and Burke 2015). The remaining cats were homozygous wild type at this locus. However, there were 14 other nonsense mutations present within the DNA sequences of these cats. As seven of these cats had reportedly developed neurologic manifestations after being given an avermectin or avermectin combination type of anthelmintic, it is presumed that more than one polymorphism may result in dysfunction of this protein.

A mouse model, which was produced prior to identification of the canine gene polymorphism, where homozygous mutant *ABCB1* mice were exquisitely sensitive to ivermectin therapies, were also found to be susceptible to the side effects of other drugs which may be administered to animals (Schinkel et al. 1995). As such, several reports have gradually appeared in the literature demonstrating sensitivity to a number of other drugs in *ABCB1Δ* dogs. Loperamide, vincristine, vinblastine, doxorubicin, digoxin, and mexiletine sensitivities were reported in collies which were either heterozygous or homozygous for the *ABCB1Δ* gene (Sartor et al. 2004; Mealey et al. 2003, Henik et al. 2006).

Lind and coworkers, studying gene polymorphisms in border collies affected by vincristine associated myelosuppression demonstrated a normal sequence in the region of *ABCB1-1Δ* mutation, with eight additional SNPs in this gene (Lind et al. 2013). One such polymorphism, an insertion mutation, has been associated with sensitivity to ivermectin toxicity (Han et al. 2010). Like avermectin-sensitive cats, these intronic and DNA-binding region SNPs could alter gene transcription leading to dysfunction of these enzymes (Court 2007).

P-gp is present and functions in the intestine, biliary, and renal epithelium and modifies drug disposition. Studies indicate that there are few differences between a homozygous mutant *ABCB1Δ* dog or wild-type dog administered an inhibitor of P-gp. Dogs administered P-gp inhibitors (such as ketoconazole) would have similar drug disposition as observed in the *ABCB1Δ* dog. As mentioned previously, ketoconazole administration augments the absorption of cyclosporine by inhibiting CYP3A and P-gp in the gut.

Other mutations of the *ABCB1* gene indicate an association with an intronic SNP (c.-6-180T>G) of the *ABCB1* gene in phenobarbital-resistant idiopathic epilepsy of border collies (Mizukami et al. 2013; Alves et al. 2011). In this mutation, it is proposed that gene transcription may be modified by the mutation resulting in altered responsiveness to drug therapy. Some investigators speculate this altered transcription associated with over-expression of P-gp in the brain of epileptic dogs may be responsible for uncontrollable seizures. Their proposal suggests that medications prescribed to prevent seizures do not achieve adequate concentrations within brain cells (Pekcec et al. 2009). A similar proposal has been proposed in humans with intractable epilepsy (Tishler et al. 1995). Their theory involves excess P-gp limits exposure of neurons to anti-epileptic drugs by their removal from this tissue. In other studies, seizuring collies possessing two copies of the *ABCB1Δ* mutation, had fewer seizures, were managed with fewer drugs achieving similar plasma concentrations with fewer adverse events than heterozygous dogs and wild-type dogs at this gene locus, suggesting that brain concentrations of anti-epilepsy drugs would be higher in the *ABCB1-1Δ* mutants (Munana et al. 2012). This controversy remains to be resolved as homozygous, *ABCB1-1Δ* dogs should have equal or higher brain concentrations of anti-epileptic drugs and more commonly used anti-seizure medications are not strong substrates for P-gp (West and Mealey 2007).

In large animals, most studies have evaluated the impacts of P-gp and inhibition of this pump on drug disposition. *ABCG2* has been shown to be upregulated in lactation in cows (Otero et al. 2015). In this location, it is apparent these pumps function to add drugs and dietary components to the milk. While increased drug concentrations within the milk may be advantageous therapeutically, increased milk drug levels could result in violative residues (Otero et al. 2015). In this study, the reported *ABCG2* mutation is a gain of function change in which the heterozygous animals had higher drug danofloxacin concentrations in the milk of animals receiving parenteral danofloxacin (Otero et al. 2015). Likewise, milk concentrations of drugs are decreased when animals ate feed containing inhibitors of ABC-cassette transporters (Perez et al. 2013). Drugs used in food animals have also been shown to be inhibitors of *ABCG2* and may alter the disposition of drugs to the udder (Barrera et al. 2012; Wassermann et al. 2013). Antibiotics (cephalexin, enrofloxacin, lincomycin, tilmicosin), other drugs (eprinomectrin, albendazole, flunixin, sodium salicylate) and dietary flavinoids (equol and quercetin) appear to be substrates of *ABCG2 in vitro* (Wassermann et al. 2013). Disposition of drugs to the udder of lactating animals may be modulated by drugs or dietary components and produce alterations in drug disposition. In the GI tract, inhibitors of transporters have been used to augment the parasite tissue concentrations of avermectin thereby improving the efficacy of their use against drug-resistant *Haemonchus* spp. and other parasites (Lifschitz et al. 2010). It is not known whether inhibition of the *ABCG2* function in the lactating mammary gland would impact plasma concentrations of a drug. Future studies should evaluate these questions as well as characterize differences between species and breeds to evaluate the impact of these ABC-transporters in animals.

Feline Hypokalemia

Periodic hypokalemic polymyopathy in cats was originally described in Burmese kittens (Blaxter et al. 1986). These, and other authors, characterized the weakness as episodic myalgia, generalized weakness and, in some cases, weakness of the neck and forelimb muscles (Blaxter et al. 1986). In more recent studies in the Burmese and Tonkinese breeds of cats, a nonsense mutation causing the production of a truncated version of lysine-deficient 4 protein kinase (WNK4) was detected (Gandolfi et al. 2012). This kinase regulates the activity or inactivity of other kinases in the kidney and has an autophosphorylation site that regulates the activity of itself. The function of WNK4 is to down regulate a variety of sodium-chloride co-transporters, sodium channels and renal outer medullary potassium channels (Gandolfi et al. 2012). The activity of WNK4 regulates the relative status of renal regulation of volume versus potassium wasting. In the mutated form, potassium loss is severe enough to cause hypokalemia in these cats. Knowledge of the breed of cat and the clinical signs in this case would be important to recognize early on in planning for a specific procedure.

Inherited Ventricular Arrhythmias and Sudden Death of German Shepherd Dogs

Ventricular arrhythmias leading to sudden cardiac death in German Shepherd dogs were first described in 1994 (Mosie et al. 1994). Animals known to be from lines of affected dogs did not possess structural or functional indications of cardiac disease, were active and apparently free of significant disease. Several died before their first year of age, often while sleeping or shortly after exercise. Of those dogs evaluated that died suddenly, each was observed to have intermittent episodes of polymorphic ventricular tachycardia. All affected dogs were related to a single sire. Recently, Jesty and coworkers demonstrated that affected German Shepherd dogs demonstrated electrophysiologic alterations due to abnormal calcium cycling within the affected dog's myocardial cells (Jesty et al. 2013). Lowered expression of the gene *ATP2A2* (Calcium transporting, ATPase) and the protein product transcribed (SERCA2a) was observed in severely affected German Shepherd dogs compared to unaffected dogs (Jesty et al. 2013). There was an inverse correlation between severity of cardiac dysfunction and *ATP2A2a* expression. Further, analysis of the affected and control expressed sequences demonstrated several polymorphisms within the affected GSD cDNA. At present, there is no information regarding change of function SNPs. Future studies should analyze the potential significance for polymorphisms expressed in this dog phenotype as well as evaluate genomic DNA for the presence of non-coding (intronic) SNPs to determine whether promotors or other DNA binding sites are altered.

Opioids and Other Polymorphisms

Opioids are commonly used to treat moderate-to-severe, acute, and chronic pain. Opioid receptors are widely distributed in animals and both endogenous opioid-like compounds and exogenous (drugs) act at these receptors. The majority of these drugs are relatively inexpensive but potent, and the side effects well recognized. In spite of their common incorporation into analgesic protocols, variability in response between patients and their diseases are also common. Wide variation in both analgesic efficacy and the generation of intolerable side effects is of major concern for the patient.

Multi-modal approaches to pain management allow the use of smaller quantities of opioids, thereby reducing opioid-associated adverse effects. Combinations of an opioid with a phenothiazine, benzodiazepine or α-adrenergic agents are commonly utilized. Common adverse effects observed with rapid IV dosing and prolonged dosing such as constipation, nausea, vomiting, anxiousness, respiratory depression are often clinically relevant.

In humans, variability in responses have been associated with variability in cytochrome P450 and phase II metabolism and variation in genetic sequences of opioid receptors (Cregg et al. 2013). A number of other factors have been shown to be associated with decreased or increased efficacy or incidence of adverse effects with the use of some opioids in humans (Cregg et al. 2013). Mu opioid receptor polymorphisms (*OPRM1*) in humans have been associated with increased dose requirements in acute and chronic pain subjects (Klepstad et al. 2004; Chou et al. 2006). Those individuals possessing the normal A allele at this location require less opioid for cancer-associated pain. In addition, individuals with variant mu opioid receptors (118 A>G variants) have fewer side effects (sedation, nausea, vomiting) suggesting this variant receptor has lowered sensitivity to opioid binding (Cregg et al. 2013).

The transcription factor regulating expression of the mu opioid receptor gene (OPRM1) STAT6, and the β-arrestin (*ARRB2*) gene modulate the responses to opioids and opioid switching (Ross et al. 2005). Cytochrome P450 metabolism in humans, is involved in conversion of codeine to morphine (CYP450 2D6), oxycodone to oxymorphone (CYP450 2D6), and tramadol to O-desmethyltramadol (CYP450 2D6). Polymorphisms in human CYP450 2D6 are associated with variation in codeine metabolism from little analgesia (poor metabolizers) to high proportions of side effects (extensive metabolizers). Human CYP450 3A enzymes involved in metabolism of some opioids were associated with clinically relevant adverse events (Cregg et al. 2013). In humans, with over 100 known polymorphisms in CYP4502D6, phenotypic classification into poor, intermediate, extensive, and ultra-rapid metabolizers is possible. In dogs, metabolism of opiates differs significantly from humans. Codeine is poorly absorbed in dogs, who produce little morphine via P-450 metabolism; rather, the major elimination pathway appears to be via glucuronidation to the codeine-6

glucuronide (Kukanich 2009). In humans, phase II metabolism of morphine is primarily via UGT2B7. Morphine is converted to morphine 3-glucuronide (M3G) and morphine 6-glucuronide (M6G). Morphine 3-glucuronide does not bind to opioid receptors and has been incriminated in excitation, hyperalgesia and allodynia in some patients. In contrast, M6G binds to opioid receptors and has significant analgesic effects. Animal differences in conjugation reactions could contribute to adverse reactions observed clinically.

Little is known about the impact of these polymorphisms in animals. Opioid receptor polymorphisms have been reported in cattle, dogs, horses and swine (Hawley and Wetmore 2010; Li et al. 2003). In dogs, one polymorphism is predicted to be associated with "dysphoria." Whereas, in swine, the two reported polymorphisms were observed in breeds displaying stereotypical behavior (Li et al. 2003). A greater understanding of these polymorphisms should prove valuable in guiding the use of opioids clinically. This may lead to better understanding of how adverse drug reactions occur and potentially interactions between these and other receptors.

Polymorphisms in the *ABCB1* gene have been shown to alter the patient's opioid response phenotype. For some variants, reduced morphine doses can be used resulting in less opioid-associated nausea and have been reported (Cregg et al. 2013). In contrast, in children, opioid-induced respiratory depression has been associated with polymorphisms in *ABCB1* (Sadhasivam et al. 2015). Like those polymorphisms present in humans, the well-characterized *ABCB1-1Δ* mutation in dogs is associated with central sedation and anesthesia after administration of loperamide (Sartor et al. 2004). To date, only two studies have documented opioid receptor polymorphisms in veterinary species.

Polymorphisms in catechol-O-methyltransferase have been shown to reduce the activity of this enzyme (>3-fold reduction) (Rakvag et al. 2005). In humans, these polymorphisms are associated with increased opioid-dose requirements and severity of nausea and vomiting (Laugsand et al. 2011). Human polymorphisms in catechol-O-methyl transferase (COMT) are associated with an individual's "sensitivity to pain" (Zhang et al. 2015). Polymorphism of the *COMT* gene at rs4680 produces a missense mutation (valine to methionine). Decreased activity of the COMT protein has been associated with accumulation of catecholamines and increased fentanyl requirements after surgery (Zhang et al. 2015). Several polymorphisms in COMT have been described in horses (Momozawa et al. 2005).

More investigation is needed to decipher the impact of polymorphisms in drug-metabolizing enzymes and transporters. With the rapid development of recombinant large- and small-animal drug metabolism and disposition enzymes, more information regarding substrate selectivity will become available. As more information becomes available on substrate selectivity, especially in polymorphic enzymes, it will become possible to tease out potential or clinical adverse reactions. Clinical observations remain critical to pharmacogenetic evaluation of these important systems. Understanding of how drugs work in individuals will provide more precise guidelines on the use of drugs. Knowledge of breed-specific polymorphisms could alert the veterinarian to potential adverse reactions prior to sedation/anesthesia.

References

Aidasani, D., Zaya, M.J., Malpas, P.B., and Locuson. (2008). In vitro drug-drug interaction screens for canine veterinary medicines: evaluation of cytochrome P450 reversible inhibition. *Drug Metab. Dispos.* 36: 1512–1518.

Alpay, F. et al. (2014). Genome-wide association study of the susceptibility to infection by *Mycobacterium avium*, subspecies paratuberculosis in Holstein cattle. *PLoS One* 9 (12): e111704. https://doi.org/10.1371/journal.pone.0111704.

Alves, L., Hulsmeyer, A., Jaggy, A. et al. (2011). Polymorphisms in the ABCB1 gene in phenobarbital responsive and resistant idiopathic epilepsy border collies. *J. Vet. Intern. Med.* 25: 484–489.

Archer, T.M., Boothe, D.M., Langston, V.C. et al. (2014). Oral cyclosporine treatment in dogs: a review of the literature. *J. Vet. Intern. Med.* 28: 1–20.

Aretz, J.S. and Geyer, J. (2010). Detection of the CYP1A2 1117C>T polymorphism in 14 dog breeds. *J. Vet. Pharmacol. Ther.* 34: 98–100.

Baratta, M.T., Zaya, M.J., White, J.A., and Locuson, C.W. (2009). Canine CYP4502B11 metabolizes and is inhibited by anesthetic agents often co-administered in dogs. *J. Vet. Pharmacol. Ther.* 33: 50–55.

Barbet, J.L., Snook, T., Gay, J.M., and Mealey, K.L. (2009). ABCB1-1 Delta (MDR1-1 Delta) genotype is associated with adverse reactions in dogs treated with milbemycin oxime for generalized demodicosis. *Vet. Dermatol.* 20: 111–114.

Barrera, B., Otero, J.A., Egido, E. et al. (2012). The anthelmintic triclabendazole and its metabolites inhibit the membrane transporter ABCG2/BCRP. *Antimicrob. Agents Chemother.* 56: 3535–3543.

Blaisdell, J., Goldstein, J.A., and Bai, S. (1998). Isolation of a new canine cytochrome P450 cDNA from the cytochrome P450 2C subfamily (CYP2C41) and evidence for polymorphic differences in its expression. *Drug Metab. Dispos.* 26: 278–283.

Blaxter, A., Livesley, P., Gruffydd-Jones, T., and Wotton, P. (1986). Periodic muscle weakness in Burmese kittens. *Vet. Rec.* 118: 619–620.

Burns, L.C., Orsini, L., and L'Italien, G. (2013). Value-based assessment of pharmacodiagnostic testing from early stage development to real-world use. *Value Health* 16: S16–S19.

Chong-Sheng, C., Lin, J.T., Goss, K.A. et al. (2004). Activation of the anticancer prodrugs cyclophosphamide and ifosfamide: identification of cytochrome P450 2B enzymes and site-specific mutants with improved enzyme kinetics. *Mol. Pharmacol.* 65: 1278–1285.

Chou, W.Y., Wang, C.H., Liu, P.H. et al. (2006). Human opioid receptor A118G polymorphism affects intravenous patient-controlled analgesia morphine consumption after total abdominal hysterectomy. *Anesthesiology* 105: 334–337.

Coelho, J.C., Tucker, R., Mattoon, J. et al. (2009). Biliary excretion of technetium-99m-sestambi in wild-type dogs and in dogs with intrinsic (ABCB1-1Δ mutation) and extrinsic (ketoconazole treated) P-glycoprotein deficiency. *J. Vet. Pharmacol. Ther.* 32: 417–421. Columbia Systems Biology systemsbiology.columbia.edu/isaec#.

Corado, C.R., McKemie, D.S., Young, A., and Kynch, H.K. (2016). Evidence for polymorphism in the cytochrome P450 2D gene in horses. *J. Vet. Pharmacol. Ther.* 39: 245–254.

Court, M.H. (2007). A pharmacogenomics primer. *J. Clin. Pharmacol.* 47: 1087–1103.

Court, M.H. (2013a). Canine cytochrome P450 (CYP) pharmacogenetics. *Vet. Clin. North Am. Small Anim. Pract.* 43: 1027–1038.

Court, M.H. (2013b). Feline drug metabolism and disposition. Pharmacokinetic evidence for species differences and molecular mechanisms. *Vet. Clin. North Am. Small Anim. Pract.* 43: 1039–1054.

Court, M.H. and Greenblatt, D.J. (2000). Molecular genetic basis for deficient acetaminophen glucuronidation by cats: UGT1A6 is a pseudogene, and evidence for reduced diversity of expressed hepatic UGT1A isoforms. *Pharmacogenetics* 10: 355–369.

Court, M.H., Von Moltke, L.L., Shader, R.I., and Greenblatt, D.J. (1997). Biotransformation of chlorzoxazone by hepatic microsomes from humans and 10 other mammalian species. *Biopharm. Drug Dispos.* 18: 213–226.

Court, M.H., Hay Kraus, B.L., Hill, D.W. et al. (1999). Propofol hydroxylation by dog liver microsomes: assay development and dog breed differences. *Drug Metab. Dispos.* 27: 1293–1299.

Cregg, R., Russo, G., Gubbay, A. et al. (2013). Pharmacogenetics of analgesic drugs. *Br. J. Pain* 7: 189–208.

Daly, A.K. (2012). Using genome-wide association studies to identify important serious adverse drug reactions. *Annu. Rev. Pharmacol. Toxicol.* 52: 21–35.

Deshpande, D., Hill, K.E., Mealey, K.L. et al. (2016). The effect of the canine ABCB1-1Delta mutation on sedation after intravenous administration of acepromazine. *JVIM* 30: 636–641.

Dhamankar, V.S., Assem, M., and Donovan, M.D. (2013). Gene expression and immunochemical localization of major cytochrome P450 drug-metabolizing enzymes in bovine nasal olfactory and respiratory mucosa. *Inhalation Toxicol.* 27: 767–777.

DiMaio Knych, H.K., DeStefano, S.C., Buckpitt, A.R., and Stanley, S.D. (2009). Equine cytochrome P450 2C92: cDNA cloning, expression and initial characterization. *Arch. Biochem. Biophys.* 485: 49–55.

DiMaio Knych, H.K., McKemie, D.S., and Stanley, S.D. (2010). Molecular cloning, expression, and initial characterization of members of the CYP3A family in horses. *Drug Metab. Dispos.* 38: 1820–1827.

Du, X., Servin, B., Womack, J.E. et al. (2014). An update of the goat genome assembly using dense radiation hybrid maps allows detailed analysis of evolutionary rearrangements in bovidae. *BMC Genomics* 15: 625. https://doi.org/10.1186/1471-2164-15-625.

Eichelbaum, M. and Gross, A.S. (1990). The genetic polymorphism of debrisoquine/sparteine metabolism – clinical aspects. *Pharmacol. Ther.* 46: 377–394.

Elsik, C.G., Bovine Genome Sequencing and Analysis Consortium et al. (2009). The genome sequence of taurine cattle: a window to ruminant biology and evolution. *Science* 324: 522–528.

Fink-Gremmels, J. (2008). Implications of hepatic cytochrome P-450-related biotransformation processes in veterinary species. *Eur. J. Pharmacol.* 585: 502–509.

Forsberg, S.K.G., Kierczak, M., Liungvall, I. et al. (2015). The Shepherds' tale: a genome-wide study across 9 dog breeds implicates two loci in the regulation of fructosamine serum concentration in Belgian shepherds. *PLoS One* 10 (5): e0123173. http://dx.doi.org/10.1371/journal.pone.0123173.

Fraser, D.J., Feyereisen, R., Harlow, G.R., and Halpert, J.R. (1997). Isolation, heterologous expression and functional characterization of a novel cytochrome P450 3A enzyme from a canine liver cDNA library. *J. Pharmacol. Exp. Ther.* 283: 1425–1432.

Gagliardi, R., Llambi, S., and Arruga, M.V. (2015). SNP genetic polymorphisms of MDR-1, CYP1A2 and CYP2B11 genes in 4 canine breeds upon toxicological evaluation. *J. Vet. Sci.* 16: 273–280.

Gandolfi, B., Gruffydd-Jones, T.J., Malik, R. et al. (2012). First WNK4-hypokalemia animal model identified by genome-wide association in Burmese cats. *PLoS One* 7 (12): e53173. https://doi.org/10.1371/journal.pone.0053173.

Garcia, E.R. (2014). Pharmacogentics in anaesthesia. *Vet. Times* 44 (15): 8–9.

Geisen, V., Wever, K., and Hartmann, K. (2009). Vitamin D-dependent hereditary rickets type I in a cat. *J. Vet. Intern. Med.* 23: 196–199.

Gonzalez, F.J., Skoda, R.C., Kimura, S. et al. (1988). Characterization of the common genetic defect in humans deficient in debrisoquine metabolism. *Nature* 331: 442–446.

Grahn, R.A., Ellis, M.R., Grahn, J.C., and Lyons, L.A. (2012). A novel CYP27B1 mutation causes a feline vitamin D-dependent rickets type IA. *J. Feline Med. Surg.* 14: 587–590.

Han, J.I., Son, H.W., and Park SCNa K-J. (2010). Novel insertion mutant of ABCB1 gene in an ivermectin-sensitive border collie. *J. Vet. Med. Sci.* 11: 341–344.

Hawley, A.T. and Wetmore, L.A. (2010). Identification of single nucleotide polymorphisms within exon 1 of the canine mu-opioid receptor gene. *Vet. Anesth. Analg.* 37: 79–82.

Hay Kraus, B.L., Greenblatt, D.J., Venkatakrishnan, K., and Court, M. (2000). Evidence for propofol hydroxylation by cytochrome P4502B11 in canine liver microsomes: breed and gender differences. *Xenobiotica* 30: 575–588.

Hendrickson, S.L. (2013). A genome wide study of genetic adaptation to high altitude in feral Andean horses of the paramo. *BMC Evol. Biol.* 13: 273. https://doi.org/10.1186/1471-2148-13-273.

Henik, R.A., Kellum, H.B., Bentjen, S.A., and Mealey, K.L. (2006). Digoxin and Mexiletine sensitivity in a collie with the MDR1 mutation. *J. Vet. Intern. Med.* 20: 415–417.

Hrycay, E.G. and Bandiera, S.M. (2015). Monooxygenase, perioxidase and peroxygenase properties and reaction mechanisms of cytochrome P450 enzymes, Chapter 1. *Adv. Exp. Med. Biol.* 851: 1–62.

Idle, J.R. and Smith, R.L. (1979). Polymorphisms of oxidation at carbon centers of drugs and their clinical significance. *Drug Metabol. Rev.* 9: 301–317.

Ingelman-Sundberg, M., Sim, S.C., Gomez, A., and Rodriguez-Antona, C. (2007). Influence of cytochrome P450 polymorphisms on drug therapies: pharmacogenetic, pharmacoepigentic and clinical aspects. *Pharmacol. Ther.* 116: 496–526.

Intorre, L., Mengozzi, G., Maccheroni, M. et al. (1995). Enrofloxacin-theophylline interactions: influence of enrofloxacin on theophylline steady-state pharmacokinetics in the beagle dog. *J. Vet. Pharmacol. Ther.* 18: 352–356.

Jesty, S.A., Jung, S.W., Cordeiro, J.M. et al. (2013). Cardiomyocyte calcium cycling in a naturally occurring German shepherd dog model of inherited ventricular arrhythmia and sudden cardiac death. *J. Vet. Cardiol.* 15: 5–14.

Jiang, Y., Xie, M., Chen, W. et al. (2014). The sheep genome illuminates biology of the rumen and lipid metabolism. *Science* 344: 1168–1173.

Kaiser, C.I., Fidel, J.L., Roos, M., and Kaser-Hotz, B. (2007). Re-evaluation of the University of Wisconsin 2-year protocol for treating canine lymphoma. *J. Am. Anim. Hosp. Assoc.* 43: 85–92.

Kalow, W. (1971). Topics in pharmacogenetics. *Ann. N. Y. Acad. Sci.* 179: 654–659.

Kennerly, E.M., Idaghdour, Y., Olby, N.J. et al. (2009). Pharmacogenetic association study of 30 genes with phenobarbital response in epileptic dogs. *Pharmacogenet. Genomics* 19: 911–922.

Klepstad, P., Rakvåg, T.T., Kaasa, S. et al. (2004). The 118 A>G polymorphism in human mu-opioid receptor gene may increase requirements in patients with pain caused by malignant disease. *Acat Anaesth. Scand.* 48: 1232–1239.

Knych, H.K., Corado, C.R., McKemie, D.S. et al. (2012). Pharmacokinetics and pharmacodynamics of tramadol in horses following oral administration. *J. Vet. Pharmacol. Ther.* 36: 389–398.

Krein, S.R., Lindsey, J.C., Blaze, C.A., and Wetmore, L.A. (2014). Evaluation of risk factors, including fluconazole administration, for prolonged anesthetic recovery times in horses undergoing general anesthesia for ocular surgery: 81 cases (2006-2013). *J. Am. Vet. Med. Assoc.* 244: 577–581.

Kukanich, B. (2009). Pharmacokinetics of acetaminophen, codeine and the codeine metabolites morphine and codeine-6-glucuronide in healthy greyhound dogs. *J. Vet. Pharmacol. Ther.* 33: 15–21.

Lankford, S.M., Bai, S.A., and Goldstein, J.A. (2000). Cloning of canine cytochrome P450 2E1 CDNA: identification and characterization of two variant alleles. *Drug Metab. Dispos.* 28: 981–986.

Laugsand, E.A., Fladvad, T., Skorpen, F. et al. (2011). Clinical and genetic factors associated with nausea and vomiting in cancer patients receiving opioids. *Eur. J. Cancer* 47: 1682–1691.

Lemley, C.O., Koch, J.M., Blemings, K.P. et al. (2008). Concommittant changes in progesterone catabolic enzymes, cytochrome P450 2C and 3A, with plasma insulin concentrations in ewes supplemented with sodium acetate or sodium propionate. *Animal* 2: 1223–1239.

Lemley, C.O., Wilmoth, T.A., Tager, L.R. et al. (2010). Effect of a high cornstarch diet on hepatic cytochrome p450 2C and 3A activity and progesterone half-life in dairy cows. *J. Dairy Sci.* 93: 1012–1021.

Li, J.H., Cui, W.G., and Bao, J. (2003). Single nucleotide polymorphism analysis in sow mu opioid receptor gene exon III. *Yi Chuan Xue Bao* 30: 30–34.

Lieber, C.S. (2004). The discovery of the microsomal ethanol oxidizing system and its physiologic and pathologic role. *Physiol. Rev.* 77: 517–544.

Lifschitz, A., Entrocasso, C., Alvarez, L. et al. (2010). Interference with P-glycoprotein improves ivermectin activity against adult resistant nematodes in sheep. *Vet. Parasitol.* 172: 291–298.

Lind, D.L., Fidel, J.L., Gay, J.M., and Mealey, K.L. (2013). Evaluation of vincristine associated myelosuppression in border collies. *Am. J. Vet. Res.* 74: 257–261.

Lindblad-Toh, K., Wade, C.M., Mikkelsen, T.S. et al. (2005). Genomic sequence, comparative analysis and haplotype structure of the domestic dog. *Nature* 431: 931–945.

Lu, P., Singh, S.B., Carr, B.A. et al. (2005). Selective inhibition of dog hepatic CYP2B11 and CYP3A12. *J. Pharmacol. Exp. Ther.* 313: 518–528.

Ludden, T.M. (1985). Pharmacokinetic interactions of the macrolide antibiotics. *Clin. Pharmacokinet.* 10: 63–79.

Madadi, P., Sistonen, J., Siverman, G. et al. (2013). Life-threatening adverse events following therapeutic opioid administration in adults: is Pharmacogenetic analysis useful? *Pain Res. Manag.* 18: 133–136.

Mahgoup, A., Dring, L., Idle, J.R. et al. (1977). Polymorphic hydroxylation of debrisoquine in man. *Lancet* 2: 584–586.

Mandsager, R.E., Clarke, C.R., Shawley, R.V., and Hague, C.M. (1995). Effects of chloramphenicol on infusion pharmacokinetics of propofol in greyhounds. *Am. J. Vet. Res.* 56: 95–99.

Martignoni, M., Groothuis, G., and de Kanter, R. (2006). Species differences between mouse, rat, dog, monkey and human CTP-mediated drug metabolism, inhibition and induction. *Expert Opin. Drug Metab. Toxicol.* 2: 875–894.

Martinez, M.N., Antonovic, L., Court, M.H. et al. (2013). Challenges in exploring the cytochrome P450 system as a source of variation in canine drug pharmacokinetics. *Drug Metabol. Rev.* 45: 218–230.

Martinez et al. (2020). Pharmacogenomics of poor drug metabolism in Greyhounds: Cytochrome P450 (CYP)2B11 genetic variation, breed distribution, and functional characterization. *Nature/Scientific Reports.* https://doi.org/10.1038/s41598-019-56660-z.

McLeod, H.L. and Yu, J. (2003). Cancer pharmacogenomics: SNPs, chips, and the individual patient. *Cancer Investig.* 21: 630–640.

Mealey, K.L. (2006). Pharmacogenetics. *Vet. Clin. North Am. Small Anim. Pract.* 36: 961–973.

Mealey, K.L. (2008). Canine ABCB1 and macrocyclic lactones: heartworm prevention and pharmacogenetics. *Vet. Parasitol.* 158: 215–222.

Mealey, K.L. and Burke, N.S. (2015). Identification of a nonsense mutation in feline ABCB1. *J. Vet. Pharmacol. Ther.* 38: 429–433.

Mealey, K.L. and Meurs, K.M. (2008). Breed distribution of the ABCB1-1Δ (multidrug sensitivity) polymorphism among dogs undergoing ABCB1 genotyping. *J. Am. Vet. Med. Assoc.* 233: 921–924.

Mealey, K.L., Bentjen, S.A., Gay, J.M., and Cantor, G.H. (2001). Ivermectin sensitivity in collies is associated with a deletion mutation of the mdr1 gene. *Pharmacogenetics* 11: 727–733.

Mealey, K.L., Northrup, N.C., and Bentjen, S.A. (2003). Increased toxicity of P-glycoprotein-substrate chemotherapeutic agents in a dog with the MDR1 mutation associated with ivermectin sensitivity. *J. Am. Vet. Med. Assoc.* 223: 1453–1455.

Mealey, K.L., Jabbes, M., Spencer, E., and Akey, J.M. (2008a). Differential expression of CYP3A12 and CYP3A26 mRNA's in canine liver and intestine. *Xenobiotica* 38: 1305–1312.

Mealey, K.L., Fidel, J., Gay, J.M. et al. (2008b). ABCB1-1Δ polymorphism can predict hematologic toxicity in dogs treated with vincristine. *J. Vet. Intern. Med.* 22: 996–1000.

Michalowska, M., Winiarczek, S., Adaszek, L. et al. (2014). Phase I/II clinical trial of encapsulated, cytochrome P450 expressing cells as local activators of cyclophosphamide to treat spontaneous canine tumors. *PLoS One* 9 (7): e102061. https://doi.org/10.137/journal.pone.0102061.

Mise, M., Yadera, S., and Matsuda, M. (2004). Polymorphic expression of CYP1A2 leading to interindividual variability in metabolism of a novel benzodiazepine receptor partial inverse agonist in dogs. *Drug Metab. Dispos.* 32: 240–245.

Miskimins Mills, B., Zaya, M.J., Walters, R.R. et al. (2010). Current cytochrome P450 phenotyping methods applied to metabolic drug-drug interaction prediction in dogs. *Drug Metab. Dispos.* 38: 396–404.

Mizukami, K., Yabuki, A., Chang, H.-S. et al. (2013). High frequency of a single nucleotide substitution (c.-6-180T>G) of the canine MDR1/ABCB1 gene associated with phenobarbital resistant idiopathic epilepsy in border collie dogs. *Dis. Markers* 35: 669–672.

Momozawa, Y., Takeuchi, Y., Tozaki, T. et al. (2005). Sequence, detection of polymorphisms and radiation hybrid mapping of the equine catechol-o-methyltransferase gene. *Anim. Genet.* 36: 160–190.

Mosher, C.M. and Court, M.H. (2010). *Comparative and Veterinary Pharmacology, Handbook of Experimental Therapeutics 199*, https://doi.org/10.1007/978-3-642-10324-7_3, 49–84. Berlin: Springer-Verlag.

Mosie, N.S., Meyers-Wallen, V., Flahive, W.J. et al. (1994). Inherited ventricular arrhythmias and sudden death in German shepherd dogs. *J. Am. Coll. Cardiol.* 24: 233–243.

Mossner, L.D., Schmitz, A., Theurillat, R. et al. (2011). Inhibition of cytochrome P450 enzymes involved in ketamine metabolism by use of liver microsomes and specific cytochrome P450 enzymes from horses, dogs and humans. *Am. J. Vet. Res.* 72: 1505–1513.

Motulsky, A.G. (1957). Drug reactions, enzymes and biochemical genetics. *J. Am. Med. Assoc.* 165: 835–857.

Mucha, S., Bunger, L., and Conington, J. (2015). Genome-wide association study of footrot in Texel sheep. *Genet. Sel. Evol.* 47: 35. https://doi.org/10.1186/s12711-015-0119-3.

Munana, K.R., Nettifee-Osborne, R.L., Bergman, R.L., and Mealey, K.L. (2012). Association between ABCB1 genotype and seizure outcome in Collies with epilepsy. *J. Vet. Intern. Med.* 26: 1358–1364.

Myre, S.A., Schoeder, T.J., Grund, V.R. et al. (1991). Critical ketoconazole dosage range for ciclosporin clearance inhibition in dogs. *Pharmacol. Ther. Part A* 43: 233–241.

Nebbia, C., Dacasto, M., Giaccherino, A.R. et al. (2003). Comparative expression of liver cytochrome P450-dependent monooxygenases in the horse and other agricultural and laboratory species. *Vet. J.* 165: 53–64.

Nebert, D.W. (1999). Pharmacogenetics and pharmacogenomics: why is this relevant to the clinical geneticist? *Clin. Genet.* 56: 247–258.

Nishibe, Y., Wakabayashi, M., Harauchi, T., and Ohno, K. (1998). Characterization of cytochrome P450 (CYP3A12) induction by rifampicin in dog liver. *Xenobiotica* 28: 549–557.

Okamatsu, G., Komatsu, T., Ono, Y. et al. (2016). Characterization of feline cytochrome P450 2B6. *Xenobiotica* https://doi.org/10.3109/00498254.2016.1145754.

Otero, J.A., Barrera, B., de la Fuente, A. et al. (2015). Short communication: the gain of function Y581S polymorphism of the ABCG2 transporter increases secretion into milk of Danofloxacin at the time of therapeutic dose for mastitis treatment. *J. Dairy Sci.* 98: 312–317.

Papich, M.G.D. (2007. Chapter 16). Interactions. In: *Veterinary Anesthesia*, 4e (ed. W.V. Lumb and E.W. Jones), 439–450. Blackwell.

Parkinson, A., Ogilvie, B.W., Buckley, D.B. et al. (2013). Biotransformation of Xenobiotics. In: *Casarett and Doull's Toxicology: The Basic Science of Poisons*, Chapter 6, 8e (ed. C. Klaassen), 185–366. New York: McGraw-Hill.

Paul, A.J., Tranquilli, W.J., Seward, R.L. et al. (1987). Clinical observations in collies given ivermectin orally. *Am. J. Vet. Res.* 48: 684–685.

Paulson, S.K., Engel, L., Reitz, B. et al. (1999). Evidence for polymorphism in the canine metabolism of the cyclooxygenase 2 inhibitor, celecoxib. *Drug Metab. Dispos.* 27: 1133–1142.

Pekcec, A., Unkruer, B., Stein, V. et al. (2009). Over-expression of P-glycoprotein in the canine brain following spontaneous status epilepticus. *Epilepsy Res.* 83: 144–151.

Perez, M., Otero, J.A., Barrera, B. et al. (2013). Inhibition of ABCG2/BCRP transporter by soy isoflavones genistein and daidzein: effect on plasma and milk levels of Danofloxacin in sheep. *Vet. J.* 196: 203–208.

Peters, L.M., Demmel, S., Pusch, G. et al. (2013). Equine cytochrome P450 2B6 - genomic identification, expression and functional characterization with ketamine. *Toxicol. Appl. Pharmacol.* 266: 101–108.

Pontius, J.U., Mullikin, J.C., Smith, D.R. et al. (2007). Initial sequence and comparative analysis of the cat genome. *Genome Res.* 17: 1675–1689.

Rakvag, T.T., Klepstad, P., Baar, C. et al. (2005). The Val158Met polymorphism of the human catehcol-O-methyltransferase (COMT) gene may influence morphine requirements in cancer pain patients. *Pain* 116: 73–78.

Regmi, N.L., Abd El-Aty, A.M., Kuroha, M. et al. (2005). Inhibitory effect of several fluoroquinolones on hepatic microsomal cytochchrome P450 1A activities in dogs. *J. Vet. Pharmacol. Ther.* 28: 553–557.

Remmer, H. and Merker, H.J. (1963). Drug-induced changes in the liver endoplasmic reticulum: association with drug-metabolizing enzymes. *Science* 142: 1657–1658.

Rieder, M.J., Reiner, A.P., Gage, B.F. et al. (2005). Effect of VKORC1 haplotypes on transcriptional regulation and warfarin dose. *N. Engl. J. Med.* 352: 2285–2293.

Riviere, J. (2009). Absorption, distribution, metabolism and elimination; Chapter 2. In: *Veterinary Pharmacology and Therapeutics*, 9e (ed. J.E. Riviere and M.G. Papich), 38–46. Ames, IA: Wiley.

Robertson, S.A., Johnston, J., and Beemsterboer, J. (1992). Cardiopulmonary, anesthetic, and postanesthetic effects of intravenous infusions of propofol in Greyhounds and non-Greyhounds. *Am. J. Vet. Res.* 53: 1027–1032.

Ross, J.R., Rutter, D., Welsh, K. et al. (2005). Clinical response to morphine in cancer patients and genetic variation in candidate genes. *Pharmacogenomics J.* 5: 324–336.

Roussel, F., Duignan, D.B., Obach, R.S. et al. (1998). Expression and characterization of canine CYP 2D15. *Arch. Biochem. Biophys.* 357 (Supplement 1): 27–36.

Sadhasivam, S., Chidambaran, V., Zhang, X. et al. (2015). Opioid-induced respiratory depression: ABCB1 transporter pharmacogenetics. *Pharmacogenomics J.* 15: 119–126.

Sams, R.A. and Muir, W.W. (1988). Effects of phenobarbital on thiopental pharmacokinetics in Greyhounds. *Am. J. Vet. Res.* 49: 245–249.

Sams, R.A., Muir, W.W., Detra, R.L., and Robinson, E.P. (1985). Comparative pharmacokinetics and anesthetic effects of methohexital, pentobarbital, thiamylal and thiopental in greyhound dogs and non-greyhound, mixed-breed dogs. *Am. J. Vet. Res.* 46: 1677–1683.

Sartor, L.L., Bentjen, S.A., Trepanier, L., and Mealey, K.L. (2004). Loperamide toxicity in a collie with MDR1 mutation associated with ivermectin sensitivity. *J. Vet. Intern. Med.* 18: 117–118.

Scherr, M.C., Lourenco, G.J., Albuquerque, D.M., and Lima, C.S. (2010). Polymorphism of cytochrome P450 A2 (CYP1A2)

in pure and mixed breed dogs. *J. Vet. Pharmacol. Ther.* 34: 184–186.

Schinkel, A.H., Wagenaar, E., van Deemter, L. et al. (1995). Absence of the mdr1a P-glycoprotein in mice affects tissue distribution and pharmacokinetics of dexamethasone, digoxin and cyclosporine A. *J. Clin. Investig.* 96: 1698–1705.

Schmitz, A., Demmel, S., Peters, L.M. et al. (2010). Comparative human-horse sequence analysis of the CYP3A subfamily gene cluster. *Animal Genet.* 41 (Suppl 2): 72–79.

Shou, M., Norcross, R., Sandig, G. et al. (2003). Substrate specificity and kinetic properties of seven heterologously expressed dog cytochromes p450. *Drug Metab. Dispos.* 31: 1161–1169.

Sivapathasundaram, S., Magnisali, P., Coldham, N.G. et al. (2001). A study of the expression of xenobiotic-metabolising cytochrome P450 proteins and of testosterone metabolism in bovine liver. *Biochem. Pharmacol.* 62: 635–645.

Smith, R. (2001). The discovery of the debrisoquine hydroxylation polymorphism: scientific and clinical impact and consequences. *Forensic Toxicol.* 168: 11–19.

Spier, S.J., Carlson, G.P., Pickar, J., and Snyder, J.R. (1989). Hyperkalemnic periodic paresis in horses. *Proc. Am. Coll. Vet. Intern. Med.* 7: 499–500.

Steward, D.J., Haining, R.L., Henne, K.R. et al. (1997). Genetic association between sensitivity to warfarin and expression of CYP2C9*3. *Pharmacogenetics* 7: 361–367.

Tanaka, N., Shinkyo, R., Sakaki, T. et al. (2005). Cytochrome P450 2E polymorphism in feline liver. *Biochem. Biophys. Acta* 1726: 194–205.

Tanaka, N., Miyasho, T., Shinkyo, R. et al. (2006). cDNA cloning and characterization of feline CYP1A1 and CYP1A2. *Life Sci.* 79: 2463–2473.

Tenmizu, D., Noguchi, K., Kamimura, H. et al. (2006). The canine CYP1A2 deficiency polymorphism dramatically affects the pharmacokinetics of 4-cyclohexyl-1-ethyl-7-methylpyrido[2,3-D]-pyrimidine-2-(1H)-one (YM-64227), a phosphodiesterase type 4 inhibitor. *Drug Metab. Dispos.* 34: 800–806.

Tishler, D.M., Weinberg, K.T., Hinton, D.R. et al. (1995). MDR1 gene expression in brain of patients with medically intractable epilepsy. *Epilepsia* 36: 1–6.

Tonomura, N., Elvers, I., Thomas, R. et al. (2015). Genome-wide association study identifies shared risk loci common to 2 malignancies in Golden retrievers. *PLos Genet.* 11 (2): e1004922. https://doi.org/10.1371/journal.pgen.1004922.

Trepanier, L.A. (2006). Cytochrome P450 and its role in veterinary drug interactions. *Vet. Clin. North Am. Small Anim. Pract.* 36: 975–985.

Tyden, E., Lofgren, M., Hakhverdyan, M. et al. (2012). The genes of all seven CYP3A isoenzymes identified in equine genome are expressed in the airways of horses. *J. Vet. Pharmacol. Ther.* 36: 370–375.

Tyden, E., Tjalve, H., and Larsson, P. (2014). Gene and protein expression and cellular localization of cytochrome P450 enzymes of the 1A, 2A, 2C, 2D and 2E subfamilies in equine intestine and liver. *Acta Veterinaria Scandinavica* 56: 69.

Vesell, E.S. (1969). Recent progress in pharmacogenetics. *Adv. Pharmacol. Chemother.* 7: 1–52.

Virkel, G., Carletti, M., Cantiello, M. et al. (2009). Characteriazation of xenobiotic metabolizing enzymes in bovine small intestinal mucosa. *J. Vet. Pharmacol. Ther.* 33: 295–304.

Wade, C.M., Giulotto, E., Sigurdsson, S. et al. (2009). Genome sequence, comparative analysis, and population genetics of the domestic horse. *Science* 326: 865–867.

Wassermann, L., Halwachs, S., Lindner, S. et al. (2013). Deterimination of functional ABCG2 activity and assessment of drug - ABCG2 interactions in dairy animals using a novel MDCKII in vitro model. *J. Pharm. Sci.* 102: 772–784.

West, C.L. and Mealey, K.L. (2007). Assessment of antiepileptic drugs as substrates for canine P-glycoprotein. *Am. J. Vet. Res.* 68: 1106–1110.

Whiterock, V.J., Morgan, D.G., Lentz, K.A. et al. (2012). Phenacetin pharmacokinetics in CYP1A2-deficient beagle dogs. *Drug Metab. Dispos.* 40: 228–231.

Zhang, K., Kohno, S., Kuroha, M. et al. (2006). Clinical oral doses of dexamethasone decreases intrinsic clearance of quinidine, a cytochrome P450 3A substrate in dogs. *J. Vet. Med. Sci.* 68: 903–907.

Zhang, F., Tong, J., Hu, J. et al. (2015). COMT haplotypes are closely associated with post-operative fentanyl dose in patients. *Anesth. Analg.* 120: 933–940.

Zimin, A.V., Delcher, A.L., Florea, L. et al. (2009). A whole genome assembly of the domestic cow, Bos Taurus. *Genome Biol.* http://genomebiology.com/2009/10/4/R42.

Zoran, D., Riedesel, D.H., and Dyer, D.C. (1993). Pharmacokinetics of propofol in mixed-breed dogs and Greyhounds. *Am. J. Vet. Res.* 54: 755–760.

3

Veterinary Regulatory Concerns Associated with Anesthesia and Analgesia for Food Animals

Jeffrey Lakritz

Introduction

There are currently few "FDA approved" analgesic ("Banamine®," Banamine Transdermal® – (flunixin), Resflor Gold® (florfenicol + flunixin), Draxxin KP® (tulathromycin + ketoprofen)) and anesthetic drugs (lidocaine) approved by the FDA for **use in farm animals**.

Drugs from other classes commonly used in anesthesia and analgesia protocols (opiates butorphanol; morphine; fentanyl; buprenorphine), dissociative (ketamine; tilet-amine), α2 agonists (xylazine; detomidine; dexmedetomidine), benzodiazepines (diazepam; midazolam), phenothiazines (acepromazine), propofol, barbiturates (Surital; thiamylal), guaifenesin, tolazoline (α-adrenergic receptor antagonist), yohimbine (α-2 adrenergic receptor blocker), and Telazol (combination of tiletamine [dissociative] and zolazepam [benzodiazepine]) are used, and are generally safe for food animal patients. However, most have not been approved for use in farm animals, which means there is no established drug or drug-metabolite tolerance and no established WDTs. As such, there is limited data regarding the time interval required before the harvest of tissues or consumption of milk, eggs etc. in food animals.

When using FDA-approved drugs in an **extra-label manner**, the prescribing veterinarian has legal, moral, and ethical obligations to ensure food safety (there are no tissue residues at the time of harvest in the food animal species that have undergone 3.2 anesthetic procedures or provision of pain management protocols) (Heavner and Teske 1986). This makes provision of a suitable amount of time prior to consuming food products (WDI) that is based upon scientific evidence.

The Drug Approval Process and Animals

In food animals, drug approval for marketing involves specific interactions between the sponsor (pharmaceutical company) and the FDA Center for Veterinary Medicine. This approval process requires the evaluation of (i) animal safety, (ii) efficacy of proposed drug in animals, (iii) human food safety (evaluation of residues, concentrations in edible tissues), (iv) drug chemistry, (v) drug manufacture (identity, strength and purity of drug, consistency of drug product marketed and drug stability), (vi) environmental impacts of livestock drug use, (vii) all other information, and (viii) product labeling. These studies comprise the sections required for evaluation of a New Animal Drug Application (NADA). Total drug quantitation (parent drug and drug metabolites in tissues), and residence of these compounds within the injection site, and other edible parts of the animal are critical to define the time required for tissue residues to deplete to concentrations known to be safe for human consumption. Metabolite identification is important to develop analytical assays used to follow tissue residues in food as well as defining whether metabolites may have concerns (toxicological) for food safety.

Extra-Label Drug Use

Extra-label drug use (ELDU) simply means a licensed veterinarian who possesses a valid veterinary client-patient relationship (VCPR) with a client and who chooses to use a drug(s) in a manner which is not in accordance with the approved drug label (21 CFR 530 subpart A General provisions Definitions). This includes use for a disease/disorder not listed on the label, species not listed on label, doses, dose frequency or routes of administration not listed on the label and deviation from the label WDT (21 CFR Subpart A 530.3 Definitions). The requirements for ELDU in food animals are promulgated by the FDA to limit the use of drugs to animals whose health is diminished to the point where suffering or death may occur without intervention. In emergent cases, ELDU is allowed when:

1) The ELDU is by the order of a licensed veterinarian in the context of a valid VCPR.

2) There is no animal drug approved for this condition in food animals.

3) There is an approved drug, but it does not contain the active pharmaceutical ingredient required.

4) There is an approved drug for the intended use, but it is not prepared in the appropriate formulation (pill vs. suspension vs. parenteral dosage form).

5) There is an approved animal drug, but it is provided in an excessive or inadequate dosage form.

6) The practitioner has found in the context of a valid VCPR, that the approved dosage form is not clinically effective as labeled.

7) FDA requirements for food animals require that approved human drugs may not be used if there is an approved drug for use in one species, in another species requiring treatment.

8) The veterinarian must ensure accurate records of use of this drug in an extra-label manner in one or more food animals.

9) The veterinarian must provide follow up to ensure adverse reactions or failure of therapy.

10) The veterinarian must also document:

   a) The condition treated
   b) Animal (species) treated
   c) Dosage administered
   d) Treatment duration
   e) Number of animals treated
   f) Provide a scientifically sound WDI prior to harvest (meat, eggs, other edible tissues or milk discard interval for milk) (https://www.fda.gov/animal-veterinary/resources-you/ins-and-outs-extra-label-drug-use-animals-resource-veterinarians#General_Conditions_for_Extra-Label_Drug_Use) (FDA 2020).

The extra-label use of FDA-approved anesthetics and analgesic drugs in food animals requires that the prescribing veterinarian has legal responsibility to ensure the drugs are safe to use in the food animal species and that the drug (or drug metabolites) do not persist in tissues eventually consumed by humans. ELDU is only allowed when the licensed DVM has established a valid VCPR. Further, ELDU by a lay person (not supervised by a DVM), ELDU in or on animal feed, ELDU that produces residues that may be harmful to the consumer and any residues present that exceed the safe level, safe concentration or established tolerance are not permitted (21 CFR 530.11). In addition to appropriate labeling of the medication used for ELDU, labeling must include the veterinarian's specific WDT for meat, milk, eggs, or other food consumed by humans.

Having few analgesic, sedative, and anesthetic agents approved for use in food animals makes their use contingent upon establishing suitable WDIs (WDI; the withdrawal interval is the time required for plasma, tissue drug levels to decline to below detectable levels and is assigned by the Veterinarian) for meat, milk or other food products to prevent the presence of drug residues in farm animals. Prior to 1994, the Federal Food, Drug and Cosmetic Act (FFDCA) prohibited veterinarians from using new animal drugs in a manner not stated on the drugs approved label. This requirement prohibited the use of approved drugs in an animal species that was not listed on the label, for an indication not included in the label and at dosages higher than provided on the label. This limited the veterinarian's ability to prescribe drugs for species not included on the label, for altering the dosage form to be useful in small animals and for animals not considered major food-producing species (small ruminants, cervids, exotic animals, pocket pets, etc.). Prior to the Animal Medical Drug Use Clarification Act (AMDUCA) of 1994, human labeled (FDA-approved) drugs were also not legally available for animals. In 1996, Title 21 of the code of federal regulations was amended to provide for ELDU in animals. This provided the framework for implementation of the AMDUCA of 1994. While a major advancement in availability of drugs and flexibility in prescribing drugs in an extra-label manner, there are a number of requirements to be fulfilled when using drugs extra-label in a food-producing animal (See ELDU above). The veterinarian (undertaking ELDU) is legally responsible for ensuring the drug(s) are safe, efficacious and are not associated with the presence of drug residues that may be harmful if consumed by humans.

ELDU is only appropriate when the health of the animal is threatened or suffering, or death may occur without the treatment with these drugs. ELDU is not permitted when the drug used is meant to augment growth. In addition, ELDU by a lay person (unless supervised by a licensed veterinarian), ELDU when a drug is delivered to animals in feed, when the treatment results in a drug residue that produces a risk to human health, or produces residue concentrations which exceed the established safe level, safe concentration, or tolerance is prohibited. For example, sedating an unmanageable animal by adding the drug to feed would not be allowed. Further, it would be very difficult to estimate the oral bioavailability of a drug and provide a suitable WDI if an injectable drug were given when mixed with the feed provided to a patient.

The Withdrawal Time, Tolerance and Withdrawal Interval

WDT withdrawal time – The WDT is derived from the data collected in the sponsor's NADA. In food animals, the study is conducted with approximately 20–25 animals (mainly cattle) that are administered the sponsored compound at one single time and groups of four to five animals are sampled at the site of the injection, as well as a wide variety of other tissues (organ, meat, organs [liver, kidney, etc.], fat and skin among other tissues) and the tissue concentrations of drug and drug metabolites are determined in these four to five animals over a period of time. The data are subjected to regression analysis through the drug concentration versus time points. The decline of concentration versus time points when log transformed should be linear. The WDT is taken as the point on the log-linear decline where statistical confidence is at least 95%. At this point, the residue levels in tissues of 99% of the study animals will have decreased to below the tolerance set for this drug. The result is an **interval of time required for the concentration of the residue in target tissue(s) to decline below a concentration known to be safe for consumption. The time required for the concentrations to fall below the Tolerance, is established as the label WDT.**

Drug tolerance – The maximum concentration of a marker residue, or other residue indicated for monitoring that can legally remain in a specific edible tissue of a treated animal (CFR Part 556 subpart B specific tolerances).

WDI – In ELDU, there is no safe concentration, drug tolerance or WDT. The WDI is a period which the veterinarian assigns for the animal(s) to deplete tissue-drug levels to a safe concentration prior to sale of milk, meat, eggs or other foods. The WDI is not the same as the WDT, which is determined by the FDA in consultation with the drug sponsor and appears upon the FDA-approved drug label.

Establishment of the Extended Withdrawal Interval

The use of anesthetic, sedative, tranquilizing, and analgesic drugs in food animals is problematic for the veterinarian because there is no established safe concentration or drug tolerance for most of these drugs in food animals. Likewise, while the Food Animal Residue Avoidance Databank (FARAD) is a valuable resource for the practitioner, since there are few approved products (anesthetic, analgesic) for FARAD to utilize, their recommendations are not uncommonly conservative. When using a drug in an extra-label manner, developing a WDI or time required for an animal to clear the drug to below the safe/detectable level is one of the factors that must be provided to prevent residues in food. In the US, the FARAD program is an online resource containing a variety of options for ELDU, including "request advice," "WDI look-up," "withdrawal date calculator" and the FARAD bibliographic database of citations among other features (www.FARAD.org). The "request advice" for ELDU requires your contact information, the

species of animal being treated, number of animals treated, average body weight, whether you are interested in meat, milk, egg WDT, the number of drugs administered, the drug or tradename, the route of administration, the total dose of the drug administered, and the number of doses administered. You will also have space for free-text composition of the rationale for drug use. Once submitted, you will receive a confirmation of submission via email and a proposed WDI from FARAD within approximately 72 hours. Obtaining a scientifically developed WDI from FARAD may also protect the prescriber (Riviere et al. 1998). In its current position, FARAD recommendations may be the most-timely resource that utilizes data obtained from a wide variety studies of drug classes in current use.

Establishing a WDI for anesthetic and analgesic drugs has been associated with several well-described methods. First, Riviere et al. (1998) provided several examples of how using the elimination half-life (and slope of terminal portion of the concentration versus time curve) to provide an approximate time interval after which drug concentrations decline to near zero in the animal. Drugs that follow "first-order" kinetics decline by 50% of the total dose administered in one half-life (dose-independent kinetics). Essentially, if you administer 10 g of drug to an animal, after one half-life (definition: time required for half of the drug to be eliminated) there is only 5 g remaining. After ten half-lives, there would only be 19.53 mg remaining (99.9% of drug is eliminated). Using the rate of drug elimination from the plasma, and the knowledge that the half-life of elimination is five hours, ten half-lives would be 50 hours. After ten half-lives, less than 0.2% of drug remains and 99.9% has been eliminated. The time required for the drug to decline to below the drug tolerance would be two days + 2 hours. Rounding up to three days will create a conservative estimate of the WDI. The assignment of a WDI in the examples provided above, may also be scientifically valid if the dose of a drug is increased (doubled) to treat a disease process not included in the approved label. In cases where the drug is known to decline from tissue in a linear fashion, it would take one additional half-life for drug concentrations to decline to the original dose of 10 g. Unfortunately, for most anesthetic agents used in food animals, there is little information regarding the half-life of a drug in tissue. Thus, making an estimate more conservative is important.

Martin-Jimenez et al. (2002) demonstrated an algorithm to calculate WDI using the drug label WDT and the slope of the terminal tissue depletion profile. While the results of the comparison of approved WDT and calculated WDI were similar, the computer software is available to FARAD and software available on Android phones (Martin-Jimenez et al. 2002).

Baynes et al. (1999) developed the provisional acceptable residue (PAR) strategy to produce safe concentrations (PAR) to develop drug WDIs. Using health-based metrics, one could calculate a PAR that would not allow consumption of residues above the safe level (Baynes et al. 1999). Likewise, the calculation of a provisional acceptable tolerance is derived from similar approaches to construction of the WDT intervals. The impetus for this health-based study was that any residue present in tissue, milk, etc. from an ELDU, would violate law if there are no tolerance or safe concentrations established. Like Martin-Jimenez et al. (2002), Baynes et al. created Provisional Acceptable Residue for milk and tissues based upon average daily intake (ADI) and food consumption values (FCVs).

Feasibility of establishing a WDI based on tissue half-lives (half-life multipliers) was later proposed by Gehring et al. (2004). In this study, the authors used the approved label WDT as it is the time required for drug residues to decline to drug tolerance levels. As such, if one were to conduct a tissue residue study for a specific drug, how many half-lives would be required prior to declining to the established drug tolerance? In terms of the half-life multiplier, the ratio of the extra-label WDI/label WDI is evaluated in terms of the half-life multipliers to define the time required for tissue-drug concentrations to fall below the drug tolerance level. In this study, half-life multipliers (smaller numbers) result in longer residence of tissue residues. This makes the WDI more conservative in terms of residues. The authors used the slope of the tissue residue decline curve to calculate a tissue residue half-life. Their results indicated that there is some merit to the use of the WDT (calculated by defining the 95% confidence that 99% of the animals would have cleared the drug) which is superior to using half-lives derived from pharmacokinetic studies. The investigators also suggested that the use of smaller half-life multipliers will provide more conservative estimates of the WDI.

Since practitioners and anesthesiologists are often asked to anesthetize animals whose health status may be severely compromised, significant illness with the possibility of having altered metabolism and drug clearance would likely be associated with altered drug kinetics in these patients. Recent studies document alteration of kinetic parameters of drugs used in clinically sick animals. Several studies document prolonged elimination associated with clinical mastitis in dairy animals. Gordon et al. 2018 demonstrated altered plasma Ceftiofur Crystalline Free Acid elimination slope and half-life of the elimination phase in cattle with experimentally induced *Escherichia coli* mastitis. Their data supported an increase in the bioavailability corrected apparent volume of distribution in diseased cows compared with control cows (Gordon et al. 2018). The same group of investigators also described altered kinetics of drugs in cattle with severe clinical mastitis after natural infection (Gordon et al. 2016). When ruminants are significantly compromised (anorexic, dehydrated, hepato-renal

compromise) resulting in prolongation of the elimination half-life, increasing the WDI may be necessary.

Anesthetic Drugs – General Characteristics

Anesthetic drugs are not commonly reported as a cause of drug residues that violate the FFDCA in food animals. This might be associated with a limited submission of samples for anesthetic drugs or limited analysis of these drugs when samples are submitted. Papich noted that anesthetic drugs are less likely to cause residues for a number of reasons (Papich 1996). First, anesthetic protocols are often short term and this would be associated with limited drug accumulation during the procedure compared with daily doses of an antibiotic to treat a bacterial infection. Another reason cited by Papich was that the half-lives of many anesthesia-related drugs are short. This would be associated with more rapid clearance of drugs in a healthy animal. Further, when animals undergo surgical procedures, the surgical wounds and the recovery of the animal may be prolonged, such that the animal may not be useful to a sale barn until these wounds have healed and the animal's physiology has normalized. The prolonged healing and recovery would provide ample time prior to marketability. Most of the drugs used in cattle, sheep and goats are given via intravenous (IV) administration. This would limit the tissue residues in animals undergoing surgical procedures in comparison to administration of the drug into the muscle or via sub-cutaneous routes. The drugs used are often very potent. Using more potent drugs would require much smaller doses and reduce the impact of drug residues in tissue. Finally, these procedures are always accompanied by the input of a veterinarian. This limits the actual exposure to tissue residues under most circumstances.

Analgesic Drugs

There are few drugs approved for use in pain management of food animals in the US. Those few drugs which are approved for fever, or in endotoxic crises, can be used in an extra-label manner as indicated on the drug label. While the public often demands the use of some of these agents, the FDA has remained steadfast in their reluctance to approve the use of analgesic and anesthesia agents based upon human health concerns (Smith 2013). Analgesic drugs of the NSAID classes are available in many countries. Flunixin, ketoprofen, carprofen, tolfenamic acid, meloxicam, and phenylbutazone and are approved for use in food as well as other species. Carprofen, tolfenamic acid, while used in other countries, is not approved for use in food animals in the US. Since flunixin is approved in the US for the same or similar indications, AMDUCA would indicate that one must use the approved drug. This would require a scientifically sound WDI.

Phenylbutazone has long been used in livestock for pain management. However, drug residues in tissue and milk products have highlighted some concerns by the FDA. There are significant concerns about residues of this NSAID and the FDA banned the use of this drug in dairy animals 20 months of age or older (after lactation starts). Residues in beef cattle became evident after studies showed the half-life of this drug in cattle is prolonged (36–60 hours) (Smith 2013). Ketoprofen is currently approved for use in the US in livestock in combination with tulathromycin (Draxxin KP®). Likewise, florphenicol (antibiotic) was combined with flunixin in one injection (Resflor Gold®).

Meloxicam, while not approved for use in the US, is commonly used for pain management in food animals.

Precautionary Comments – Euthanasia

One exception to the limited exposure of humans or animals to anesthetic drugs is the use of pentobarbital or related drugs for the process of euthanasia (Payne et al. 2015). Whenever pentobarbital is used for euthanasia, the animal should be digested, buried deeply or composted in a manner which prevents scavenging. Because pentobarbital is used in very large quantities and not degraded in the dead animal, scavenging animals may consume significant, even fatal quantities of pentobarbital (Payne et al. 2015). Thus, the veterinarian should supervise the disposal process ensuring their instructions are followed (O'Connor et al. 1985).

References

Baynes, R.E., Martin-Jimenez, T., Craigmill, A.L., and Riviere, J.E. (1999). Estimating provisional acceptable residues for extralabel drug use in livestock. *Regul. Toxicol. Pharmacol.* 29: 287–299.

FDA (2020). The Ins and Outs of Extra-Label Drug Use in Anumals: A Resoure for Veterinarians. https://www.fda.gov/animal-veterinary/resources-you/ins-and-outs-extra-label-drug-use-animals-resource-veterinarians#General_Conditions_for_Extra-Label_Drug_Use (accessed 28 June 2022).

Gehring, R., Baynes, R.E., Craigmill, A.L., and Riviere, J.E. (2004). Feasibility of using half-life multipliers to estimate extended withdrawal intervals following extralabel use of drugs in food producing animals. *J. Food Prot.* 67: 555–560.

Gordon, P.J., Kleinhenz, M.D., Wulf, L.W. et al. (2016). Altered plasma pharmacokinetics of ceftiofur hydrochloride in cows affected with severe clinical mastitis. *J. Dairy Sci.* 99: 505–514.

Gordon, P.J., Ydstie, J.A., Kleinhenz, M.D. et al. (2018). Comparative plasma and interstitial fluid pharmacokinetics and tissue residues of ceftiofur crystalline-free acid in cattle with induced coliform mastitis. *J. Vet. Pharmacol. Therap.* 41: 848–860.

Heavner, J.E. and Teske, R.H. (1986). Legal implications of the extra-label use of drugs in food animals. *Vet. Clin. North Am. Food Anim. Pract.* 2 (3): 517–525.

Lin, H. (2015). Comparative Anesthesia and Analgesia of Ruminants and Swine. In: *Veterinary Anesthesia and Analgesia: the Fifth Edition of Lumb and Jones* (ed. K.A. Grimm, L.A. Lamont, W.J. Tranquilli, et al.), 743–753. Chichester: Wiley.

Martin-Jimenez, T., Baynes, R.E., Craigmill, A., and Riviere, J.E. (2002). Extrapolated withdrawal-interval estimator (EWE) algorithm: a quantitative approach to establishing extralabel withdrawal times. *Regul. Toxicol. Pharmacol.* 36: 131–137.

O'Connor, J.J., Stowe, C.M., and Robinson, R.R. (1985). Fate of sodium pentobarbital in rendered products. *Am. J. Vet. Res.* 46: 1721–1724.

Papich, M.G. (1996). Drug residue considerations for anesthetics and adjunctive drugs in food-producing animals. *Vet. Clin. North Am. Food Animal Pract.* 12: 693–705.

Passler, T. (2014). Regulatory and legal considerations of anesthetics and analgesics used in food-producing animals. In: *Farm Animal Anesthesia; Cattle, Small Ruminants, Camelids and Pigs*, 1e (ed. H. Lin and P. Walz), 228–247. Chichester: Wiley.

Payne, J., Farris, R., Parker, G. et al. (2015). Quantification of sodium pentobarbital residues from equine mortality compost piles. *J. Anim. Sci.* 93: 1824–1829.

Riviere, J.E. (1991). Pharmacologic principles of residue avoidance for veterinary practitioners. *J. Am. Vet. Med. Assoc.* 198: 809–816.

Riviere, J.E., Webb, A.I., and Craigmill, A.L. (1998). FARAD digest: primer on estimating withdrawal times after extralabel drug use. *J. Am. Vet. Med. Assoc.* 213: 966–968.

Rollin, B.E. (2004). Annual meeting keynote address: animal agriculture and emerging social ethics for animals. *J. Anim. Sci.* 82: 955–964.

Smith, G. (2013). Extralabel use of anesthetic and analgesic compounds in cattle. *Vet. Clin. North Am. Food Anim. Pract.* 29: 29–45.

4

α_2 Receptor Agonists and Antagonists

Lydia Love

Introduction

α_2 receptor agonists provide reversible sedation, anxiolysis, analgesia, and muscle relaxation and have been clinically used in a variety of species for more than four decades. Xylazine, clonidine, detomidine, medetomidine, dexmedetomidine, and romifidine are currently available for use in veterinary patients. The available α_2 antagonists, including yohimbine, tolazoline, and atipamezole, reverse the desired and adverse effects of α_2 agonists, whereas the peripherally restricted α_2 antagonist, vatinoxan, interferes mainly with the initial cardiovascular effects of α_2 agonists.

α_2 Receptors

Adrenergic receptors are intermediaries of the sympathetic nervous system, binding catecholamines resulting in tissue- and cell-specific effects. α receptors were originally differentiated from β-adrenergic receptors by their catecholamine-binding profiles (Ahlquist 1967). Further pharmacologic and molecular techniques, including production of genetically modified mice, have identified two primary classifications of α receptors: α_1 and α_2, and three substantially homologous α_2-adrenergic receptor subtypes: α_{2A}, α_{2B}, and α_{2C} receptors. The α_{2D} receptor is a species-specific (rat, mouse, cow, guinea pig, and chicken) ortholog of α_{2A} receptors (identified in humans, pigs, rabbits, and dogs) that displays an identical agonist-binding profile but dissimilar antagonist pharmacology (Bond et al. 2014). This receptor will be referred to as α_{2A} throughout.

α_2 receptors belong to the large class of G-protein coupled receptors (GPCRs) that span the cell membrane and are intimately associated with intracellular signal transducers known as G proteins. "G" refers to the guanine diphosphate (GDP) bound by these heterotrimeric proteins in the inactive state. Extracellular binding of catecholamines causes the G protein to exchange GDP for guanine triphosphate (GTP) and split into various subunits that interact with downstream cellular mediators. All subtypes of α_2 receptor are coupled to inhibitory G proteins that result in inhibition of adenyl cyclase-mediated production of cyclic adenosine monophosphate (cAMP), inhibition of voltage-gated Ca^{2+} channels, and stimulation of inwardly rectifying K^+ channels, thus hyperpolarizing the cell and dampening cellular activity.

Distributed throughout the central and peripheral nervous system, and in many other tissues, α_2 receptors occupy pre- and post-synaptic positions. A minority of α_2 receptors are located extra-synaptically, e.g. on platelets. Pre-synaptic α_2 receptors are grouped into autoreceptors and heteroreceptors. Autoreceptors, largely of the α_{2A} subtype, form an inhibitory feedback loop on adrenergic neurons, managing the release of their own endogenous agonist, norepinephrine (Figure 4.1). Pre-synaptic α_2 receptors that regulate neurotransmitter release (e.g. serotonin, gamma aminobutyric acid [GABA], acetylcholine) on non-adrenergic neurons are termed heteroreceptors (Feuerstein et al. 1993).

The α_{2A} receptor is the principal mediator of central sedative and sympatholytic effects of α_2-agonist drugs (Lakhlani et al. 1997). Initial evidence indicated that α_{2A} autoreceptors mediated these effects (Lakhlani et al. 1997; Link et al. 1996). Interestingly, a recent study suggests that many of the pharmacodynamic effects of α_2 agonists are a result of activation of α_{2A} heteroreceptors on nonadrenergic neurons. Transgenic mice that do not express α_{2A} heteroreceptors (but do have functional α_{2A} autoreceptors) do not experience the sedative, antinociceptive, anesthetic-sparing, or hypothermic effects of dexmedetomidine (Gilsbach et al. 2009).

Sedative and Analgesic Effects

The sedative effects of α_2-agonist drugs have been localized to the locus coeruleus (LC), a pontine nucleus involved in arousal and vigilance (Correa-Sales et al. 1992). Sedation is

Pharmacology in Veterinary Anesthesia and Analgesia, First Edition. Edited by Turi Aarnes and Phillip Lerche.
© 2024 John Wiley & Sons, Inc. Published 2024 by John Wiley & Sons, Inc.

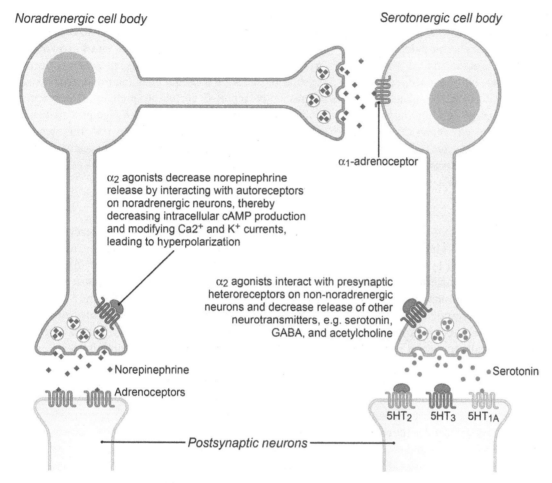

Noradrenergic cell body

Serotonergic cell body

α_1-adrenoceptor

α_2 agonists decrease norepinephrine release by interacting with autoreceptors on noradrenergic neurons, thereby decreasing intracellular cAMP production and modifying Ca2+ and K+ currents, leading to hyperpolarization

α_2 agonists interact with presynaptic heteroreceptors on non-noradrenergic neurons and decrease release of other neurotransmitters, e.g. serotonin, GABA, and acetylcholine

◆ Norepinephrine

Adrenoceptors

● Serotonin

5HT$_2$ 5HT$_3$ 5HT$_{1A}$

— *Postsynaptic neurons* —

Figure 4.1 α_2-agonists interact with pre-synaptic receptors on noradrenergic and non-noradrenergic neurons to decrease neurotransmitter release.

thought to be due to activation of an endogenous sleep-promoting pathway, involving inhibition of the LC and subsequent disinhibition of the ventrolateral preoptic nucleus in the hypothalamus (Nelson et al. 2003). Separation of the loss of righting reflex from sedation in genetically modified mice implicates the preoptic hypothalamus as the primary mediator of sedation generated by low-dose dexmedetomidine (Zhang et al. 2015).

The profound analgesic effects of α_2 agonists are predominantly mediated by α_{2A} receptors in the brainstem and the dorsal horn of the spinal cord through pre- and post-synaptic mechanisms. Stimulation of α_2 receptors in the LC by systemic administration of low doses of dexmedetomidine results in descending pontospinal inhibition of post-synaptic transmission in the substantia gelatinosa (SG) (Funai et al. 2014). Activation of α_{2A} heteroreceptors on C-fiber afferents in the SG decreases release of substance P and glutamate, contributing to the analgesic effects of α_2 agonists (Kawasaki et al. 2003; Chen et al. 2007; Gilsbach et al. 2009). In addition, activation of

post-synaptic α_{2A} and α_{2C} receptors inhibits nociceptive transmission in spinal interneurons and projection neurons (Stone et al. 1998; Fairbanks et al. 2002; Nazarian et al. 2008; Ishii et al. 2008).

Synergistic analgesic effects between opioids and α_2 agonists occur at the level of the spinal cord: α_{2A} and α_{2C} receptors co-localize with μ and δ opioid receptors on nociceptive primary afferents and spinal interneurons in the superficial layers of the dorsal horn. Formation of α_2-opioid heteromers augments downstream signaling pathways, including production of protein kinase C and calcitonin gene-related peptide (Schuster et al. 2013; Chabot-Doré et al. 2015).

Peripheral nerve injury leads to increased expression of α_2 receptors on primary nociceptive afferents and enhances G protein coupling (Bantel et al. 2005) and α_2 agonists can interrupt the resultant exaggerated nociceptive signaling. Activation of inhibitory cholinergic interneurons by α_2 agonists and resulting increases in spinal acetylcholine concentrations have been documented in experimental neuropathic pain states (Kimura et al. 2012). In addition, microglial activation, which significantly contributes to the development and maintenance of chronic pain, is reduced by α_2 agonists (Xu et al. 2010; Li et al. 2014).

Many α_2 agonists also engage with imidazoline binding sites in the central nervous system (CNS), platelets, pancreas, and liver. Imidazoline receptors inhibit monoamine oxidase activity, increasing concentrations of serotonin and norepinephrine (Lanza et al. 2014) and may be involved in some of the clinical effects of α_2 agonists, including cardiovascular effects and analgesia.

Cardiovascular Effects

Parenteral administration of α_2 agonists induces a biphasic hemodynamic response characterized by initial vasoconstriction, bradycardia and reduced cardiac output, followed eventually by a vasodilation, hypotension, and continued bradycardia and reduced cardiac output.

Activation of post-synaptic α_{2B} receptors on arterial smooth-muscle cells results initially in arterial and venous vasoconstriction and a baroreceptor-mediated decrease in heart rate and cardiac output that is only partially dose-dependent and exhibits a ceiling effect (Link et al. 1996; Sarazan et al. 1989; Pypendop and Verstegen 1998). The vasoconstrictive effects of α_2 agonists extend to the coronary, cerebral, and pulmonary circulation (Zornow et al. 1990; Flacke et al. 1993; Pypendop et al. 2011). A direct effect of α_2 agonists on cardiac muscle does not occur (Schmeling et al. 1991; Flacke et al. 1992).

The initial reflex bradycardia caused by α_2 agonists can be mitigated by the administration of anticholinergics. However, the combination of α_2 agonist and an anticholinergic results in hypertension, increased myocardial work, and increased incidence of arrhythmias without causing a significant increase in cardiac output compared to an α_2 agonist alone (Congdon et al. 2011). If unstable bradycardia occurs closely following α_2 agonist administration, reversal of the drug may be the best choice. However, this may lead to an unwanted decrease in sedation. In dogs, another course of action can be administration of a lidocaine bolus to increase heart rate and cardiac output (Tisotti et al. 2021).

Eventually, a reduction in sympathetic tone mediated by hypothalamic pre- and post-synaptic α_{2A} receptors predominates, leading to continued bradycardia, reduced cardiac output and peripheral vasodilation (Guyenet and Cabot 1981; Bloor et al. 1992b). It is this central sympatholysis, which appears to predominate at low doses, that is the basis for the use of oral α_2 agonists as antihypertensives in humans.

The magnitude of the cardiovascular responses and how long the initial phase lasts are dependent on the specific drug, dose, route of administration and species in which it is used (Bloor et al. 1992a, 1992b; Ringer et al. 2013).

In addition to sinus bradycardia and sinus arrhythmia, α_2 agonists may cause first- and second-degree atrioventricular block. More consequential abnormal rhythms are occasionally reported including premature ventricular contractions and asystole. However, α_2 agonists are generally identified as anti-dysrhythmic in that they tend to increase the dose of epinephrine required to cause ventricular arrhythmias (Hayashi et al. 1991; Lemke et al. 1993).

Respiratory Effects

The respiratory effects of α_2 agonists include decreases in respiratory rate with no or minimal development of hypercarbia (Wagner et al. 1991; Kuo and Keegan 2004; Ringer et al. 2013). However, the ventilatory response to carbon dioxide is depressed by α_2 agonists (Lerche and Muir 2004).

Hypoxemia, thought to be related to ventilation-perfusion mismatching, may develop but is generally absent or mild when α_2 agonists are administered alone to healthy dogs, horses, cats, and pigs (Wagner et al. 1991; Tendillo et al. 1996; Lamont et al. 2001; Kuo and Keegan 2004). Ruminants, including goats (Kutter et al. 2006) and cattle (Rioja et al. 2008), appear to be more sensitive to the respiratory side effects of α_2 agonists and, in sheep, severe hypoxemia that may not be completely reversed by the administration of α_2 antagonists can develop. This has been attributed to the activation of pulmonary intravascular macrophages and the subsequent development of interstitial edema as well as changes in pulmonary mechanics (Celly et al. 1997b; Kutter et al. 2006). Overt hypoxemia may also develop in rabbits following administration of α_2 agonists (Cardoso et al. 2020). α_2 agonists cause a decrease in thoracic compliance and increases in airway resistance and dead space in anesthetized sheep and goats (Kutter et al. 2006). Upper airway resistance increases with xylazine sedation in standing horses (Tomasic et al. 1997) and this likely occurs in other species as well. Patients administered α_2 agonists should be monitored carefully for airway patency and decreases in hemoglobin saturation. In addition, oxygen supplementation should be provided, especially when α_2 agonists are combined with other sedatives and analgesics.

Other Organ Effects

Renal blood flow (RBF) tends to decrease after administration of α_2 agonists (Lawrence et al. 1996; Talke et al. 2000). Diuresis can be expected following α_2-agonist administration, due to decreases in production of antidiuretic hormone, increases in atrial natriuretic peptide, and activation of renal sympathetic nerves (Burton et al. 1998; Menegaz et al. 2001; Saleh et al. 2005; Murahata et al. 2014).

The endocrine effects of α_2 agonists include a decrease in the stress response (Flacke et al. 1993; Rizk et al. 2012) and decreased insulin release. In addition to a centrally mediated decrease in sympathetic outflow, regulation of catecholamine release from the adrenal medulla occurs via activation of all three α_2-receptors subtypes on adrenal chromaffin cells (Moura et al. 2006). This effect has been manipulated clinically to promote hemodynamic stability in the management of pheochromocytoma patients. Agonism of α_{2A} receptors on pancreatic β cells decreases insulin release and can cause hyperglycemia (Burton et al. 1997; Guedes and Rude 2013; Kodera et al. 2013). This effect has been suggested as beneficial in the perioperative management of dogs with insulinomas (Guedes and Rude 2013).

Gastrointestinal (GI) effects of α_2 agonists include relaxation of the lower esophageal sphincter (Strombeck and Harrold 1985), inhibition of gastric emptying (Doherty et al. 1999), decreased intestinal contractility (Merritt et al. 1998; Zullian et al. 2011) and increased intestinal transit time (Hsu and McNeel 1983). A gastroprotective effect has been suggested as α_2 agonists reduce gastric-acid production and inhibit ulcerogenic actions of nonsteroidal anti-inflammatory agents (Gyires et al. 2000; Zádori et al. 2011).

Hypothermia and decreased febrile responses occur following administration of α_2 agonists and are mediated by central α_{2A} receptors (Szreder 1997; Lähdesmäki et al. 2003; Kendall et al. 2010). Blockade of excitatory adrenergic output from the medulla prevents thermogenesis in brown adipose tissue as well as skeletal-muscle shivering (Madden et al. 2013). The initial peripheral vasoconstriction caused by α_2 agonist administration may lessen cutaneous heat loss (Sinclair 2003). Indeed, heat loss was faster and greater when the peripheral α_2 antagonist MK-467 was added to medetomidine/butorphanol sedation (Vainionpää et al. 2013a). However, temperature should be monitored and precautions should be taken to prevent heat loss whenever heavy sedation occurs as a result of α_2 agonists.

Contraindications

Caution should be exercised with administration of α_2 agonists to patients that are hemodynamically unstable and when administered in conjunction with other sedatives and analgesics, dose reduction is warranted as sedative and cardiopulmonary effects may be compounded. Contraindications to the use of α_2 agonists include co-existing disease in which systemic or pulmonary vasoconstriction could be detrimental and when vomiting, diuresis, or hyperglycemia could be problematic.

Specific α₂ Receptor Agonists

Clonidine

Originally designed as a nasal decongestant, clonidine was introduced commercially as an anti-hypertensive agent for humans in 1966 (van Zweiten 1980; Stähle 2000). It is an imidazoline derivative, displays weak activity at α_1 receptors, and is a partial agonist at α_2 receptors (Guyenet 1997) (Table 4.1).

Clonidine is a highly lipid soluble drug with a large volume of distribution (Dirikolu et al. 2006). A two-compartment model was the best fit for the pharmacokinetic data in rats and cats with a rapid distribution phase and elimination half-life of 49–77 minutes. The volume of distribution at steady state was quite large, although increasing the dose resulted in a decreased volume of distribution and a higher percentage of clonidine in the central compartment (Paalzow and Edlund 1979).

Clonidine is most commonly used as an oral anxiolytic in dogs and it can be administered at home prior to transport to sedate and calm anxious patients. A parenteral form is available and intravenous (IV) and epidural use in animal species is reported. Clonidine is identified as a Class 3 agent by the Association of Racing Commissioners International and it may be illegally administered prior to a race to reduce pulmonary arterial pressure and exercise-induced pulmonary hemorrhage in horses (Dirikolu et al. 2006).

Epidural administration has been reported in dogs (Ghignone et al. 1987), pigs (Gordh and Hartvig 1986), sheep (Castro and Eisenach 1989), horses (Dória et al. 2008), and cattle (de Rossi et al. 2003). Although plasma concentrations are low after epidural administration, systemic side effects such as sedation and hypotension can result. IV clonidine reduces the minimum alveolar concentration of halothane in dogs (Bloor and Flacke 1982). The central hypotensive effects tend to predominate after administration of clonidine (Hood et al. 1995). Clonidine, like other α_2 agonists, causes severe hypoxemia in sheep (Celly et al. 1997a).

Table 4.1 $\alpha_2{:}\alpha_1$ selectivity of various α_2 receptor agonists.

Drug	$\alpha_2{:}\alpha_1$ selectivity
Xylazine	160 : 1
Clonidine	220 : 1
Detomidine	260 : 1
Romifidine	340 : 1
(Dex)Medetomidine	1620 : 1

Xylazine

Xylazine was first used in veterinary practice in the late 1960s. It does not have an imidazole ring and displays the lowest $\alpha_2 : \alpha_1$ selectivity of the commonly available α_2 agonists (Table 4.1). Interestingly, cattle are more sensitive to the sedative effects than are dogs or pigs and this may be related to species differences in efficiency of coupling of the α_{2A} receptor to its G proteins (Törneke et al. 2003).

The pharmacokinetic profile of xylazine is similar among dogs, cattle, horses, and sheep, with rapid distribution into a large volume and a half-life between 1.2 and 6 minutes (Garcia-Villar et al. 1981). Absorption after intramuscular (IM) administration is rapid and bioavailability is 38–45% in the horse and sheep whereas it is approximately 74% in dogs (Garcia-Villar et al. 1981; Kaukinen et al. 2011). Plasma concentrations were not detectable in cattle although sedative effects were documented (Garcia-Villar et al. 1981). Pharmacokinetic variables after intraosseous administration in horses do not differ significantly from IV administration (Santonastaso et al. 2014).

Xylazine undergoes extensive and rapid hepatic metabolism with phase I transformation mediated by CYP3A microsomes (LaVoie et al. 2013).

Xylazine is most commonly used in horses and cattle as a sedative for standing procedures, an analgesic for acute colic, sedation prior to general anesthesia, and as an infusion during general anesthesia to reduce inhalant requirements. It is also used to delay and improve recovery from inhalant anesthetics in the horse. Xylazine may be administered in the epidural space or as an IV infusion in the standing large animal patient for analgesia. Xylazine, in combination with other drugs, is used extensively in laboratory species such as rats, mice, and rabbits to induce and maintain anesthesia. It is occasionally used in small-animal patients as a premedication or part of a total IM or IV anesthetic protocol, although more α_2-specific agents are usually chosen for dogs and cats. Indeed, an increased risk of general anesthesia-related mortality has been documented with the administration of xylazine to dogs (Dyson et al. 1998). Activation of α_2 receptors in the chemoreceptor trigger zone can cause emesis and xylazine is considered by many to be the emetic of choice for cats.

During general anesthesia, IV xylazine reduces the minimal alveolar concentration (MAC) of halothane in dogs (Tranquilli et al. 1984) and of isoflurane in horses in a dose-dependent manner (Steffey et al. 2000). Epidural administration of xylazine to dogs reduces the MAC of isoflurane with minimal systemic cardiopulmonary effects (Soares et al. 2004) and, by this route in horses, it reduces the MAC of halothane without causing ataxia in recovery (Doherty et al. 1997). Post-anesthetic administration of xylazine improves recovery characteristics in horses after general anesthesia (Ida et al. 2013).

Cardiopulmonary effects of xylazine are as expected of α_2 agonists, with an initial increase in systemic vascular resistance (SVR) accompanied by bradycardia and reduced cardiac output (Haskins et al. 1986; Carter et al. 1990). This is followed quickly by a long-lasting hypotension, continued bradycardia, and reduced oxygen delivery (Wagner et al. 1991; Rioja et al. 2008; Ringer et al. 2013). Xylazine tends to be arrhythmogenic in nature (Wright et al. 1987) and it has been suggested that this is due to the relatively high α_1 receptor affinity (Grimsrud et al. 2015). In healthy horses, IV xylazine decreases cerebrospinal fluid (CSF) pressure (Moore and Trim 1992) and GI motility (Nakamura et al. 1997; Merritt et al. 1998). IM doses of xylazine up to 4.0 mg/kg do not affect intraocular pressure in dogs and changes in pupil size do not occur (Kanda et al. 2015). Xylazine administration increases uterine tone and can decrease uterine blood flow (Sakamoto et al. 1996).

Detomidine

Detomidine is an α_2-receptor agonist with an imidazole ring, introduced into clinical practice in the 1980s as a sedative and analgesic for horses and cows. In these species, detomidine is rapidly absorbed and distributed, with IV administration resulting in higher plasma concentrations with a shorter half-life than IM administration (Salonen et al. 1989; Grimsrud et al. 2009; Mama et al. 2009). Maximal exercise increases the volume of distribution, leading to lower peak plasma concentrations and slower elimination in horses (Hubbell et al. 2009). Sublingual detomidine gel exhibits a bioavailability of 22% in horses with wide individual variability. The peak plasma concentration following sublingual administration was higher than that reported for IV administration; however, collection of samples for detomidine assays from the jugular vein may have affected these results (Kaukinen et al. 2011). Detomidine undergoes extensive and rapid hepatic metabolism in horses and rats (Salonen and Suolinna 1988; Salonen et al. 1989).

Detomidine is most commonly used as an analgesic and sedative in horses and cattle when a longer duration of action than xylazine is required. It results in a dose-dependent duration, but not intensity, of sedation and analgesia in horses (Kamerling et al. 1988). IV infusions are also described in the horse for standing procedures. Epidural administration is reported in horses (Fischer et al. 2009), cattle (Prado et al. 1999), dogs (Pohl et al. 2012), and buffalo (Tiwari et al. 1998). In conscious cattle, epidural detomidine at 40 mcg/kg produced similar systemic effects as the same dose administered IM and did not appear to offer an analgesic advantage (Prado et al. 1999). A sublingual formulation is labeled for use in horses, with maximal sedative effects occurring approximately 45 minutes after administration. Detomidine gel is occasionally used to facilitate handling of anxious dogs (Hopfensberger et al. 2013). Detomidine use in injectable combinations for total IM anesthesia has been reported in a variety of wild species.

Detomidine reduces the minimum alveolar concentration of isoflurane in horses in a dose-dependent manner (Steffey and Pascoe 2002). However, one group was unable to identify a reduction in isoflurane requirements in horses with administration of detomidine at 5 mcg/kg/hr (Schauvliege et al. 2011).

The cardiovascular effects of detomidine are similar to other α_2-receptors agonists (Still et al. 1996) but, in horses, are more pronounced and longer lasting than those caused by xylazine or medetomidine (Yamashita et al. 2000). During general anesthesia, IV detomidine increases SVR and mean arterial pressure and decreases heart rate, cardiac index, and arterial oxygen content (Still et al. 1996; Schauvliege et al. 2011).

Mild hypoxemia develops after detomidine administration in horses and is the result of VQ mismatching. In addition, respiratory rate decreases, and arterial carbon dioxide concentrations increase slightly (Nyman et al. 2009). As with other α_2 agonists, detomidine can induce severe hypoxemia in sheep (Celly et al. 1997b).

Horses receiving 20 mcg/kg detomidine IV experienced reductions in intraocular pressure of approximately 15–20% (Holve 2012). Detomidine decreased myometrial tone in pregnant mares (Jedruch et al. 1989) but increased intrauterine pressure has been documented in nonpregnant mares (Schatzmann et al. 1994). In horses with insulin dysregulation, as part of equine metabolic syndrome, detomidine administration causes less rebound hyperinsulinemia when compared to xylazine (Kritchevsky et al. 2020).

Medetomidine

A lipophilic derivative of detomidine, medetomidine exhibits a strong affinity for α_2 receptors (Table 4.1). It is a racemic mixture of the pharmacologically active dextrorotary enantiomer and the inactive levorotary enantiomer (Kuusela et al. 2000). The sedative and analgesic effects are mediated by central α_{2A} receptors whereas initial cardiovascular effects are due to peripheral α_{2B} activation (Scheibner et al. 2001).

IV medetomidine in ponies can be fitted to a two-compartment model with a distribution half-life of 7.6 minutes (Bettschart-Wolfensberger et al. 1999; Grimsrud et al. 2015). IM medetomidine is rapidly absorbed with peak plasma concentrations occurring within 30 minutes in sheep (Kästner et al. 2003). Medetomidine experiences a large volume of distribution of approximately 3 L/kg in dogs, cats, and sheep. The elimination half-life of IM medetomidine in sheep and horses is approximately 40 minutes whereas longer half-lives of approximately 1–1.5 hours are found in dogs and cats (Kästner et al. 2003; Grimsrud et al. 2012; Salonen et al. 1989; Muge et al. 1996; Duhamel et al. 2010).

Extensive hepatic hydroxylation with subsequent conjugation of medetomidine occurs in the dog and rat. As cats are deficient in glucuronidation capacity, the hydroxylated metabolite is the major product recovered from the urine in this species (Salonen 1989; Duhamel et al. 2010). Cytochrome p450 enzymes, mainly CYP3A with minor contributions from CYP2D and CYP2E, are responsible for metabolism of medetomidine in the dog. These hepatic microsomes display a high affinity for medetomidine and metabolism can be saturated at fairly low concentrations (Duhamel et al. 2010). Differences in microsome activity between strains of laboratory rabbits are correlated with disparities in clinical response to medetomidine (Avsaroglu et al. 2008).

Medetomidine is used in dogs and cats as a sedative prior to general anesthesia. Combinations of medetomidine and other classes of drugs can produce chemical restraint or total injectable anesthesia and this use is common in cats, dogs, pigs, and a variety of wildlife species. Medetomidine is also used as an IV infusion to reduce inhalational anesthetic requirements in dogs. Extremely low doses are employed in dogs and cats during anesthetic recovery to minimize emergence delirium. Epidural administration of medetomidine is reported in several species but may be associated with systemic effects of sedation and hemodynamic depression. In general, other α_2 agonists that are less expensive and/or specifically marketed for large animals are used in these species.

The sedative effects of medetomidine are at least partially dose-dependent (Pypendop and Verstegen 1998). There appears to be a ceiling effect where higher doses do not deepen sedation but do extend the duration (Ansah et al. 1998; Lamont et al. 2012; Grimsrud et al. 2015). At extremely high doses, lessened sedation is evident with medetomidine, and this could be due to α_1 agonism (Ansah et al. 2000). As expected, medetomidine reduces the MAC of isoflurane and halothane in dogs (Lerche and Muir 2006) and of desflurane in ponies (Bettschart-Wolfensberger et al. 2001). In horses, 5 mcg/kg/hr medetomidine with 1.4% end-tidal isoflurane results in greater depth of anesthesia with higher blood pressures compared to intermittent bolus administration of xylazine and 1.7% end-tidal isoflurane (Creighton et al. 2012).

Cardiovascular effects typical of α_2 agonists are noted following administration of medetomidine in a partially dose-dependent manner, including bradycardia, increased SVR, and reductions in cardiac output. At very low doses, the central sympatholytic effects predominate (Pypendop and Verstegen 1998).

Respiratory effects of medetomidine are generally mild in dogs, cats, and horses (Bueno et al. 1999; Kuusela et al. 2000; Lamont et al. 2001). During halothane or isoflurane anesthesia, administration of 5 mcg/kg of medetomidine to dogs results in minor differences in respiratory rate, respiratory drive, and sensitivity of the respiratory centers to carbon dioxide (Lerche and Muir 2006). Medetomidine, like other α_2 agonists, can cause severe hypoxemia in sheep (Celly et al. 1997b).

RBF is decreased by administration of medetomidine (Lawrence et al. 1996; Talke et al. 2000). However, RBF and glomerular filtration rate (GFR) may follow changes in systemic arterial pressure, with IV medetomidine increasing and IM administration decreasing RBF and GFR (Saleh et al. 2005). Typical of its class, medetomidine causes diuresis via suppression of anti-diuretic hormone (Saleh et al. 2005). Medetomidine inhibits intestinal motility in all species studied (Maugeri et al. 1994; Scheibner et al. 2002; Zullian et al. 2011). Although medetomidine decreases cerebral blood flow (Talke et al. 2000), intracranial pressure is unaffected in isoflurane-anesthetized dogs (Keegan et al. 1995). Medetomidine inhibits insulin secretion and causes hyperglycemia (Guedes et al. 2013).

Dexmedetomidine

The pharmacologically active dextrorotary enantiomer of medetomidine, dexmedetomidine displays the highest $\alpha_2:\alpha1$ selectivity in its class. The levorotary enantiomer of medetomidine is essentially without effect, although supraclinical doses can reduce sedation and analgesia (MacDonald et al. 1991; Kuusela et al. 2001; Ansah et al. 2000).

Pharmacokinetic data for dexmedetomidine is best described by noncompartmental analysis in horses (Bettschart-Wolfensberger et al. 2005) whereas in rats and cats, two- and three-compartment models have been defined (Bol et al. 1997; Pypendop and Ilkiw 2014). The distribution half-life is one to three minutes in cats, rats, goats, and sheep (Bol et al. 1997; Kästner et al. 2006; Pypendop and Ilkiw 2014) whereas, in dogs, a large variation in distribution half-life is documented (Honkavaara et al. 2012). The volume of distribution in dogs and cats is less than 1 L/kg (Kuusela et al. 2000; Pypendop and Ilkiw 2014), whereas it is much larger in rats at >3 L/kg (Bol et al. 1997). The elimination half-life in cats is quite rapid at approximately five to six minutes (Pypendop and

Ilkiw 2014). In horses, the elimination half-life is 8–30 minutes (Bettschart-Wolfensberger et al. 1999, 2005; Rezende et al. 2015) and is 21 minutes following an infusion of dexmedetomidine at 8 mcg/kg/hr for 150 minutes (Ranheim et al. 2015). The elimination half-life in sheep and goats is similar, 33 and 39 minutes, respectively (Kästner et al. 2006). A relatively long elimination half-life is reported in rats and dogs at close to one hour (Bol et al. 1997; Kuusela et al. 2000). In comparison to an equivalent dose of racemic medetomidine, dexmedetomidine has a shorter half-life in dogs (Kuusela et al. 2000).

Inhalant anesthesia affects the PK parameters of dexmedetomidine by affecting hemodynamics and organ blood flow. One group reported the PK data for dexmedetomidine during isoflurane anesthesia in cats (Escobar et al. 2012a). However, direct comparisons cannot be made between this study and the one available for conscious cats because dosing strategies were quite different, with the anesthetized cats receiving 10 mcg/kg IV over five minutes and conscious cats receiving 5, 20, or 50 mcg/kg as an IV bolus (Escobar et al. 2012a; Pypendop and Ilkiw 2014). A two-compartment model is the best fit to describe the pharmacokinetic data of dexmedetomidine in anesthetized cats. The distribution half-life is 5.4 minutes; the volume of distribution at steady state is fairly large at 1.7 L/kg; clearance is 6.3 mL/kg/min; and the elimination half-life is quite long at 198 minutes (Escobar et al. 2012a).

Dexmedetomidine undergoes extensive hepatic hydroxylation (Salonen 1991). Subsequent glucuronidation occurs with significant species differences in efficiency (Kaivosaari et al. 2002).

Dexmedetomidine is used in dogs and cats as a sedative for minimally invasive procedures or prior to general anesthesia, usually in combination with an opioid. It may be incorporated into total IM anesthetic protocols, especially for uncooperative pets and wildlife. Dexmedetomidine can be infused IV to reduce inhalational anesthetic requirements in dogs although this practice in cats results in more cardiovascular depression than an equipotent dose of inhalant alone (Pypendop et al. 2011). Very low doses of dexmedetomidine can minimize emergence delirium in small-animal patients. Dexmedetomidine can be placed in the epidural space but this route may produce systemic side effects. Less expensive α_2 agonists marketed for large animals are typically chosen for use in these species.

Dexmedetomidine decreases the MAC of halothane in rats and cats (Segal et al. 1988; Schmeling et al. 1999), sevoflurane in ponies (Gozalo-Marcilla et al. 2013), and isoflurane in pigs, dogs, cats, and rats (Vainio and Bloor 1994; Pascoe et al. 2006; Rioja et al. 2006; Escobar et al. 2012b). Infusion of dexmedetomidine at 0.5 mcg/kg/hr reduced the MAC of isoflurane in dogs by 30% and the combination of dexmedetomidine with morphine, lidocaine, and ketamine infusions reduced isoflurane MAC by 90% (Ebner et al. 2013).

The cardiovascular effects of dexmedetomidine are similar to an equipotent dose of medetomidine (Kuusela et al. 2000). Dexmedetomidine decreases the incidence of epinephrine-induced arrhythmias in halothane-anesthetized dogs likely due to the central sympatholytic effects (Hayashi et al. 1991).

The respiratory effects of dexmedetomidine are similar to other α₂ agonists, with decreases in respiratory rate but minimal changes in oxygenation or ventilation when administered alone to healthy animals (Bettschart-Wolfensberger et al. 2005).

Dexmedetomidine decreases cerebral blood flow in the isoflurane-anesthetized dog without reducing cerebral metabolic oxygen requirements (Zornow et al. 1990). The central sympatholytic effects of dexmedetomidine contribute to neuroprotection in ischemia-reperfusion injury of the spinal cord and brain (Engelhard et al. 2002).

GI motility is inhibited by dexmedetomidine (Asai et al. 1997). Dexmedetomidine is reported to induce ocular hypotension and mydriasis (Vartiainen et al. 1992; Horváth et al. 1994). Dexmedetomidine reduces RBF but increases urine output and has been shown to protect the kidneys against ischemic-reperfusion injury in experimental settings (Lawrence et al. 1996; Gonullu et al. 2014). Moreover, anti-ischemic and anti-inflammatory effects of dexmedetomidine have been documented in the CNS, heart, and liver (Sahin et al. 2013; Goyagi and Tobe 2014; Ueki et al. 2014). In experimental sepsis, dexmedetomidine reduces mortality, possibly by inhibiting inflammatory pathways (Wu et al. 2013).

Romifidine

Marketed for use in horses, romifidine became clinically available in the early 1990s. Romifidine produces long-lasting sedation, analgesia, and cardiovascular effects typical of α₂ agonists. Romifidine is an imidazole derivative with partial-agonist activity at α₂ receptors that is structurally very similar to clonidine (Wojtasiak-Wypart et al. 2012). It displays an α₂:α₁ selectivity greater than detomidine but less than medetomidine (Table 4.1).

Available pharmacokinetic data for romifidine is limited. Plasma concentration versus time data is best fit to a two-compartment model in horses administered 80 mcg/kg IV over two minutes. The median distribution half-life is 15.1 minutes whereas the median elimination half-life is 138.2 minutes. The volume of distribution at steady state is large at 4.56 L/kg (Wojtasiak-Wypart et al. 2012). Following administration to horses of a loading dose (0.08 mg/kg) and an infusion (0.03 mg/kg/hr), a two-compartment model

best fit the data, with marked hysteresis between the nociceptive withdrawal reflex and plasma concentrations (Diez Bernal et al. 2020). Plasma elimination half-lives of 1.5 and 2 hours are reported in rats and dogs, respectively (Committee for Veterinary Medicinal Products 2009).

As with other α₂ agonists, romifidine undergoes extensive hepatic metabolism and subsequent renal excretion of the hydroxylated metabolite (Committee for Veterinary Medicinal Products 2009).

Romifidine is marketed for sedation and analgesia in horses to facilitate handling and minor surgical procedures. IV administration of 80 mcg/kg results in sedation in horses equivalent to that produced by 1 mg/kg IV xylazine and 20 mcg/kg IV detomidine, but with less ataxia and longer duration (England et al. 1992). It is also used as a sedative prior to induction of general anesthesia and in the recovery period to delay emergence. Romifidine may be infused IV to supplement inhalational anesthesia or as part of a total IV anesthetic protocol. Use of romifidine as a premedication before general anesthesia for cats and dogs, in total IM anesthetic protocols in pigs and cats, and in the epidural space in dogs and cattle is reported.

No formal studies evaluating MAC reduction by romifidine have been published. A clinical study in horses receiving 40 mcg/kg/hr romifidine IV during isoflurane anesthesia was unable to detect a difference in inhalant requirements compared with saline infusion (Devisscher et al. 2010).

Improved recovery scores have been reported with 20 mcg/kg of romifidine IV upon discontinuation of inhalational anesthetics, compared with a lower dose of romifidine (10 mcg/kg) or xylazine at either 100 or 200 mcg/kg IV (Woodhouse et al. 2013). Romifidine is generally purported to result in less ataxia in equine recovery than other α₂ agonists.

Biphasic cardiovascular effects typical of α₂ agonists are produced in dogs, cats, and horses by romifidine (Pypendop and Verstegen 2001; Freeman et al. 2002; Muir and Gadawski 2002). Compared to premedication with detomidine 20 mcg/kg, romifidine 100 mcg/kg resulted in more severe hypotension and more frequent use of dobutamine in horses during halothane anesthesia (Taylor et al. 2001).

During infusion of romifidine in standing horses, slight hypercapnia develops but no change in arterial oxygen concentration occurs (Ringer et al. 2013). In sheep, as with administration of other α₂ agonists, romifidine can induce severe hypoxemia without changes in arterial CO_2 concentrations. Compared with xylazine, detomidine, and medetomidine, increases in respiratory rate and pleural pressure lasted longer after administration of romifidine (Celly et al. 1997b).

Centrally mediated sedation, analgesia, and ataxia occur in horses after administration of romifidine, and these effects may be more persistent than equivalent doses of xylazine or detomidine (England et al. 1992; López-Sanromán et al. 2013; Costa et al. 2015).

As expected, romifidine decreases GI motility (Freeman and England 2001). IV romifidine reduces intraocular pressure in horses (Stine et al. 2014).

α_2 Receptor Antagonists

The availability of reversal agents for α_2 agonists allows for greater control over the duration of sedation. The currently available α_2 antagonists reverse all effects of α_2 agonists, including sedation, analgesia, and cardiovascular effects, although in some species, cardiopulmonary consequences may not be completely ameliorated by reversal.

Yohimbine

Yohimbine is an indole alkaloid derived from various plant sources that displays an $\alpha_2{:}\alpha_1$ selectivity of approximately 40 : 1 (Doxey et al. 1983; Virtanen et al. 1989; Tam et al. 2001).

Following IV administration of yohimbine to horses, pharmacokinetic analysis is best fit to a two-compartment model. Maximum plasma concentrations are reached very quickly, within 5.5 minutes (Dimaio Knych et al. 2011a). Whether administered as a sole agent or following detomidine, yohimbine displays a large volume of distribution of >2–3 L/kg (Dimaio Knych et al. 2011a, 2011b; Knych and Stanley 2014). A large steady state volume of distribution is also reported in cattle and dogs (Jernigan et al. 1988). A mean elimination half-life of three hours is reported when yohimbine is administered as a sole agent to horses and this is consistent with the large volume of distribution and slow clearance (13.5 mL/min/kg) (Dimaio Knych et al. 2011a). The volume of distribution and clearance of yohimbine are lower following detomidine administration than when it is administered as a sole agent. Following administration of detomidine in horses, a mean elimination half-life of two hours is reported in horses (Knych et al. 2012). A hydroxylated metabolite of yohimbine can be identified in horse urine (DiMaio Knych et al. 2011a).

Yohimbine effectively reverses the sedative and cardiovascular effects of xylazine in horses (Kollias-Baker et al. 1993). However, yohimbine reversal of the sedative effects of detomidine may be incomplete or may allow for sedation to reoccur (DiMaio Knych et al. 2012; Knych and Stanley 2014). In addition, yohimbine appears to partially antagonize the effects of ketamine (Hatch and Ruch 1974) and barbiturates (Hatch 1973) in cats. When administered to horses without prior α_2-agonist exposure, a variety of behavioral effects may result, including no change, sedation, or excitation (Dimaio Knych et al. 2011a, 2011b). Yohimbine reversal of xylazine sedation in cats can cause agitation and vocalization (Hartsfield et al. 1991) and sole administration of yohimbine to dogs can result in agitation, tremoring, and hypersalivation (Jernigan et al. 1988).

Elevations in heart rate are documented with administration of yohimbine either as a sole agent or after exposure to xylazine (Kollias-Baker et al. 1993; DiMaio Knych et al. 2011b) and this is likely due to increased sympathetic activity.

Yohimbine administration increases GI sounds in horses when administered as a sole agent (DiMaio Knych et al. 2011b). Plasma-insulin concentrations increase in dogs and horses and xylazine-induced hyperglycemia in dogs is reversed with administration of yohimbine (Hsu 1988; DiMaio Knych et al. 2011b). Yohimbine reverses the diuretic effect of medetomidine in cats and dogs (Talukder et al. 2009; Murahata et al. 2014).

Respiratory distress, tachycardia, and death have been anecdotally reported following IV administration of yohimbine in horses (Scofield et al. 2010) and excitation is a possibility in all species. IM administration is recommended unless an emergent situation exists.

Tolazoline

The α_2 antagonist tolazoline displays the lowest affinity for α_2 receptors compared with yohimbine and atipamezole (Schwartz and Clark 1998).

Limited pharmacokinetic data for tolazoline is available. A two-compartment model was the best fit for the pharmacokinetic data following IV administration of 4 mg/kg to adult horses (Casbeer and Knych 2013). The volume of distribution at steady state ranged from 1.3 to 2.4 L/kg. The elimination half-life is 2.75 hours when administered as a sole agent and 3.37 hours following detomidine sedation (Knych and Stanley 2014; Casbeer and Knych 2013). Tolazoline is excreted intact in the urine.

Tolazoline reverses the CNS and cardiovascular effects of xylazine in horses (Kollias-Baker et al. 1993). However, reversal of detomidine sedation may be incomplete and/or short-lived (Hubbell and Muir 2006; Knych and Stanley 2014).

Both tachycardia and bradycardia have been demonstrated following administration of tolazoline (FDA Report n.d.; Casbeer and Knych 2013). Tolazoline can result in hypotension and decreases in cerebral blood blow and oxygen delivery (Balsan et al. 1990). During isoflurane anesthesia, tolazoline antagonism of detomidine in horses resulted in improvements in blood pressure and heart rate but further deterioration in arterial oxygenation.

Following sedation with xylazine, two horses died when administered a five-fold overdose of tolazoline. Hypertension, tachycardia, and cardiac conduction disturbances were noted in the horses that survived (FDA Report n.d.). A two- to three-fold overdose of tolazoline in mule deer resulted in apnea and muscle fasciculations (Mortenson and Robison 2011). Anecdotal reports of New World camelid deaths following tolazoline administration to reverse xylazine sedation exist. In addition, a published case report of toxicosis in a llama that received 8.6 mg/kg tolazoline described anxiety, tachypnea, hypotension, diarrhea, and seizures that responded to supportive treatment (Read et al. 2000). IM or slow IV administration is recommended.

Atipamezole

Atipamezole displays the highest α_2:α_1 selectivity of the available α_2 antagonists at 8526 : 1 (Virtanen et al. 1989). The affinity of atipamezole for α_{2A}, α_{2B}, and α_{2C} receptors is comparable to yohimbine but its affinity for the species-specific α_{2D} homolog of α_{2A} receptors found in cows, rats, and sheep is 100-fold higher (Haapalinna et al. 1997; Schwartz and Clark 1998).

A one-compartment model best describes the pharmacokinetics of atipamezole administered alone to dogs; however, the study design included long intervals between sampling times that may have affected detection of a distribution phase. Rapid absorption from IM deposition occurs and peak plasma concentrations are reached within one hour. A large volume of distribution is apparent, at approximately 2.3 L/kg. The elimination half-life was approximately one hour. Atipamezole increases the clearance and decreases the elimination half-life of medetomidine in dogs (Salonen et al. 1995). In reindeer, administration of atipamezole increases medetomidine concentrations in plasma and the elimination half-life of atipamezole was faster than medetomidine, resulting in resedation (Ranheim et al. 1997). Similar pharmacokinetic and sedative profiles were determined for the combination of medetomidine and atipamezole in dairy calves and cows (Ranheim et al. 1998, 1999). In sheep, IV atipamezole resulted in excitation and, at the same time, increased plasma medetomidine concentrations. In contrast to reports in other ruminants, resedation did not occur (Ranheim et al. 2000). In horses following sublingual detomidine, clearance of atipamezole was slower and the elimination half-life longer than reported for ruminants (Knych and Stanley 2014). In pigs, a similar pharmacokinetic profile for atipamezole has been identified with rapid absorption and occurrence of peak plasma concentrations, a large volume of distribution, and an elimination half-life of approximately one hour (Kanazawa et al. 1995).

Atipamezole undergoes hydroxylation and subsequent renal excretion of the water-soluble metabolite (Salonen et al. 1995; Kaivosaari et al. 2002).

Atipamezole is marketed for the reversal of medetomidine and dexmedetomidine; and it can also effectively reverse the effects of other α_2 agonists. However, in horses, atipamezole may only transiently and incompletely reverse detomidine sedation (Hubbell and Muir 2006; Knych and Stanley 2014).

Hypotension, tachycardia, and hyperactivity can occur with IV administration of atipamezole and IM injection is generally recommended.

Vatinoxan

Vatinoxan is a peripheral α_2 antagonist that does not cross the blood–brain barrier, preventing the initial vasoconstrictive and hypertensive response to administration of α_2 agonists while preserving the central sedative and sympatholytic effects (Pagel et al. 1998; Honkavaara et al. 2011). Zenalpha, a combination drug product of medetomidine (0.5 mg/mL) and vatinoxan (10 mg/mL) hydrochlorides was brought to the market in the US in 2022.

The co-administration of dexmedetomidine and vatinoxan increases the volume of distribution of dexmedetomidine and reduces plasma dexmedetomidine concentrations, compared to dexmedetomidine alone, likely due to avoidance of the initial cardiovascular effects of the α_2 agonist (Honkavaara et al. 2012; Vainionpää et al. 2013b). No changes in the elimination half-life occur (Honkavaara et al. 2012).

A slight decrease in sedation occurs with co-administration of dexmedetomidine and vatinoxan and this is thought to be due to the decreased plasma concentrations that occur compared with administration of dexmedetomidine alone (Honkavaara et al. 2011). At the doses studied in anesthetized cats so far, the overall hemodynamic state did not improve or was worsened due to profound hypotension incited by vatinoxan (Jaeger et al. 2019). In horses, vatinoxan prevented detomidine induced bradycardia and ileus. The degree of sedation was similar to detomidine alone but duration was reduced (Vainionpää et al. 2013b). In anesthetized horses, vatinoxan lead to more hypotension and higher dobutamine requirements than medetomidine alone (Tapio et al. 2019). Vatinoxan prevents hypoinsulinemia and hyperglycemia caused by dexmedetomidine (Restitutti et al. 2012).

References

Ahlquist, R.P. (1967). Development of the concept of α₂ and beta adrenotropic receptors. *Ann. N. Y. Acad. Sci.* 139 (3): 549–552.

Ansah, O.B., Raekallio, M., and Vainio, O. (1998). Comparison of three doses of dexmedetomidine with medetomidine in cats following intramuscular administration. *J. Vet. Pharmacol. Therap.* 21 (5): 380–387.

Ansah, O.B., Raekallio, M., and Vainio, O. (2000). Correlation between serum concentrations following continuous intravenous infusion of dexmedetomidine or medetomidine in cats and their sedative and analgesic effects. *J. Vet. Pharmacol. Therap.* 23 (1): 1–8.

Asai, T., Mapleson, W.W., and Power, I. (1997). Differential effects of clonidine and dexmedetomidine on gastric emptying and gastrointestinal transit in the rat. *Br. J. Anaesth.* 78 (3): 301–307.

Avsaroglu, H., Bull, S., Maas-Bakker, R.F. et al. (2008). Differences in hepatic cytochrome P450 activity correlate with the strain-specific biotransformation of medetomidine in AX/JU and IIIVO/JU inbred rabbits. *J. Vet. Pharmacol. Therap.* 31 (4): 368–377.

Balsan, M.J., Cronin, C.M., and Shaw, M.D. (1990). Blood flow distribution and brain metabolism during tolazoline-induced hypotension in newborn dogs. *Pediatr. Res.* 28 (2): 111–115.

Bantel, C., Eisenach, J.C., Duflo, F. et al. (2005). Spinal nerve ligation increases alpha2-adrenergic receptor G-protein coupling in the spinal cord. *Brain Res.* 1038 (1): 76–82.

Bettschart-Wolfensberger, R., Clarke, K.W., Vainio, O. et al. (1999). Pharmacokinetics of medetomidine in ponies and elaboration of a medetomidine infusion regime which provides a constant level of sedation. *Res. Vet. Sci.* 67 (1): 41–46.

Bettschart-Wolfensberger, R., Jäggin-Schmucker, N., Lendl, C. et al. (2001). Minimal alveolar concentration of desflurane in combination with an infusion of medetomidine for the anaesthesia of ponies. *Vet. Rec.* 148 (9): 264–267.

Bettschart-Wolfensberger, R., Freeman, S.L., Bowen, I.M. et al. (2005). Cardiopulmonary effects and pharmacokinetics of i.v. dexmedetomidine in ponies. *Equine Vet. J.* 37 (1): 60–64.

Bloor, B.C. and Flacke, W.E. (1982). Reduction in halothane anesthetic requirement by clonidine, an alpha-adrenergic agonist. *Anesth. Analg.* 61 (9): 741–745.

Bloor, B.C., Frankland, M., Alper, G. et al. (1992a). Hemodynamic and sedative effects of dexmedetomidine in dog. *J. Pharmacol. Exp. Therap.* 263 (2): 690–697.

Bloor, B.C., Ward, D.S., Belleville, J.P. et al. (1992b). Effects of intravenous dexmedetomidine in humans II. Hemodynamic changes. *Anesthesiology* 77 (6): 1134–1142.

Bol, C.J.J.G., Danhof, M., Stanski, D.R. et al. (1997). Pharmacokinetic-pharmacodynamic characterization of the cardiovascular, hypnotic, EEG and ventilatory responses to dexmedetomidine in the rat. *J. Pharmacol. Exp. Therap.* 283 (3): 1051–1058.

Bond, R.A., Bylund, D.B., Eikenburg, D.C. et al. (2014). Adrenoceptors: α₂ₐ-adrenoceptor. http://www. guidetopharmacology.org/GRAC/ObjectDisplayForward?objectId=25 (accessed 4 April 2015).

Bueno, A.C., Cornick-Seahorn, J., Seahorn, T.L. et al. (1999). Cardiopulmonary and sedative effects of intravenous administration of low doses of medetomidine and xylazine to adult horses. *Am. J. Vet. Res.* 60 (11): 1371–1376.

Burton, S.A., Lemke, K.A., Ihle, S.L. et al. (1997). Effects of medetomidine on serum insulin and plasma glucose concentrations in clinically normal dogs. *Am. J. Vet. Res.* 58 (12): 1440–1442.

Burton, S., Lemke, K.A., Ihle, S.L. et al. (1998). Effects of medetomidine on serum osmolality; urine volume, osmolality and pH; free water clearance; and fractional clearance of sodium, chloride, potassium, and glucose in dogs. *Am. J. Vet. Res.* 59 (6): 756–761.

Cardoso, C.G., Ayer, I.M., Jorge, A.T. et al. (2020). A comparative study of the cardiopulmonary and sedative effects of a single intramuscular dose of ketamine anesthetic combinations in rabbits. *Res. Vet. Sci.* 128: 177–182.

Carter, S.W., Robertson, S.A., Steel, C.J. et al. (1990). Cardiopulmonary effects of xylazine sedation in the foal. *Equine Vet. J.* 22 (6): 384–388.

Casbeer, H.C. and Knych, H.K. (2013). Pharmacokinetics and pharmacodynamic effects of tolazoline following intravenous administration to horses. *Vet. J.* 196 (3): 504–509.

Castro, M.I. and Eisenach, J.C. (1989). Pharmacokinetics and dynamics of intravenous, intrathecal, and epidural clonidine in sheep. *Anesthesiology* 71 (3): 418–425.

Celly, C.S., McDonell, W.N., Black, W.D. et al. (1997a). Cardiopulmonary effects of clonidine, diazepam and the peripheral alpha 2 adrenoceptor agonist ST-91 in conscious sheep. *J. Vet. Pharmacol. Therap.* 20 (6): 472–478.

Celly, C.S., McDonell, W.N., Young, S.S. et al. (1997b). The comparative hypoxaemic effect of four alpha 2 adrenoceptor agonists (xylazine, romifidine, detomidine and medetomidine) in sheep. *J. Vet. Pharmacol. Therap.* 20 (6): 464–471.

Chabot-Doré, A.J., Schuster, D.J., Stone, L.S. et al. (2015). Analgesic synergy between opioid and α2-adrenoceptors. *Br. J. Pharmacol.* 172 (2): 388–402.

Chen, S.R., Pan, H.M., Richardson, T.E. et al. (2007). Potentiation of spinal alpha(2)-adrenoceptor analgesia in rats deficient in TRPV1-expressing afferent neurons. *Neuropharmacology* 52 (8): 1624–1630.

Committee for Veterinary Medicinal Products (2009). Romifidine. Summary Report. http://www.ema.europa.eu/docs/en_GB/document_library/Maximum_Residue_Limits_-_Report/2009/11/WC500015833.pdf (accessed 25 March2015).

Congdon, J.M., Marquez, M., Niyom, S. et al. (2011). Evaluation of the sedative and cardiovascular effects of intramuscular administration of dexmedetomidine with and without concurrent atropine administration in dogs. *J. Am. Vet. Med. Assoc.* 239 (1): 81–89.

Correa-Sales, C., Rabin, B.C., and Maze, M. (1992). A hypnotic response to dexmedetomidine, an alpha 2 agonist, is mediated in the locus coeruleus in rats. *Anesthesiology* 76 (6): 948–952.

Costa, G.L., Cristarella, S., Quartuccio, M. et al. (2015). Anti-nociceptive and sedative effects of romifidine, tramadol and their combination administered intravenously slowly in ponies. *Vet. Anaesth. Analg.* 42 (2): 220–225.

Creighton, C.M., Lemke, K.A., Lamont, L.A. et al. (2012). Comparison of the effects of xylazine bolus versus medetomidine constant rate infusion on cardiopulmonary function and depth of anesthesia in horses anesthetized with isoflurane. *J. Am. Vet. Med. Assoc.* 240 (8): 991–997.

De Rossi, R., Bucker, G.V., and Varela, J.V. (2003). Perineal analgesic actions of epidural clonidine in cattle. *Vet. Anaesth. Analg.* 30 (2): 64–71.

Devisscher, L., Schauvliege, S., Dewulf, J. et al. (2010). Romifidine as a constant rate infusion in isoflurane anaesthetized horses: a clinical study. *Vet. Anaesth. Analg.* 37 (5): 425–433.

Diez Bernal, S., Studer, N., Thormann, W. et al. (2020). Pharmacokinetic-pharmacodynamic modelling of the antinociceptive effect of a romifidine infusion in standing horses. *Vet. Anaesth. Analg.* 47 (1): 129–136.

Dimaio Knych, H.K., Steffey, E.P., Deuel, J.L. et al. (2011a). Pharmacokinetics of yohimbine following intravenous administration to horses. *J. Vet. Pharmacol. Therap.* 34 (1): 58–63.

Dimaio Knych, H.K., Steffey, E.P., and Stanley, S.D. (2011b). Pharmacokinetics and pharmacodynamics of three intravenous doses of yohimbine in the horse. *J. Vet. Pharmacol. Therap.* 34 (4): 359–366.

DiMaio Knych, H.K., Covarrubias, V., and Steffey, E.P. (2012). Effect of yohimbine on detomidine induced changes in behavior, cardiac and blood parameters in the horse. *Vet. Anaesth. Analg.* 39 (6): 574–583.

Dirikolu, L., McFadden, E.T., Ely, K.J. et al. (2006). Clonidine in horses: identification, detection, and clinical pharmacology. *Vet. Therap.* 7 (2): 141–155.

Doherty, T.J., Geiser, D.R., and Rohrbach, B.W. (1997). The effect of epidural xylazine on halothane minimum alveolar concentration in ponies. *J. Vet. Pharmacol. Therap.* 20 (3): 246–248.

Doherty, T.J., Andrews, F.M., Provenza, M.K. et al. (1999). The effect of sedation on gastric emptying of a liquid marker in ponies. *Vet. Surg.* 28 (5): 375–379.

Dória, R.G., Valadão, C.A., Duque, J.C. et al. (2008). Comparative study of epidural xylazine or clonidine in horses. *Vet. Anaesth. Analg.* 35 (2): 166–172.

Doxey, J.C., Roach, A.G., and Smith, C.F. (1983). Studies on RX 781094: a selective, potent and specific antagonist of alpha 2-adrenoceptors. *Br. J. Pharmacol.* 78 (3): 489–505.

Duhamel, M.C., Troncy, E., and Beaudry, F. (2010). Metabolic stability and determination of cytochrome P450 isoenzymes' contribution to the metabolism of medetomidine in dog liver microsomes. *Biomed. Chromatogr.* 24 (8): 868–877.

Dyson, D.H., Maxie, M.G., and Schnurr, D. (1998). Morbidity and mortality associated with anesthetic management in small animal veterinary practice in Ontario. *J. Am. Anim. Hosp. Assoc.* 34 (4): 325–335.

Ebner, L.S., Lerche, P., Bednarski, R.M. et al. (2013). Effect of dexmedetomidine, morphine-lidocaine-ketamine, and dexmedetomidine-morphine-lidocaine-ketamine constant rate infusions on the minimum alveolar concentration of isoflurane and bispectral index in dogs. *Am. J. Vet. Res.* 74 (7): 963–970.

Engelhard, K., Werner, C., Kaspar, S. et al. (2002). Effect of the alpha2-agonist dexmedetomidine on cerebral neurotransmitter concentrations during cerebral ischemia in rats. *Anesthesiology* 96 (2): 450–457.

England, G.C., Clarke, K.W., and Goossens, L. (1992). A comparison of the sedative effects of three alpha 2-adrenoceptor agonists (romifidine, detomidine and xylazine) in the horse. *J. Vet. Pharmacol. Therap.* 15 (2): 194–201.

Escobar, A., Pypendop, B.H., Siao, K.T. et al. (2012a). Pharmacokinetics of dexmedetomidine administered intravenously in isoflurane-anesthetized cats. *Am. J. Vet. Res.* 73 (2): 285–289.

Escobar, A., Pypendop, B.H., Siao, K.T. et al. (2012b). Effect of dexmedetomidine on the minimum alveolar concentration of isoflurane in cats. *J. Vet. Pharmacol. Therap.* 35 (2): 163–168.

Fairbanks, C.A., Stone, L.S., Kitto, K.F. et al. (2002). Alpha(2C)-adrenergic receptors mediate spinal analgesia and adrenergic-opioid synergy. *J. Vet. Pharmacol. Therap.* 300 (1): 282–290.

FDA Report (n.d.). Tolazoline [Online]. https://fda.report/Dai lyMed/7d44e15d-4ac7-49ca-900f-13916aeea247 (Accessed 03/26/2015).

Feuerstein, T.J., Mutschler, A., Lupp, A. et al. (1993). Endogenous noradrenaline activates alpha 2-adrenoceptors on serotonergic nerve endings in human and rat neocortex. *J. Neurochem.* 61 (2): 474–480.

Fischer, B.L., Ludders, J.W., Asakawa, M. et al. (2009). A comparison of epidural buprenorphine plus detomidine with morphine plus detomidine in horses undergoing bilateral stifle arthroscopy. *Vet. Anaesth. Analg.* 36 (1): 67–76.

Flacke, W.E., Flacke, J.W., Blow, K.D. et al. (1992). Effect of dexmedetomidine, an alpha 2-adrenergic agonist, in the isolated heart. *J. Cardiothorac. Vasc. Anesth.* 6 (4): 418–423.

Flacke, W.E., Flacke, J.W., Bloor, B.C. et al. (1993). Effects of dexmedetomidine on systemic and coronary hemodynamics in the anesthetized dog. *J. Cardiothorac. Vasc. Anesth.* 7 (1): 41–49.

Freeman, S.L. and England, G.C. (2001). Effect of romifidine on gastrointestinal motility, assessed by transrectal ultrasonography. *Equine Vet. J.* 33 (6): 570–576.

Freeman, S.L., Bowen, I.M., Bettschart-Wolfensberger, R. et al. (2002). Cardiovascular effects of romifidine in the standing horse. *Res. Vet. Sci.* 72 (2): 123–129.

Funai, Y., Pickering, A.E., Uta, D. et al. (2014). Systemic dexmedetomidine augments inhibitory synaptic transmission in the superficial dorsal horn through activation of descending noradrenergic control: an in vivo patch-clamp analysis of analgesic mechanisms. *Pain* 155 (3): 617–628.

Garcia-Villar, R., Toutain, P.L., Alvinerie, M. et al. (1981). The pharmacokinetics of xylazine hydrochloride: an interspecific study. *J. Vet. Pharmacol. Therap.* 4 (2): 87–92.

Ghignone, M., Calvillo, O., Quintin, L. et al. (1987). Haemodynamic effects of clonidine injected epidurally in halothane-anaesthetized dogs. *Can. J. Anaesth.* 34 (1): 46–50.

Gilsbach, R., Röser, C., Beetz, N. et al. (2009). Genetic dissection of alpha2-adrenoceptor functions in adrenergic versus nonadrenergic cells. *Mol. Pharmacol.* 75 (5): 1160–1170.

Gonullu, E., Ozkardesler, S., Kume, T. et al. (2014). Comparison of the effects of dexmedetomidine administered at two different times on renal ischemia/reperfusion injury in rats. *Braz. J. Anesth.* 64 (3): 152–158.

Gordh, T. and Hartvig, P. (1986). Cerebrospinal fluid and plasma concentrations of clonidine in pigs after epidural, intravenous and intramuscular administration. *Upsala J. Med. Sci.* 91 (3): 311–315.

Goyagi, T. and Tobe, Y. (2014). Dexmedetomidine improves the histological and neurological outcomes 48 h after transient spinal ischemia in rats. *Brain Res.* 1566: 24–30.

Gozalo-Marcilla, M., Hopster, K., Gasthuys, F. et al. (2013). Effects of a constant-rate infusion of dexmedetomidine on the minimal alveolar concentration of sevoflurane in ponies. *Equine Vet. J.* 45 (2): 204–208.

Grimsrud, K.N., Mama, K.R., Thomasy, S.M. et al. (2009). Pharmacokinetics of detomidine and its metabolites following intravenous and intramuscular administration in horses. *Equine Vet. J.* 41 (4): 361–365.

Grimsrud, K.N., Mama, K.R., Steffey, E.P. et al. (2012). Pharmacokinetics and pharmacodynamics of intravenous medetomidine in the horse. *Vet. Anaesth. Analg.* 39 (1): 38–48.

Grimsrud, K.N., Ait-Oudhia, S., Durbin-Johnson, B.P. et al. (2015). Pharmacokinetic and pharmacodynamic analysis comparing diverse effects of detomidine, medetomidine, and dexmedetomidine in the horse: a population analysis. *J. Vet. Pharmacol. Therap.* 38 (1): 24–34.

Guedes, A.G. and Rude, E.P. (2013). Effects of pre-operative administration of medetomidine on plasma insulin and glucose concentrations in healthy dogs and dogs with insulinoma. *Veterinary Anaesthesia and Analgesia* 40 (5): 472–481.

Guedes, A.G., Rude, E.P., and Kannan, M.S. (2013). Potential role of the CD38/cADPR signaling pathway as an underlying mechanism of the effects of medetomidine on insulin and glucose homeostasis. *Vet. Anaesth. Analg.* 40 (5): 512–516.

Guyenet, P.G. (1997). Is the hypotensive effect of clonidine and related drugs due to imidazoline binding sites? *Am. J. Phys* 273 (5 part 2): r1580–r1584.

Guyenet, P.G. and Cabot, J.B. (1981). Inhibition of sympathetic preganglionic neurons by catecholamines and clonidine: mediation by an alpha-adrenergic receptor. *Journal of Neuroscience* 1 (8): 908–917.

Gyires, K., Müllner, K., Fürst, S. et al. (2000). Alpha-2 adrenergic and opioid receptor-mediated gastroprotection. *J. Physiol.* 94 (2): 117–121.

Haapalinna, A., Viitamaa, T., and MacDonald, E. (1997). Evaluation of the effects of a specific alpha 2-adrenoceptor antagonist, atipamezole, on alpha 1- and alpha 2-adrenoceptor subtype binding, brain neurochemistry and behaviour in comparison with yohimbine. *Naunyn-Schmiedeberg's Arch. Pharmacol.* 356 (5): 570–582.

Hartsfield, S.M., Matthews, N.S., Miller, S. et al. (1991). Comparison of the effects of tolazoline, yohimbine, and doxapram in cats medicated with xylazine. *Vet. Anaesth. Analg.* 18 (s1): 71–73.

Haskins, S.C., Patz, J.D., and Farver, T.B. (1986). Xylazine and xylazine-ketamine in dogs. *Am. J. Vet. Res.* 47 (3): 636–641.

Hatch, R.C. (1973). Experiments on antagonism of barbiturate anesthesia with adrenergic, serotonergic, and cholinergic stimulants given alone and in combination. *Am. J. Vet. Res.* 34 (10): 1321–1331.

Hatch, R.C. and Ruch, T. (1974). Experiments on antagonism of ketamine anesthesia in cats given adrenergic, serotonergic, and cholinergic stimulants alone and in combination. *Am. J. Vet. Res.* 35 (1): 35–39.

Hayashi, Y., Sumikawa, K., Maze, M. et al. (1991). Dexmedetomidine prevents epinephrine-induced arrhythmias through stimulation of central alpha 2 adrenoceptors in halothane-anesthetized dogs. *Anesthesiology* 75 (1): 113–117.

Holve, D.L. (2012). Effect of sedation with detomidine on intraocular pressure with and without topical anesthesia in clinically normal horses. *J. Am. Vet. Med. Assoc.* 240 (3): 308–311.

Honkavaara, J.M., Restitutti, F., Raekallio, M.R. et al. (2011). The effects of increasing doses of MK-467, a peripheral alpha(2)-adrenergic receptor antagonist, on the cardiopulmonary effects of intravenous dexmedetomidine in conscious dogs. *J. Vet. Pharmacol. Therap.* 34 (4): 332–337.

Honkavaara, J., Restitutti, F., Raekallio, M. et al. (2012). Influence of MK-467, a peripherally acting α2-adrenoceptor antagonist on the disposition of intravenous dexmedetomidine in dogs. *Drug Metab. Dispos.* 40 (3): 445–449.

Hood, D.D., Eisenach, J.C., Tong, C. et al. (1995). Cardiorespiratory and spinal cord blood flow effects of intrathecal neostigmine methylsulfate, clonidine, and their combination in sheep. *Anesthesiology* 82 (2): 428–435.

Hopfensberger, M.J., Messenger, K.M., Papich, M.G. et al. (2013). The use of oral transmucosal detomidine to facilitate handling in dogs. *J. Vet. Behav. Clin. Appl. Res.* 8 (3): 114–123.

Horváth, G., Kovács, M., Szikszay, M. et al. (1994). Mydriatic and antinociceptive effects of intrathecal dexmedetomidine in conscious rats. *Eur. J. Pharmacol.* 253 (1, 2): 61–66.

Hsu, W.H. (1988). Yohimbine increases plasma insulin concentrations and reverses xylazine-induced hypoinsulinemia in dogs. *Am. J. Vet. Res.* 49 (2): 242–244.

Hsu, W.H. and McNeel, S.V. (1983). Effect of yohimbine on xylazine-induced prolongation of gastrointestinal transit in dogs. *J. Am. Vet. Med. Assoc.* 183 (3): 297–300.

Hubbell, J.A. and Muir, W.W. (2006). Antagonism of detomidine sedation in the horse using intravenous tolazoline or atipamezole. *Equine Vet. J.* 38 (3): 238–241.

Hubbell, J.A., Sams, R.A., Schmall, L.M. et al. (2009). Pharmacokinetics of detomidine administered to horses at rest and after maximal exercise. *Equine Vet. J.* 41 (5): 419–422.

Ida, K.K., Fantoni, D.T., Ibiapina, B.T. et al. (2013). Effect of postoperative xylazine administration on cardiopulmonary function and recovery quality after isoflurane anesthesia in horses. *Vet. Surg.* 42 (7): 877–884.

Ishii, H., Kohno, T., Yamakura, T. et al. (2008). Action of dexmedetomidine on the substantia gelatinosa neurons of the rat spinal cord. *Eur. J. Neurosci.* 27 (12): 3182–3190.

Jaeger, A.T., Pypendop, B.H., Ahokoivu, H. et al. (2019). Cardiopulmonary effects of dexmedetomidine, with and without vatinoxan, in isoflurane-anesthetized cats. *Vet. Anaesth. Analg.* 46 (6): 753–764.

Jedruch, J., Gajewski, Z., and Kuussaari, J. (1989). The effect of detomidine hydrochloride on the electrical activity of uterus in pregnant mares. *Acta Vet. Scand.* 30 (3): 307–311.

Jernigan, A.D., Wilson, R.C., Booth, N.H. et al. (1988). Comparative pharmacokinetics of yohimbine in steers, horses and dogs. *Can. J. Vet. Res.* 52 (2): 172–176.

Kaivosaari, S., Salonen, J.S., and Taskinen, J. (2002). N-Glucuronidation of some 4-arylalkyl-1H-imidazoles by rat, dog, and human liver microsomes. *Drug Metab. Dispos.* 30 (3): 295–300.

Kamerling, S.G., Cravens, W.M., and Bagwell, C.A. (1988). Objective assessment of detomidine-induced analgesia and sedation in the horse. *Eur. J. Pharmacol.* 151 (1): 1–8.

Kanazawa, H., Nishimura, R., Sasaki, N. et al. (1995). Determination of medetomidine, atipamezole and midazolam in pig plasma by liquid chromatography-mass spectrometry. *Biomed. Chromatogr.* 9 (4): 188–191.

Kanda, T., Iguchi, A., Yoshioka, C. et al. (2015). Effects of medetomidine and xylazine on intraocular pressure and pupil size in healthy Beagle dogs. *Vet. Anaesth. Analg.* 2015 42 (6): 623–628.

Kästner, S.B.R., Wapf, P., Feige, K. et al. (2003). Pharmacokinetics and sedative effects of intramuscular medetomidine in domestic sheep. *J. Vet. Pharmacol. Therap.* 26 (4): 271–276.

Kästner, S.B., Pakarinen, S.M., Ramela, M.P. et al. (2006). Comparative pharmacokinetics of medetomidine enantiomers in goats and sheep during sevoflurane anaesthesia. *J. Vet. Pharmacol. Therap.* 29 (1): 63–66.

Kaukinen, H., Aspegrén, J., Hyyppä, S. et al. (2011). Bioavailability of detomidine administered sublingually to horses as an oromucosal gel. *J. Vet. Pharmacol. Therap.* 34 (1): 76–81.

Kawasaki, Y., Kumamoto, E., Furue, H. et al. (2003). Alpha 2 adrenoceptor-mediated presynaptic inhibition of primary afferent glutamatergic transmission in rat substantia gelatinosa neurons. *Anesthesiology* 98 (3): 682–689.

Keegan, R.D., Greene, S.A., Bagley, R.S. et al. (1995). Effects of medetomidine administration on intracranial pressure and cardiovascular variables of isoflurane-anesthetized dogs. *Am. J. Vet. Res.* 56 (2): 193–198.

Kendall, A., Mosley, C., and Bröjer, J. (2010). Tachypnea and antipyresis in febrile horses after sedation with alpha-agonists. *J. Vet. Int. Med.* 24 (4): 1008–1011.

Kimura, M., Saito, S., and Obata, H. (2012). Dexmedetomidine decreases hyperalgesia in neuropathic pain by increasing acetylcholine in the spinal cord. *Neurosci. Lett.* 529 (1): 70–74.

Knych, H.K. and Stanley, S.D. (2014). Effects of three antagonists on selected pharmacodynamic effects of sublingually administered detomidine in the horse. *Vet. Anaesth. Analg.* 41 (1): 36–47.

Knych, H.K., Steffey, E.P., and Stanley, S.D. (2012). The effects of yohimbine on the pharmacokinetic parameters of detomidine in the horse. *Vet. Anaesth. Analg.* 39 (3): 221–229.

Kodera, S.Y., Yoshida, M., Dezaki, K. et al. (2013). Inhibition of insulin secretion from rat pancreatic islets by dexmedetomidine and medetomidine, two sedatives frequently used in clinical settings. *Endocr. J.* 60 (3): 337–346.

Kollias-Baker, C.A., Court, M.H., and Williams, L.L. (1993). Influence of yohimbine and tolazoline on the cardiovascular, respiratory, and sedative effects of xylazine in the horse. *J. Vet. Pharmacol. Therap.* 16 (3): 350–358.

Kritchevsky, J.E., Muir, G.S., Leschke, D. et al. (2020). Blood glucose and insulin concentrations after alpha-2-agonists administration in horses with and without insulin dysregulation. *J. Vet. Int. Med.* 34 (2): 902–908.

Kuo, W.C. and Keegan, R.D. (2004). Comparative cardiovascular, analgesic, and sedative effects of medetomidine, medetomidine-hydromorphone, and medetomidine-butorphanol in dogs. *Am. J. Vet. Res.* 65 (7): 931–937.

Kutter, A.P., Kästner, S.B., Bettschart-Wolfensberger, R. et al. (2006). Cardiopulmonary effects of dexmedetomidine in goats and sheep anaesthetised with sevoflurane. *Vet. Rec.* 159 (19): 624–629.

Kuusela, E., Raekallio, M., Anttila, M. et al. (2000). Clinical effects and pharmacokinetics of medetomidine and its enantiomers in dogs. *J. Vet. Pharmacol. Therap.* 23 (1): 15–20.

Kuusela, E., Vainio, O., Kaistinen, A. et al. (2001). Sedative, analgesic, and cardiovascular effects of levomedetomidine alone and in combination with dexmedetomidine in dogs. *Am. J. Vet. Res.* 62 (4): 616–621.

Lähdesmäki, J., Sallinen, J., MacDonald, E. et al. (2003). Alpha2-adrenergic drug effects on brain monoamines, locomotion, and body temperature are largely abolished in mice lacking the alpha2A-adrenoceptor subtype. *Neuropharmacology* 44 (7): 882–892.

Lakhlani, P.P., MacMillan, L.B., Guo, T.Z. et al. (1997). Substitution of a mutant alpha2a-adrenergic receptor via "hit and run" gene targeting reveals the role of this subtype in sedative, analgesic, and anesthetic-sparing responses in vivo. *Proc. Natl. Acad. Sci. U.S.A.* 94 (18): 9950–9955.

Lamont, L.A., Bulmer, B.J., Grimm, K.A. et al. (2001). Cardiopulmonary evaluation of the use of medetomidine hydrochloride in cats. *Am. J. Vet. Res.* 62 (11): 1745–1749.

Lamont, L.A., Burton, S.A., Caines, D. et al. (2012). Effects of 2 different infusion rates of medetomidine on sedation score, cardiopulmonary parameters, and serum levels of medetomidine in healthy dogs. *Can. J. Vet. Res.* 76 (4): 308–316.

Lanza, M., Ferrari, F., Menghetti, I. et al. (2014). Modulation of imidazoline I2 binding sites by CR4056 relieves postoperative hyperalgesia in male and female rats. *Br. J. Pharmacol.* 171 (15): 3693–3701.

Lavoie, D.S., Pailleux, F., Vachon, P. et al. (2013). Characterization of xylazine metabolism in rat liver microsomes using liquid chromatography-hybrid triple quadrupole-linear ion trap-mass spectrometry. *Biomed. Chromatogr.* 27 (7): 882–888.

Lawrence, C.J., Prinzen, F.W., and de Lange, S. (1996). The effect of dexmedetomidine on nutrient organ blood flow. *Anesth. Analg.* 83 (6): 1160–1165.

Lemke, K.A., Tranquilli, W.J., Thurmon, J.C. et al. (1993). Alterations in the arrhythmogenic dose of epinephrine after xylazine or medetomidine administration in isoflurane-anesthetized dogs. *American Journal of Veterinary Research* 54 (12): 2139–2144.

Lerche, P. and Muir, W.W. (2004). Effect of medetomidine on breathing and inspiratory neuromuscular drive in conscious dogs. *Am. J. Vet. Res.* 65 (6): 720–724.

Lerche, P. and Muir, W.W. (2006). Effect of medetomidine on respiration and minimum alveolar concentration in halothane- and isoflurane-anesthetized dogs. *Am. J. Vet. Res.* 67 (5): 782–789.

Li, S.S., Zhang, W.S., Ji, D. et al. (2014). Involvement of spinal microglia and interleukin-18 in the anti-nociceptive effect of dexmedetomidine in rats subjected to CCI. *Neurosci. Lett.* 560: 21–25.

Link, R.E., Desai, K., Hein, L. et al. (1996). Cardiovascular regulation in mice lacking alpha2-adrenergic receptor subtypes b and c. *Science* 273 (5276): 803–805.

López-Sanromán, F.J., Holmbak-Petersen, R., Varela, M. et al. (2013). Accelerometric comparison of the locomotor pattern of horses sedated with xylazine hydrochloride, detomidine hydrochloride, or romifidine hydrochloride. *Am. J. Vet. Res.* 74 (6): 828–834.

MacDonald, E., Scheinin, M., Scheinin, H. et al. (1991). Comparison of the behavioral and neurochemical effects of the two optical enantiomers of medetomidine, a selective alpha-2-adrenoceptor agonist. *J. Pharmacol. Exp. Therap.* 259 (2): 848–854.

Madden, C.J., Tupone, D., Cano, G. et al. (2013). α2 adrenergic receptor-mediated inhibition of thermogenesis. *J. Neurosci.* 33 (5): 2017–2028.

Mama, K.R., Grimsrud, K., Snell, T. et al. (2009). Plasma concentrations, behavioural and physiological effects following intravenous and intramuscular detomidine in horses. *Equine Vet. J.* 41 (8): 772–777.

Maugeri, S., Ferre, I.P., Intorre, L. et al. (1994). Effects of medetomidine on intestinal and colonic motility in the dog. *J. Vet. Pharmacol. Therap.* 17 (2): 148–154.

Menegaz, R.G., Kapusta, D.R., Mauad, H. et al. (2001). Activation of alpha(2)-receptors in the rostral ventrolateral medulla evokes natriuresis by a renal nerve mechanism. *Am. J. Physiol. Regul. Integr. Comp. Physiol.* 281 (1): R98–R107.

Merritt, A.M., Burrow, J.A., and Hartless, C.S. (1998). Effect of xylazine, detomidine, and a combination of xylazine and butorphanol on equine duodenal motility. *Am. J. Vet. Res.* 59 (5): 619–623.

Moore, R.M. and Trim, C.M. (1992). Effect of xylazine on cerebrospinal fluid pressure in conscious horses. *Am. J. Vet. Res.* 53 (9): 1558–1561.

Mortenson, J.A. and Robison, J.A. (2011). Tolazoline-induced apnea in mule deer (*Odocoileus hemionus*). *J. Zoo Wildl. Med.* 42 (1): 105–107.

Moura, E., Afonso, J., Hein, L. et al. (2006). Alpha2-adrenoceptor subtypes involved in the regulation of catecholamine release from the adrenal medulla of mice. *Br. J. Pharmacol.* 149 (8): 1049–1058.

Muge, D.K., Chambers, J.P., and Livingston, A. (1996). Single dose pharmacokinetics of medetomidine in sheep. *J. Vet. Pharmacol. Therap.* 19 (2): 109–112.

Muir, W.W. 3rd and Gadawski, J.E. (2002). Cardiovascular effects of a high dose of romifidine in propofol-anesthetized cats. *Am. J. Vet. Res.* 63 (9): 1241–1246.

Murahata, Y., Yamamoto, A., Miki, Y. et al. (2014). Antagonistic effects of atipamezole, yohimbine and prazosin on medetomidine-induced diuresis in healthy cats. *J. Vet. Med. Sci.* 76 (2): 173–182.

Nakamura, K., Hara, S., and Tomizawa, N. (1997). The effects of medetomidine and xylazine on gastrointestinal motility and gastrin release in the dog. *J. Vet. Pharmacol. Therap.* 20 (4): 290–295.

Nazarian, A., Christianson, C.A., Hua, X.Y. et al. (2008). Dexmedetomidine and ST-91 analgesia in the formalin model is mediated by alpha2A-adrenoceptors: a mechanism of action distinct from morphine. *Br. J. Pharmacol.* 155 (7): 1117–1126.

Nelson, L.E., Lu, J., Guo, T. et al. (2003). The alpha2-adrenoceptor agonist dexmedetomidine converges on an endogenous sleep-promoting pathway to exert its sedative effects. *Anesthesiology* 98 (2): 428–436.

Nyman, G., Marntell, S., Edner, A. et al. (2009). Effect of sedation with detomidine and butorphanol on pulmonary gas exchange in the horse. *Acta Vet. Scand.* 51: 22.

Paalzow, L.K. and Edlund, P.O. (1979). Pharmacokinetics of clonidine in the rat and cat. *J. Pharmacokinet. Biopharm.* 7 (5): 481–494.

Pagel, P.S., Proctor, L.T., Devcic, A. et al. (1998). A novel alpha 2-adrenoceptor antagonist attenuates the early, but preserves the late cardiovascular effects of intravenous dexmedetomidine in conscious dogs. *J. Cardiothorac. Vasc. Anesth.* 12 (4): 429–434.

Pascoe, P.J., Raekallio, M., Kuusela, E. et al. (2006). Changes in the minimum alveolar concentration of isoflurane and some cardiopulmonary measurements during three continuous infusion rates of dexmedetomidine in dogs. *Vet. Anaesth. Analg.* 33 (2): 97–103.

Pohl, V.H., Carregaro, A.B., Lopes, C. et al. (2012). Epidural anesthesia and postoperative analgesia with alpha-2 adrenergic agonists and lidocaine for ovariohysterectomy in bitches. *Can. J. Vet. Res.* 76 (3): 215–220.

Prado, M.E., Streeter, R.N., Mandsager, R.E. et al. (1999). Pharmacologic effects of epidural versus intramuscular administration of detomidine in cattle. *Am. J. Vet. Res.* 60 (10): 1242–1247.

Pypendop, B.H. and Ikiw, J.E. (2014). Pharmacokinetics of dexmedetomidine after intravenous administration of a bolus to cats. *Am. J. Vet. Res.* 75 (5): 441–445.

Pypendop, B.H. and Verstegen, J.P. (1998). Hemodynamic effects of medetomidine in the dog: a dose titration study. *Vet. Surg.* 27 (6): 612–622.

Pypendop, B.H. and Verstegen, J.P. (2001). Cardiovascular effects of romifidine in dogs. *Am. J. Vet. Res.* 62 (4): 490–495.

Pypendop, B.H., Barter, L.S., Stanley, S.D. et al. (2011). Hemodynamic effects of dexmedetomidine in isoflurane-anesthetized cats. *Vet. Anaesth. Analg.* 38 (6): 555–567.

Ranheim, B., Horsberg, T.E., Nymoen, U. et al. (1997). Reversal of medetomidine-induced sedation in reindeer (*Rangifer tarandus tarandus*) with atipamezole increases the medetomidine concentration in plasma. *J. Vet. Pharmacol. Therap.* 20 (5): 350–354.

Ranheim, B., Søli, N.E., and Ryeng, K.A. (1998). Pharmacokinetics of medetomidine and atipamezole in dairy calves: an agonist-antagonist interaction. *J. Vet. Pharmacol. Therap.* 21 (6): 428–432.

Ranheim, B., Arnemo, J.M., Ryeng, K.A. et al. (1999). A pharmacokinetic study including some relevant clinical effect of medetomidine and atipamezole in lactating dairy cows. *J. Vet. Pharmacol. Therap.* 22 (6): 368–373.

Ranheim, B., Arnemo, J.M., Stuen, S. et al. (2000). Medetomidine and atipamezole in sheep: disposition and clinical effects. *J. Vet. Pharmacol. Therap.* 23 (6): 401–404.

Ranheim, B., Risberg, Å.I., Spadavecchia, C. et al. (2015). The pharmacokinetics of dexmedetomidine administered as a constant rate infusion in horses. *J. Vet. Pharmacol. Therap.* 38 (1): 93–96.

Read, M.R., Duke, T., and Toews, A.R. (2000). Suspected tolazoline toxicosis in a llama. *J. Am. Vet. Med. Assoc.* 216 (2): 227–229.

Restitutti, F., Raekallio, M., Vainionpää, M. et al. (2012). Plasma glucose, insulin, free fatty acids, lactate and cortisol concentrations in dexmedetomidine-sedated dogs with or without MK-467: a peripheral α-2 adrenoceptor antagonist. *Vet. J.* 193 (2): 481–485.

Rezende, M.L., Grimsrud, K.N., Stanley, S.D. et al. (2015). Pharmacokinetics and pharmacodynamics of intravenous dexmedetomidine in the horse. *J. Vet. Pharmacol. Therap.* 38 (1): 15–23.

Ringer, S.K., Schwarzwald, C.C., Portier, K.G. et al. (2013). Effects on cardiopulmonary function and oxygen delivery of doses of romifidine and xylazine followed by constant rate infusions in standing horses. *Vet. J.* 195 (2): 228–234.

Rioja, E., Santos, M., Martínez Taboada, F. et al. (2006). Cardiorespiratory and minimum alveolar concentration sparing effects of a continuous intravenous infusion of dexmedetomidine in halothane or isoflurane-anaesthetized rats. *Lab. Anim.* 40 (1): 9–15.

Rioja, E., Kerr, C.L., Enouri, S.S. et al. (2008). Sedative and cardiopulmonary effects of medetomidine hydrochloride and xylazine hydrochloride and their reversal with atipamezole hydrochloride in calves. *Am. J. Vet. Res.* 69 (3): 319–329.

Rizk, A., Herdtweck, S., Meyer, H. et al. (2012). Effects of xylazine hydrochloride on hormonal, metabolic, and cardiorespiratory stress responses to lateral recumbency and claw trimming in dairy cows. *J. Am. Vet. Med. Assoc.* 240 (10): 1223–1230.

Sahin, T., Begeç, Z., Toprak, H.İ. et al. (2013). The effects of dexmedetomidine on liver ischemia-reperfusion injury in rats. *J. Surg. Res.* 183 (1): 385–390.

Sakamoto, H., Misumi, K., Nakama, M. et al. (1996). The effects of xylazine on intrauterine pressure, uterine blood flow, maternal and fetal cardiovascular and pulmonary function in pregnant goats. *J. Vet. Med. Sci.* 58 (3): 211–217.

Saleh, N., Aoki, M., Shimada, T. et al. (2005). Renal effects of medetomidine in isoflurane-anesthetized dogs with special reference to its diuretic action. *J. Vet. Med. Sci.* 67 (5): 461–465.

Salonen, J.S. (1989). Pharmacokinetics of medetomidine. *Acta Vet. Scand.* 85: 49–54.

Salonen, J.S. (1991). Tissue-specificity of hydroxylation and N-methylation of arylalkylimidazoles. *Pharmacol. Toxicol.* 69 (1): 1–4.

Salonen, J.S. and Suolinna, E.M. (1988). Metabolism of detomidine in the rat. I. Comparison of 3H-labelled metabolites formed in vitro and in vivo. *Eur. J. Drug Metab. Pharmacokinet.* 13 (1): 53–58.

Salonen, J.S., Vähä-Vahe, T., Vainio, O. et al. (1989). Single-dose pharmacokinetics of detomidine in the horse and cow. *J. Vet. Pharmacol. Therap.* 12 (1): 65–72.

Salonen, S., Vuorilehto, L., Vainio, O. et al. (1995). Atipamezole increases medetomidine clearance in the dog: an agonist-antagonist interaction. *J. Vet. Pharmacol. Therap.* 18 (5): 328–332.

Santonastaso, A., Hardy, J., Cohen, N. et al. (2014),). Pharmacokinetics and pharmacodynamics of xylazine administered by the intravenous or intra-osseous route in adult horses. *J. Vet. Pharmacol. Therap.* 37 (6): 565–570.

Sarazan, R.D., Starke, W.A., Krause, G.F. et al. (1989). Cardiovascular effects of detomidine, a new alpha 2-adrenoceptor agonist, in the conscious pony. *J. Vet. Pharmacol. Therap.* 12 (4): 378–388.

Schatzmann, U., Jossfck, H., Stauffer, J.L. et al. (1994). Effects of alpha 2-agonists on intrauterine pressure and sedation in horses: comparison between detomidine, romifidine and xylazine. *Zentralblatt für Veterinärmedizin* 41 (7): 523–529.

Schauvliege, S., Marcilla, M.G., Verryken, K. et al. (2011),). Effects of a constant rate infusion of detomidine on cardiovascular function, isoflurane requirements and recovery quality in horses. *Vet. Anaesth. Analg.* 38 (6): 544–554.

Scheibner, J., Trendelenburg, A.U., Hein, L. et al. (2001). Alpha2-adrenoceptors modulating neuronal serotonin release: a study in alpha2-adrenoceptor subtype-deficient mice. *Br. J. Pharmacol.* 32 (4): 925–933.

Scheibner, J., Trendelenburg, A.U., Hein, L. et al. (2002). Alpha 2-adrenoceptors in the enteric nervous system: a study in alpha 2A-adrenoceptor-deficient mice. *Br. J. Pharmacol.* 35 (3): 697–704.

Schmeling, W.T., Kampine, J.P., Roerig, D.L. et al. (1991). The effects of the stereoisomers of the alpha 2-adrenergic agonist medetomidine on systemic and coronary hemodynamics in conscious dogs. *Anesthesiology* 75 (3): 499–511.

Schmeling, W.T., Ganjoo, P., Staunton, M. et al. (1999). Pretreatment with dexmedetomidine: altered indices of anesthetic depth for halothane in the neuraxis of cats. *Anesth. Analg.* 88 (3): 625–632.

Schuster, D.J., Kitto, K.F., Overland, A.C. et al. (2013). Protein kinase Cε is required for spinal analgesic synergy between delta opioid and alpha-2A adrenergic receptor agonist pairs. *J. Neurosci.* 33 (33): 13538–13546.

Schwartz, D.D. and Clark, T.P. (1998). Selectivity of atipamezole, yohimbine, and tolazoline for alpha-2 adrenergic receptor subtypes: implications for clinical reversal of alpha 2 adrenergic receptor mediated sedation in sheep. *J. Vet. Pharmacol. Therap.* 21 (5): 342–347.

Scofield, D.B., Alexander, D.L., Franklin, R.P. et al. (2010). Review of fatalities and adverse reactions after administration of α-2 adrenergic agonist reversal agents in the horse. *Proceedings of the 56th American Association of Equine Practitioners*, Baltimore, USA (8 December 2010). American Association of Equine Practitioners.

Segal, I.S., Vickery, R.G., Walton, J.K. et al. (1988). Dexmedetomidine diminishes halothane anesthetic requirements in rats through a postsynaptic alpha 2 adrenergic receptor. *Anesthesiology* 69 (6): 818–823.

Sinclair, M.D. (2003). A review of the physiological effects of alpha2-agonists related to the clinical use of medetomidine in small animal practice. *Can. Vet. J.* 44 (11): 885–897.

Soares, J.H., Ascoli, F.O., Gremiao, I.D. et al. (2004). Isoflurane sparing action of epidurally administered xylazine hydrochloride in anesthetized dogs. *Am. J. Vet. Res.* 65 (6): 854–859.

Stähle, H. (2000). A historical perspective: development of clonidine. *Best Pract. Res. Clin. Anesth.* 14 (2): 237–246.

Steffey, E.P. and Pascoe, P.J. (2002). Detomidine reduces isoflurane anesthetic requirement (MAC) in horses. *Vet. Anaesth. Analg.* 29 (4): 223–227.

Steffey, E.P., Pascoe, P.J., Woliner, M.J. et al. (2000). Effects of xylazine hydrochloride during isoflurane-induced anesthesia in horses. *Am. J. Vet. Res.* 61 (10): 1225–1231.

Still, J., Serteyn, D., and van der Merwe, C.A. (1996). Cardiovascular and respiratory effects of detomidine in isoflurane-anaesthetised horses. *J. S. Afr. Vet. Assoc.* 67 (4): 199–203.

Stine, J.M., Michau, T.M., Williams, M.K. et al. (2014). The effects of intravenous romifidine on intraocular pressure in clinically normal horses and horses with incidental ophthalmic findings. *Vet. Ophthalmol.* 17 (s1): 134–139.

Stone, L.S., Broberger, C., Vulchanova, L. et al. (1998). Differential distribution of alpha2A and alpha2C adrenergic receptor immunoreactivity in the rat spinal cord. *J. Neurosci.* 18 (15): 5928–5937.

Strombeck, D.R. and Harrold, D. (1985). Effects of atropine, acepromazine, meperidine, and xylazine on gastroesophageal sphincter pressure in the dog. *Am. J. Vet. Res.* 46 (4): 963–965.

Szreder, Z. (1997). Do cardiovascular mechanisms participate in thermoregulatory activity of alpha 2-adrenoceptor agonists and antagonists in rabbits? *Ann. N. Y. Acad. Sci.* 813: 512–525.

Talke, P.O., Traber, D.L., Richardson, C.A. et al. (2000). The effect of alpha(2) agonist-induced sedation and its reversal with an alpha(2) antagonist on organ blood flow in sheep. *Anesth. Analg.* 90 (5): 1060–1066.

Talukder, M.H., Hikasa, Y., Takahashi, H. et al. (2009). Antagonistic effects of atipamezole and yohimbine on medetomidine-induced diuresis in healthy dogs. *Can. J. Vet. Res.* 73 (4): 260–270.

Tam, S.W., Worcel, M., and Wyllie, M. (2001). Yohimbine: a clinical review. *Pharmacol. Therap.* 91 (3): 215–243.

Tapio, H.A., Raekallio, M.R., Mykkänen, A.K. et al. (2019). Effects of vatinoxan on cardiorespiratory function, fecal output and plasma drug concentrations in horses anesthetized with isoflurane and infusion of medetomidine. *Vet. J.* 251: 105345.

Taylor, P.M., Bennett, R.C., Brearley, J.C. et al. (2001). Comparison of detomidine and romifidine as premedicants before ketamine and halothane anesthesia in horses undergoing elective surgery. *Am. J. Vet. Res.* 62 (3): 359–363.

Tendillo, F.J., Mascías, A., Santos, M. et al. (1996). Cardiopulmonary and analgesic effects of xylazine, detomidine, medetomidine, and the antagonist atipamezole in isoflurane-anesthetized swine. *Lab. Anim. Sci.* 46 (2): 215–219.

Tisotti, T., Valverde, A., Hopkins, A. et al. (2021). Use of intravenous lidocaine to treat dexmedetomidine-induced bradycardia in sedated and anesthetized dogs. *Vet. Anaesth. Analg.* 48 (2): 174–186.

Tiwari, S.K., Kumar, A., and Vainio, O. (1998). Reversal of sedative and clinicophysiological effects of epidural xylazine and detomidine with atipamezole and yohimbine in buffaloes (*Bubalus bubalis*). *Vet. Rec.* 143 (19): 529–532.

Tomasic, M., Mann, L.S., and Soma, L.R. (1997). Effects of sedation, anesthesia, and endotracheal intubation on respiratory mechanics in adult horses. *Am. J. Vet. Res.* 58 (6): 641–646.

Törneke, K., Bergström, U., and Neil, A. (2003). Interactions of xylazine and detomidine with alpha2-adrenoceptors in brain tissue from cattle, swine and rats. *J. Vet. Pharmacol. Therap.* 26 (3): 205–211.

Tranquilli, W.J., Thurmon, J.C., Corbin, J.E. et al. (1984). Halothane-sparing effect of xylazine in dogs and subsequent reversal with tolazoline. *J. Vet. Pharmacol. Therap.* 7 (1): 23–28.

Ueki, M., Kawasaki, T., Habe, K. et al. (2014). The effects of dexmedetomidine on inflammatory mediators after cardiopulmonary bypass. *Anaesthesia* 69 (7): 693–700.

Vainio, O.M. and Bloor, B.C. (1994). Relation between body temperature and dexmedetomidine-induced minimum alveolar concentration and respiratory changes in isoflurane-anesthetized miniature swine. *Am. J. Vet. Res.* 55 (7): 1000–1006.

Vainionpää, M., Salla, K., Restitutti, F. et al. (2013a). Thermographic imaging of superficial temperature in dogs sedated with medetomidine and butorphanol with and without MK-467 (L-659′066). *Vet. Anaesth. Analg.* 40 (2): 142–148.

Vainionpää, M.H., Raekallio, M.R., Pakkanen, S.A. et al. (2013b). Plasma drug concentrations and clinical effects of a peripheral alpha-2-adrenoceptor antagonist, MK-467, in horses sedated with detomidine. *Vet. Anaesth. Analg.* 40 (3): 257–264.

Van Zweiten, P.A. (1980). Pharmacology of centrally acting hypotensive drugs. *Br. J. Pharmacol.* 10 (S1): 13s–20s.

Vartiainen, J., MacDonald, E., Urtti, A. et al. (1992). Dexmedetomidine-induced ocular hypotension in rabbits with normal or elevated intraocular pressures. *Investigative Ophthalmology & Visual Science* 33 (6): 2019–2023.

Virtanen, R., Savola, J.M., and Saano, V. (1989). Highly selective and specific antagonism of central and peripheral alpha 2-adrenoceptors by atipamezole. *Arch. Int. Pharmacodyn. Thér.* 297: 190–204.

Wagner, A.E., Muir, W.W. 3rd, and Hinchcliff, K.W. (1991). Cardiovascular effects of xylazine and detomidine in horses. *Am. J. Vet. Res.* 52 (5): 651–657.

Wojtasiak-Wypart, M., Soma, L.R., Rudy, J.A. et al. (2012). Pharmacokinetic profile and pharmacodynamic effects of romifidine hydrochloride in the horse. *J. Vet. Pharmacol. Therap.* 35 (5): 478–488.

Woodhouse, K.J., Brosnan, R.J., Nguyen, K.Q. et al. (2013). Effects of postanesthetic sedation with romifidine or xylazine on quality of recovery from isoflurane anesthesia in horses. *J. Am. Vet. Med. Assoc.* 242 (4): 533–539.

Wright, M., Heath, R.B., and Wingfield, W.E. (1987). Effects of xylazine and ketamine on epinephrine-induced arrhythmia in the dog. *Vet. Surg.* 16 (5): 398–403.

Wu, Y., Liu, Y., Huang, H. et al. (2013). Dexmedetomidine inhibits inflammatory reaction in lung tissues of septic rats by suppressing TLR4/NF-κB pathway. *Mediators Inflamm.* 2013: 562154.

Xu, B., Zhang, W.S., Yang, J.L. et al. (2010). Evidence for suppression of spinal glial activation by dexmedetomidine in a rat model of monoarthritis. *Clin. Exp. Pharmacol. Physiol.* 37 (10): e158–e166.

Yamashita, K., Tsubakishita, S., Futaok, S. et al. (2000). Cardiovascular effects of medetomidine, detomidine and xylazine in horses. *J. Vet. Med. Sci.* 62 (10): 1025–1032.

Zádori, Z.S., Shujaa, N., Brancati, S.B. et al. (2011). Both α2B- and α2C-adrenoceptor subtypes are involved in the mediation of centrally induced gastroprotection in mice. *Eur. J. Pharmacol.* 669 (1–3): 115–120.

Zhang, Z., Ferretti, V., Güntan, İ. et al. (2015). Neuronal ensembles sufficient for recovery sleep and the sedative actions of α2 adrenergic agonists. *Nat. Neurosci.* 18 (4): 553–561.

Zornow, M.H., Fleischer, J.E., Scheller, M.S. et al. (1990). Dexmedetomidine, an alpha 2-adrenergic agonist, decreases cerebral blood flow in the isoflurane-anesthetized dog. *Anesth. Analg.* 70 (6): 624–630.

Zullian, C., Menozzi, A., Pozzoli, C. et al. (2011). Effects of α2-adrenergic drugs on small intestinal motility in the horse: an in vitro study. *Vet. J.* 187 (3): 342–346.

5

Phenothiazines and Butyrophenones

John A.E. Hubbell

Phenothiazine and butyrophenone drugs have been used to produce apparent calming, tranquilization, or sedation in a wide variety of animals, including humans. Historically, both phenothiazines and butyrophenones have been classified as "major tranquilizers" because they have been used to treat "major" incidents of psychoses in humans. This is in contrast to the term, "minor tranquilizer" which refers to drugs used as anxiolytic drugs in humans. Such descriptions are antiquated and should be removed from the veterinary lexicon.

Phenothiazine drugs were initially used in veterinary medicine as antihistamines. Acepromazine is currently the most commonly used drug but the use of chlorpromazine, fluphenazine, promazine, and triflupromazine have been reported in the literature. Butyrophenone drugs are less commonly used with no drug currently marketed for animals in the United States. Previously marketed drugs include droperidol (as a component of Innovar-Vet), lenperone, and azaperone, a drug initially marketed for control of aggression in swine. Azaperone and haloperidol can be obtained from compounding pharmacies.

Mechanism of Action

The central nervous system (CNS) (neuroleptic) effects of phenothiazines and butyrophenones are thought to be mediated via inhibition of the activity of dopamine at the level of subcortical structures including the basal ganglia and limbic system. Specific receptors have not been identified, thus, no specific antagonists have been developed. In addition to the neuroleptic actions, phenothiazines produce α_1-adrenoreceptor blockade and have varying degrees of antihistaminic, anticholinergic, and antispasmodic activity. Butyrophenones have α_1-adrenoreceptor blocking effects and prevent the development of malignant hyperthermia in susceptible pigs.

Pharmacokinetics of Acepromazine in Major Species (Awake and Under Anesthesia)

Dogs

Acepromazine: Sedation after oral dosing lasts approximately four hours. The $t_{1/2}\,\alpha$ after IV administration in the dog is 54 minutes and the $t_{1/2}\,\beta$ is 7.1 hours (Hashem et al. 1992). After oral administration, the $t_{1/2}\,\alpha$ is 2.5 hours with a $t_{1/2}\,\beta$ of 15.9 hours. The volume of distribution is 18.3 l/kg with a bioavailability of 20% after oral administration. Total clearance is 2.9 l/kg/hr.

Horses

There are varied estimations of pharmacokinetic values for acepromazine in horses. The pharmacokinetics of acepromazine are usually described in a two-compartment model with values for $t_{1/2}\,\alpha$ ranging from less than three minutes (Ballard et al. 1982) to six minutes (Schneiders et al. 2012) and values for $t_{1/2}\,\beta$ ranging from 2 (Hashem and Keller 1993; Schneiders et al. 2012) to 3.5 hours (Ballard et al. 1982). Acepromazine is relatively highly protein bound with over 50% bound to erythrocytes (Ballard et al. 1982). The V_D is estimated at 1.3 (Schneiders et al. 2012) to 6.6 l/kg (Ballard et al. 1982) and clearance is estimated at 4.6 (Schneiders et al. 2012) to 24 l/kg/hr (Ballard et al. 1982). 2-(1-hydroxyethyl) promazine sulphoxide is a primary metabolite with a $t_{1/2}\,\beta$ of 1.98 hours, a clearance of 1.34 l/kg/hr and a V_D of 2.3 l/kg (Schneiders et al. 2012). The pharmacokinetics of oral acepromazine are described by a two-compartment open model with first-order absorption. Oral bioavailability has been estimated at 55% (Hashem and Keller 1993).

Metabolism

Acepromazine is metabolized by the liver in the horse and excreted via the kidneys in two-conjugated and one-unconjugated form (Dewey et al. 1981). Data from other species are not available. Azaperone is rapidly absorbed after intramuscular (IM) administration. Azaperone is oxidized by the liver resulting in at least three metabolites which are rapidly excreted via the kidneys (Porter and Slusser 1984).

Clinical Use

Dogs and Cats

Acepromazine produces reliable tranquilization when administered IM or subcutaneously to socialized dogs and cats. Oral administration produces less reliable results. Animals appear calm and resistance to handling is reduced. Peak action is enhanced if the animals are placed in a quiet environment for 15–20 minutes after drug administration. Unsocialized or aggressive dogs and cats do not uniformly become tractable after acepromazine administration. Sedation and tranquilization from acepromazine is enhanced by coadministration with a number of opioids and α_2-adrenoreceptor agonists, which also provide analgesia (Muir 2013). Acepromazine is anti-emetic but reduces lower esophageal sphincter tone so regurgitation may be facilitated. Acepromazine should be avoided in animals in shock due to any cause due to the vasodilatory effects of acepromazine. Although there is conflicting evidence about its effects on platelets and the clotting cascade, acepromazine should be avoided in patients with bleeding disorders, particularly those that are hypotensive (Muir and Hubbell 1985; Barr et al. 1992; Connor et al. 2012). The administration of acepromazine to patients with intracranial disease should be avoided because it limits the ability to reduce intracranial pressure via hyperventilation.

Butyrophenone tranquilizers have not gained sufficient popularity to sustain the economics of production and distribution. A combination of droperidol and fentanyl (Innovar-Vet) was marketed for IM use in the dog (Buckhold et al. 1977). Administration of the combination was associated with profound sedation, bradycardia, and self-limiting watery diarrhea. Droperidol-fentanyl administration to cats was associated with increased tractability but not profound sedation (Grandy and Heath 1987). Apparent central nervous system (CNS) excitation has been reported after administration of the combination to cats (Yelnosky and Field 1964). Lenperone was marketed for use in dogs, cats, and swine (Cloyd and Gilbert 1973). Hypotension after lenperone is less marked than after acepromazine (Muir and Hubbell 1985) but the drug was not used widely.

Horses

A number of phenothiazine tranquilizers have been investigated in the horse. Chlorpromazine produced inconsistent effects ranging from no appreciable effect to recumbency

with some horses evidencing hypersensitivity (Martin and Beck 1956; Owen and Neal 1957). Promazine produced satisfactory sedation in 72% of horses when administered IV (Gorman 1959). Acepromazine causes sedation and reduces motor activity while minimally affecting coordination when administered to horses (Ballard et al. 1982). The onset of action after parenteral administration occurs within 15–30 minutes but peak effects may not be seen for up to 45 minutes. The duration of sedation depends on the dose administered but frequently lasts for 6–10 hours. Acepromazine does not produce analgesia but may make analgesic drugs more effective. In general, acepromazine administration will not make an aggressive horse a malleable patient but it will reduce the horse's reaction to stimuli. Increasing the dose of acepromazine does not usually produce a greater effect but the duration of action is prolonged. Acepromazine can be used to reduce awareness as an aid to breaking and training or prior to transportation. The best index of the degree of sedation with acepromazine is the presence of protrusion of the penis in male horses. In addition, the eyelids will droop and the third eyelid will protrude. The degree and duration of penile protrusion is thought to be dose dependent. The incidence of persistent penile protrusion (also referred to as penile paralysis, paraphimosis, priapism, erection and penile prolapse) is unknown but is frequent enough for some to suggest that the use of acepromazine in breeding stallions is contraindicated (Pauwels et al. 2005). Sedation with acepromazine does not appear to be accompanied by somatic analgesia although it has been stated that it can potentiate the effects of other analgesics (Love et al. 2012).

Butyrophenones are not suitable for sedation in the horse. Initial investigations of the use of azaperone as a sedative in ponies and horses showed promise but later investigations reported paradoxical excitement following intravenous (IV) administration (Dodman and Waterman 1979). Sedation was judged as good to excellent in ponies given azaperone with an onset of action within 10 minutes and a duration of action of two to six hours (Serrano and Lees 1976). Body temperature and arterial blood pressures were reduced. A mild tachycardia was noted. In a study in horses, azaperone reduced packed cell volume 5–10% and mean arterial blood pressure for at least four hours (Lees and Serrano 1976). Azaperone in combination with metomidate was investigated as a method to produce short-term anesthesia in the horse. While most horses recovered from anesthesia free from excitement, a significant number evidenced excitement and one horse was hyperexcitable (Hillidge et al. 1973). Another group of investigators noted muscle tremors and seizure-like activity in horses administered metomidate (hypnodil) and azaperone sedation (Roztocil et al. 1972).

Pigs

Azaperone is an effective tranquilizer in swine and reduces the incidence of malignant hyperthermia in stress susceptible patients. Peak sedation after IM azaperone administration occurs with 15 minutes in young pigs with a duration of action of one to two hours. Both droperidol (another butyrophenone) and acepromazine prevent or delay the induction of malignant hyperthermia but acepromazine does not consistently produce useful sedation (McGrath et al. 1981).

Ruminants

Azaperone increased distance traveled, urination, and time spent walking when administered to sheep (Hughes et al. 1977). Grazing behavior and investigatory activities increased and vocalization decreased. Acepromazine administered in similar circumstances only decreased vocalization.

Effect in Patients Under General Anesthesia

Acepromazine reduces the anesthetic requirement of halothane and isoflurane in the dog (Heard et al. 1986; Webb and O'Brien 1988). Acepromazine decreases arterial blood pressure in a dose-dependent manner when administered to halothane-anesthetized dogs because of α-adrenergic antagonism that can be partially reversed by infusing phenylephrine (Ludders et al. 1983).

Effects on Organ Systems

Cardiovascular System

The cardiovascular effects of lenperone have been assessed in dogs. Lenperone administered in combination with glycopyrrolate induced decreases in systemic vascular resistance, mean arterial blood pressure and rate-pressure product and increased cardiac index (Benson et al. 1987). The hypotension associated with lenperone administration can be offset by infusing phenylephrine indicating $α_1$-adrenergic blockade as a contributing mechanism (Muir and Hubbell 1985).

Promazine and acepromazine reduce packed cell volume and plasma protein concentration in a number of species in part due to induced sequestration of erythrocytes in the spleen (De Moor et al. 1978; Robertson et al. 2001). Phenothiazines have antiarrhythmic activity with regard to ventricular arrhythmias via reduction in sympathetic tone and potentially, myocardial depression (Sato and Tanabe 1962; Dyson and Pettifer 1997). Horses given acepromazine IV had decreased mean aortic pressures and decreased central venous pressures within 15 minutes of administration (Muir et al. 1979). Arterial blood pressures, stroke volume, and left ventricular work decreased in dogs given acepromazine IV (Popovic et al. 1972; Farver et al. 1986).

Respiratory System

Acepromazine given IV reduces respiratory rate in cattle accompanied by a transient small decrease in the arterial partial pressure of oxygen and no change in the arterial partial pressure of carbon dioxide (Hodgson et al. 2002). Horses given acepromazine IV experienced decreased respiratory rates but arterial blood gases were not altered. Breathing rate, minute ventilation, and oxygen consumption decreased after acepromazine administration to dogs but arterial blood gas values were not changed (Popovic et al. 1979; Farver et al. 1986).

Central Nervous System

Acepromazine produces sedation within 10 minutes of IM administration in dogs with effects lasting four to six hours (Hofmeister et al. 2010). Controversy exists with regard to the effects of acepromazine on the seizure threshold. Many texts caution against the use of phenothiazine tranquilizers, particularly acepromazine, in dogs with a seizure history, although the recommendations are generally extrapolated from evidence acquired with the use of another phenothiazine; chlorpromazine in humans (Baldessarini 1985). The risk has not been verified with retrospective studies suggesting that there is either no effect or potentially, antiepileptic effects (Tobias et al. 2006; McConnell et al. 2007). Aggression is reported as a rare, idiosyncratic reaction to acepromazine administration in dogs (Meyer 1997).

Renal System

Renal blood flow and glomerular filtration rate remained high despite deceases in mean arterial blood pressure when acepromazine was administered to anesthetized dogs (Bostrom et al. 2003). Urine output in anesthetized dogs premedicated with acepromazine averaged 1.8 ml/kg/hr (Robertson et al. 2001).

Other Effects

Acepromazine causes penile protrusion in the horse and cow and has been associated with persistent protrusion requiring treatment. A variety of pharmacologic and surgical approaches have been attempted (Wilson et al. 1991).

Acepromazine and droperidol (as a component of fentanyl-droperidol) reduce gastroesophageal sphincter pressure in dogs (Hall et al. 1987). Prior administration of acepromazine reduces the incidence of vomiting associated with opioid administration in dogs (Valverde et al. 2004).

Acepromazine is reported to transiently reduce adenosine diphosphate-induced platelet aggregation in dogs but the same effect was not seen when assessed using thromboelastography (Barr et al. 1992; Connor et al. 2012).

References

Baldessarini, R.J. (1985). Drugs and the treatment of psychiatric disorders. In: *Goodman and Gilman's The Pharmacologic Basis of Therapeutics*, 7e (ed. A.G. Gilman, L.S. Goodman, T.W. Rail, et al.), 387–445. New York: Macmillan Publishing.

Ballard, S., Shults, T., Kownacki, A.A. et al. (1982). The pharmacokinetics, pharmacological responses and behavioral effects in the horse. *J. Vet. Pharmacol. Therap.* 5: 21–31.

Barr, S.C., Ludders, J.W., Looney, A.L. et al. (1992). Platelet aggregation in dogs after sedation with acepromazine and atropine and during subsequent general anesthesia and surgery. *Am. J. Vet. Res.* 53: 2067–2070.

Benson, G.J., Thurmon, J.C., Tranquilli, W.J. et al. (1987). Intravenous administration of lenperone and glycopyrrolate followed by continuous infusion of sufentanil in dogs. *Am. J. Vet. Res.* 48: 1372–1375.

Bostrom, I., Nyman, G., Kampa, N. et al. (2003). Effects of acepromazine on renal function in anesthetized dogs. *Am. J. Vet. Res.* 64: 590–598.

Buckhold, D.K., Erickson, H.H., and Lumb, W.V. (1977). Cardiovascular response to fentanyl-droperidol and atropine in the dog. *Am. J. Vet. Res.* 38: 479–482.

Cloyd, G.D. and Gilbert, D.L. (1973). Dose calibration studies of lenperone, a new tranquilizer for dogs, cats, and swine. *Vet. Med. Small Anim. Clin.* 68: 344–348.

Connor, B.J., Hanel, R.M., Hansen, B.D. et al. (2012). Effects of acepromazine maleate on platelet function assessed by use of adenosine disphosphate activated and arachidonic acid-activated modified thromboelastography in healthy dogs. *Am. J. Vet. Res.* 73: 595–601.

De Moor, A., Desmet, P., Van Den Hende, C., and Moens, Y. (1978). Influence of promazine on the venous haematocrit and plasma protein concentration in the horse. *Zbl. Vet. Med.* 25: 189–197.

Dewey, E.A., Maylin, G.A., Ebel, J.G., and Henlon, J.D. (1981). The metabolism of promazine and acetylpromazine in the horse. *Drug Metab. Dispos.* 9: 30–36.

Dodman, N.H. and Waterman, A.E. (1979). Paradoxical excitement following the intravenous administration of azaperone in the horse. *Equine Vet. J.* 11: 33–35.

Dyson, D.H. and Pettifer, G.R. (1997). Evaluation of the arrhythmogenicity of a low dose of acepromazine: comparison with xylazine. *Can. J. Vet. Res.* 61: 241–245.

Farver, T.B., Haskins, S.C., and Parz, J.D. (1986). Cardiopulmonary effects of acepromazine and the subsequent administration of ketamine in the dog. *Am. J. Vet. Res.* 47: 631–641.

Gorman, T.N. (1959). Promazine hydrochloride in equine practice. *J. Am. Vet. Med. Assoc.* 134: 464–466.

Grandy, J.L. and Heath, R.B. (1987). Cardiopulmonary and behavioral effects of fentanyl-droperidol in cats. *J. Am. Vet. Med. Assoc.* 191: 59–61.

Hall, J.A., Magne, M.L., and Twedt, D.C. (1987). Effect of acepromazine, diazepam, fentanyl-droperidol, and oxymorphone on gastroesophageal sphincter pressure in health dogs. *Am. J. Vet. Res.* 48: 556–557.

Hashem, A., Kietzmann, M., and Scherkl, R. (1992). The pharmacokinetics and bioavailability of acepromazine in the plasma of dogs. *Dtsch. Tierarztl. Wocehenschr.* 99: 396–398.

Hashem, A. and Keller H. (1993). Disposition, bioavailability and clinical efficacy of orally administered acepromazine in the horse. *J. Vet. Pharmacol. Therap.* 16: 359–368.

Heard, D.J., Webb, A.I., and Daniels, R.T. (1986). Effect of acepromazine on the anesthetic requirement of halothane in the dog. *Am. J. Vet. Res.* 47: 2113–2115.

Hillidge, C.J., Lees, P., and Serrano, L. (1973). Investigations of azaperone/metomidate anaesthesia in the horse. *Vet. Rec.* 93: 307–311.

Hodgson, D.S., Dunlop, C.I., Chapman, P.L., and Smith, J.A. (2002). Cardiopulmonary effects of xylazine and acepromazine in pregnant cows in late gestation. *Am. J. Vet. Res.* 63: 1695–1699.

Hofmeister, E.H., Chandler, M.J., and Read, M.R. (2010). Effects of acepromazine, hydromorphone, or an acepromazine-hydromorphone combination on the degree of sedation in clinically normal dogs. *J. Am. Vet. Med. Assoc.* 237: 1155–1159.

Hughes, R.N., Syme, L.A., and Syme, G.J. (1977). Open-field behavior in sheep following treatment with the neuroleptics azaperone and acetylpromazine. *Psychopharmacology* 52: 107–109.

Lees, P. and Serrano, L. (1976). Effects of azaperone on cardiovascular and respiratory functions in the horse. *Br. J. Pharmacol.* 56: 263–269.

Love, E.J., Taylor, P.M., Murrell, J., and Whay, H.R. (2012). Effects of acepromazine, butorphanol and buprenorphine on thermal and mechanical nociceptive thresholds in horses. *Equine Vet. J.* 44: 221–225.

Ludders, J.W., Reitan, J.A., Martucci, R. et al. (1983). Blood pressure response to phenylephrine infusion in halothane-anesthetized dogs given acetylpromazine maleate. *Am. J. Vet. Res.* 44: 996–999.

Martin, J.E. and Beck, J.D. (1956). Some effects of chlorpromazine hydrochloride in horses. *Am. J. Vet. Res.* 17: 678–686.

McConnell, J., Kirby, R., and Rudloff, E. (2007). Administration of acepromazine maleate to 31 dogs with a history of seizures. *J. Vet. Emerg. Crit. Care* 17: 262–267.

McGrath, C.J., Rempel, W.E., Addis, P.B., and Crimi, A.J. (1981). Acepromazine and droperidol inhibition of halothane-induced malignant hyperthermia (porcine stress syndrome) in swine. *Am. J. Vet. Res.* 42: 195–198.

Meyer, E.K. (1997). Rare, idiosyncratic reaction to acepromazine in dogs. *J. Am. Med. Assoc.* 210: 1114–1115.

Muir, W.W. (2013). Preanesthetic and perioperative medications. In: *Handbook of Veterinary Anesthesia*, 5e (ed. W.W. Muir and J.A.E. Hubbell), 22–57. St. Louis: Elsevier.

Muir, W.W. and Hubbell, J.A.E. (1985). Blood pressure response to acetylpromazine and lenperone in halothane anesthetized dogs. *J. Am. Anim. Hosp. Assoc.* 21: 285–289.

Muir, W.W., Skarda, R.T., and Sheehan, W. (1979). Hemodynamic and respiratory effects of a xylazine-acetylpromazine drug combination in horses. *Am. J. Vet. Res.* 40: 1518–1522.

Owen, L.N. and Neal, P.A. (1957). Sedation with chlorpromazine in the horse. *Vet. Rec.* 70: 413–417.

Pauwels, F., Schumacher, J., and Varner, D. (2005). Priapism in horses. *Compend. Contin. Educ. Pract. Vet.* 27 (4): 311–315.

Popovic, N.A., Mullane, J.F., and Yhap, E.O. (1972). Effects of acetylpromazine maleate on certain cardiorespiratory responses in dogs. *Am. J. Vet. Res.* 33 (9): 1819–1824.

Porter, D.B. and Slusser, C.A. (1984). Stresnil (Azaperone), a new neuroleptic for swine. Presented at the Annual Meeting of the American Association of Swine Practitioners, Kansas City, USA.

Robertson, S.A., Hauptman, J.G., Nachreiner, R.F., and Richter, M.A. (2001). Effects of acetylpromazine or morphine on urine production in halothane-anesthetized dogs. *Am. J. Vet. Res.* 62: 1922–1927.

Roztocil, V., Nemecek, L., Pavlica, J. et al. (1972). Effects of the combination of stressnil and hypnodil in the horse. *Acta Vet. Brno* 41: 271–280.

Sato, T. and Tanabe, Y. (1962). The antiarrhythmic action of phenothiazine derivatives. *Jpn. Circ. J.* 26: 216–224.

Schneiders, F.I., Noble, G.K., Boston, R.C. et al. (2012). Acepromazine pharmacokinetics: a forensic perspective. *Vet J.* 194: 48–54.

Serrano, L. and Lees, P. (1976). The applied pharmacology of azaperone in ponies. *Res. Vet. Sci.* 20: 316–323.

Tobias, K.M., Marioni-Henry, K., and Wagner, R. (2006). A retrospective study on the use of acepromazine maleate in dogs with seizures. *J. Am. Anim. Hosp. Assoc.* 42: 283–289.

Valverde, A., Cantwell, S., Hernandez, J., and Brotherson, C. (2004). Effects of acepromazine on the incidence of vomiting associated with opioid administration in dogs. *Vet. Anesth. Analg.* 31: 40–45.

Webb, A.I. and O'Brien, J.M. (1988). The effect of acepromazine maleate on the anesthetic potency of halothane and isoflurane. *J. Am. Anim. Hosp. Assoc.* 24: 609–613.

Wilson, D.V., Nickels, F.A., and Williams, M.A. (1991). Pharmacologic treatment of priapism in two horses. *J. Am. Vet. Med. Assoc.* 199: 1183–1184.

Yelnosky, J. and Field, W.E. (1964). A preliminary report on the uses of a combination of droperidol and fentanyl citrate in veterinary medicine. *Am. J. Vet. Res.* 25: 1751–1756.

6

Benzodiazepines

Sébastien Hyacinthe Bauquier

Introduction

Benzodiazepines produce hypnotic, anxiolytic, anticonvulsant, myorelaxant, and amnesic effects. Although they are species-specific and dose-dependent, those effects confer the ability to the prescriber to use them in a wide range of pathologies. In veterinary medicine, benzodiazepines are used primarily for their anticonvulsant and centrally mediated muscle relaxant actions. They can increase hypnotic and anxiolytic actions of general anesthetics; however, in some species (e.g. horses) and when administered as a single therapy, some animals will become more anxious and agitated. Benzodiazepines can also be used to manage behavior pathologies, although a review of those effects is outside the scope of this anesthesia-focused chapter. Zolazepam is a benzodiazepine only available combined with tiletamine, and it is used as an anesthetic induction agent. In consequence, Zolazepam will be discussed in the intravenous (IV) anesthetic chapter. The new benzodiazepine remimazolam will be mentioned; however, there is no report on its use in companion animals at the time of writing.

Benzodiazepine agonists (e.g. diazepam, midazolam, lorazepam) depress the central nervous system (CNS) by facilitating the binding of its primary inhibitory neurotransmitter (i.e. gamma-aminobutyric acid [GABA]) on the GABA receptors, resulting in the hyperpolarization of post-synaptic cell membranes. Benzodiazepine inverse agonists (e.g. beta-carboline alkaloids) produce opposite effects such as seizures and anxiety, and benzodiazepine antagonists (e.g. flumazenil) have little intrinsic activity but reverse the effects of both benzodiazepine agonists and inverse agonists, making the benzodiazepines a unique class of drug acting on the CNS that can be fully reversed. Flumazenil is commercially available in many countries, including the US.

Structures and Mechanisms of Action

Molecular Structure of Benzodiazepines

The fundamental structure of a benzodiazepine is constituted of a benzene ring joined to a seven-membered 1,4-diazepine ring (Goodchild 1993). The radical at the 5th carbon of the diazepine ring is a 5-aryl in most benzodiazepines, and molecules such as diazepam, midazolam and lorazepam have a 5-aryl-1,4-benzodiazepine structure (Figure 6.1). This common structure is responsible for diazepam's, midazolam's, and lorazepam's similar molecular weights (284.7, 325.8, and 321.1 respectively) and melting points (132, 159, and 167 °C respectively) (Riviere and Papich 2009).

The diazepine ring can be hydrolyzed to form open-ring benzophenone in a middle acidic environment (Figure 6.2). This reaction does not occur with all benzodiazepines but allows some molecules like midazolam to be water-soluble in pH ranging from 1 to 4 and lipid soluble at pH > 4 (Andersin 1991). The pH of the midazolam's commercial preparation is between 3 and 3.6 allowing a water solubility at 25 °C of 1030 mg/l compared to 50 and 80 mg/l for diazepam and lorazepam respectively (Table 6.1) (Riviere and Papich 2009). In strong acidic environments, all benzodiazepines will irreversibly degrade to aminobenzophenones (Andersin 1991).

Benzodiazepine Interaction with GABAA Receptors

Benzodiazepines bind to the GABA (gamma-aminobutyric acid) type A receptors, ligand-gated chloride channels, to produce their pharmacologic effects (Figure 6.3) (Goodchild 1993). Like many other receptors, the GABA$_A$ receptors are constituted of several protein subunits (commonly two α, two β and one γ with many combinations of those subunits being possible) and, in consequence, have

Pharmacology in Veterinary Anesthesia and Analgesia, First Edition. Edited by Turi Aarnes and Phillip Lerche.
© 2024 John Wiley & Sons, Inc. Published 2024 by John Wiley & Sons, Inc.

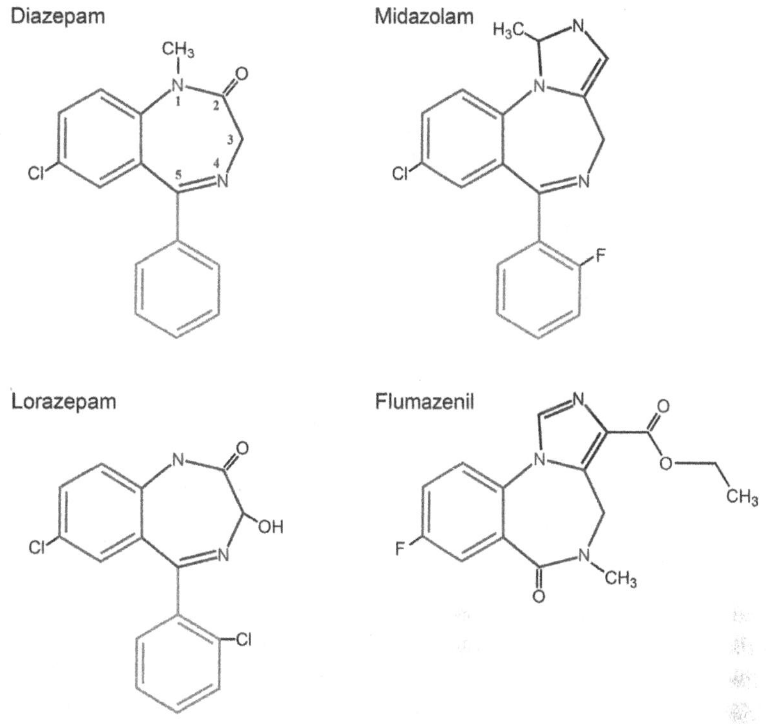

Figure 6.1 The fundamental structure of a benzodiazepine is constituted of a benzene ring (red) joined to a seven-membered 1,4-diazepine ring (purple). The most commonly used benzodiazepines (i.e. diazepam, midazolam and lorazepam) have a 5-aryl-1,4-benzodiazepine structure as the radical at the 5th carbon of the diazepine ring is a 5-aryl (green). Flumazenil is a benzodiazepine antagonist that has little intrinsic activity but reverses the effects of both benzodiazepine agonists and antagonists.

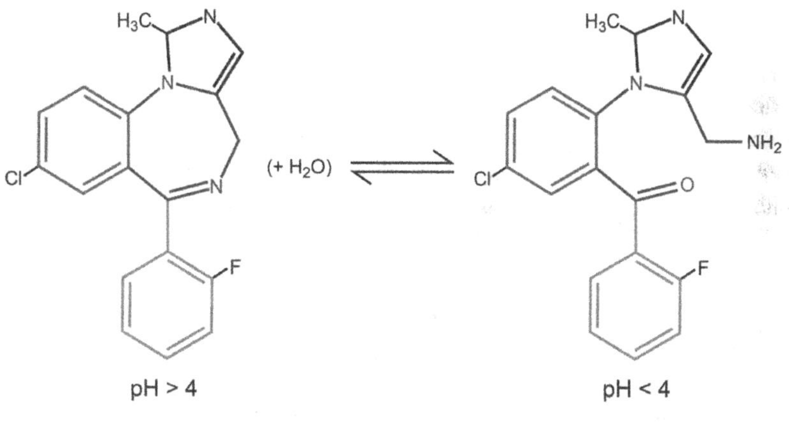

Diazepam

Midazolam

Lorazepam

Flumazenil

Figure 6.2 The diazepine ring (purple) of midazolam can hydrolyzed to form open-ring benzophenone in a middle acidic environment. The molecule becomes water-soluble in pH ranging from 1 to 4 (commercial preparation) but reverses to lipid-soluble at physiological pH.

$(+ H_2O)$

pH > 4

pH < 4

Table 6.1 pKa, pH and water solubility of the most commonly used benzodiazepines.

	Midazolam	Diazepam	Lorazepam
pKa	6.15	3.45	13
pH of commercial preparation	3 to 3.6	6.2 to 6.9	
Water solubility of the commercial preparation at 25 °C (mg/l)	1030	50	80

four levels of structure: primary structure – linear sequence of amino acids; secondary structure – α-helix or β-sheets; tertiary structure – the three-dimensional structure of a subunit; and quaternary structure – the three-dimensional structure of multiple subunits linked together. Benzodiazepines are part of a group of ligands called allosteric modulators that increase the efficiency of a receptor without directly activating them. Those allosteric modulators change mainly the tertiary and quaternary structure of the protein receptors improving the potency of the endogenous ligands (i.e. GABA for the $GABA_A$ receptor). GABA is the principal inhibitory transmitter of the CNS and allows the chloride anions to flow into the cell hyperpolarizing the neuron and thus inhibiting subsequent depolarization (Goodchild 1993). The lack of intrinsic activity of benzodiazepines limits their pharmacologic activity (e.g. CNS depression) but offer a wide therapeutic window.

(a) (b)

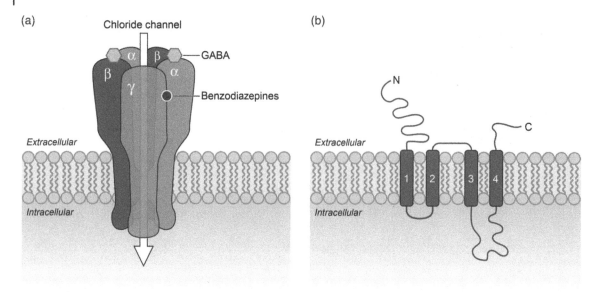

Figure 6.3 **(a)** Benzodiazepines are part of ligands called allosteric modulators that increase the efficiency of the GABA (gamma-aminobutyric acid) type A receptors, ligand-gated chloride channels, to produce their pharmacologic effects. Like many other receptors, the GABA$_A$ receptors are constituted of several protein subunits (commonly two α, two β and one γ with many combinations of those subunits being possible). The binding site of the benzodiazepine is situated between an α and the γ subunits. **(b)** Also, each subunit has four transmembrane spanning (alpha-helix) segments creating the chloride channel.

The GABA$_A$ receptors are large macromolecules to which several ligands can bind to simultaneously at different sites. GABA binds between the α and β subunits. The binding site of the benzodiazepine is situated on the α subunits subtype 1 and subtype 2 between the γ subunit and α subunits (Figure 6.3). GABA$_A$ receptors α-1 subtype (approximately 60% of the GABA$_A$) are mainly situated in the cerebral cortex, cerebellar cortex and thalamus and are thought to produce sedation. However, GABA$_A$ receptors α-2 subtype are primarily located in the hippocampus and amygdala and produce anxiolysis (Low et al. 2000; McKernan et al. 2000). Commonly used IV anesthetics such as propofol, barbiturates (e.g. thiopental) and neurosteroids (e.g. alfaxalone) act by binding to the β subunits. If administered simultaneously with a benzodiazepine, they may produce synergistic pharmacologic effects, leading to life-threatening CNS depression if overdosed.

Pharmacokinetic Properties

Routes of Administration

As previously mentioned, at physiologic pH, all benzodiazepines are highly lipid-soluble, allowing them to cross the blood–brain barrier easily and to enter the CNS rapidly. They have been administered via different routes, including (IV), intramuscular (IM), per rectum (PR), submucosal, sublingual and intranasal, with an overall good bioavailability (Tables 6.2 and 6.3). The IV route is preferred peri-operatively when a catheter is available, although midazolam can be used IM. IM diazepam is not recommended as its eluent propylene glycol induces pain at injection. The efficacy of the PR route is species-specific and depends on the hepatic portal system of the species. Compared to humans, some animal species (e.g. dogs) have a higher percentage of blood drainage from the rectum that passes through hepatic filtration before joining the systemic circulation (Wagner et al. 1998). In those species, submucosal, sublingual or intranasal delivery of diazepam for the treatment of convulsions may be advantageous. The administration of intranasal diazepam (0.5 mg/kg of body weight) in dogs resulted in a mean bioavailability of 80%, a mean peak plasma concentration 50% superior to the suggested therapeutic index and a time-to-peak plasma concentration (Tmax) of 4.5 minutes (only 90 seconds longer than IV administration) (Platt et al. 2000). Interestingly, intracavernous application of diazepam has been reported as an alternative route of administration of the seizure treatment in rabbits (Dundaroz et al. 2002). In that study, diazepam blood levels were not significantly different when comparing IV and intracavernous administration, and no significant side effects were reported.

When administered through those routes, commercial preparations of midazolam have shown lower bioavailability than diazepam in the dog. However, lipid solubility is the main factor influencing benzodiazepine distribution to the CNS (brain/plasma partition coefficient of 2.67 for

Table 6.2 Diazepam pharmacokinetics in various species.

Species	Parent drug and metabolites	Route of administration	Terminal half-life (hours)	Time of maximal concentration (hours)	Apparent volume of distribution (l/kg)	Clearance (ml/kg/min)	Total bioavailability (%)	References
Dog	Diazepam	IV	0.25–3.2		0.29–6.1			Löscher and Frey (1981), Papich and Alcorn (1995), Musulin et al. (2011), Kukanich and Nauss (2012), Probst et al. (2013). (Loscher and Frey 1981; Papich and Alcorn 1995; Musulin et al. 2011; Kukanich and Nauss 2012; Probst et al. 2013)
		Oral					74–100	Löscher and Frey (1981). (Loscher and Frey 1981)
		Rectal	1.7–2.0	3–8 min			66–79	Papich and Alcorn (1995). (Papich and Alcorn 1995)
		Nasal	2.2–6.6	0.2–0.6			41–42	Musulin et al. (2011). (Musulin et al. 2011)
	Nordiazepam	IV						Löscher and Frey (1981), Papich and Alcorn (1995), Musulin et al. (2011), Probst et al. (2013). (Loscher and Frey 1981; Papich and Alcorn 1995; Musulin et al. 2011; Probst et al. 2013)
		Rectal	3.2	1.75				Probst et al. (2013). (Probst et al. 2013)
		Nasal	7.2–9.6	0.9				Musulin et al. (2011). (Musulin et al. 2011)
	Oxazepam	IV	3.5–6.4	2–2.1				Löscher and Frey (1981), Papich and Alcorn (1995), Musulin et al. (2011), Kukanich and Nauss (2012). (Loscher and Frey 1981; Papich and Alcorn 1995; Musulin et al. 2011; Kukanich and Nauss 2012)
		Nasal	6.9–7.8	1.8–2.1				Musulin et al. (2011). (Musulin et al. 2011)
Cat	Diazepam	IV	5.5			4.7		Cotler et al. (1984). (Cotler et al. 1984)
	Nordiazepam	IV	21			0.85		Cotler et al. (1984). (Cotler et al. 1984)
Horse Adult	Diazepam	IV	6.5–22					Muir et al. (1982). (Muir et al. 1982)
Foal 4 d old	Diazepam	IV			1.6	5.1		Norman et al. (1997). (Norman et al. 1997)
Foal 21 d old	Diazepam	IV			2.7	8.6		Norman et al. (1997). (Norman et al. 1997)
Foal 42 d old	Diazepam	IV			3	7.3		Norman et al. (1997). (Norman et al. 1997)
Foal 84 d old	Diazepam	IV			2.5	8.4		Norman et al. (1997). (Norman et al. 1997)

Table 6.3 Midazolam and lorazepam pharmacokinetic in various species.

Drug	Species	Route of administration	Terminal half-life (hours, ±SD)	Time of maximal concentration (min, ±SD)	Apparent volume of distribution (l/kg, ±SD)	Clearance (ml/kg/min, ±SD)	Total bioavailability (%)	References
Midazolam	Dog	IV	1–1.6	1	1.1–100	10.1–27		Court and Greenblatt (1992), Henry et al. (1998), Podell et al. (1998b), Schwartz et al. (2013). (Court and Greenblatt 1992; Henry et al. 1998; Schwartz et al. 2013)
		IM		7–15			90	Court and Greenblatt (1992), Schwartz et al. (2013). (Court and Greenblatt 1992; Schwartz et al. 2013)
		Oral (1 dog)		10			50–67	Court and Greenblatt (1992). (Court and Greenblatt 1992)
		Rectal	Most midazolam plasmatic concentrations were below the limit of quantification					Schwartz et al. (2013). (Schwartz et al. 2013)
		Nasal atomizer		9.5 (plasma)			7.3 (plasma); 27.8 (CSF)	Henry et al. (1998) (Henry et al. 1998)
		Nasal drops		10.8 (plasma)			7.1 (plasma); 16.3 (CSF)	Henry et al. (1998). (Henry et al. 1998)
Midazolam	Horse Adult	IV	3.6–6.8		2.1–2.8	10.4–10.6		Hubbell et al. (2013). (Hubbell et al. 2013)
Midazolam	Sheep	IV	0.79±0.44		0.84±0.33	21.2±5.2		Simon et al. (2017). (Simon et al. 2017)
		IM		27.6±15.6			352±148	Simon et al. (2017). (Simon et al. 2017)
Lorazepam	Dog	IV		5				(Podell et al. 1998b)
		Nasal		3–9				Mariani et al. (2003). (Mariani et al. 2003)
		Rectal	Lorazepam plasmatic concentration was below the limit of quantification					Podell et al. 1998b

diazepam and 0.27 for midazolam). Combined with the differences in metabolism, it explains how midazolam can have a longer Tmax than diazepam while still having a faster onset of action (Buhrer et al. 1990; Upton et al. 2001). Further, intranasal bioavailability of midazolam can be improved using an atomizer and, in theory, when administrating midazolam in its lipid-soluble form (Henry 1998; Zhang et al. 2002). A more recent study evaluated the clinical efficacy of intranasal midazolam via a mucosal atomization device and compared it to rectal administration of diazepam for controlling status epilepticus before IV access is available (Charalambous et al. 2017). The study concluded that the midazolam via mucosal atomization is a quick, safe and effective first-line medication for controlling status epilepticus in dogs and appears superior to rectal diazepam (Charalambous et al. 2017).

Protein Binding

Benzodiazepines are highly protein bound (e.g. midazolam 96%). However, a direct correlation between unwanted CNS depression and low plasma protein concentrations (i.e. hypoalbuminemia) has only been demonstrated with benzodiazepines that have active metabolites also highly bound to plasma proteins (e.g. diazepam) (Muller 1977; Court and Greenblatt 1992). In those cases, a direct correlation between the plasma protein binding and the biological half-life was also established (Muller 1977).

Metabolism

Most benzodiazepines need to be metabolized to a more water-soluble compound for efficient elimination. Metabolic pathways for benzodiazepines are drug and species-specific (see diazepam below). Diazepam and midazolam undergo reduction (phase 1 metabolism – cytochrome P450) and glucuronidation (phase 2 metabolism) before being excreted in the urine. In contrast, lorazepam mainly undergoes only glucuronidation (Elliott 1976; Reves et al. 1985; Johnson et al. 2002; Vanderk et al. 1971). In consequence, benzodiazepine metabolites may or may not be active, and the metabolite of a particular benzodiazepine may be active in one species and inactive in another. This variability in metabolite activity will significantly affect the duration of the benzodiazepines' clinical effects.

Metabolism of benzodiazepines that undergo phase 1 metabolism (i.e. diazepam and midazolam) is affected by the co-administration of some drugs that will affect the cytochrome P450. Those drugs include (but are not limited to) cimetidine, erythromycin, isoniazid, ketoconazole, propranolol, and valproic acid. They will partially inhibit the metabolism of diazepam and midazolam, potentially exacerbating pharmacologic effects (Hiller et al. 1990; Long

et al. 1997). Fentanyl can also reduce midazolam hepatic clearance and elimination half-life in humans by up to 30% and 50%, respectively (Hase et al. 1997). On the other hand, rifampin will accelerate the metabolism of diazepam in rabbits (Long et al. 1997).

Excretion

Midazolam renal clearance doesn't seem to be affected by renal failure in humans (Vinik et al. 1983). However, chronic use of diazepam can result in the accumulation of its active metabolites as the metabolites' elimination half-life exceeds that of the parent drug.

Indications and Pharmacodynamic Effects

Hypnotic and Anxiolytic

Sedative effects are, at best, mild in most adult dogs, cats, and horses, and paradoxical effects such as excitement dysphoria and ataxia can be seen due to reduction in inhibition. In a few species (e.g. ruminants, swine, ferrets, rabbits, and many birds), benzodiazepines will produce excellent sedation as well as in the very young (e.g. foal of less than a month old), very sick (e.g. septic dog) and very old animals that will also show signs of CNS depression. In all cases, the sedative effects are more reliable when the benzodiazepine is administered as part of a balanced anesthesia protocol potentiating the effects of opioids and/or α-2 adrenergic agonists.

Anesthetic Sparing

Benzodiazepines decrease the minimum alveolar concentration (MAC) of inhalant anesthetics (e.g. isoflurane, halothane) in multiple species as well as potentiating the MAC reduction resulting from opioid administration (Hellyer et al. 2001; Matthews et al. 1990; Seddighi et al. 2011). It also decreases the drug (e.g. propofol, alfaxalone) requirements to induce anesthesia, although there are conflicting results in the literature in species in which benzodiazepines can induce excitement (Hopkins et al. 2014; Covey-Crump and Murison 2008; Dzikiti et al. 2014; Santos Gonzalez et al. 2013; Robinson and Borer-Weir 2015; Italiano and Robinson 2018; Liao et al. 2017; Muñoz et al. 2017; Zapata et al. 2018). In healthy dogs, administering midazolam after alfaxalone for co-induction of anesthesia lowers the incidence of excitement while still reducing the alfaxalone dose requirement (Zapata et al. 2018).

Anticonvulsant and Central Nervous System Effects

Benzodiazepines are anticonvulsants; they block arousal and decrease seizure propagation and are the drug of choice in status epilepticus as they cross the blood–brain barrier rapidly (Wauquier et al. 1979; Podell 1995; Podell 1996; Bassett et al. 2014). Preferably, benzodiazepines will be administered IV, although rectal administration has been used historically to control cluster seizures (Podell et al. 1998a). Newer evidence indicates that intranasal administration of midazolam controls seizures better than rectal administration of diazepam (Holsti et al. 2007; Charalambous et al. 2017).

Most CNS-depressant drugs decrease oxygen consumption and have an associated auto-regulated proportional decrease in cerebral blood flow. With benzodiazepines, the reduction in oxygen consumption is even more significant, making the drug of particular interest in patients with intracranial diseases (Reves et al. 1985; Hoffman et al. 1986).

Diazepam administered at clinical doses to dogs undergoing isoflurane anesthesia decreased the absolute power of their electroencephalogram (EEG) in theta, delta, alpha, and beta frequencies for at least three hours. As expected, the use of flumazenil antagonized this effect in all frequencies (Greene et al. 1992).

Muscle Relaxation

Benzodiazepines provide reliable centrally mediated muscle relaxation in veterinary medicine, and they are often co-administered with other anesthetic drugs that induce muscle rigidity (i.e. ketamine) (Riviere and Papich 2009). At supra-clinical (2 mg/kg) doses IV diazepam even caused ataxia and recumbency in dogs (Platt et al. 2000). The same can be seen in horses at doses around 0.2 mg/kg IV and above. However, they do not induce myorelaxation to the extent of neuromuscular blockers, and they are not considered adequate muscle relaxants for surgical procedures in human anesthesia (Stoelting et al. 2006). Neuromuscular blockers act at the neuromuscular junction level, allowing complete blockade, whereas benzodiazepines "only" potentiate GABA-mediated muscle relaxation at the level of the spinal internuncial neurons (Dretchen et al. 1971). There is conflicting evidence as to whether or not benzodiazepines potentiate the effects of neuromuscular blockers (Driessen et al. 1987; Hepaguslar et al. 2002).

Amnesic Effects

Benzodiazepines are consistently associated with a dose-dependent amnesic and non-amnestic cognitive impairment in humans (Tannenbaum et al. 2012). They induce severe anterograde amnesia (acquisition impairment) and affect retrograde amnesia altering retrieval processes in both humans and animals (Beracochea 2006). Judicious use of benzodiazepines during hospitalization could improve patient welfare, although benzodiazepines can, paradoxically, enhance retrieval memory processes in rats under stress (Harris and Westbrook 1998; Obradovic et al. 2004).

Appetite Stimulation

Benzodiazepines stimulate the intake of food, water, and salt, whereas inverse agonists have anorectic effects (Cooper and Estall 1985). Those effects have not been intensely studied in companion animals; however, they have been demonstrated in human and laboratory animals, and reports in some domestic species exist (e.g. cats, goats) (Center et al. 1996; Mereu et al. 1976; Van Miert et al. 1989). There is conflicting evidence regarding gastric emptying time, and they probably should not be used to treat anorexia due to gastrointestinal (GI) stasis (Chandler et al. 1999; Steyn et al. 1997).

Side Effects

Respiratory and Cardiovascular

Benzodiazepines have few respiratory and cardiovascular side effects. Ventilation is not affected at clinical doses, even although the respiratory rate may decrease. In dogs at clinical or supra-clinical doses, systemic arterial, pulmonary arterial and central venous pressures, cardiac output, heart rate and regional coronary blood flow were not or were mildly affected by the administration of diazepam or midazolam (Jones et al. 1979). Indirectly, by decreasing the amount of their co-induction anesthetic drugs necessary to induce anesthesia, they may benefit the cardiovascularly unstable patient. However, they will not mask and may exacerbate anesthetics' respiratory and cardiovascular side effects (Hopkins et al. 2014).

Analgesic Effects

Although it has been demonstrated that GABA plays a role in mediating the transmission and perception of pain, there is no conclusive evidence for any analgesic effect of benzodiazepines (Enna and McCarson 2006). Further, enhancing activation of the $GABA_A$ receptor at the supraspinal level will inhibit descending anti-nociceptive pathways and exacerbate the response to nociceptive stimuli. Indeed, benzodiazepines can decrease the analgesic efficacy of opioids and antagonism of the benzodiazepines with flumazenil enhances the opioid-induced analgesia (Gross et al. 1996; Gear et al. 1997; Kissin et al. 1990).

Hepatic Necrosis

Acute fulminant hepatic necrosis has been associated with repeated oral administration of diazepam in cats. Although idiosyncratic hepato-toxicosis was suspected due to the rarity of this complication, testing of serum transaminase activity within five days of treatment initiation of repeated diazepam administration is recommended (Center et al. 1996). In another report, the hepatic failure, secondary to oral diazepam administration, in a two-year-old cat for behavioral problems was treated successfully with intensive supportive care and five days of hospitalization (Park 2012).

Drug Interaction

Lidocaine metabolism is non-competitively inhibited by midazolam (Nagashima et al. 2005). In consequence, the combination of the two drugs could prolong the effects of lidocaine. The clinical significance of such interaction is unclear.

Dependence

The chronic use of benzodiazepines in animals can produce dependence. In dogs, studies have shown that withdrawal from diazepam can induce many signs ranging from tremor, hot foot walking, rigidity and decreased food intake to tonic-clonic convulsions that were lethal in some dogs (McNicholas et al. 1983). The severity of those symptoms is dependent on the benzodiazepine used and its metabolites (Martin et al. 1990). Because benzodiazepine metabolism is species-specific, signs are also likely to vary depending on the species (Martin et al. 1990).

Aging

The long-term use of benzodiazepines in elderly human patients has been associated with an increased incidence of confusion in the post-operative period (Kudoh et al. 2004). Also, age-associated decreased liver function affects phase one metabolism (oxidation) more than phase two (glucuronidation), and in this regard, lorazepam may be advantageous.

Laryngeal Function

No differences in arytenoid cartilage motion were seen immediately after induction of anesthesia with diazepam (or midazolam) plus ketamine, propofol, alfaxalone or thiopental in dogs or cats (Nelissen et al. 2012; Jackson et al. 2004). Nevertheless, the arytenoid motion may recover more quickly following thiopental induction compared to the diazepam-ketamine combination in dogs (Jackson et al. 2004).

Propylene Glycol

The injectable formulations of diazepam and lorazepam include 40% and 79% propylene glycol, respectively. Propylene glycol is a hyperosmotic molecule that can induce pain and thrombophlebitis when administered IM and IV (in peripheral veins), respectively (Doenicke et al. 1994). It can also cause hemolysis when diazepam or lorazepam are administered at large doses or as a constant rate infusion (CRI). Lorazepam should also be diluted with an equal volume in sterile water, saline or dextrose 5% immediately before slow IV administration to decrease the incidence of phlebitis (Ativan®, Baxter Healthcare Corporation product information notice). However, less commonly used benzodiazepines have an antihemolytic effect on human erythrocytes (Terhaag and Bockisch 1976). Indeed, chlordiazepoxide, medazepam and oxazepam have a similar effect to chlorpromazine on human erythrocytes placed in hypotonic NaCl solution.

Pregnancy

The FDA classifies benzodiazepines as category D. There is an increased risk of congenital malformations associated with benzodiazepines during the first trimester of pregnancy; however, the potential benefits from its use may outweigh the risk. Also, the chronic use of benzodiazepines during late pregnancy increases the risk of CNS depressant effects and withdrawal symptoms during the post-natal period in newborns. Benzodiazepines and their metabolites will distribute into milk (Plumb 2015). The implications for veterinary patients are not fully understood, and those effects may be less with lorazepam (Plumb 2015).

Diazepam Hydrochloride

Empirical formula: $C_{16}H_{13}ClN_2O$

Chemical name (International Union of Pure and Applied Chemistry [IUPAC]): 7-chloro-1,3-dihydro-1-methyl-5-phenyl-2H-1,4-benzodiazepin-2-one. Structure: see Figure 6.1.

US veterinary labeled products: none. US human labeled products: Available as an oral tablet, oral solution, injectable solution and rectal gel.

Legal status: AU: S4, CA: Schedule IV, DE: Anlage III, NZ: Class C, UK: Schedule 4 (Subclass Controlled Drug Benz), US: Schedule IV. Diazepam is not intended for food-producing animals (no established withdrawal time) and is classified as a class-2 substance by the Racing Commissioners International (Association of Racing Commissioners International [ARCI]).

Diazepam is often considered the benzodiazepine of reference. It is a colorless to light yellow crystalline compound. It is poorly water-soluble (Table 6.1) and, as previously mentioned, it requires propylene glycol to be solubilized. Most of the limitations of diazepam are due to its hyperosmotic vehicle (unreliable absorption in any route other than

IV and pain on injection). It also has a much shorter duration of action in dogs and cats compared to horses (Table 6.2) and humans (elimination half-time of 20–50 hours), requiring more frequent dosing (Barash 2009). In cats, repeated administration of diazepam has been associated with hepatic failure and death, and the authors recommended frequent testing of the serum transaminase activity (Center et al. 1996). In dogs, diazepam anticonvulsant tolerance occurs after one week of continuous administration and diazepam serum concentrations are not directly related to its anticonvulsant effects. Its main metabolites (in decreasing importance) nordiazepam (also known as desmethyldiazepam, 50% in cats), oxazepam and temazepam are active metabolites, although their anticonvulsant potency is around one third that of diazepam (Table 6.2) (Katzung 2004; Morgan et al. 2006). In horses, diazepam can induce excitement, ataxia and recumbency. However, in the author's experience, accidental administration of 0.1 mg/kg IV diazepam to a horse diagnosed with West Nile virus induced sedation. The posology of diazepam in various species is summarized in Table 6.4.

Plastic bags and tubes commonly made with plasticized poly(vinyl chloride) (PVC) are often used for the administration of drugs. These plastics can absorb diazepam and a partition coefficient of 300 has been reported (Treleano et al. 2009). In another study, the sorption of diazepam by infusion sets reached 80% during slow infusion (Winsnes et al. 1981). Consequently, injectable solutions of diazepam should be stored in glass or polyolefin containers protected from light and stored at room temperature. This sorption phenomenon is seen with diazepam but not with midazolam or lorazepam (Martens et al. 1990).

Diazepam precipitates when combined with most other drugs, although diazepam and ketamine are often mixed before induction of anesthesia. There is no evidence if this combination is safe or leads to the formation of microcrystals invisible to the naked eye.

Midazolam Maleate

Empirical formula: $C_{18}H_{13}ClFN_3$

Chemical name (IUPAC): 8-chloro-6-(2-fluorophenyl)-1-methyl-4H-imidazo[1,5-a][1,4]benzodiazepine. Structure: see Figure 6.1.

Table 6.4 Posology of the most commonly used benzodiazepines in the perioperative period.

Effects	Species	Diazepam (mg/kg)	Midazolam (mg/kg)	Lorazepam (mg/kg)
Sedation				
	Dogs and cats	0.1–0.5 IV	0.1–0.5 IV, IM, SQ 0.2–1.0 intranasal	0.2–0.3 IV
	Ruminants	0.3–1.0 IV	0.2–1.0 IV, IM	
	Foals (<1 month)	0.1–0.3 IV	0.1–0.3 IV	
	Pigs	0.3–1.0 IV	0.2–1.0 IV, IM	
	Rabbits, ferrets		0.5–1.0 IM	
	Birds		0.5–1.0 IM	
Co-induction agent				
	Dogs and cats	0.1–0.5 IV	0.1–0.3 IV	
	Ruminants	0.1–0.5 IV	0.1–0.3 IV	
	Horses	0.05–0.1 IV	0.05–0.1 IV	
	Pigs	0.1–0.3 IV	0.1–0.3 IV	
	Rabbits, ferrets	0.1–0.5 IV	0.1–0.3 IV	
	Birds	0.1–0.5 IV		
Anticonvulsant				
	Dogs and cats	0.5–2.0 IV, per rectum	0.5–1.0 IV	0.2 IV, intranasal
	Horses	0.05–0.4 IV	0.05–0.4 IV	
Appetite stimulant				
	Cats	0.05 IV		
	Goat	0.06 IV		

US veterinary labeled products: none. US human labeled products: Available as syrup or an injectable solution.

Legal status: AU: S4, CA: Schedule IV, DE: Anlage III, NZ: Class C, UK: Schedule 3, US: Schedule IV. Midazolam is not intended for food-producing animals (no established withdrawal time) and is classified as a class-2 substance by the Racing Commissioners International (ARCI).

Although midazolam is often reported to be twice as potent as diazepam, its main advantage resides in the ability of its diazepine ring to reversibly hydrolyze and form open-ring benzophenone in mildly acidic environments (Figure 6.2). The good hydro-solubility seen at a pH ranging from 3 to 4 (commercial preparation) allows the molecule to be solubilized without propylene glycol and can be used more reliably IM or intranasally. The high lipid-solubility of midazolam at physiologic pH also means rapid transfer across the blood–brain barrier for a fast onset of action. Combined with the fact that midazolam has very similar pharmacodynamics and is cheaper in certain countries than diazepam, midazolam has become very popular in veterinary medicine. The posology of midazolam in various species is summarized in Table 6.4. Rectal administration of midazolam is not recommended as it results in undetectable midazolam plasma concentration (Table 6.3) (Schwartz et al. 2013).

Lorazepam

Empirical formula: $C_{15}H_{10}Cl_2N_2O_2$

Chemical name (IUPAC): 7-chloro-5-(2-chlorophenyl)-3-hydroxy-1,3-dihydro-1,4-benzodiazepin-2-one. Structure: see Figure 6.1.

US veterinary labeled products: none. US human labeled products: Available as an oral tablet, oral solution or injectable solution.

Legal status: AU: S4, CA: Schedule IV, DE: Anlage III, UK: Schedule 4 (Subclass Controlled Drug Benz), US: Schedule IV. Lorazepam is not intended for food-producing animals (no established withdrawal time) and is classified as class-2 substance by the Racing Commissioners International (ARCI).

Lorazepam is rarely used in veterinary medicine and, to the author's knowledge, is not used as part of a balanced anesthesia protocol. Although it is a more potent sedative and amnesic than diazepam or midazolam, it has a lower lipid solubility and a more prolonged onset of action (Stoelting et al. 2006; Barr et al. 2001; Healey et al. 1983). In humans, postoperative sedation with a continuous infusion of lorazepam resulted in significant delays in emergence compared to midazolam (Barr et al. 2001).

Lorazepam has been used as an adjunctive agent for treating separation anxiety in dogs (Sherman 2008). Its use as an anticonvulsant has been reported in small animals due to its increased duration of action and potential for better bioavailability (when administered intranasally) compared to diazepam (Mariani et al. 2003). However, like midazolam, rectal administration of lorazepam resulted in immeasurable plasmatic concentration levels (Table 6.3) (Podell et al. 1998b). The posology of lorazepam in various species is summarized in Table 6.4.

In most species, Lorazepam metabolism differs from diazepam and midazolam. The principal metabolite in man, dogs, pigs, and cats is the glucuronide metabolite, but the rat produces other metabolites after small doses of lorazepam (Elliott 1976). Because the formation of lorazepam metabolites is mostly independent from hepatic microsomal enzymes, decreases in hepatic function or aging are less likely to prolong lorazepam elimination half-time when compared to diazepam or midazolam (Stoelting et al. 2006). Also, a decrease in renal function will not affect the lorazepam metabolite effects as they are inactive byproducts.

Due to the high content of propylene glycol and benzyl alcohol in the injectable formulation, lorazepam should be diluted before administration, and repeated high doses or infusion should be used with caution.

Remimazolam (also Known as CNS 7056)

Empirical formula: $C_{21}H_{19}BrN_4O_2$

Chemical name (IUPAC): methyl 3-[(4S)-8-bromo-1-methyl-6-(pyridin-2-yl)-4H-imidazo[1,2-a][1,4]benzodiazepin-4-yl]propanoate.

US veterinary labeled products: none. US human labeled products: Available as an injectable solution.

Legal status: CA: Schedule IV, DE: Anlage III, EU: Rx-only, UK: Under Psychoactive Substances Act, US: R-Only. Lorazepam is not intended for food-producing animals (no established withdrawal time).

Remimazolam is a newer benzodiazepine that has recently been approved in human medicine (USA and Japan in 2020, and EU in 2021) for induction and maintenance of procedural sedation. As its name indicates, remimazolam combined the properties of two well-known sedative/anesthetic drugs (i.e. midazolam and remifentanil) (Goudra and Singh 2014). Remimazolam has similar pharmacodynamic effects to other benzodiazepines, with reported significantly reduced times to onset of sedation and recovery in phase 3 clinical trials compared to midazolam (Lee and Shirley 2021). Remimazolam has an organ-independent metabolism similar to remifentanil. It is degraded by tissue carboxylesterases (predominantly type 1A) to CNS7054, which is subsequently metabolized by hydroxylation and glucuronidation.

However, the pharmacokinetics of remimazolam are altered in patients with hepatic impairment, despite the limited metabolism by cytochrome P450 (Lee and Shirley 2021).

Remimazolam is a promising drug. However, to the author's knowledge, there are no reports of the use of remimazolam in companion animals.

Flumazenil

Empirical formula: $C_{15}H_{14}FN_3O_3$

Molecular weight: 303.3 g/mol

Chemical name (IUPAC): Ethyl 8-fluoro-5-methyl-6-oxo-5,6-dihydro-4H-benzo[f]imidazo[1,5-a][1,4]diazepine-3-carboxylate. Structure: see Figure 6.1.

US veterinary labeled products: none. US human labeled products: Available as an injectable solution.

Legal status: Flumazenil is not an Food and Drug Administration (FDA) scheduled drug. Flumazenil is not intended for food-producing animals (no established withdrawal time). Flumazenil has been shown to have an adverse effect on the developing fetus, but potential benefits may warrant use during pregnancy despite potential risks.

Flumazenil is a benzodiazepine derivative with a high affinity for benzodiazepine sites on the $GABA_A$ receptors. It has little intrinsic activity but reverses the effects of both benzodiazepine agonists and inverse agonists in a dose-dependent manner. It does not reverse the effects of other drugs that bind to the $GABA_A$ receptor, such as propofol, alfaxalone and barbiturates. Still, it can improve the outcome of animal and human patients with hepatic encephalopathy (Grimm et al. 1988; Laccetti et al. 2000; Baraldi et al. 1984; Bassett et al. 1987). In humans, flumazenil undergoes extensive metabolism in the liver (phase one and phase two) with less than 0.2% recovered unchanged in the urine (Klotz 1988). Its relatively short duration of action is explained by its short half-life (0.7–1.3 hour), high plasma clearance (520–1300 ml/min) and the fact that its three known metabolites are inactive (Klotz 1988). Flumazenil also has a relatively low plasma protein binding (40%) when compared to other benzodiazepines (Klotz 1988).

In dogs, flumazenil serum levels reached a plateau within 4 minutes of submucosal administration of 0.2 mg of flumazenil (Oliver et al. 2000). In that study, the average maximum flumazenil serum level achieved was 8.5 ng/ml and decreased to −2 ng/ml by two hours. The bioavailability of submucosal flumazenil was 101 ± 14% (Oliver et al. 2000).

In rabbits previously medicated with midazolam, IV flumazenil terminal half-life, plasma clearance and volume of distribution were 26.3 minutes [95%CI: 23.3–29.3], 18.74 ml/minutes/kg [16.47–21.00] and 0.63 l/kg [0.55–0.71], respectively (Rousseau-Blass et al. 2021). However, the duration of flumazenil action was not long enough to avoid a return of sedation in the majority of rabbits (Rousseau-Blass et al. 2021).

Flumazenil is usually administered as an antagonist for benzodiazepines; however, its relatively high price often prevents routine clinical use. It is administered to effect IV, and most patients respond to doses between 0.01 and 0.04 mg/kg in dogs and cats and 0.01 to 0.02 in horses. In dogs, the IM, rectal, submucosal, and sublingual routes have been shown to be viable alternatives; however, the onset of response following administration of flumazenil IV was significantly faster (1.7 minute) followed by the submucosal route (2.3 minutes) (Unkel et al. 2006; Heniff et al. 1997). Oral administration is not recommended as peak plasma concentrations are reached after one hour and decrease rapidly (Wala et al. 1988).

Flumazenil reverses EEG changes and the centrally mediated muscle relaxation induced by the benzodiazepines but doesn't impair cerebral blood flow autoregulation (Greene et al. 1992; Keegan et al. 1993; Artru 1989). The administration of flumazenil is not associated with excitement, dysphonia, alterations in cardiorespiratory functions, or increased MAC (Schwieger et al. 1989). However, flumazenil antagonizes the respiratory depression seen when combining benzodiazepine and opioids and antagonizes the fall of arterial blood pressure seen in cats after the administration of benzodiazepines (Gross et al. 1996; Driessen et al. 1987).

Flumazenil should be used with caution in patients with a history of seizures or chronic administration of benzodiazepine as it can precipitate seizures and trigger withdrawal symptoms, respectively (Spivey 1992; Martin et al. 1990).

References

Andersin, R. (1991). Solubility and acid–base behaviour of midazolam in media of different pH, studied by ultraviolet spectrophotometry with multicomponent software. *J. Pharm. Biomed. Anal.* 9: 451–455.

Artru, A.A. (1989). Flumazenil reversal of midazolam in dogs: dose-related changes in cerebral blood flow, metabolism, EEG, and CSF pressure. *J. Neurosurg. Anesthesiol.* 1: 46–55.

Baraldi, M., Zeneroli, M.L., Ventura, E. et al. (1984). Supersensitivity of benzodiazepine receptors in hepatic encephalopathy due to fulminant hepatic failure in the rat: reversal by a benzodiazepine antagonist. *Clin. Sci. (Lond.)* 67: 167–175.

Barash, P.G. (2009). *Clinical Anesthesia*. Philadelphia: Wolters Kluwer/Lippincott Williams & Wilkins.

Barr, J., Zomorodi, K., Bertaccini, E.J. et al. (2001). A double-blind, randomized comparison of IV lorazepam versus midazolam for sedation of ICU patients via a pharmacologic model. *Anesthesiology* 95: 286–298.

Bassett, M.L., Mullen, K.D., Skolnick, P., and Jones, E.A. (1987). Amelioration of hepatic encephalopathy by pharmacologic antagonism of the GABA$_A$-benzodiazepine receptor complex in a rabbit model of fulminant hepatic failure. *Gastroenterology* 93: 1069–1077.

Bassett, L., Troncy, E., Pouliot, M. et al. (2014). Telemetry video-electroencephalography (EEG) in rats, dogs and non-human primates: methods in follow-up safety pharmacology seizure liability assessments. *J. Pharmacol. Toxicol. Methods* 70: 230–240.

Beracochea, D. (2006). Anterograde and retrograde effects of benzodiazepines on memory. *ScientificWorldJournal* 6: 1460–1465.

Buhrer, M., Maitre, P.O., Crevoisier, C., and Stanski, D.R. (1990). Electroencephalographic effects of benzodiazepines. II. Pharmacodynamic modeling of the electroencephalographic effects of midazolam and diazepam. *Clin. Pharmacol. Ther.* 48: 555–567.

Center, S.A., Elston, T.H., Rowland, P.H. et al. (1996). Fulminant hepatic failure associated with oral administration of diazepam in 11 cats. *J. Am. Vet. Med. Assoc.* 209: 618–625.

Chandler, M.L., Guilford, W.G., Lawoko, C.R., and Whittem, T. (1999). Gastric emptying and intestinal transit times of radiopaque markers in cats fed a high-fiber diet with and without low-dose intravenous diazepam. *Vet. Radiol. Ultrasound* 40: 3–8.

Charalambous, M., Bhatti, S.F.M., Van Ham, L. et al. (2017). Intranasal midazolam versus rectal diazepam for the Management of Canine Status Epilepticus: a multicenter randomized parallel-group clinical trial. *J. Vet. Intern. Med.* 31: 1149–1158.

Cooper, S.J. and Estall, L.B. (1985). Behavioural pharmacology of food, water and salt intake in relation to drug actions at benzodiazepine receptors. *Neurosci. Biobehav. Rev.* 9: 5–19.

Cotler, S., Gustafson, J.H., and Colburn, W.A. (1984). Pharmacokinetics of diazepam and nordiazepam in the cat. *J. Pharm. Sci.* 73: 348–351.

Court, M.H. and Greenblatt, D.J. (1992). Pharmacokinetics and preliminary observations of behavioral changes following administration of midazolam to dogs. *J. Vet. Pharmacol. Ther.* 15: 343–350.

Covey-Crump, G.L. and Murison, P.J. (2008). Fentanyl or midazolam for co-induction of anaesthesia with propofol in dogs. *Vet. Anaesth. Analg.* 35: 463–472.

Doenicke, A., Roizen, M.F., Nebauer, A.E. et al. (1994). A comparison of two formulations for etomidate, 2-hydroxypropyl-beta-cyclodextrin (HPCD) and propylene glycol. *Anesth. Analg.* 79: 933–939.

Dretchen, K., Ghoneim, M.M., and Long, J.P. (1971). The interaction of diazepam with myoneural blocking agents. *Anesthesiology* 34: 463–468.

Driessen, J.J., Van Egmond, J., Van Der Pol, F., and Crul, J.F. (1987). Effects of two benzodiazepines and a benzodiazepine antagonist on neuromuscular blockade in the anaesthetized cat. *Arch. Int. Pharmacodyn. Ther.* 286: 58–70.

Dundaroz, R., Degim, T., Sizlan, A. et al. (2002). Intracavernous application of diazepam: an alternative route of the seizure treatment – an experimental study in rabbits. *Pediatr. Int.* 44: 163–167.

Dzikiti, T.B., Zeiler, G.E., Dzikiti, L.N., and Garcia, E.R. (2014). The effects of midazolam and butorphanol, administered alone or combined, on the dose and quality of anaesthetic induction with alfaxalone in goats. *J. S. Afr. Vet. Assoc.* 85: 1047.

Elliott, H.W. (1976). Metabolism of lorazepam. *Br. J. Anaesth.* 48: 1017–1023.

Enna, S.J. and McCarson, K.E. (2006). The role of GABA in the mediation and perception of pain. *Adv. Pharmacol.* 54: 1–27.

Gear, R.W., Miaskowski, C., Heller, P.H. et al. (1997). Benzodiazepine mediated antagonism of opioid analgesia. *Pain* 71: 25–29.

Goodchild, C.S. (1993). GABA receptors and benzodiazepines. *Br. J. Anaesth.* 71: 127–133.

Goudra, B.G. and Singh, P.M. (2014). Remimazolam: the future of its sedative potential. *Saudi J. Anaesth.* 8: 388–391.

Greene, S.A., Moore, M.P., Keegan, R.D., and Gallagher, L.V. (1992). Quantitative electroencephalography for measurement of central nervous system responses to diazepam and the benzodiazepine antagonist, flumazenil, in isoflurane-anaesthetized dogs. *J. Vet. Pharmacol. Ther.* 15: 259–266.

Grimm, G., Ferenci, P., Katzenschlager, R. et al. (1988). Improvement of hepatic encephalopathy treated with flumazenil. *Lancet* 2: 1392–1394.

Gross, J.B., Blouin, R.T., Zandsberg, S. et al. (1996). Effect of flumazenil on ventilatory drive during sedation with midazolam and alfentanil. *Anesthesiology* 85: 713–720.

Harris, J.A. and Westbrook, R.F. (1998). Benzodiazepine-induced amnesia in rats: reinstatement of conditioned performance by noxious stimulation on test. *Behav. Neurosci.* 112: 183–192.

Hase, I., Oda, Y., Tanaka, K. et al. (1997). I.v. fentanyl decreases the clearance of midazolam. *Br. J. Anaesth.* 79: 740–743.

Healey, M., Pickens, R., Meisch, R., and Mckenna, T. (1983). Effects of clorazepate, diazepam, lorazepam, and placebo on human memory. *J. Clin. Psychiatry* 44: 436–439.

Hellyer, P.W., Mama, K.R., Shafford, H.L. et al. (2001). Effects of diazepam and flumazenil on minimum alveolar concentrations for dogs anesthetized with isoflurane or a combination of isoflurane and fentanyl. *Am. J. Vet. Res.* 62: 555–560.

Heniff, M.S., Moore, G.P., Trout, A. et al. (1997). Comparison of routes of flumazenil administration to reverse midazolam-induced respiratory depression in a canine model. *Acad. Emerg. Med.* 4: 1115–1118.

Henry, R.J. (1998). A pharmacokinetic study of midazolam in dogs: nasal drop vs. atomizer administration. *Pediatr. Dentist.* 20: 321.

Henry, R.J., Ruano, N., Casto, D., and Wolf, R.H. (1998). A pharmacokinetic study of midazolam in dogs: nasal drop vs. atomizer administration. *Pediatr. Dent.* 20: 321–326.

Hepaguslar, H., Oztekin, S., Mavioglu, O. et al. (2002). The effect of midazolam pre-medication on rocuronium-induced neuromuscular blockade. *J. Int. Med. Res.* 30: 318–321.

Hiller, A., Olkkola, K.T., Isohanni, P., and Saarnivaara, L. (1990). Unconsciousness associated with midazolam and erythromycin. *Br. J. Anaesth.* 65: 826–828.

Hoffman, W.E., Miletich, D.J., and Albrecht, R.F. (1986). The effects of midazolam on cerebral blood-flow and oxygen-consumption and its interaction with nitrous-oxide. *Anesth. Anal.* 65: 729–733.

Holsti, M., Sill, B.L., Firth, S.D. et al. (2007). Prehospital intranasal midazolam for the treatment of pediatric seizures. *Pediatr. Emerg. Care* 23: 148–153.

Hopkins, A., Giuffrida, M., and Larenza, M.P. (2014). Midazolam, as a co-induction agent, has propofol sparing effects but also decreases systolic blood pressure in healthy dogs. *Vet. Anaesth. Analg.* 41: 64–72.

Hubbell, J.A., Kelly, E.M., Aarnes, T.K. et al. (2013). Pharmacokinetics of midazolam after intravenous administration to horses. *Equine Vet. J.* 45: 721–725.

Italiano, M. and Robinson, R. (2018). Effect of benzodiazepines on the dose of alfaxalone needed for endotracheal intubation in healthy dogs. *Vet. Anaesth. Analg.* 45: 720–728.

Jackson, A.M., Tobias, K., Long, C. et al. (2004). Effects of various anesthetic agents on laryngeal motion during laryngoscopy in normal dogs. *Vet. Surg.* 33: 102–106.

Johnson, T.N., Rostami-Hodjegan, A., Goddard, J.M. et al. (2002). Contribution of midazolam and its 1-hydroxy metabolite to preoperative sedation in children: a pharmacokinetic-pharmacodynamic analysis. *Br. J. Anaesth.* 89: 428–437.

Jones, D.J., Stehling, L.C., and Zauder, H.L. (1979). Cardiovascular responses to diazepam and midazolam maleate in the dog. *Anesthesiology* 51: 430–434.

Katzung, B.G. (2004). *Basic & Clinical Pharmacology*. New York: Lange Medical Books/McGraw Hill.

Keegan, R.D., Greene, S.A., Moore, M.P., and Gallagher, L.V. (1993). Antagonism by flumazenil of midazolam-induced changes in quantitative electroencephalographic data from isoflurane-anesthetized dogs. *Am. J. Vet. Res.* 54: 761–765.

Kissin, I., Brown, P.T., and Bradley, E.L. Jr. (1990). Morphine and fentanyl anesthetic interactions with diazepam: relative antagonism in rats. *Anesth. Analg.* 71: 236–241.

Klotz, U. (1988). Drug interactions and clinical pharmacokinetics of flumazenil. *Eur. J. Anaesthesiol. Suppl.* 2: 103–108.

Kudoh, A., Takase, H., Takahira, Y., and Takazawa, T. (2004). Postoperative confusion increases in elderly long-term benzodiazepine users. *Anesth. Analg.* 99: 1674–1678. table of contents.

Kukanich, B. and Nauss, J.L. (2012). Pharmacokinetics of the cytochrome P-450 substrates phenytoin, theophylline, and diazepam in healthy Greyhound dogs. *J. Vet. Pharmacol. Ther.* 35: 275–281.

Laccetti, M., Manes, G., Uomo, G. et al. (2000). Flumazenil in the treatment of acute hepatic encephalopathy in cirrhotic patients: a double blind randomized placebo controlled study. *Dig. Liver Dis.* 32: 335–338.

Lee, A. and Shirley, M. (2021). Remimazolam: a review in procedural sedation. *Drugs* 81: 1193–1201.

Liao, P., Sinclair, M., Valverde, A. et al. (2017). Induction dose and recovery quality of propofol and alfaxalone with or without midazolam coinduction followed by total intravenous anesthesia in dogs. *Vet. Anaesth. Analg.* 44: 1016–1026.

Long, C.F., Zhang, Y., and Lou, Y.C. (1997). Effects of rifampin and isoniazid on the pharmacokinetics of diazepam in rabbits. *Yao Xue Xue Bao* 32: 481–484.

Loscher, W. and Frey, H.H. (1981). Pharmacokinetics of diazepam in the dog. *Arch. Int. Pharmacodyn. Ther.* 254: 180–195.

Low, K., Crestani, F., Keist, R. et al. (2000). Molecular and neuronal substrate for the selective attenuation of anxiety. *Science* 290: 131–134.

Mariani, C.L., Clemmons, R.M., Lee-Ambrose, L. et al. (2003). *A Comparison of Intransal and Intravenous Lorazepam in Normal Dogs*. Charlotte, NC, USA: ACVIM.

Martens, H.J., De Goede, P.N., and Van Loenen, A.C. (1990). Sorption of various drugs in polyvinyl chloride, glass, and polyethylene-lined infusion containers. *Am. J. Hosp. Pharm.* 47: 369–373.

Martin, W.R., Sloan, J.W., and Wala, E. (1990). Precipitated abstinence in orally dosed benzodiazepine-dependent dogs. *J. Pharmacol. Exp. Ther.* 255: 744–755.

Matthews, N.S., Dollar, N.S., and Shawley, R.V. (1990). Halothane-sparing effect of benzodiazepines in ponies. *Cornell Vet.* 80: 259–265.

McKernan, R.M., Rosahl, T.W., Reynolds, D.S. et al. (2000). Sedative but not anxiolytic properties of benzodiazepines are mediated by the GABA(A) receptor alpha1 subtype. *Nat. Neurosci.* 3: 587–592.

McNicholas, L.F., Martin, W.R., and Cherian, S. (1983). Physical dependence on diazepam and lorazepam in the dog. *J. Pharmacol. Exp. Ther.* 226: 783–789.

Mereu, G.P., Fratta, W., Chessa, P., and Gessa, G.L. (1976). Voraciousness induced in cats by benzodiazepines. *Psychopharmacology (Berl.)* 47: 101–103.

Morgan, G.E., Mikhail, M.S., and Murray, M.J. (2006). *Clinical Anesthesiology*. New York: Lange Medical Books/McGraw Hill, Medical Pub. Division.

Muir, W.W., Sams, R.A., Huffman, R.H., and Noonan, J.S. (1982). Pharmacodynamic and pharmacokinetic properties of diazepam in horses. *Am. J. Vet. Res.* 43: 1756–1762.

Muller, W.E. (1977). The influence of plasma protein binding on distribution and pharmacological activity of tranquilizers of the benzodiazepine group (author's transl). *Klin. Wochenschr.* 55: 105–110.

Muñoz, K.A., Robertson, S.A., and Wilson, D.V. (2017). Alfaxalone alone or combined with midazolam or ketamine in dogs: intubation dose and select physiologic effects. *Vet. Anaesth. Analg.* 44: 766–774.

Musulin, S.E., Mariani, C.L., and Papich, M.G. (2011). Diazepam pharmacokinetics after nasal drop and atomized nasal administration in dogs. *J. Vet. Pharmacol. Ther.* 34: 17–24.

Nagashima, A., Tanaka, E., Inomata, S. et al. (2005). A study of the in vitro interaction between lidocaine and premedications using human liver microsomes. *J. Clin. Pharm. Ther.* 30: 185–188.

Nelissen, P., Corletto, F., Aprea, F., and White, R.A. (2012). Effect of three anesthetic induction protocols on laryngeal motion during laryngoscopy in normal cats. *Vet. Surg.* 41: 876–883.

Norman, W.M., Court, M.H., and Greenblatt, D.J. (1997). Age-related changes in the pharmacokinetic disposition of diazepam in foals. *Am. J. Vet. Res.* 58: 878–880.

Obradovic, D.I., Savic, M.M., Andjelkovic, D.S. et al. (2004). The influence of midazolam on active avoidance retrieval and acquisition rate in rats. *Pharmacol. Biochem. Behav.* 77: 77–83.

Oliver, F.M., Sweatman, T.W., Unkel, J.H. et al. (2000). Comparative pharmacokinetics of submucosal vs. intravenous flumazenil (Romazicon) in an animal model. *Pediatr. Dent.* 22: 489–493.

Papich, M.G. and Alcorn, J. (1995). Absorption of diazepam after its rectal administration in dogs. *Am. J. Vet. Res.* 56: 1629–1636.

Park, F.M. (2012). Successful treatment of hepatic failure secondary to diazepam administration in a cat. *J. Feline Med. Surg.* 14: 158–160.

Platt, S.R., Randell, S.C., Scott, K.C. et al. (2000). Comparison of plasma benzodiazepine concentrations following intranasal and intravenous administration of diazepam to dogs. *Am. J. Vet. Res.* 61: 651–654.

Plumb, D.C. (2015). *Plumb's Veterinary Drug Handbook*. Stockholm, Wisconsin: Wiley.

Podell, M. (1995). The use of diazepam per rectum at home for the acute management of cluster seizures in dogs. *J. Vet. Intern. Med.* 9: 68–74.

Podell, M. (1996). Seizures in dogs. *Vet. Clin. North Am. Small Anim. Pract.* 26: 779–809.

Podell, M., Smeak, D., and Lord, L.K. (1998a). Diazepam used to control cluster seizures in dogs. *J. Vet. Intern. Med.* 12: 120–121.

Podell, M., Wagner, S.O., and Sams, R.A. (1998b). Lorazepam concentrations in plasma following its intravenous and rectal administration in dogs. *J. Vet. Pharmacol. Ther.* 21: 158–160.

Probst, C.W., Thomas, W.B., Moyers, T.D. et al. (2013). Evaluation of plasma diazepam and nordiazepam concentrations following administration of diazepam intravenously or via suppository per rectum in dogs. *Am. J. Vet. Res.* 74: 611–615.

Reves, J.G., Fragen, R.J., Vinik, H.R., and Greenblatt, D.J. (1985). Midazolam: pharmacology and uses. *Anesthesiol.* 62: 310–324.

Riviere, J.E. and Papich, M.G. (2009). *Veterinary Pharmacology and Therapeutics*. Ames, Iowa: Wiley-Blackwell.

Robinson, R. and Borer-Weir, K. (2015). The effects of diazepam or midazolam on the dose of propofol required to induce anaesthesia in cats. *Vet. Anaesth. Analg.* 42: 493–501.

Rousseau-Blass, F., Cribb, A.E., Beaudry, F., and Pang, D.S. (2021). A pharmacokinetic-pharmacodynamic study of intravenous midazolam and flumazenil in adult New Zealand White-Californian rabbits (*Oryctolagus cuniculus*). *J. Am. Assoc. Lab. Anim. Sci.* 60: 319–328.

Santos Gonzalez, M., Bertran De Lis, B.T., and Tendillo Cortijo, F.J. (2013). Effects of intramuscular alfaxalone

alone or in combination with diazepam in swine. *Vet. Anaesth. Analg.* 40: 399–402.

Schwartz, M., Munana, K.R., Nettifee-Osborne, J.A. et al. (2013). The pharmacokinetics of midazolam after intravenous, intramuscular, and rectal administration in healthy dogs. *J. Vet. Pharmacol. Ther.* 36: 471–477.

Schwieger, I.M., Szlam, F., and Hug, C.C. Jr. (1989). Absence of agonistic or antagonistic effect of flumazenil (Ro 15-1788) in dogs anesthetized with enflurane, isoflurane, or fentanyl-enflurane. *Anesthesiol.* 70: 477–480.

Seddighi, R., Egger, C.M., Rohrbach, B.W. et al. (2011). The effect of midazolam on the end-tidal concentration of isoflurane necessary to prevent movement in dogs. *Vet. Anaesth. Analg.* 38: 195–202.

Sherman, B.L. (2008). Separation anxiety in dogs. *Compend. Contin. Educ. Vet.* 30: 27–42.

Simon, B.T., Scallan, E.M., Odette, O. et al. (2017). Pharmacokinetics and pharmacodynamics of midazolam following intravenous and intramuscular administration to sheep. *Am. J. Vet. Res.* 78: 539–549.

Spivey, W.H. (1992). Flumazenil and seizures: analysis of 43 cases. *Clin. Ther.* 14: 292–305.

Steyn, P.F., Twedt, D., and Toombs, W. (1997). The effect of intravenous diazepam on solid phase gastric emptying in normal cats. *Vet. Radiol. Ultrasound* 38: 469–473.

Stoelting, R.K., Hillier, S., and Stoelting, R.K. (2006). *Handbook of Pharmacology & Physiology in Anesthetic Practice*. Philadelphia: Lippincott Williams & Wilkins.

Tannenbaum, C., Paquette, A., Hilmer, S. et al. (2012). A systematic review of amnestic and non-amnestic mild cognitive impairment induced by anticholinergic, antihistamine, GABAergic and opioid drugs. *Drugs Aging* 29: 639–658.

Terhaag, B. and Bockisch, A. (1976). Antihemolytic effect of various benzodiazepines on human erythrocytes. *Acta Biol. Med. Ger.* 35: 1415–1417.

Treleano, A., Wolz, G., Brandsch, R., and Welle, F. (2009). Investigation into the sorption of nitroglycerin and diazepam into PVC tubes and alternative tube materials during application. *Int. J. Pharm.* 369: 30–37.

Unkel, J.H., Brickhouse, T.H., Sweatman, T.W. et al. (2006). A comparison of 3 routes of flumazenil administration to reverse benzodiazepine-induced desaturation in an animal model. *Pediatr. Dent.* 28: 357–362.

Upton, R.N., Ludbrook, G.L., Grant, C., and Martinez, A. (2001). In vivo cerebral pharmacokinetics and pharmacodynamics of diazepam and midazolam after short intravenous infusion administration in sheep. *J. Pharmacokinet. Pharmacodyn.* 28: 129–153.

Van Miert, A.S., Koot, M., and Van Duin, C.T. (1989). Appetite-modulating drugs in dwarf goats, with special emphasis on benzodiazepine-induced hyperphagia and its antagonism by flumazenil and RO 15-3505. *J. Vet. Pharmacol. Ther.* 12: 147–156.

Vanderk, L.E., Vanrossu, J.M., Muskens, E.T.J., and Rijntjes, N.V. (1971). Pharmacokinetics of diazepam in dogs, mice and humans. *Acta Pharmacol. Toxicol.* 29: 109–127.

Vinik, H.R., Reves, J.G., Greenblatt, D.J. et al. (1983). The pharmacokinetics of midazolam in chronic renal failure patients. *Anesthesiol.* 59: 390–394.

Wagner, S.O., Sams, R.A., and Podell, M. (1998). Chronic phenobarbital therapy reduces plasma benzodiazepine concentrations after intravenous and rectal administration of diazepam in the dog. *J. Vet. Pharmacol. Ther.* 21: 335–341.

Wala, E., McNicholas, L.F., Sloan, J.W., and Martin, W.R. (1988). Flumazenil oral absorption in dogs. *Pharmacol. Biochem. Behav.* 30: 945–948.

Wauquier, A., Ashton, D., and Melis, W. (1979). Behavioral analysis of amygdaloid kindling in beagle dogs and the effects of clonazepam, diazepam, phenobarbital, diphenylhydantoin, and flunarizine on seizure manifestation. *Exp. Neurol.* 64: 579–586.

Winsnes, M., Jeppsson, R., and Sjoberg, B. (1981). Diazepam adsorption to infusion sets and plastic syringes. *Acta Anaesthesiol. Scand.* 25: 93–96.

Zapata, A., Laredo, F.G., Escobar, M. et al. (2018). Effects of midazolam before or after alfaxalone for co-induction of anaesthesia in healthy dogs. *Vet. Anaesth. Analg.* 45: 609–617.

Zhang, J., Niu, S., Zhang, H., and Streisand, J.B. (2002). Oral mucosal absorption of midazolam in dogs is strongly pH dependent. *J. Pharm. Sci.* 91: 980–982.

7

Opioid Agonists and Antagonists

Phillip Lerche

Introduction

Opioids are considered to be the most effective class of drugs that provide analgesia in the face of severe pain, including the acute pain associated with surgery. They are commonly used in veterinary anesthesia to provide analgesia to treat preoperative, intraoperative, and postoperative pain, as well as to treat the intense pain caused by some disease processes, e.g. pleuritis, peritonitis and pancreatitis. Opioids are also frequently used in combination with sedatives for enhanced sedation, known as neuroleptanalgesia, or, with the addition of drugs like ketamine, as part of total injectable anesthetic techniques. Ultrapotent opioids are used to sedate and/or immobilize free-roaming wildlife.

Mechanism of Action

Opioids act at opioid receptors which are found in many of the body's tissues, including the central nervous system (CNS), the peripheral nervous system (sensory nerves), gastrointestinal (GI) system, urinary system, synovial membranes and macrophages. Opioid receptors are part of the G protein-coupled receptor family. Endogenous (e.g. endorphins) and exogenous (e.g. opioid drugs like morphine) ligands bind to opioid receptors, activating the Gα and Gβγ subunits which exert effects via second messenger systems. These effects lead to decreases in intracellular ionized calcium and inhibition of release of excitatory neurotransmitters like glutamate and substance P. Additionally, activation of G protein-coupled with inwardly rectifying potassium channels results in hyperpolarization of neurons and increased activation thresholds of nociceptive receptors. The overall impact is a reduction in the excitatory signal in the nociceptive pathway (Che et al. 2021).

Three main subtypes of opioid receptors have been identified. The mu, kappa, and delta subtypes correspond to the endogenous ligands endorphins, dynorphins, and enkephalins. A fourth opioid receptor subtype, the orphanin or nociceptin opioid receptor, that nociceptin binds to, has also been identified. The investigation of compounds that act as agonists at nociceptin receptors is ongoing, as they may produce analgesia with fewer side effects and decreased potential for addiction in people (El Daibani and Che 2022).

In dogs, polymorphism of the mu opioid receptor gene has been demonstrated (Hawley and Wetmore 2010). The impact of this has not been fully elucidated, however, it may be associated with dysphoria seen in certain breeds (Alaskan malamute, Siberian husky, Labrador retriever). Genetic polymorphism of the mu opioid receptor has also been found in horses, which is associated with increased opioid-induced locomotor side effects (Wetmore et al. 2016).

Opioid drugs are classified based on their activity at the opioid receptors (Table 7.1). They can be classified as agonists (e.g. morphine), partial agonists (buprenorphine), agonist-antagonists, (e.g. butorphanol), or antagonists (e.g. naloxone).

Pharmacokinetics

Opioids are typically administered parenterally in the perianesthetic period. Opioids can be given by intravenous (IV), intramuscular (IM), and by subcutaneous (SC) injection. Additionally, some opioids are available in formulations that allow for transdermal (TD) application (topical buprenorphine for use in cats; fentanyl patches). Opioids are lipophilic drugs, and therefore well-absorbed from these routes, including when administered by mouth (PO). Orally administered opioids are subject to first-pass metabolism by the liver in animals, making this route of administration much less effective, and therefore

Table 7.1 Opioid receptors and their endogenous and exogenous ligands.

	Mu opioid receptor	Kappa opioid receptor	Delta opioid receptor
Endogenous agonists	Endorphins Dynorphins Enkephalins	Dynorphins	Enkephalins
Agonists	Morphine Hydromorphone Methadone Meperidine Oxymorphone Fentanyl Sufentanil Alfentanil Remifentanil Etorphine Carfentanil Thiafentanil	Butorphanol Nalbuphine Pentazocine Meperidine Etorphine	Morphine Fentanyl Pentazocine Etorphine
Partial agonist	Buprenorphine		
Antagonists	Naloxone Naltrexone Methylnaltrexone Butorphanol Nalbuphine Pentazocine	Naloxone Naltrexone	Naloxone Naltrexone

infrequently used in veterinary anesthesia. Buprenorphine has been shown to be relatively well-absorbed in cats after oral transmucosal (OTM) administration between the cheek and the teeth, although bioavailability will be altered if it is swallowed or if some exits via the mouth, and can be impacted by mucosal intracellular enzymes and local pH. Buprenorphine and naloxone have been administered via the intranasal (IN) route in dogs. The large surface area and vascularity of the nasal mucosa promotes absorption, although drug can be lost due to sneezing or swallowing. Opioids can also be administered into joints. Lastly, opioids can be administered into the epidural space or intrathecally.

Distribution of opioids is a function of drug lipophilicity and regional blood flow. Lipophilicity of fentanyl, sufentanil, and meperidine are significantly higher than for morphine and hydromorphone, thus contributing to the more rapid onset and shorter duration of action of the former compared to the latter (Lötsch et al. 2013). The lower lipophilicity of a drug like morphine makes it a suitable option for epidural administration, as it will equilibrate with the systemic circulation at a relatively slow rate, thus remaining effective in the epidural space longer with fewer systemic side effects compared to parenteral administration.

Additionally, P-glycoprotein (P-gp) transporters that form part of the blood-brain barrier are responsible for returning some opioids from the CNS to the systemic circulation against a concentration gradient (Tournier et al. 2011). A mutation of the *ABCB1-1Δ* (formerly *MDR1*) gene that can decrease the function of the ABCB1-1Δ P-gp transporter in affected dogs of sheep-herding breeds may result in prolonged effects of butorphanol (Gramer et al. 2011; Grubb et al. 2020). Opioids readily cross the placental barrier.

Opioids undergo hepatic biotransformation via phase 1 and/or phase 2 processes. Morphine, for example, is metabolized in dogs via glucuronidation, with the major metabolite being morphine-3-glucuronide. In cats, only a small amount of morphine undergoes glucuronidation, and the major metabolite via sulfate conjugation is morphine-3-ethereal sulfate (Garrett and Jackson 1979; Yeh et al. 1971). Unique among the opioids, remifentanil undergoes hydrolysis by plasma esterases (Egan et al. 1993).

Elimination of opioid parent compounds and their metabolites occurs via renal and biliary excretion.

Pharmacokinetic parameters are given below in the section on individual drugs.

Note that limited pharmacokinetic information is available for opioids in ruminants and pigs. Clinically, doses similar to those used in horses are often used for acute pain management. Clinicians should always consider whether use of drugs that do not have published withdrawal times is appropriate in animals that may enter the food supply.

Pharmacodynamics

Opioids are considered to be the most effective class of drugs to manage severe pain, including perioperative pain. In general, opioids that are full mu opioid receptor agonists are associated with providing the greatest degree of analgesia, however, agonism of the mu opioid receptor is also associated with greater side effects. Many effects are common to most opioid agonists and are summarized in Table 7.2.

Nervous System Effects – Analgesia

As previously mentioned, opioid agonism at all opioid receptors decreases nociceptive signaling in the nervous system, both in the spinal cord and in supraspinal structures (periaqueductal grey matter, locus ceruleus, rostral ventromedial medulla), resulting in an antinociceptive, i.e. analgesic, effect (Stein 2018). The antinociceptive effects of opioids are well documented in animals (Houghton et al. 1991; Pieper et al. 2011; Chiavaccini et al. 2017; Love et al. 2015; Reed et al. 2019; Adami and Spadavecchia 2020). Administration of opioids peripherally, e.g. by intra-articular (IA) injection, is also effective in producing analgesia (Lindegaard et al. 2010; Day et al. 1995).

Table 7.2 Effects of opioid receptor agonists.

Body system	Mu opioid receptor	Kappa opioid receptor	Delta opioid receptor
Central nervous system and pupil	• Supraspinal and spinal analgesia • Euphoria • Sedation • Dysphoria • Excitement • Miosis (dog) • Midriasis (cat, horse) • Increased locomotor activity (horse)	• Supraspinal and spinal analgesia • Sedation • Miosis (dog) • Midriasis (cat, horse)	• Supraspinal and spinal analgesia
Cardiovascular system	• Bradycardia • Vasodilation due to histamine release (morphine, meperidine)		
Respiratory system	• Depression • Panting (dogs) • Antitussive	• Antitussive	
Gastrointestinal system	• Emesis • Anti-emesis • Decreased motility • Decreased secretions • Increased pyloric sphincter tone • Colic (horses)	• Anti-emesis • Decreased motility • Decreased secretions	• Emesis
Urinary effects	• Urinary retention • Increased bladder sphincter tone		
Thermoregulation	• Hypothermia • Hyperthermia (cats)		
Integumentary	• Pruritus		

CNS Sedation and Excitation

Systemically administered opioids most commonly produce sedation (Monteiro et al. 2008). Dysphoria and excitement can also occur, with some breed prevalence in dogs (e.g. so-called northern breeds, like the Siberian husky) (Hawley and Wetmore 2010). Horses and cats are more likely to show excitement than other species (Pascoe et al. 1991; Benson and Thurmon 1987). At clinically effective doses of opioids, excitement is not commonly seen in cats (Steagall et al. 2006). Combining a sedative with an opioid (neuroleptanalgesia) minimizes excitement.

Opioids can cause increased locomotor activity in horses (Pascoe et al. 1991). Administration of a sedative (e.g. ace-promazine) or opioid antagonist (naloxone) diminishes or abolishes this behavior (Combie et al. 1981).

Ocular Effects

Opioids can cause miosis or midriasis. Miosis is the most common effect in dogs, with midriasis being more commonly seen in cats and horses (Sharpe and Pickworth 1985; Hamra et al. 1993). This is thought to be due to species differences in effect at the Edinger-Westphal nucleus, which lies dorsal to the oculomotor nucleus in the midbrain. There is also conflicting evidence as to whether peripheral opioid receptors on the iris can impact pupil size (Murray et al. 1983).

Cardiovascular Effects

The most common effect of opioids on the cardiovascular system is bradycardia. This is a central effect, shown in dogs to be due to opioid receptor agonism in the nucleus ambiguus, located in the medulla oblongata, with resultant increased vagal output (Laubie et al. 1979). Opioid-induced bradycardia is therefore typically responsive to anticholinergic therapy.

In dogs, morphine at doses of 0.6 mg/kg and higher when given IV, particularly if administered rapidly, causes histamine release from mast cells which can lead to hypotension (Guedes et al. 2006; Schurig et al. 1978). The magnitude of histamine release is not consistent among individual dogs (Guedes et al. 2006). The mechanism for histamine release is unclear. Administration of naloxone does not prevent histamine release, thus is not due to activity at opioid receptors. Morphine (0.5 mg/kg IM) administered to dogs with mast cell tumor disease did not result in cardiovascular changes compared to dogs with soft-tissue sarcomas (Curley et al. 2021). Meperidine and codeine also have the potential to cause histamine release (Blunk et al. 2004). Morphine (0.15 mg/kg IV followed by 0.1 mg/kg/h IV) and butorphanol (0.05 mg/kg IV followed by 0.01 mg/kg/h IV) cause a similar amount of histamine release in horses (Duke-Novakovski et al. 2021).

Respiratory Effects

Supraspinal opioid receptor agonism results in respiratory depression. This is characterized by a decreased sensitivity of the ventilatory centers to $PaCO_2$. For example, fentanyl (15 µg/kg IV) given to awake dogs and dogs sedated with a medetomidine infusion (1.5 µg/kg/h) resulted in an increase in $PaCO_2$ and a decrease in pH in both groups, with a significant decrease in pO_2 in the sedated dogs (Grimm et al. 2005). Inhalant anesthetics and most injectable general anesthetics decrease minute ventilation, therefore concomitant opioid administration can be expected to exacerbate respiratory depression. Most patients under general anesthesia breathe an increased fraction of inspired oxygen, often with $FiO_2 = 1$, therefore pCO_2 may be elevated while pO_2 remains within clinically acceptable limits. Opioids have also been shown to cause marked panting in dogs (Ryan et al. 2022).

Opioids have antitussive effects via depression of medullary cough centers. Oral formulations of codeine, hydrocodone, and butorphanol can be used to suppress coughing in dogs. Butorphanol given SC was 100 and 4 times more effective at reducing cough compared to codeine and morphine respectively (Cavanagh et al. 1976). In the same study, orally administered butorphanol was 15–20 times more effective than morphine, likely due to the significant first-pass effect when morphine is given enterally. In horses, neither codeine (0.6 mg/kg PO) nor butorphanol (0.02 mg/kg IV) were effective in reducing coughing in response to bronchoalveolar lavage when given 2 hours and 20 minutes respectively prior to the procedure (Westermann et al. 2005).

Gastrointestinal Effects

Opioids can cause nausea and vomiting and can also have anti-emetic effects (Blancquaert et al. 1986). This can be explained due to different effects at the chemoreceptor trigger zone (CTZ) located in the floor of the fourth ventricle, which has emetic effects and lies partly outside the blood-brain barrier (BBB), and the vomiting center (VC), which has anti-emetic function and lies within the BBB. Several mechanisms have been suggested as being responsible for nausea and vomiting, including increased vestibular sensitivity possibly mediated by kappa and delta opioid receptors in the inner ear, delayed gastric emptying and decreased intestinal motility, as well as stimulation of

dopamine, mu opioid and delta opioid receptors in the CTZ (Smith and Laufer 2014). For example, opioid-induced nausea and vomiting can be ameliorated by prior administration of acepromazine, a dopamine antagonist and naloxone, an opioid antagonist at all opioid receptors (Valverde et al. 2004; Takahashi et al. 2007). Methadone causes less vomiting than morphine in dogs. This is likely due to it being more lipophilic than morphine, and therefore it distributes rapidly across the BBB to the VC. Morphine's lower lipophilicity will result in it distributing more slowly across the BBB, with emetic effects mediated via the CTZ occurring before it penetrates to the VC (Blancquaert et al. 1986). Despite this difference in the two drugs, methadone can cause nausea and vomiting in dogs (Ryan et al. 2022). Methadone given every four hours to dogs after tibial plateau leveling osteotomy (TPLO) also caused nausea and vomiting, however, when methadone was given based on pain-scoring criteria, vomiting was decreased (Bini et al. 2018). This supports the clinical observation that emesis is more commonly seen when administering opioids to non-painful animals vs those that are painful (Pascoe 2000; KuKanich and Weise 2015b). Mu opioid agonists decrease the tone of the lower esophageal sphincter (LES), although meperidine resulted in a lower incidence of gastro-esophageal reflux compared to morphine in isoflurane-anesthetized dogs (Wilson et al. 2007). Many non-opioid factors decrease LES tone in cats and dogs, including administration of sedatives, atropine, IV anesthetic induction agents and inhalant anesthetics, as well as patient and procedure factors (Figueiredo 2022). Diminishing perioperative nausea and vomiting and regurgitation is an important goal in veterinary anesthesia, and the pharmacology of anti-nausea, anti-emetic, and prokinetic drugs used in the perioperative period are discussed in Chapter 27.

Opioids that are mu opioid receptor agonists increase pyloric sphincter tone in dogs (McFadzean et al. 2017). This contrasts with cats, where butorphanol and hydromorphone did not impact the passage of an endoscope through the pylorus (Smith et al. 2004).

Many factors can contribute to post-operative ileus, including the stress associated with anesthesia and surgery causing endogenous opioid release, duration of surgery, and type of surgery, with abdominal surgery more likely to result in ileus, and opioid administration (de Boer et al. 2017).

Systemic administration of mu opioid receptor agonists decreases propulsive peristalsis in the GI tract, resulting in delayed gastric emptying and ileus, which can lead to constipation. These effects are mediated by central as well as peripheral opioid receptors. In rats, mu opioid receptors in the lateral cerebral ventricle are associated with decreased gastric motility (Tsuchida et al. 2004). Opioid receptors are present throughout the GI tract and are found in submucosal and mesenteric nerve plexuses (Sternini et al. 2004). Agonism of opioid receptors at these sites interferes with normal propulsive activity by decreasing the release of the neurotransmitters acetyl choline and substance P.

Post-operative ileus has been shown to last up to 72 hours in people, and clinical experience suggests that this is similar and well-tolerated in healthy cats and dogs (de Boer et al. 2017; KuKanich and Weise 2015b). In an experimental model of intestinal surgery without opioid use, dogs, and sheep had post-operative ileus for 24 and 72 hours (Bueno et al. 1978). Epidural administration of morphine resulted in shorter times to return to normal contractile activity in the proximal GI tract compared to IV morphine (Nakayoshi et al. 2007). In equids, opioid agonists (meperidine) and agonist/antagonists (butorphanol, pentazocine) decrease intestinal motility (Sojka et al. 1988). Other factors contribute to the development of postoperative ileus in horses including presence of a small intestinal lesion, preoperative nasogastric reflux, and duration of anesthesia, as well as use of alpha$_2$ agonists (Cohen et al. 2004; Merritt et al. 1998). The scientific literature presents conflicting information as to the risk of opioids, particularly full agonists, resulting in colic in horses. In one study, the risk of colic occurring after orthopedic surgery in horses was four times greater than when butorphanol or no opioids were given (Senior et al. 2004). Another study showed no increased risk when morphine was given to horses anesthetized for MRI or non-abdominal surgery (Andersen et al. 2006). As with ileus, the risk of horses developing colic is multifactorial, and includes intrinsic factors (e.g. sex, age, and breed), use of antibiotics, recent changes in housing or diet and abdominal surgery (Gonçalves et al. 2002; Andersen et al. 2006; Cohen et al. 1999; Proudman et al. 2002). Despite this, it is prudent when using mu agonist opioids in equine anesthesia to closely monitor horses for signs of postoperative ileus and colic.

Urinary Effects

Epidural and intrathecal administration of morphine can lead to urinary retention, increased urinary sphincter tone and inhibition of micturition. Post-operative urinary retention after epidural morphine was observed in 7 of 242 dogs (2.9%) and 2 of 23 cats (8.7%) (Troncy et al. 2002). In another study in dogs undergoing orthopedic surgery, urinary retention was lower with epidural (3%) compared to systemic administration of morphine (8%) (Peterson et al. 2014). Mu opioid receptor agonists decreased urine output (Anderson and Day 2008). This may be due to increased release of vasopressin (antidiuretic hormone) in the case of fentanyl, however, this was not the case with morphine (Biswai et al. 1976; Robertson et al. 2001). Agonism of kappa opioid receptors suppressed release of vasopressin leading to increased urine output (Leander et al. 1985).

Integumentary Effects

Intrathecal administration of morphine caused discomfort that the authors attributed to pruritus in 8% of dogs undergoing orthopedic surgery (Sarotti et al. 2013). Epidural morphine did not result in pruritus in dogs (Naganobu et al. 2004). Pruritus after intrathecal and epidural morphine has been reported in cats, as well as after epidural morphine in horses (Gent et al. 2013; Burford and Corley 2006). Signs of pruritus have also been noted following intrathecal morphine administration in sheep (Wagner et al. 1996).

Thermoregulatory Effects

Opioids interrupt thermoregulatory processes via direct action at the hypothalamus, commonly resulting in hypothermia in domestic animals. Post-operative hyperthermia can occur in cats after opioid administration (Posner et al. 2007; Posner et al. 2010). Morphine and hydromorphone have been shown to increase temperature in horses (Figueiredo et al. 2012, Reed et al. 2019).

Effect on Inhalant Anesthetic Requirement

Opioids have been shown to reduce the minimum alveolar concentration (MAC) of inhalant anesthetics in dogs in a dose-dependent fashion (Reed and Doherty 2018). Greater MAC reduction is seen with mu opioid receptor agonists compared to partial mu opioid receptor agonists, and kappa opioid receptor agonists produce only mild decreases in MAC. Mu opioid receptor agonists have also been shown to reduce MAC in cats, ruminants, and pigs (Machado et al. 2018; Sayre et al. 2015; Dzikiti et al. 2011; Greene et al. 2004). In horses, morphine does not consistently have the same effect on MAC that is seen in other species, and at higher doses (2 mg/kg) increased MAC by 11% (Steffey et al. 2003).

Interactions with Sedatives

Combining sedatives like acepromazine and alpha$_2$ agonists with opioids (neuroleptanalgesia) enhances sedation (Gomes and Marques 2022; Corletto et al. 2005). Applying the principle of neuroleptanalgesia allows lower doses of both sedative and opioid to be used for sedation, which may decrease side effects of each individual drug used. However, when sedatives share similar side effects with opioids they may be exacerbated, e.g. bradycardia, respiratory depression and changes to GI motility seen with alpha$_2$ agonists. Opioids are commonly used as part of combinations with ketamine and alpha$_2$ agonists that, when administered IV or IM, produce heavy sedation or general anesthesia in cats, dogs, and pigs (Posner et al. 2020; De Monte et al. 2015). The degree of sedation and anesthesia produced in individuals of a species can vary considerably with these combinations, therefore, close monitoring is advised so that interventions to support ventilation and cardiovascular function can be carried out in a timely manner.

Interactions with Selective Serotonin Reuptake Inhibitors

Selective serotonin reuptake inhibitors (SSRIs), e.g. fluoxetine, are used to treat a variety of behavioral disorders in animals. Meperidine, fentanyl and fentanyl derivatives act as weak SSRIs (Greenier et al. 2014). The use of these opioids in patients receiving SSRIs is not contra-indicated, however, they could contribute to development of serotonin syndrome (see Chapter 22).

Opioid Agonists

Opioid agonists have the ability to fully agonize the mu opioid receptor, and they may also act as agonists at kappa and delta opioid receptors. They are frequently referred to as mu agonists, or full agonists.

Morphine

Morphine was isolated from opium over 200 years ago, with the analgesic benefits of opium having been known for thousands of years (Wicks et al. 2021). The discovery of morphine's structure and the ability to synthesize it led to the development of other opioid drugs (Figure 7.1). Pharmacokinetic data for morphine are presented in

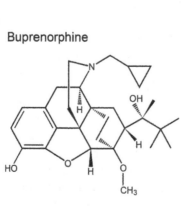

Figure 7.1 Chemical structures of selected opioids.

Table 7.3 Selected pharmacokinetic parameters for morphine in cats, dogs, and horses.

Species	Dose (mg/kg)	Route	F (%)	C_{max} (ng/ml)	T_{max} (h)	$t_{1/2}$ (h)	V (l/kg)	Cl (ml/min/kg)	References
Dog	0.5	IV	—	135 (C_0)	—	1.2	4.6	62.5	KuKanich et al.
	1.6	Oral (extended release tablets)	5	5	2	1.4	—	—	(2005b)
	0.5	IV	—	—	—	1.6	7.2	85.2	Barnhart et al. (2000)
	1	IM	119	185	0.08	1.4	6.8	91.2	
	5	Rectal	19	51	0.5	1.6	7.5	92.6	
Cat	0.2	IV	—	—	—	1.3	2.6	24.1	Taylor et al. (2001)
	0.2	IM	—	120	0.25	1.6	1.7	13.9	
Horse	0.05	IV	—	—	—	8.2	12.1	24.3	Hamamoto-Hardman
	0.1	IV	—	—	—	9.5	11.5	27.4	et al. (2019)
	0.1	IM	—	31	0.31	1.5	4.5	34.9	Devine et al. (2013)

F, bioavailability, C_{max}, maximum plasma concentration, T_{max}, time to reach C_{max}, $t_{1/2}$, terminal elimination half-life, V, apparent volume of distribution, Cl, clearance, C_0, concentration at time zero.

Table 7.3. As discussed earlier, morphine's lipophilicity is relatively low, which can lead to a lag time (slower onset time) of up to 15 minutes, making it ideal for epidural administration as duration of action will be prolonged, e.g. 10–24 hours in dogs (Torske and Dyson 2000). A pharmacokinetic/pharmacodynamic study assessing dose/response to nociception using von Frey filaments in dogs showed that response to noxious stimulus was decreased for four hours following morphine 1 mg/kg IV (KuKanich et al. 2005a). An oral formulation of extended-release morphine had a bioavailability of 5.3% in dogs, therefore, this route of administration of morphine is not recommended (KuKanich et al. 2005b). Volume of distribution is lower in cats compared to dogs, and lower doses can be used (Table 7.4). In horses, elimination half-life is longer than in cats and dogs, therefore the recommended dosing interval is every eight hours. Morphine pharmacokinetics have been determined in calves receiving a 24 hour co-infusion of morphine, lidocaine, and ketamine (MLK) (Hartnack et al. 2020). Steady state serum concentration for morphine given at 4.8 μg/kg/h IV as part of the MLK co-infusion was likely not achieved in all calves in the study, due to the half-life being 4.1 hours. Morphine has been used as part of an MLK co-infusion in dogs and horses (Muir et al. 2003; Villalba et al. 2011). The loading dose of morphine prior to MLK in horses was 0.15 mg/kg IV. No significant side effects were noted in either study. In dogs, MAC reduction with morphine infusion alone and MLK were comparable, however in horses, MAC reduction from MLK in horses was not different from MAC reduction with lidocaine and ketamine. Morphine has also been placed into joints following arthroscopy in dogs and horses. Analgesia from IA morphine was similar to epidural morphine after stifle arthrotomy in dogs, and similar to IA bupivacaine (Day et al. 1995; Sammarco et al. 1996). After elbow arthroscopy, IA morphine was not shown to improve outcome based on post-operative gait analysis (Gurney et al. 2012). OTM (buccal) administration of 0.5 mg/kg morphine in cats had an average bioavailability of 36.6%, however, individual variation was high (range: 12.7–49.5) (Pypendop et al. 2014).

Hydromorphone

Hydromorphone is a derivative of morphine (Figure 7.1), and by comparison has increased potency with generally similar effects but shorter elimination half-life in dogs, which may warrant more frequent dosing (Table 7.5)

Table 7.4 Commonly used morphine dosages in cats, dogs, and horses.

Species	IV bolus (mg/kg)	CRI (mg/kg/h)	IM (mg/kg)	IA (mg/kg)	Epidural[a] (mg/kg)
Dog	0.25–0.5 q 2–4 h	0.1–0.2	0.25–1 q 2–4 h	0.1 mg/kg	0.1
Cat	0.1–0.3 q 2–4 h	0.05–0.1	0.1–0.25 q 2–4 h	—	0.1
Horse	0.1–0.15 q 8 h	0.1	0.1–0.2 q 8 h	0.05 mg/kg	0.05–0.2[b]

IV, intravenous, CRI, IV constant rate infusion, IM, intramuscular, IA, intra-articular.

[a] Preservative-free morphine should be used for epidural administration; dose should be reduced to 1/3–1/2 of epidural dosage for intrathecal injection.

[b] Standard morphine preparation can be diluted in sterile saline to a volume of 10–30 ml to allow forward spread (Adapted from Natalini 2010 © Elsevier).

Table 7.5 Selected pharmacokinetic parameters of hydromorphone in dogs, cats, and horses.

Species	Dose (mg/kg)	Route	F (%)	C_{max} (ng/ml)	T_{max} (h)	$t_{1/2}$ (h)	V (l/kg)	Cl (ml/min/kg)	References
Dog	0.1	IV	—	32 (C_0)	—	0.57	4.2	106.3	KuKanich et al.
	0.1	SC	—	33	0.19	0.66	3.3	57.4	(2008a)
Cat	0.1	IV	—	—	—	1.6	2.9	24.6	Wegner and Robertson (2004)
Horse	0.04	IV	—	75 (C_0)	—	0.32	1.1	79	Reed et al.
	0.04	IM	155	20	0.13	0.45	—	—	(2020)

F, bioavailability, C_{max}, maximum plasma concentration, T_{max}, time to reach C_{max}, $t_{1/2}$, terminal elimination half-life, V, apparent volume of distribution, Cl, clearance, C_0, plasma concentration at time zero.

(KuKanich et al. 2008a). In horses, the active metabolite hydromorphone-3-glucuronide has a much longer $t_{1/2}$ than its parent compound after both IV (3.5 vs 0.32 hours) and IM (4.3 vs 0.45 hours) (Reed et al. 2020). This was also associated with evidence of analgesia (increased thermal threshold) for 7–12 hours, and side effects such as excitement for 1–2 hours and decreased fecal output for 8 hours. Commonly used clinical dosages are presented in Table 7.6.

Methadone

Methadone is a synthetic opioid (Figure 7.1) with similar potency to morphine, and exists as a racemic mixture. The D-enantiomer is an antagonist at N-methyl-D-aspartate receptors with possible weak agonism of opioid receptors, and the L-enantiomer is associated with opioid receptor agonism (Davis and Inturrisi 1999). Pharmacokinetics of methadone in dogs, cats, and horses are presented in Table 7.7. Elimination half-life in dogs was longer after IV methadone compared to IV morphine, although in horses, elimination half-life was shorter at one hour (Ingvast-Larsson et al. 2010). Pharmacokinetics for IV dosing of methadone in cats have not been directly studied. Elimination half-life calculated for IV methadone in cats was similar to dogs, with a longer elimination half-life (10.4 hours) after IM dosing, and antinociception present for up to 6 hours (Slingsby et al. 2016). Chloramphenicol

Table 7.6 Dosages for selected mu agonist opioids in cats and dogs.

Opioid	Species	Dosage (mg/kg) q 2–4 h	CRI rate
Hydromorphone	Dog	0.1–0.2 (IV or IM)	0.02–0.04 mg/kg/h
	Cat	0.1 (IV or IM)	0.02–0.03 mg/kg/h
Methadone	Dog	0.2–0.4 (IV) 0.2–1 (IM)	0.05–0.2 mg/kg/h
	Cat	0.2–0.4 (IV) 0.2–0.6 (IM) 0.6 (OTM)	0.05–0.1 mg/kg/h
Meperidine	Dog	5–10 (IM) q 1–3 h	—
	Cat	3–5 (IM)	—

IV, intravenous, CRI, IV constant rate infusion, IM, intramuscular.

decreases hepatic metabolism of methadone via inhibition of cytochrome P450 in dogs (KuKanich and KuKanich 2015a). Bioavailability in cats after OTM administration of 0.75 mg/kg methadone was 44.2% with a wide individual range (18.7–70.5%) (Ferreira et al. 2011). Methadone has similar side effects to other mu opioid receptor agonists and is less likely to cause vomiting in dogs (Blancquaert et al. 1986).

Table 7.7 Selected pharmacokinetic parameters of methadone in dogs, cats and horses.

Species	Dose (mg/kg)	Route	F (%)	C_{max} (ng/ml)	T_{max} (h)	$t_{1/2}$ (h)	V (l/kg)	Cl (ml/min/kg)	References
Dog	0.4	IV	—	—	—	3.9	9.2	27.9	Ingvast-Larsson et al. (2010)
		SC	79	19	1.2	9.2	—	—	
Cat	0.3	IV[a]	—	—	—	4.6[a]	—	4.3[a]	Slingsby et al. (2016)
	0.6	IM	—	105	1.1	10.4	8	9.1	
Horse	0.15	IV	—	—	—	1	0.7	8	Linardi et al. (2012)

F, bioavailability, C_{max}, maximum plasma concentration, T_{max}, time to reach C_{max}, $t_{1/2}$, terminal elimination half-life, V, apparent volume of distribution, Cl, clearance.
[a] Slingsby et al. (2016) calculated the values for $t_{1/2}$ and V from data presented in work by Ferreira et al. (2011) (Adapted from Ferreira et al. 2011).

Meperidine

Meperidine (pethidine) is a synthetic opioid (Figure 7.1) with mu and kappa opioid receptor agonist activity (Trescot et al. 2008). Additionally, meperidine has been shown to have possible agonist activity at alpha$_2$ receptors and antagonist activity at sodium channels (Höcker et al. 2008; Wagner et al. 1999). Pharmacokinetics have been studied in cats, dogs, and horses. Elimination half-life was less than 1 hour in dogs, and 3.4 hours in cats (Taylor et al. 2001; Ritschel et al. 1987). In horses, half-life after IM administration was 3.1 hours, and antinociception to mechanical and thermal thresholds was not present (Hanafi et al. 2021). Meperidine causes histamine release more frequently in people than morphine, and histamine release has been shown to occur in dogs given meperidine (Flacke et al. 1987; Akcasu et al. 2009). In people, meperidine has been shown to precipitate serotonin syndrome when given with SSRIs (Tissot 2003). Unlike other mu opioid receptor agonists, meperidine has been shown to decrease cardiac output in dogs, with increases in heart rate seen due to an anticholinergic effect (Priano and Vatner 1981). Dosages for cats and dogs are given in Table 7.6.

Oxymorphone

Oxymorphone is a derivative of hydromorphone. It is more potent than morphine, with similar duration of action and side effects in cats and dogs. Pharmacokinetics in cats showed a relatively short terminal half-life (1.5 hours) (Siao et al. 2011). Bioavailability of oxymorphone after OTM administration was low (18.8%) (Pypendop et al. 2014). In dogs, the elimination half-life was 0.8 hours, and the incidence of vomiting was low (KuKanich et al. 2008a,b). At the time of writing the injectable form is no longer available in the USA.

Fentanyl

Fentanyl is a synthetic opioid with a similar chemical structure to meperidine (Figure 7.1) and is approximately 100 times more potent than morphine. It generally has a short half-life compared to previously discussed mu opioid receptor agonist and is frequently administered clinically as a continuous rate infusion (CRI). Pharmacokinetics of fentanyl given as a single IV bolus in cats, dogs, and horses are given in Table 7.8. Terminal elimination half-life was generally short, although slightly longer in cats. The same IV dose of fentanyl (4 µg/kg) given to conscious and isoflurane-anesthetized horses produced similar elimination half-life and volume of distribution, with a reduction in clearance of approximately 30% (Thomasy et al. 2007). Pharmacokinetics have also been reported in calves, pigs, alpacas, sheep, and goats, with plasma fentanyl concentrations declining rapidly after administration of a single IV

Table 7.8 Selected pharmacokinetic parameters for fentanyl in dogs, cats, and horses.

Species	Dose (µg/kg)	Route	$t_{1/2}$ (h)	V (l/kg)	Cl (ml/min/kg)	References
Dog	10	IV	0.8	10.5	77.9	Sano et al. (2006)
Cat	7.2	IV	2.4	2.6	19.8	Lee et al. (2000)
Horse	4	IV	1	0.37	9.2	Thomasy et al. (2007)

IV, intravenous, $t_{1/2}$, terminal elimination half-life, V, apparent volume of distribution, Cl, clearance.

Table 7.9 Dosages for fentanyl and remifentanil* in dogs, cats, and horses.

Opioid	Species	IV bolus (µg/kg)	CRI (µg/kg/h)	References
Fentanyl	Dog	1–3	1–40[a]	Grubb et al. (2020), KuKanich and Wiese (2015b)
	Cat	1–3	1–40[a]	
	Horse	2–4	0.3–0.5	
Remifentanil	Dog	—	10–20	Seddighi et al. (2023), Machado et al. (2018), Benmansour and Duke-Novakovski (2013), Pallarols et al. (2020)
	Cat	—	12–24	
	Horse	—	3–6	

IV, intravenous, CRI, IV constant rate infusion.
[a] Dosage will vary depending on degree of pain, with acute surgical pain requiring higher doses, and post-operative pain requiring lower doses.

bolus (Smith et al. 2018a,b; Egan et al. 1999; Lovasz et al. 2017; Ahern et al. 2010; Carroll et al. 1999). Recommended clinical dosages for fentanyl are given in Table 7.9. Fentanyl (2 µg/kg IV) can be used for co-induction of anesthesia in dogs, allowing the induction dose of propofol to be reduced by 17% (Covey-Crump and Murison 2008). Fentanyl (2–5 µg/kg IV) can be co-administered with midazolam (0.2 mg/kg IV) to induce anesthesia in compromised small animal patients, e.g. dogs in severe shock due to gastric dilatation/volvulus (Wong 1992; Figueiredo 2022).

Fentanyl is also available as a transdermal delivery system, or patch, in people, and it is frequently used in animals. Fentanyl patches are designed to deliver a specific dose of fentanyl per hour, ranging from 12 to 100 µg/h. Pharmacokinetics have been studied in dogs, cats, horses, pigs, calves, sheep, goats, llamas, and alpacas (Kyles et al. 1998; Lee et al. 2000; Skrzypczak et al. 2022;

Osorio Lujan et al. 2017; Smith et al. 2018a,b). In general, a lag time exists from placement of a fentanyl patch to reaching steady state plasma concentration, ranging from 12 to 24 hours, with steady state concentrations lasting for 2–3 days, and considerable individual variability in time-to-peak plasma concentration. As with CRIs, once plasma concentrations have reached steady state, kinetics will be zero order, i.e. the amount of drug absorbed equals the amount of drug cleared per unit time. In dogs, the rate of delivery from fentanyl patches was lower than predicted, and resulted in plasma concentrations considered to be analgesic for 1–3 days (Kyles et al. 1998). Sedation scores were higher, vocalization occurred more frequently, and salivation and anorexia lasted longer after fentanyl patch placement compared to morphine epidural in dogs undergoing ovariohysterectomy (Pekcan and Koc 2010). No side effects were observed in cats when pharmacokinetics of a 25 µg/h patch (equivalent to delivery of 4.5–11.2 µg/kg/h of fentanyl) was conducted (Lee et al. 2000). Fentanyl was readily absorbed by the TD route in horses and was detected for up to 4 days in plasma, with no side effects (Skrzypczak et al. 2022). In another equine study of TD fentanyl, side effects included increases in heart rate and respiratory rate (Thomasy et al. 2004). In pigs, TD fentanyl resulted in peak- plasma concentrations occurring between 6 and 36 hours, with no side effects being observed. Interestingly, placement of a subsequent patch in pigs did not result in consistent plasma concentrations, thus this modality may not be effective for providing analgesia longer than 2 days (Osorio Lujan et al. 2017). Time-to-peak plasma concentration in calves varied widely (4–48 hours). Side effects (vocalization, recumbency, excitement, tachycardia, hyperthermia, panting) were severe in two of four calves when delivery of TD fentanyl was 2 µg/kg/h, and moderate in two of three calves when delivery was 1 µg/kg/h. Removing the patch or administering naloxone resulted in the effects diminishing (Smith et al. 2018a,b).

Fentanyl Derivatives and Remifentanil

Alfentanil and sufentanil are fentanyl analogs. Alfentanil is less potent than fentanyl and has a shorter onset time. Sufentanil has a greater affinity for the mu opioid receptor compared to fentanyl with a similar onset time and is approximately 10 times more potent than fentanyl. Remifentanil has similar potency to fentanyl, with a rapid onset time similar to alfentanil. Its chemical structure is unique among the opioids in that it has an ester linkage and is degraded rapidly by plasma and tissue esterases to inactive compounds (Cohen and Royston 2001). Clinically, these opioids are given by CRI due to their short onset and offset. In the case of remifentanil and alfentanil, the

short-offset means that, for animals likely to be in pain after surgery, additional analgesia will be required when the infusion is turned off.

Alfentanil reduces propofol requirements for maintenance of anesthesia in dogs, and inhalant MAC in dogs, cats, and horses (Auckburally et al. 2008; Hall et al. 1987a,b; Ilkiw et al. 1997; Pascoe et al. 1993). Similarly, sufentanil reduces MAC in cats and dogs, as does remifentanil (Brosnan et al. 2020; Hall et al. 1987a,b; Seddighi et al. 2023; Ferreira et al. 2009; Benmansour and Duke-Novakovski 2013).

Ultra-Potent Agonists

Etorphine, carfentanil, and thiafentanil are extremely potent opioids used alone, or in combination, with sedatives for sedation and immobilization of wild animals. These drugs should be handled with extreme caution, and safety precautions include never working alone with these drugs, and having antagonists available, as well as being able to communicate with medical personnel should inadvertent self-injection occur. Their use in anesthesia of wildlife is reviewed elsewhere (Caulkett and Arnemo 2015).

Oral Opioid Agonist Drugs

Oral bioavailability of opioids is poor in animals due to high first-pass hepatic metabolism. As such, they have limited use in the peri-anesthetic period in veterinary anesthesia. Codeine (methylmorphine) has a structure similar to morphine with a methyl substitution (for hydroxyl) on the number 3 carbon atom which decreases first-pass metabolism in people, however, this is not the case in dogs, where a bioavailability of 4% is reported (KuKanich 2010). Hydrocodone is a codeine derivative opioid agonist used in dogs mostly as an antitussive. Bioavailability in dogs is 19%, with some hydrocodone being metabolized to hydromorphone (KuKanich and Spade 2013). In another pharmacokinetic study, metabolism to the active M1 metabolite was low, and metabolism to hydromorphone was limited (Benitez and Roush 2015b). Orally administered extended-release hydrocodone provided inadequate analgesia in dogs undergoing TPLO, with 9/18 dogs requiring rescue analgesia compared to 2/18 dogs that received oral firocoxib (Heffernan et al. 2018). Hydrocodone is available as a combined product with acetaminophen. This combination given orally, prior to TPLO surgery resulted in rescue analgesia being required in 5/19 dogs (Benitez and Roush 2015a).

Opioid Partial Agonist
Buprenorphine

Buprenorphine is a semi-synthetic opioid derived from thebaine, an opium alkaloid (Figure 7.1). It is about 25 times more potent than morphine. Buprenorphine has a high affinity for the mu opioid receptor, however, does not produce the maximal effects seen with full opioid agonists (Lewis 1985). Due to its high affinity, buprenorphine can prevent binding of full agonists and antagonists to the mu opioid receptor. Buprenorphine has a longer duration of action than morphine (four to eight hours), and co-administration of buprenorphine with full agonists is not recommended. Buprenorphine is available in an injectable form (0.3 mg/ml). Additionally, injectable buprenorphine at a high concentration (1.8 mg/ml) (Simbadol®) and transdermal buprenorphine solution combined with a permeation enhancer (Zorbium®) are licensed in cats. Zorbium is available in two sizes, 0.4 ml containing 8 mg buprenorphine, and 1 ml containing 20 mg, with effects lasting up to four days. Special handling and wearing of protective equipment to avoid accidental skin or eye exposure to Zorbium is essential, given the high concentration.

The pKa of buprenorphine is 8.24, and therefore in a more basic environment, such as the feline oral mucosa, OTM absorption is promoted due to more of the drug existing in its non-ionized state. Side effects of buprenorphine are similar to and generally less marked when compared to morphine.

Pharmacokinetics of buprenorphine given by IV, IM, and SC routes have been studied in several species (see Table 7.10). In general, elimination half-life is longer than morphine in cats and dogs, leading to longer dosing intervals in small animal patients which can have advantages for post-operative care. In dogs, buprenorphine has also been given via the OTM and IN routes (Enomoto et al. 2022). Bioavailability was 41% and 58% respectively, with a wide individual range. In cats, OTM bioavailability was 116%, although this may be inaccurate based on later findings that jugular sampling after OTM administration may overestimate true plasma concentration (Robertson et al. 2003). The

mean elimination half-life after 10, 30, or 50 mg/kg transdermal buprenorphine solution was 78–90 hours, with peak-plasma concentration occurring between 2 and 72 hours, and bioavailability was 16–22% (Freise et al. 2022). The extended half-life is attributed to the fact that the drug absorbed into the skin acts as a slow-release depot. In horses, pharmacokinetics of sublingual administration of buprenorphine (0.006 mg/kg) resulted in a longer elimination half-life and a similar duration of decreased intestinal borborygmi compared to IV administration (8.8 hours), with no horses showing signs of colic (Messenger et al. 2011). In an equine model of lipopolysaccharide-induced synovitis, buprenorphine was still detectable in synovial fluid 24 hours after intra-articular administration of 0.005 mg/kg (Steagall et al. 2020). Analgesic efficacy was not evaluated in that study, and *in vitro*, buprenorphine had dose-dependent cytotoxic effects on chondrocytes (Castro-Cuellar et al. 2023). Clinically used dosages for buprenorphine are presented in Table 7.11.

Table 7.11 Dosages for buprenorphine in dogs, cats, and horses.

Species	IV or IM bolus (mg/kg)	OTM	SC	References
Dog	0.01–0.03 q 4–8 h	—	—	Grubb et al. (2020), KuKanich and Wiese (2015b)
Cat	0.01–0.03 q 4–8 h	0.03–0.05 q 8–12 h	0.24 mg/kg[a] q 24 h	
Horse	0.005–0.01	—	—	

IV, intravenous, IM, intramuscular, OTM, oral transmucosal, SC, subcutaneous.
[a] Buprenorphine 1.8 mg/ml (Simbadol®).

Table 7.10 Selected pharmacokinetic parameters for buprenorphine in dogs, cats, and horses.

Species	Dose (mg/kg)	Route	F (%)	C_{max} (ng/ml)	T_{max} (h)	$t_{1/2}$ (h)	V (l/kg)	Cl (ml/min/kg)	References
Dog	0.02	IV	—	—	—	4	3.5	10.3	KuKanich and Allen (2014), Steagall et al. (2020)
	0.02[a]	IV	—	35.9 (C_0)	—	3.7	6.8	21.5	
	0.02[a]	IM	63	6.2	0.14	5.7	14.2	27.5	
	0.02[a]	SC	40	1.4	0.04	22	40.1	23.3	
Cat	0.01	IV	—	—	—	6.9	7.1	16.7	Taylor et al. (2001), Robertson et al. (2003)
	0.01	IM	—	8.7	0.05	6.3	8.9	23.6	
	0.01	OTM	—	7.5	0.25	5.8	3.4	8.5	
Horse	0.005	IV	—	—	—	3.6	3	8	Davis et al. (2012)
	0.005	IM	65	1.7	0.9	4.2	—	—	

F, bioavailability, C_{max}, maximum plasma concentration, T_{max}, time to reach C_{max}, $t_{1/2}$, terminal elimination half-life, V, apparent volume of distribution, Cl, clearance, IV, intravenous, IM, intramuscular, SC, subcutaneous, OTM, oral transmucosal, IN, intranasal.
[a] Buprenorphine 1.8 mg/ml was used (Simbadol®).

Opioid Agonist-Antagonists

Agonist-antagonist opioids, sometimes referred to as "mixed" agonists, have agonist activity at kappa opioid receptors and antagonist activity at mu opioid receptors (Trescot et al. 2008).

Butorphanol

Butorphanol is a synthetic opioid with kappa opioid receptor agonist and mu opioid receptor antagonist activity (Figure 7.1). Butorphanol pharmacokinetics are presented in Table 7.12. In general, elimination half-life and therefore duration of action is shorter compared to morphine. Butorphanol may cause side effects typical of the opioid class of drugs, however, the effects tend to be mild.

In cats and dogs, butorphanol was not effective at providing sufficient analgesia after ovariohysterectomy (Warne et al. 2014; Gültiken et al. 2022). Butorphanol was also not effective as an analgesic for pain associated with shoulder arthrotomy in dogs (Mathews et al. 1996). In contrast, in a canine thermal nociceptive escape model, butorphanol (0.4 mg/kg IV) provided greater antinociception than buprenorphine (0.03 mg/kg IV). It is possible that thermal nociception does not truly represent pain associated with acute post-operative pain. It is also possible that butorphanol may have weak partial agonist activity at the mu opioid receptor rather than being an antagonist (Trescot et al. 2008). Additionally, the short duration of action and frequent dosing interval for butorphanol argues against using it to manage moderate-to-severe peri-anesthetic pain in small animals (Bednarski 2015; Pascoe 2000). Bioavailability after administration of butorphanol 0.4 mg/kg OTM to cats was relatively low at 37%, and plasma concentrations consistent with analgesic effect were not reached (Wells et al. 2008). Butorphanol has been identified as a substrate of the P-glycoprotein (P-gp)

transporter in the CNS, and mutation of the *ABCB1 P-gp* gene may result in sedation that is more pronounced and of longer duration in affected dogs (mostly sheep herding breeds) (Mealey et al. 2023). A 25% dose reduction is recommended for heterozygous dogs, and 50% reduction for homozygous dogs.

Elimination half-life after butorphanol 0.1 mg/kg IV is longer in horses compared to cats and dogs, with side effects (increased locomotor activity/excitement, increased heart rate, decreased intestinal borborygmi) lasting as long as six hours (Knych et al. 2013). In goats, pharmacokinetics are similar to small animas (Carroll et al. 2001). Lower dosages and increased dosing intervals are therefore prudent in horses compared to other species (Table 7.13). Butorphanol has been shown to be efficacious for treating visceral pain in horses (Muir and Robertson 1985; Sellon et al. 2004). In another study, a single dose of butorphanol (0.1 mg/kg IV), as part of preanesthetic medication, provided insufficient analgesia after castration, with 19/20 ponies requiring additional analgesia (Love et al. 2009).

Butorphanol (0.4 mg/kg IV) reduced isoflurane MAC in dogs by 20%, however, butorphanol 0.2 mg/kg IM did not

Table 7.13 Dosages for butorphanol in dogs, cats, and horses.

Opioid	Species	IV or IM bolus (mg/kg)	CRI (mg/kg/h)	References
Butorphanol	Dog	0.2–0.4 q1–4 h	0.1–0.2	KuKanich and Weise (2015b)
	Cat	0.2–0.4 q1–4 h	0.1–0.2	
	Horse	0.01–0.04 q 2–6 h	0.01–0.025	

IV, intravenous, CRI, IV continuous rate infusion, IM, intramuscular.

Table 7.12 Selected pharmacokinetic parameters for butorphanol in dogs, cats, and horses.

Species	Dose (mg/kg)	Route	F (%)	C_{max} (ng/ml)	T_{max} (h)	$t_{1/2}$ (h)	V (l/kg)	Cl (ml/min/kg)	References
Dog	0.4	IV	—	—	—	1.8	3.5	46.5	Springfield et al. (2022), Pfeffer et al. (1980)
	0.25	IM	—	25	0.7	1.5	7.5	56.8	
	0.25	SC	—	33	0.5	1.7	8.4	58.3	
Cat	1	IV	—	—	—	2.9	3.9	18.4	Pypendop and Shilo-Benjamini (2021)[a], Wells et al. (2008)
	0.4	IM	—	132	0.35	6.3	7.6	12.9	
	0.4	OTM	24	34	1.1	5.2	15.6	35.3	
Horse	0.1	IV	—	—	—	5.9	1.4	11.5	Knych et al. (2013), Sellon et al. (2009)
	0.08	IV	—	—	—	7.8	1.1	4.6	
	0.08	IM	37	99	0.11	0.6	0.6	12.4	

IV, intravenous, IM, transdermal, SC, subcutaneous, F, bioavailability, C_{max}, maximum plasma concentration, T_{max}, time to reach C_{max}, $t_{1/2}$, terminal elimination half-life, V, apparent volume of distribution, Cl, clearance.
[a] Study performed in isoflurane-anesthetized cats.

(Ko et al. 2000; Grimm et al. 2000). Doses of butorphanol from 0.2 to 0.8 mg/kg IV did not decrease halothane MAC in dogs (Quandt et al. 1994). In cats, IV doses of butorphanol (0.08 mg/kg and 0.8 mg/kg) both decreased isoflurane MAC by 19% 60 minutes after administration, evidence that MAC reduction is likely not dose dependent (Ilkiw et al. 2002). A later study found a dose-dependent effect on isoflurane MAC when butorphanol was given at three different IV bolus doses/CRI rates, with reduction in MAC between 23% and 68% (Pypendop et al. 2022). In ponies, butorphanol (0.022 and 0.044 mg/kg IV) tended to decrease MAC by a similar amount (10%), however, this decrease was not statistically significantly different from MAC of halothane alone (Matthews and Lindsay 1990). Goats given butorphanol 0.2 mg/kg IM prior to anesthesia had minimal cardiorespiratory or sedative effects and the induction dose of propofol was reduced by 22% (Dzikiti et al. 2009). Trace residues of butorphanol in bovine milk were present for 36 hours after a 0.045 mg/kg IV dose (Court et al. 1992).

Butorphanol can be used to reverse sedative (and other) effects of mu opioid agonists (Dyson et al. 1990).

Nalbuphine

Nalbuphine is a semisynthetic opioid with relatively low lipophilicity and similar potency to morphine. Structurally, it is related to oxymorphone and naloxone (de Oliviera Frazílio et al. 2014). Like butorphanol, it is a kappa opioid receptor agonist and mu opioid receptor antagonist (Trescot et al. 2008). Pharmacologic studies in animals are relatively limited. Nalbuphine 0.5 mg/kg IV provided less sedation than an equipotent dose of butorphanol in dogs (Lester et al. 2003). Nalbuphine doses between 1 and 2 mg/kg produced mild sedation in dogs that was not dose-dependent, and was enhanced by acepromazine, with minimal cardiorespiratory effects (Gomes and Marques 2022). Epidural administration of 0.3 and 0.6 mg/kg nalbuphine decreased isoflurane MAC by 26% and 38% respectively (de Oliviera Frazílio et al. 2014). In cats, IM sedation with nalbuphine (0.5 mg/kg) and acepromazine (0.05 mg/kg) was mild, and similar to that seen with butorphanol (0.4 mg/kg) and acepromazine (Costa et al. 2021). Pharmacokinetics have been described in conscious horses after 0.3 mg/kg nalbuphine (0.3 mg/kg) combined with xylazine (0.55 mg/kg) was given IV (Hammad et al. 2022). Nalbuphine had a large volume of distribution and an elimination half-life of 3.5 hours in that study. When given with xylazine, nalbuphine extended the duration of sedation (45 minutes) compared to xylazine alone (30 minutes). Xylazine and nalbuphine together produced antinociceptive effects as assessed by response to needle prick and electrical stimulation for 15 minutes compared to xylazine alone (8 minutes).

Pentazocine

Pentazocine is a derivative of benzomorphan and has antagonist (or possibly weak agonist) activity at mu opioid receptors while acting as an agonist at kappa and delta opioid receptors.

The pharmacokinetics of pentazocine (2.5, 5, and 10 mg/kg IM) during halothane anesthesia have been studied and fit a two-compartment model (Arakawa et al. 1979). Half-life (1.2 hours) was similar regardless of dose and was not different from awake dogs that received 2.5 mg/kg IM. In dogs premedicated with atropine and pentazocine, the induction dose of propofol was reduced by 11% compared to atropine alone (Anandmay et al. 2016). Pentazocine increases cardiac contractility in dogs, likely due to stimulation of catecholamines from the adrenal medulla (Levitsky S 1971; Fukumitsu et al. 1991). A few minutes after IV injection of pentazocine (1 or 2 mg/kg IV), renal blood flow decreased by approximately 80% with both doses, an effect which lasted for up to 15 minutes (Yamashiro 1978).

In horses, pentazocine (1 mg/kg IV) has a large volume of distribution (3 L/kg) and reached maximum plasma concentrations after 30 minutes. The elimination half-life is 2.3 hours, with duration of effect being approximately 30 minutes (Tobin and Miller 1979). It is metabolized via glucuronidation and hydrolysis and excreted in the urine. In a cecal balloon colic model in horses, pentazocine provided analgesia for approximately 30 minutes that was inferior to xylazine's analgesic effects (Muir and Robertson 1985). Pentazocine had a minimal effect on the cardiorespiratory changes induced by the colic model. In another study, pentazocine (2.2 mg/kg IV) had an antinociceptive effect lasting 15–30 minutes. Side effects include increased locomotor activity and increased blood pressure in conscious horses. Similar to butorphanol, pentazocine decreased small intestinal motility in ponies (Sojka et al. 1988).

Opioid Antagonists

Opioid antagonists are used to reverse unwanted side effects of opioid agonists, and, at higher doses, the analgesia provided by opioid drugs as well as endogenous opioids will be reversed. Administering butorphanol may offer the advantage of reversing side effects (mu opioid receptor antagonism) while providing some analgesia (via kappa opioid receptor agonism).

Naloxone

Naloxone acts as an antagonist at all opioid receptors. Elimination half-life is relatively short at 0.62 hours, and renarcotization was observed in 2/6 dogs two hours after naloxone was given IV to reverse oxymorphone

(Wahler et al. 2019; Dyson et al. 1990). Bioavailability of IN administration of naloxone using a single-dose commercial atomizer (4 mg total dose) was 32%, and lag time was short at 2.3 minutes. In the case of an emergency i.e. during cardiopulmonary resuscitation, naloxone should be given at the full dose of 0.04 mg/kg IV (Fletcher et al. 2012). In non-emergent situations, it is prudent to administer antagonists to effect, which may result in reversal of side effects while maintaining some analgesia. Incremental doses of naloxone, e.g. 0.001 mg/kg q 1–5 minutes can be titrated until the desired effect is reached (KuKanich and Wiese 2015b).

Naltrexone

Like naloxone, naltrexone is non-specific opioid antagonist. It has a longer duration of action and is most commonly used to reverse potent opioids used for wildlife immobilization. In cats, the duration of action of naltrexone was 1–2 hours, with a dose of 0.3 mg/kg IV

reversing adverse behavior resulting from very high doses of remifentanil, while a dose of 0.6 mg/kg reversed dysphoria while maintaining antinociception (Pypendop et al. 2011).

Other Antagonists

Methylnaltrexone, a derivative of naltrexone, has peripheral opioid antagonist activity. This offers advantages of decreasing peripheral side effects, e.g. decreased incidence of vomiting and GI motility, while maintaining central analgesic effects. Methylnaltrexone antagonized the GI effects of morphine in horses, and decreased morphine-induced emesis in a dose-dependent fashion in dogs, although central effects of morphine were not reported (Boscan and Hoogmoed 2006; Foss et al. 1993).

Nalmefene, an opioid antagonist with long duration (elimination half-life of 8–11 hours in people and 3.6 hours in dogs) is no longer available (Wang et al. 1998; Veng-Pedersen et al. 1995).

References

Adami, C. and Spadavecchia, C. (2020). Use of nociceptive threshold testing in cats in experimental and clinical settings: a qualitative review. *Vet. Anaesth. Analg.* 47: 419–436.

Ahern, B.J., Soma, L.R. et al. (2010). Pharmacokinetics of fentanyl administered transdermally and intravenously in sheep. *Am. J. Vet. Res.* 71: 1127–1132.

Akcasu, A., Yillar, D.O. et al. (2009). The role of mast cells in the genesis of acute manifestations following the intravenous injection of meperidine in dogs. *J. Basic Clin. Physiol. Pharmacol.* 20: 67–72.

Anandmay, A.K., Dass, L.L. et al. (2016). Clinico-anesthetic changes following administration of propofol alone and in combination of meperidine and pentazocine lactate in dogs. *Vet. World* 9: 1178–1183.

Andersen, M.S., Clark, L. et al. (2006). Risk factors for colic in horses after general anaesthesia for MRI or nonabdominal surgery: absence of evidence of effect from perianaesthetic morphine. *Equine Vet. J.* 38: 368–374.

Anderson, M.K. and Day, T.K. (2008). Effects of morphine and fentanyl constant rate infusion on urine output in healthy and traumatized dogs. *Vet. Anaesth. Analg.* 35: 528–536.

Arakawa, Y., Bandoh, M. et al. (1979). Pharmacokinetics of pentazocine in dogs under halothane anesthesia. *Chem. Pharm. Bull.* 27: 2217–2220.

Auckburally, A., Pawson, P., and Flaherty, D. (2008). A comparison of induction of anaesthesia using a target-controlled infusion device in dogs with propofol or a

propofol and alfentanil admixture. *Vet. Anaesth. Analg.* 35: 319–325.

Barnhart, M.D., Hubbell, J.A. et al. (2000). Pharmacokinetics, pharmacodynamics, and analgesic effects of morphine after rectal, intramuscular, and intravenous administration in dogs. *Am. J. Vet. Res.* 61: 24–28.

Bednarski, R.M. (2015). Dogs and cats. In: *Veterinary Anesthesia and Analgesia*, 5e (ed. K.A. Grimm, L.A. Lamont, W.J. Tranquilli, et al.), 819–826. Ames IA: Wiley Blackwell.

Benitez, M.E., Roush, J.K. et al. (2015a). Clinical efficacy of hydrocodone-acetaminophen and tramadol for control of postoperative pain in dogs following tibial plateau leveling osteotomy. *Am. J. Vet. Res.* 76: 755–762.

Benitez, M.E., Roush, J.K. et al. (2015b). Pharmacokinetics of hydrocodone and tramadol administered for control of postoperative pain in dogs following tibial plateau leveling osteotomy. *Am. J. Vet. Res.* 76: 763–770.

Benmansour, P. and Duke-Novakovski, T. (2013). Prolonged anesthesia using sevoflurane, remifentanil and dexmedetomidine in a horse. *Vet. Anaesth. Analg.* 40: 521–526.

Benson, G.J. and Thurmon, J.C. (1987). Species difference as a consideration in alleviation of animal pain and distress. *J. Am. Vet. Med. Assoc.* 191: 1227–1230.

Bini, G., Vettorato, E. et al. (2018). A retrospective comparison of two analgesic strategies after uncomplicated tibial plateau levelling osteotomy in dogs. *Vet. Anaesth. Analg.* 45: 557–565.

Biswai, A.V., Liu, W.S. et al. (1976). The effects of large doses of fentanyl and fentanyl with nitrous oxide on renal function in the dog. *Can. Anaesth. Soc. J.* 23: 296–302.

Blancquaert, J.P., Lefebvre, R.A., and Willems, J.L. (1986). Emetic and antiemetic effects of opioids in the dog. *Eur. J. Pharmacol.* 128: 143–150.

Blunk, J.A., Schmelz, M. et al. (2004). Opioid-induced mast cell activation and vascular responses is not mediated by mu-opioid receptors: an in vivo microdialysis study in human skin. *Anesth. Analg.* 98: 364–370.

de Boer, H.D., Detriche, O., and Forget, P. (2017). Opioid-related side effects: postoperative ileus, urinary retention, nausea and vomiting, and shivering. A review of the literature. *Best Pract. Res. Clin. Anaesthesiol.* 31: 499–504.

Boscan, P. and Van Hoogmoed, L.M. (2006). Pharmacokinetics of the opioid antagonist N-methylnaltrexone and evaluation of its effects on gastrointestinal tract function in horses treated or not treated with morphine. *Am. J. Vet. Res.* 67: 998–1004.

Brosnan, R.J., Pypendop, B.H., and Stanley, S.D. (2020). Phenylpiperidine opioid effects on isoflurane minimum alveolar concentration in cats. *J. Vet. Pharmacol. Ther.* 43: 533–537.

Bueno, L., Fioramonti, J., and Ruckebusch, Y. (1978). Postoperative intestinal motility in dogs and sheep. *Am. J. Dig. Dis.* 23: 682–689.

Burford, J.H. and Corley, K.T. (2006). Morphine-associated pruritus after single extradural administration in a horse. *Vet. Anaesth. Analg.* 33: 193–198.

Carroll, G.L., Hooper, R.N. et al. (1999). Pharmacokinetics of fentanyl after intravenous and transdermal administration in goats. *Am. J. Vet. Res.* 60: 986–991.

Carroll, G.L., Boothe, D.M. et al. (2001). Pharmacokinetics and selected behavioral responses to butorphanol and its metabolites in goats following intravenous and intramuscular administration. *Vet. Anaesth. Analg.* 28: 188–195.

Castro-Cuellar, G., Cremer, J. et al. (2023). Buprenorphine has a concentration-dependent cytotoxic effect on equine chondrocytes in vitro. *Am. J. Vet. Res.* 84: https://doi.org/10.2460/ajvr.22.08.0143. PMID: 36662607.

Caulkett, N.A. and Arnemo, J.M. (2015). Comparative anesthesia and analgesia of zoo animals and wildlife. In: *Veterinary Anesthesia and Analgesia*, 5e (ed. K.A. Grimm, L.A. Lamont, W.J. Tranquilli, et al.), 764–776. Ames, IA: Wiley Blackwell.

Cavanagh, R.L., Gylys, J.A., and Bierwagen, M.E. (1976). Antitussive properties of butorphanol. *Arch. Int. Pharmacodyn. Ther.* 220: 258–268.

Che, T., Dwivedi-Agnihotri, H. et al. (2021). Biased ligands at opioid receptors: current status and future directions. *Sci. Signal.* 14: eaav0320. https://doi.org/10.1126/scisignal.aav0320.

Chiavaccini, L., Claude, A.K. et al. (2017). Comparison of morphine, morphine-lidocaine, and morphine-lidocaine-ketamine infusions in dogs using an incision-induced pain model. *J. Am. Anim. Hosp. Assoc.* 53: 65–72.

Cohen, J. and Royston, D. (2001). Remifentanil. *Curr. Opin. Crit. Care* 7: 227–231.

Cohen, N.D., Gibbs, P.G., and Woods, A.M. (1999). Dietary and other management factors associated with colic in horses. *J. Am. Vet. Med. Assoc.* 215: 53–60.

Cohen, N.D., Lester, G.D. et al. (2004). Evaluation of risk factors associated with development of postoperative ileus in horses. *J. Am. Vet. Med. Assoc.* 225: 1070–1078.

Combie, J., Shults, T. et al. (1981). Pharmacology of narcotic analgesics in the horse: selective blockade of narcotic-induced locomotor activity. *Am. J. Vet. Res.* 42: 716–721.

Corletto, F., Raisis, A.A., and Brearley, J.C. (2005). Comparison of morphine and butorphanol as pre-anaesthetic agents in combination with romifidine for field castration in ponies. *Vet. Anaesth. Analg.* 32: 16–22.

Costa, G.P., Monteiro, E.R. et al. (2021). Sedative effects of acepromazine in combination with nalbuphine or butorphanol, intramuscularly or intravenously, in healthy cats: a randomized, blinded clinical trial. *J. Feline Med. Surg.* 23: 540–548.

Court, M.H., Dodman, N.H. et al. (1992). Pharmacokinetics and milk residues of butorphanol in dairy cows after single intravenous administration. *J. Vet. Pharmacol. Ther.* 15: 28–35.

Covey-Crump, G.L. and Murison, P.J. (2008). Fentanyl or midazolam for co-induction of anaesthesia with propofol in dogs. *Vet. Anaesth. Analg.* 35: 463–472.

Curley, T.L., Thamm, D.H. et al. (2021). Effects of morphine on histamine release from two cell lines of canine mast cell tumor and on plasma histamine concentrations in dogs with cutaneous mast cell tumor. *Am. J. Vet. Res.* 82: 1013–1018.

Davis, A.M. and Inturrisi, C.E. (1999). d-Methadone blocks morphine tolerance and N-methyl-D-aspartate-induced hyperalgesia. *J. Pharmacol. Exp. Ther.* 289: 1048–1053.

Davis, J.L., Messenger, K.M. et al. (2012). Pharmacokinetics of intravenous and intramuscular buprenorphine in the horse. *J. Vet. Pharmacol. Ther.* 35: 52–58.

Day, T.K., Pepper, W.T. et al. (1995). Comparison of intra-articular and epidural morphine for analgesia following stifle arthrotomy in dogs. *Vet. Surg.* 24: 522–530.

De Monte, V., Staffieri, F. et al. (2015). Comparison of ketamine-dexmedetomidine-methadone and tiletamine-zolazepam-methadone combinations for short-term anaesthesia in domestic pigs. *Vet. J.* 205: 364–368.

Devine, E.P., KuKanich, B., and Beard, W.L. (2013). Pharmacokinetics of intramuscularly administered morphine in horses. *J. Am. Vet. Med. Assoc.* 243: 105–112.

Duke-Novakovski, T., Jimenez, C.P. et al. (2021). Plasma histamine concentrations in horses administered sodium penicillin, guaifenesin-xylazine-ketamine and isoflurane with morphine or butorphanol. *Vet. Anaesth. Analg.* 48: 17–25.

Dyson, D.H., Doherty, T. et al. (1990). Reversal of oxymorphone sedation by naloxone, nalmefene, and butorphanol. *Vet. Surg.* 19: 398–403.

Dzikiti, T.B., Stegmann, G.F. et al. (2009). Sedative and cardiopulmonary effects of acepromazine, midazolam, butorphanol, acepromazine-butorphanol and midazolam-butorphanol on propofol anaesthesia in goats. *J. S. Afr. Vet. Assoc.* 80: 10–16.

Dzikiti, T.B., Stegmann, G.F. et al. (2011). Effects of fentanyl on isoflurane minimum alveolar concentration and cardiovascular function in mechanically ventilated goats. *Vet. Rec.* 168: 429.

Egan, T.D., Lemmens, H.J. et al. (1993). The pharmacokinetics of the new short-acting opioid remifentanil (GI87084B) in healthy adult male volunteers. *Anesthesiology* 79: 881–892.

Egan, T.D., Kuramkote, S. et al. (1999). Fentanyl pharmacokinetics in hemorrhagic shock: a porcine model. *Anesthesiology* 91: 156–166.

El Daibani, A. and Che, T. (2022). Spotlight on nociceptin/orphanin FQ receptor in the treatment of pain. *Molecules* 27: 595.

Enomoto, H., Love, L. et al. (2022). Pharmacokinetics of intravenous, oral transmucosal, and intranasal buprenorphine in healthy male dogs. *J. Vet. Pharmacol. Ther.* 45: 358–365.

Ferreira, T.H., Aguiar, A.J. et al. (2009). Effect of remifentanil hydrochloride administered via constant rate infusion on the minimum alveolar concentration of isoflurane in cats. *Am. J. Vet. Res.* 70: 581–588.

Ferreira, T.H., Rezende, M.L., and Mama, K.R. (2011). Plasma concentrations and behavioral, antinociceptive, and physiologic effects of methadone after intravenous and oral transmucosal administration in cats. *Am. J. Vet. Res.* 72: 764–771.

Figueiredo, J.P. (2022). Gastrointestinal disease. In: *Canine and Feline Anesthesia and Co-Existing Disease*, 2e (ed. R.A. Johnson, L.B.C. Snyder, and C.A. Schroeder), 155–201. Hoboken NJ: Wiley Blackwell.

Figueiredo, J.P., Muir, W.W., and Sams, R. (2012). Cardiorespiratory, gastrointestinal, and analgesic effects of morphine sulfate in conscious healthy horses. *Am. J. Vet. Res.* 73: 799–808.

Flacke, J.W., Flacke, W.E. et al. (1987). Histamine release by four narcotics: a double-blind study in humans. *Anesth. Analg.* 66: 723–730.

Fletcher, D.J., Boller, M. et al. (2012). RECOVER evidence and knowledge gap analysis on veterinary CPR. Part 7: clinical guidelines. *J. Vet. Emerg. Crit. Care* 22 (Suppl): S102–S131.

Foss, J.F., Bass, A.S., and Goldberg, L.I. (1993). Dose-related antagonism of the emetic effect of morphine by methylnaltrexone in dogs. *J. Clin. Pharmacol.* 33: 747–751.

Freise, K.J., Reinemeyer, C. et al. (2022). Single-dose pharmacokinetics and bioavailability of a novel extended duration transdermal buprenorphine solution in cats. *J. Vet. Pharmacol. Ther.* 45 (Suppl): S31–S39.

Fukumitsu, K., Sumikawa, K. et al. (1991). Pentazocine-induced catecholamine efflux from the dog perfused adrenals. *J. Pharm. Pharmacol.* 43: 331–336.

Garrett, E.R. and Jackson, A.J. (1979). Pharmacokinetics of morphine and its surrogates. III: morphine and morphine 3-monoglucuronide pharmacokinetics in the dog as a function of dose. *J. Pharm. Sci.* 68: 753–771.

Gent, T., Bettschart-Wolfensberger, R., and Mosing, M. (2013). Neuraxial morphine induced pruritus in two cats and treatment with sub anaesthetic doses of propofol. *Vet. Anaesth. Analg.* 40: 517–520.

Gomes, V.H. and Marques, J.L.R. (2022). Comparison of the sedative effects of three nalbuphine doses, alone or combined with acepromazine, in dogs. *Am. J. Vet. Res.* 83: ajvr.21.12.0214 https://doi.org/10.2460/ajvr.21.12.0214.

Gonçalves, S., Julliand, V., and Leblond, A. (2002). Risk factors associated with colic in horses. *Vet. Res.* 33: 641–652.

Gramer, I., Leidolf, R. et al. (2011). Breed distribution of the nt230(del4) MDR1 mutation in dogs. *Vet. J.* 189: 67–71.

Greene, S.A., Benson, G.J. et al. (2004). Effect of isoflurane, atracurium, fentanyl, and noxious stimulation on bispectral index in pigs. *Comp. Med.* 54: 397–403.

Greenier, E.L., Lukyanova, V., and Reede, L. (2014). Serotonin syndrome: fentanyl and selective serotonin reuptake inhibitor interactions. *AANA J.* 82: 340–345.

Grimm, K.A., Tranquilli, W.J. et al. (2000). Duration of nonresponse to noxious stimulation after intramuscular administration of butorphanol, medetomidine, or a butorphanol-medetomidine combination during isoflurane administration in dogs. *Am. J. Vet. Res.* 61: 42–47.

Grimm, K.A., Tranquilli, W.J. et al. (2005). Cardiopulmonary effects of fentanyl in conscious dogs and dogs sedated with a continuous rate infusion of medetomidine. *Am. J. Vet. Res.* 66: 1222–1226.

Grubb, T., Sager, J. et al. (2020). 2020 AAHA anesthesia and monitoring guidelines for dogs and cats. *J. Am. Anim. Hosp. Assoc.* 56: 59–82.

Guedes, A.G., Rudé, E.P., and Rider, M.A. (2006). Evaluation of histamine release during constant rate infusion of morphine in dogs. *Vet. Anaesth. Analg.* 33: 28–35.

Gültiken, N., Gürler, H. et al. (2022). Antioxidant and analgesic potential of butorphanol in dogs undergoing ovariohysterectomy. *Theriogenology* 190: 1–7.

Gurney, M.A., Rysnik, M. et al. (2012). Intra-articular morphine, bupivacaine or no treatment for postoperative analgesia following unilateral elbow joint arthroscopy. *J. Small Anim. Pract.* 53: 387–392.

Hall, R.I., Murphy, M.R., and Hug, C.C. (1987a). The enflurane sparing effect of sufentanil in dogs. *Anesthesiology* 67: 518–525.

Hall, R.I., Szlam, F., and Hug, C.C. (1987b). The enflurane-sparing effect of alfentanil in dogs. *Anesth. Analg.* 66: 1287–1291.

Hamamoto-Hardman, B.D., Steffey, E.P. et al. (2019). Pharmacokinetics and selected pharmacodynamics of morphine and its active metabolites in horses after intravenous administration of four doses. *J. Vet. Pharmacol. Ther.* 42: 401–410.

Hammad, A., Gadallah, S. et al. (2022). Pharmacodynamics and pharmacokinetics of nalbuphine in xylazine-sedated horses. *Vet. Ital.* 58: https://doi.org/10.12834/VetIt.2408.16506.1.

Hamra, J.G., Kamerling, S.G. et al. (1993). Diurnal variation in plasma ir-beta-endorphin levels and experimental pain thresholds in the horse. *Life Sci.* 53: 121–129.

Hanafi, A.L., Reed, R.A. et al. (2021). Pharmacokinetics and pharmacodynamics of meperidine after intramuscular and subcutaneous administration in horses. *Vet. Surg.* 50: 410–417.

Hartnack, A.K., Niehaus, A.J. et al. (2020). Pharmacokinetics of an intravenous constant rate infusion of a morphine-lidocaine-ketamine combination in Holstein calves undergoing umbilical herniorrhaphy. *Am. J. Vet. Res.* 81: 17–24.

Hawley, A.T. and Wetmore, L.A. (2010). Identification of single nucleotide polymorphisms within exon 1 of the canine mu-opioid receptor gene. *Vet. Anaesth. Analg.* 37: 79–82.

Heffernan, A.E., Katz, E.M. et al. (2018). Once daily oral extended-release hydrocodone as analgesia following tibial plateau leveling osteotomy in dogs. *Vet. Surg.* 47: 516–523.

Höcker, J., Weber, B. et al. (2008). Meperidine, remifentanil and tramadol but not sufentanil interact with alpha(2)-adrenoceptors in alpha(2A)-, alpha(2B)- and alpha(2C)-adrenoceptor knock out mice brain. *Eur. J. Pharmacol.* 582: 70–77.

Houghton, K.J., Rech, R.H. et al. (1991). Dose-response of intravenous butorphanol to increase visceral nociceptive threshold in dogs. *Proc. Soc. Exp. Biol. Med.* 197: 290–296.

Ilkiw, J.E., Pascoe, P.J., and Fisher, L.D. (1997). Effect of alfentanil on the minimum alveolar concentration of isoflurane in cats. *Am. J. Vet. Res.* 58: 1274–1279.

Ilkiw, J.E., Pascoe, P.J., and Tripp, L.D. (2002). Effects of morphine, butorphanol, buprenorphine, and U50488H on the minimum alveolar concentration of isoflurane in cats. *Am. J. Vet. Res.* 63: 1198–1202.

Ingvast-Larsson, C., Holgersson, A. et al. (2010). Clinical pharmacology of methadone in dogs. *Vet. Anaesth. Analg.* 37: 48–56.

Knych, H.K., Casbeer, H.C. et al. (2013). Pharmacokinetics and pharmacodynamics of butorphanol following intravenous administration to the horse. *J. Vet. Pharmacol. Ther.* 36: 21–30.

Ko, J.C., Lange, D.N. et al. (2000). Effects of butorphanol and carprofen on the minimal alveolar concentration of isoflurane in dogs. *J. Am. Vet. Med. Assoc.* 217: 1025–1028.

KuKanich, B. (2010). Pharmacokinetics of acetaminophen, codeine, and the codeine metabolites morphine and codeine-6-glucuronide in healthy greyhound dogs. *J. Vet. Pharmacol. Ther.* 33: 15–21.

KuKanich, B. and Allen, P. (2014). Comparative pharmacokinetics of intravenous fentanyl and buprenorphine in healthy greyhound dogs. *J. Vet. Pharmacol. Ther.* 37: 595–597.

KuKanich, B. and KuKanich, K. (2015a). Chloramphenicol significantly affects the pharmacokinetics of oral methadone in greyhound dogs. *Vet. Anaesth. Analg.* 42 (6): 597–607.

KuKanich, B. and Spade, J. (2013). Pharmacokinetics of hydrocodone and hydromorphone after oral hydrocodone in healthy greyhound dogs. *Vet. J.* 196: 266–268.

KuKanich, B. and Weise, A. (2015b). Opioids. In: *Veterinary Anesthesia and Analgesia*, 5e (ed. K.A. Grimm, L.A. Lamont, W.J. Tranquilli, et al.), 207–226. Ames IA: Wiley Blackwell.

KuKanich, B., Lascelles, B.D., and Papich, M.G. (2005a). Assessment of a von Frey device for evaluation of the antinociceptive effects of morphine and its application in pharmacodynamic modeling of morphine in dogs. *Am. J. Vet. Res.* 66: 1616–1622.

KuKanich, B., Lascelles, B.D., and Papich, M.G. (2005b). Pharmacokinetics of morphine and plasma concentrations of morphine-6-glucuronide following morphine administration to dogs. *J. Vet. Pharmacol. Ther.* 28: 371–376.

KuKanich, B., Hogan, B.K. et al. (2008a). Pharmacokinetics of hydromorphone hydrochloride in healthy dogs. *Vet. Anaesth. Analg.* 35: 256–264.

KuKanich, B., Schmidt, B.K. et al. (2008b). Pharmacokinetics and behavioral effects of oxymorphone after intravenous and subcutaneous administration to healthy dogs. *J. Vet. Pharmacol. Ther.* 31: 580–583.

Kyles, A.E., Hardie, E.M. et al. (1998). Comparison of transdermal fentanyl and intramuscular oxymorphone on post-operative behaviour after ovariohysterectomy in dogs. *Res. Vet. Sci.* 65: 245–251.

Laubie, M., Schmitt, H., and Vincent, M. (1979). Vagal bradycardia produced by microinjections of morphine-like drugs into the nucleus ambiguus in anaesthetized dogs. *Eur. J. Pharmacol.* 59: 287–291.

Leander, J.D., Zerbe, R.L., and Hart, J.C. (1985). Diuresis and suppression of vasopressin by kappa opioids: comparison with mu and delta opioids and clonidine. *J. Pharmacol. Exp. Ther.* 234: 463–469.

Lee, D.D., Papich, M.G., and Hardie, E.M. (2000). Comparison of pharmacokinetics of fentanyl after intravenous and transdermal administration in cats. *Am. J. Vet. Res.* 61: 672–677.

Lester, P.A., Gaynor, J.S. et al. (2003). The sedative and behavioral effects of nalbuphine in dogs. *Contemp. Top. Lab. Anim. Sci.* 42: 27–31.

Levitsky, S., Mullin, E.M. et al. (1971). Experimental evaluation of pentazocine: effect on myocardial contractility and peripheral vascular resistance. *Am. Heart J.* 81: 381–386.

Lewis, J.W. (1985). Buprenorphine. *Drug Alcohol Depend.* 14: 363–372.

Linardi, R.L., Stokes, A.M. et al. (2012). Bioavailability and pharmacokinetics of oral and injectable formulations of methadone after intravenous, oral, and intragastric administration in horses. *Am. J. Vet. Res.* 73: 290–295.

Lindegaard, C., Thomsen, M.H. et al. (2010). Analgesic efficacy of intra-articular morphine in experimentally induced radiocarpal synovitis in horses. *Vet. Anaesth. Analg.* 37: 171–185.

Lötsch, J., Walter, C. et al. (2013). Pharmacokinetics of non-intravenous formulations of fentanyl. *Clin. Pharmacokinet.* 52: 23–36.

Lovasz, M., Aarnes, T.K. et al. (2017). Pharmacokinetics of intravenous and transdermal fentanyl in alpacas. *J. Vet. Pharmacol. Ther.* 40: 663–669.

Love, E.J., Taylor, P.M. et al. (2009). Analgesic effect of butorphanol in ponies following castration. *Equine Vet. J.* 41: 552–556.

Love, E.J., Pelligand, L. et al. (2015). Pharmacokinetic-pharmacodynamic modelling of intravenous buprenorphine in conscious horses. *Vet. Anaesth. Analg.* 42: 17–29.

Machado, M.L., Soares, J.H.N. et al. (2018). Dose-finding study comparing three treatments of remifentanil in cats anesthetized with isoflurane undergoing ovariohysterectomy. *J. Feline Med. Surg.* 20: 164–171.

Mathews, K.A., Paley, D.M. et al. (1996). A comparison of ketorolac with flunixin, butorphanol, and oxymorphone in controlling postoperative pain in dogs. *Can. Vet. J.* 37: 557–567.

Matthews, N.S. and Lindsay, S.L. (1990). Effect of low-dose butorphanol on halothane minimum alveolar concentration in ponies. *Equine Vet. J.* 22: 325–327.

McFadzean, W.J., Hall, E.J., and van Oostrom, H. (2017). Effect of premedication with butorphanol or methadone on ease of endoscopic duodenal intubation in dogs. *Vet. Anaesth. Analg.* 44: 1296–1302.

Mealey, K.L., Owens, J.G. et al. (2023). Canine and feline P-glycoprotein deficiency: what we know and where we need to go. *J. Vet. Pharmacol. Ther.* 46: 1–16.

Merritt, A.M., Burrow, J.A., and Hartless, C.S. (1998). Effect of xylazine, detomidine, and a combination of xylazine and butorphanol on equine duodenal motility. *Am. J. Vet. Res.* 59: 619–623.

Messenger, K.M., Davis, J.L. et al. (2011). Intravenous and sublingual buprenorphine in horses: pharmacokinetics and influence of sampling site. *Vet. Anaesth. Analg.* 38: 374–384.

Monteiro, E.R., Figueroa, C.D. et al. (2008). Effects of methadone, alone or in combination with acepromazine or xylazine, on sedation and physiologic values in dogs. *Vet. Anaesth. Analg.* 35: 519–527.

Muir, W.W. and Robertson, J.T. (1985). Visceral analgesia: effects of xylazine, butorphanol, meperidine, and pentazocine in horses. *Am. J. Vet. Res.* 46 (10): 2081–2084.

Muir, W.W., Wiese, A.J., and March, P.A. (2003). Effects of morphine, lidocaine, ketamine, and morphine-lidocaine-ketamine drug combination on minimum alveolar concentration in dogs anesthetized with isoflurane. *Am. J. Vet. Res.* 64: 1155–1160.

Murray, R.B., Adler, M.W., and Korczyn, A.D. (1983). The pupillary effects of opioids. *Life Sci.* 33: 495–509.

Naganobu, K., Maeda, N. et al. (2004). Cardiorespiratory effects of epidural administration of morphine and fentanyl in dogs anesthetized with sevoflurane. *J. Am. Vet. Med. Assoc.* 224: 67–70.

Nakayoshi, T., Kawasaki, N. et al. (2007). Epidural administration of morphine facilitates time of appearance of first gastric interdigestive migrating complex in dogs with paralytic ileus after open abdominal surgery. *J. Gastrointest. Surg.* 11: 648–654.

Natalini, C.C. (2010). Spinal anesthetics and analgesics in the horse. *Vet. Clin. North Am. Equine Pract.* 26: 551–564.

de Oliviera Frazílio, F., DeRossi, R. et al. (2014). Effects of epidural nalbuphine on intraoperative isoflurane and postoperative analgesic requirements in dogs. *Acta Cir. Bras.* 29: 38–46.

Osorio Lujan, S., Habre, W. et al. (2017). Plasma concentrations of transdermal fentanyl and buprenorphine in pigs (*Sus scrofa domesticus*). *Vet. Anaesth. Analg.* 44: 665–675.

Pallarols, N.B., Lamuraglia, R. et al. (2020). Behavioral and cardiopulmonary effects of a constant rate infusion of remifentanil-xylazine for sedation in horses. *J. Equine Vet.* 91: 103111. https://doi.org/10.1016/j.jevs.2020.103111.

Pascoe, P. (2000). Opioid analgesics. *Vet. Clin. North Am. Small Anim. Pract.* 30: 757–772.

Pascoe, P.J., Lamuraglia, R. et al. (1991). The pharmacokinetics and locomotor activity of alfentanil in the horse. *J. Vet. Pharmacol. Ther.* 14: 317–325.

Pascoe, P.J., Steffey, E.P. et al. (1993). Evaluation of the effect of alfentanil on the minimum alveolar concentration of halothane in horses. *Am. J. Vet. Res.* 54: 1327–1332.

Pekcan, Z. and Koc, B. (2010). The post-operative analgesic effects of epidurally administered morphine and transdermal fentanyl patch after ovariohysterectomy in dogs. *Vet. Anaesth. Analg.* 37: 557–565.

Peterson, N.W., Buote, N.J. et al. (2014). Effect of epidural analgesia with opioids on the prevalence of urinary retention in dogs undergoing surgery for cranial cruciate ligament rupture. *J. Am. Vet. Med. Assoc.* 244: 940–943.

Pfeffer, M., Smyth, R.D. et al. (1980). Pharmacokinetics of subcutaneous and intramuscular butorphanol in dogs. *J. Pharm. Sci.* 69: 801–803.

Pieper, K., Schuster, T. et al. (2011). Antinociceptive efficacy and plasma concentrations of transdermal buprenorphine in dogs. *Vet. J.* 187: 335–341.

Posner, L.P., Gleed, R.D. et al. (2007). Post-anesthetic hyperthermia in cats. *Vet. Anaesth. Analg.* 34: 40–47.

Posner, L.P., Pavuk, A.A. et al. (2010). Effects of opioids and anesthetic drugs on body temperature in cats. *Vet. Anaesth. Analg.* 37: 35–43.

Posner, L.P., Applegate, J. et al. (2020). Total injectable anesthesia of dogs and cats for remote location veterinary sterilization clinic. *BMC Vet. Res.* 16: 304. https://doi.org/10.1186/s12917-020-02525-x.

Priano, L.L. and Vatner, S.F. (1981). Generalized cardiovascular and regional hemodynamic effects of meperidine in conscious dogs. *Anesth. Analg.* 60: 649–654.

Proudman, C.J., Smith, J.E. et al. (2002). Long-term survival of equine surgical colic cases. Part 1: patterns of mortality and morbidity. *Equine Vet. J.* 34: 432–437.

Pypendop, B.H. and Shilo-Benjamini, Y. (2021). Pharmacokinetics of butorphanol in male neutered cats anesthetized with isoflurane. *J. Vet. Pharmacol. Ther.* 44: 883–887.

Pypendop, B.H., Brosnan, R.J., and Ilkiw, J.E. (2011). Use of naltrexone to antagonize high doses of remifentanil in cats: a dose-finding study. *Vet. Anaesth. Analg.* 38: 594–597.

Pypendop, B.H., Ilkiw, J.E., and Shilo-Benjamini, Y. (2014). Bioavailability of morphine, methadone, hydromorphone, and oxymorphone following buccal administration in cats. *J. Vet. Pharmacol. Ther.* 37: 295–300.

Pypendop, B.H., Goich, M., and Shilo-Benjamini, Y. (2022). Effect of intravenous butorphanol infusion on the minimum alveolar concentration of isoflurane in cats. *Vet. Anaesth. Analg.* 49: 165–172.

Quandt, J.E., Raffe, M.R., and Robinson, E.P. (1994). Butorphanol does not reduce the minimum alveolar concentration of halothane in dogs. *Vet. Surg.* 23: 156–159.

Reed, R. and Doherty, T. (2018). Minimum alveolar concentration: key concepts and a review of its pharmacological reduction in dogs. Part 2. *Res. Vet. Sci.* 118: 27–33.

Reed, R., Barletta, M. et al. (2019). The pharmacokinetics and pharmacodynamics of intravenous hydromorphone in horses. *Vet. Anaesth. Analg.* 46: 395–404.

Reed, R.A., Knych, H.K. et al. (2020). Pharmacokinetics and pharmacodynamics of hydromorphone after intravenous and intramuscular administration in horses. *Vet. Anaesth. Analg.* 47: 210–218.

Ritschel, W.A., Neub, M., and Denson, D.D. (1987). Meperidine pharmacokinetics following intravenous, peroral and buccal administration in beagle dogs. *Methods Find. Exp. Clin. Pharmacol.* 9: 811–815.

Robertson, S.A., Hauptman, J.G. et al. (2001). Effects of acetylpromazine or morphine on urine production in halothane-anesthetized dogs. *Am. J. Vet. Res.* 62: 1922–1927.

Robertson, S.A., Taylor, P.M., and Sear, J.W. (2003). Systemic uptake of buprenorphine by cats after oral mucosal administration. *Vet. Rec.* 152: 675–678.

Ryan, A.C., Murrell, J.C., and Gurney, M.A. (2022). Post-operative nausea and vomiting (PONV) observed in a clinical study designed to assess the analgesic effects of intravenous and subcutaneous methadone in dogs. *Vet. J.* 287: 105876. https://doi.org/10.1016/j.tvjl.2022.105876.

Sammarco, J.L., Conzemius, M.G. et al. (1996). Postoperative analgesia for stifle surgery: a comparison of intra-articular bupivacaine, morphine, or saline. *Vet. Surg.* 25: 59–69.

Sano, T., Nishimura, R. et al. (2006). Pharmacokinetics of fentanyl after single intravenous injection and constant rate infusion in dogs. *Vet. Anaesth. Analg.* 33: 266–273.

Sarotti, D., Rabozzi, R., and Franci, P. (2013). A retrospective study of efficacy and side effects of intrathecal administration of hyperbaric bupivacaine and morphine solution in 39 dogs undergoing hind limb orthopaedic surgery. *Vet. Anaesth. Analg.* 40: 220–224.

Sayre, R.S., Lepiz, M.A. et al. (2015). Effects of oxymorphone hydrochloride or hydromorphone hydrochloride on minimal alveolar concentration of desflurane in sheep. *Am. J. Vet. Res.* 76: 583–590.

Schurig, J.E., Cavanagh, R.L., and Buyniski, J.P. (1978). Effect of butorphanol and morphine on pulmonary mechanics, arterial blood pressure and venous plasma histamine in the anesthetized dog. *Arch. Int. Pharmacodyn. Ther.* 233: 296–304.

Seddighi, R., Geist, A. et al. (2023). The effect of remifentanil infusion on sevoflurane minimum alveolar concentration-no movement (MACNM) and bispectral index in dogs. *Vet. Anaesth. Analg.* 50: 121–128.

Sellon, D.C., Roberts, M.C. et al. (2004). Effects of continuous rate intravenous infusion of butorphanol on physiologic and outcome variables in horses after celiotomy. *J. Vet. Intern. Med.* 18: 555–563.

Sellon, D.C., Papich, M.G. et al. (2009). Pharmacokinetics of butorphanol in horses after intramuscular injection. *J. Vet. Pharmacol. Ther.* 32: 62–65.

Senior, J.M., Pinchbeck, G.L. et al. (2004). Retrospective study of the risk factors and prevalence of colic in horses after orthopaedic surgery. *Vet. Rec.* 155: 321–325.

Sharpe, L.G. and Pickworth, W.B. (1985). Opposite pupillary size effects in the cat and dog after microinjections of morphine, normorphine and clonidine in the Edinger-Westphal nucleus. *Brain Res. Bull.* 15: 329–333.

Siao, K.T., Pypendop, B.H. et al. (2011). Pharmacokinetics of oxymorphone in cats. *J. Vet. Pharmacol. Ther.* 34: 594–598.

Skrzypczak, H., Reed, R. et al. (2022). The pharmacokinetics of a fentanyl matrix patch applied at three different anatomical locations in horses. *Equine Vet. J.* 54: 153–158.

Slingsby, L.S., Sear, J.W. et al. (2016). Effect of intramuscular methadone on pharmacokinetic data and thermal and mechanical nociceptive thresholds in the cat. *J. Feline Med. Surg.* 18: 875–881.

Smith, H.S. and Laufer, A. (2014). Opioid induced nausea and vomiting. *Eur. J. Pharmacol.* 722: 67–78.

Smith, A.A., Posner, L.P. et al. (2004). Evaluation of the effects of premedication on gastroduodenoscopy in cats. *J. Am. Vet. Med. Assoc.* 225: 540–544.

Smith, J.S., Coetzee, J.F. et al. (2018a). Pharmacokinetics of fentanyl citrate and norfentanyl in Holstein calves and effect of analytical performances on fentanyl parameter estimation. *J. Vet. Pharmacol. Ther.* 41: 555–561.

Smith, J.S., Mochel, J.P. et al. (2018b). Adverse reactions to fentanyl transdermal patches in calves: a preliminary clinical and pharmacokinetic study. *Vet. Anaesth. Analg.* 45: 575–580.

Sojka, J.E., Adams, S.B. et al. (1988). Effect of butorphanol, pentazocine, meperidine, or metoclopramide on intestinal motility in female ponies. *Am. J. Vet. Res.* 49: 527–529.

Springfield, D., KuKanich, B. et al. (2022). Dosing protocols to increase the efficacy of butorphanol in dogs. *J. Vet. Pharmacol. Ther.* 45: 516–529.

Steagall, P.V., Carnicelli, P. et al. (2006). Effects of subcutaneous methadone, morphine, buprenorphine or saline on thermal and pressure thresholds in cats. *J. Vet. Pharmacol. Ther.* 29: 531–537.

Steagall, P.V., Ruel, H.L.M. et al. (2020). Pharmacokinetics and analgesic effects of intravenous, intramuscular or subcutaneous buprenorphine in dogs undergoing ovariohysterectomy: a randomized, prospective, masked, clinical trial. *BMC Vet. Res.* 16: 154. https://doi.org/10.1186/s12917-020-02364-w. PMID: 32448336.

Steffey, E.P., Eisele, J.H. et al. (2003). Interactions of morphine and isoflurane in horses. *Am. J. Vet. Res.* 64: 166–175.

Stein, C. (2018). New concepts in opioid analgesia. *Expert Opin. Investig. Drugs* 27: 765–775.

Sternini, C., Patierno, S. et al. (2004). The opioid system in the gastrointestinal tract. *Neurogastroenterol. Motil.* 16 (Suppl): 3–16.

Takahashi, T., Tsuchida, D., and Pappas, T.N. (2007). Central effects of morphine on GI motility in conscious dogs. *Brain Res.* 1166: 29–34.

Taylor, P.M., Robertson, S.A. et al. (2001). Morphine, pethidine and buprenorphine disposition in the cat. *Vet. Pharmacol. Ther.* 24: 391–398.

Thomasy, S.M., Slovis, N. et al. (2004). Transdermal fentanyl combined with nonsteroidal anti-inflammatory drugs for analgesia in horses. *J. Vet. Intern. Med.* 18: 550–554.

Thomasy, S.M., Mama, K.R. et al. (2007). Influence of general anaesthesia on the pharmacokinetics of intravenous fentanyl and its primary metabolite in horses. *Equine Vet. J.* 39: 54–58.

Tissot, T. (2003). Probable meperidine-induced serotonin syndrome in a patient with a history of fluoxetine use. *Anesthesiology* 98: 1511–1512.

Tobin, T. and Miller, J.R. (1979). The pharmacology of narcotic analgesics in the horse. I. The detection, pharmacokinetics and urinary clearance times of pentazocine. *J. Equine Med. Surg.* 3: 191–198.

Torske, K.E. and Dyson, D.H. (2000). Epidural analgesia and anesthesia. *Vet. Clin. North Am. Small Anim. Pract.* 30: 859–874.

Tournier, N., Declèves, X. et al. (2011). Opioid transport by ATP-binding cassette transporters at the blood-brain barrier: implications for neuropsychopharmacology. *Curr. Pharm. Des.* 17: 2829–2842.

Trescot, A.M., Datta, S. et al. (2008). Opioid pharmacology. *Pain Physician* 11 (2 Suppl): S133–S153.

Troncy, E., Junot, S. et al. (2002). Results of preemptive epidural administration of morphine with or without bupivacaine in dogs and cats undergoing surgery: 265 cases (1997–1999). *J. Am. Vet. Med. Assoc.* 221: 666–672.

Tsuchida, D., Fukuda, H. et al. (2004). Central effect of mu-opioid agonists on antral motility in conscious rats. *Brain Res.* 1024: 244–250.

Valverde, A., Cantwell, S. et al. (2004). Effects of acepromazine on the incidence of vomiting associated with opioid administration in dogs. *Vet. Anaesth. Analg.* 31: 40–45.

Veng-Pedersen, P., Wilhelm, J.A. et al. (1995). Duration of opioid antagonism by nalmefene and naloxone in the dog: an integrated pharmacokinetic/pharmacodynamic comparison. *J. Pharm. Sci.* 84: 1101–1106.

Villalba, M., Santiago, I., and Gomez de Segura, I.A. (2011). Effects of constant rate infusion of lidocaine and ketamine, with or without morphine, on isoflurane MAC in horses. *Equine Vet. J.* 43: 721–726.

Wagner, A.E., Dunlop, C.I., and Turner, A.S. (1996). Experiences with morphine injected into the subarachnoid space in sheep. *Vet. Surg.* 25: 256–260.

Wagner, L.E., Eaton, M. et al. (1999). Meperidine and lidocaine block of recombinant voltage-dependent Na+ channels: evidence that meperidine is a local anesthetic. *Anesthesiology* 91: 1481–1490.

Wahler, B.M., Lerche, P. et al. (2019). Pharmacokinetics and pharmacodynamics of intranasal and intravenous naloxone hydrochloride administration in healthy dogs. *Am. J. Vet. Res.* 80: 696–701.

Wang, D.S., Sternbach, G., and Varon, J. (1998). Nalmefene: a long-acting opioid antagonist. Clinical applications in emergency medicine. *J. Emerg. Med.* 16: 471–475.

Warne, L.N., Beths, T. et al. (2014). Evaluation of the perioperative analgesic efficacy of buprenorphine, compared with butorphanol, in cats. *J. Am. Vet. Med. Assoc.* 245: 195–202.

Wegner, K. and Robertson, S.A. (2004). Pharmacokinetic and pharmacodynamic evaluation of intravenous hydromorphone in cats. *J. Vet. Pharmacol. Ther.* 27: 329–336.

Wells, S.M., Glerum, L.E., and Papich, M.G. (2008). Pharmacokinetics of butorphanol in cats after intramuscular and buccal transmucosal administration. *Am. J. Vet. Res.* 69: 1548–1554.

Westermann, C.M., Laan, T.T. et al. (2005). Effects of antitussive agents administered before bronchoalveolar lavage in horses. *Am. J. Vet. Res.* 66: 1420–1424.

Wetmore, L.A., Pascoe, P.J. et al. (2016). Effects of fentanyl administration on locomotor response in horses with the G57C μ-opioid receptor polymorphism. *Am. J. Vet. Res.* 77: 828–832.

Wicks, C., Hudlicky, T., and Rinner, U. (2021). Morphine alkaloids: history, biology, and synthesis. *Alkaloids Chem. Biol.* 86: 145–342.

Wilson, D.V., Evans, T.A., and Mauer, W.A. (2007). Pre-anesthetic meperidine: associated vomiting and gastroesophageal reflux during the subsequent anesthetic in dogs. *Vet. Anaesth. Analg.* 34: 15–22.

Wong, P.L. (1992). Anesthesia for gastric dilatation/volvulus. *Vet. Clin. North Am. Small Anim. Pract.* 22: 471–474.

Yamashiro, H. (1978). Effect of pentazocine on renal blood flow. *Br. J. Anaesth.* 50: 133–137.

Yeh, S.Y., Chernov, H.I., and Woods, L.A. (1971). Metabolism of morphine by cats. *J. Pharm. Sci.* 60: 469–471.

8

Barbiturates

Bonnie L. Hay Kraus

Introduction

Barbiturates are central nervous system (CNS) depressants that can be used for sedation, anesthesia, induced coma and even death in the form of euthanasia solutions. Thiopental was first introduced into human anesthesia in 1934 and revolutionized the practice of anesthesia. Rapid barbiturate induction replaced the prolonged, unpleasant and often dangerous induction of general anesthesia with diethyl ether (Rathmell and Rosow 2015). Barbiturates have been used in human medicine for induction and maintenance of anesthesia, cerebral protection in at-risk patients and electroshock therapy (Vuyk et al. 2020). Since 2011, thiopental is no longer manufactured in the US and overseas manufacturers have stopped exporting to the US in protest at its use as part of the lethal injection "cocktail" for capital punishment (Woolston 2013). Although methohexital is still available in the US, and it provides a rapid return to consciousness, the high incidence of excitatory phenomena such as myoclonus and postoperative seizures has led to its replacement by propofol (Michic and Harris 2011). Barbiturate pharmacology is included in this textbook for several reasons, including the fact that these drugs are still widely used outside the US, exportation or US manufacture may resume, and perhaps most importantly, the pharmacokinetics and pharmacodynamics of barbiturates are the prototypes for comparison for most of the currently available IV anesthetics. Understanding the pharmacokinetics/dynamics of drugs such as propofol, alphaxalone and etomidate is enhanced if the anesthetist understands the properties of barbiturates, to which they are often compared.

There are four barbiturates used in veterinary medicine. Phenobarbital is used as an anticonvulsant and pentobarbital, thiopental and methohexital are used as anesthetic agents. Thiamylal is very similar to thiopental in anesthetic effects and chemical structure, however, it is no longer available (Berry 2015). Historically, pentobarbital was the principal anesthetic agent in veterinary medicine, however, it has been replaced by shorter-acting injectable agents and inhalants. It may still be used as a sedative/anesthetic in patients being mechanically ventilated and in rodent laboratory animal situations (Plumb 2018b). Pentobarbital is also a major ingredient in many commercial euthanasia solutions. Until recently (early 2000's), thiopental was the most commonly used injectable anesthetic used in veterinary medicine, however, cessation of manufacturing in the US has led to its replacement by other IV injectable agents such as propofol, ketamine/midazolam and alphaxalone and the use of total IM anesthesia with dexmedetomidine-based protocols. Methohexital is the only anesthetic barbiturate still available in the US, however, it has been largely replaced by propofol for clinical use.

Physicochemical Characteristics

The classification of barbiturates as ultra-short, short, intermediate and long acting is no longer recommended as it incorrectly associates a duration of action of a certain time interval, however, this nomenclature is still used in many anesthesia texts (Stoelting and Hillier 2006). Barbiturates are derived from barbituric acid, which is hypnotically inactive and formed by malonic acid and urea. The substitutions on barbituric acid determine the physiochemical properties such as lipid solubility, onset and duration of action, metabolic degradation and relative potency (Figure 8.1). Substitutions at the number 2 and 5 carbon atoms primarily result in barbiturates with CNS depressant, sedative and hypnotic effects and are used for clinical anesthesia (Berry 2015; Rathmell and Rosow 2015; Vuyk et al. 2020). Barbiturates are classified by their chemical structure as thiobarbiturates or oxybarbiturates. Thiobarbiturates (thiopental and thiamylal) have a sulfur atom at position 2 and oxybarbiturates (phenobarbital, pentobarbital, methohexital) have an oxygen atom at position 2 (Berry 2015; Rathmell and Rosow 2015; Vuyk et al. 2020). The sulfur atom imparts

Pharmacology in Veterinary Anesthesia and Analgesia, First Edition. Edited by Turi Aarnes and Phillip Lerche.
© 2024 John Wiley & Sons, Inc. Published 2024 by John Wiley & Sons, Inc.

Barbituric Acid

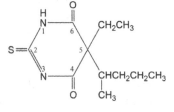

Methohexital   Thiopental

Pentobarbital   Phenobarbital

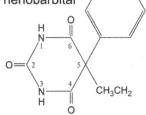

Figure 8.1 The four barbiturates currently used in veterinary medicine result from substitutions at the number two and five carbons of barbituric acid. (Created by Nickolas H. Kraus using Latexian v1.2.7 for Mac Os x by Taco Software).

greater potency and greater lipid solubility, thereby producing a more rapid onset of action and shorter duration of action. A good example of this is a comparison of thiopental with pentobarbital. Thiopental differs from pentobarbital only in the replacement of oxygen with a sulfur atom at carbon 2. However, this change results in the increased lipid solubility, faster onset of action, greater hypnotic potency and shorter duration, resulting in vast differences in the clinical use of the two drugs.

In general, modifications that increase the lipid solubility of the molecule will increase its potency while shortening the onset and duration of action. The addition of alkyl or aryl groups at position 5 of the barbituric acid ring imparts CNS depressant effects and the length of the side chain influences both potency and duration of action; longer side chains increase potency (Berry 2015; Posner 2018). Asymmetric carbon atoms in the side chains at position 5 results in D-isomers and L-isomers (twice as potent), however, barbiturates are supplied as racemic mixtures (Berry 2015; Posner 2018).

Methohexital is an oxybarbiturate that has a methyl group on the nitrogen atom which increases lipid solubility, making it more potent than thiopental and producing a faster onset of action. However, it also increases excitatory

side effects and causes myoclonus and tremors during induction (Rathmell and Rosow 2015). Pentobarbital is an oxybarbiturate identical to methohexital with the exception of the methyl group and has a duration of action 4–8 times that of thiopental in most species (Berry 2015). Phenobarbital has a phenyl group at the fifth carbon positron which increases the anticonvulsant but not hypnotic potency (Rathmell and Rosow 2015).

Barbiturates are acids, however, they are prepared as sodium salts which are very alkaline. The high alkalinity of the solution is bacteriostatic but caustic if given perivascularly and will cause sloughing of tissue (Posner 2018). Thiopental and methohexital are both supplied as crystalline powders that can be reconstituted with either sterile water, normal saline or D5W to a 2.5% solution for thiopental and a 1% solution for methohexital (Plumb's 2018a,c). Barbiturates cannot be reconstituted with lactated ringer's solution or mixed with other acidic solutions as the decrease in alkalinity will result in precipitation of the barbiturate (Vuyk et al. 2020). Although reconstituted methohexital is stable for up to 6 weeks and thiopental solution is stable at room temperature for 3 days and for 7 days when refrigerated, current label recommendations are to discard unused portions within 24 hours due to the lack of preservative (Plumb's 2018a,c). Thiopental has been used in a 1:1 mixture with propofol, however, compatibility with other drugs depends on factors such as pH, concentration, temperature and diluent used and consultation with specific references or a pharmacist is advised (Plumb's 2018c). Pentobarbital (generic) is available as a human labeled product as a 50 mg/ml injectable solution (Plumb's 2018b).

Pharmacokinetics

Physiologic and compartmental models have been used to describe barbiturate pharmacokinetics and both indicate rapid redistribution as the primary mechanism that terminates the effects of a single induction dose (Vuyk et al. 2020). In the physiologic model, the drug mixes in the central blood compartment and is delivered to the tissues according to the perfusion of the tissue, the tissue affinity and the relative concentration in the blood and tissues (Berry 2015; Vuyk et al. 2020). Rapid distribution occurs to highly perfused, low-volume tissues such as the brain, thereby inducing anesthesia (Figure 8.2). The concentration in the

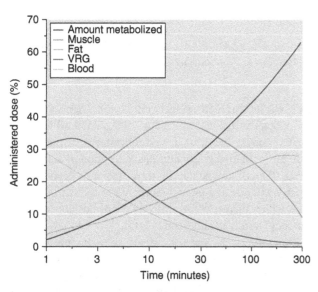

Figure 8.2 The percentage of thiopental in blood rapidly decreases as the drug moves from the blood to body tissues after an IV bolus. The time to achievement of peak tissue levels is a direct function of the tissue capacity for barbiturate relative to blood flow. A larger capacity or smaller blood flow results in a longer time-to-peak tissue levels. Most thiopental is initially taken up by the vessel-rich group (VRG) of tissues because of their high blood flow. The drug is then redistributed to muscle and, to a lesser extent, to fat. During this period, some thiopental is removed and metabolized by the liver and this removal is cumulative, unlike tissue removal. The rate of metabolism equals the early rate of removal by fat and the sum of these is similar to the amount of uptake by skeletal muscle. (From Vuyk et al. (2015) with permission).

brain and blood decreases rapidly as the drug redistributes to less perfused tissues, such as skeletal muscle, thus terminating the effect of an induction dose and allowing the patient to regain consciousness (Berry 2015; Vuyk et al. 2020). Adipose tissue uptake and metabolic clearance play only a minor role in termination of effect of a single induction dose due to the minimal perfusion ratio and slow rate of elimination (Vuyk et al. 2015). In compartmental models, a single dose of thiopental or methohexital exhibits first-order kinetics where a constant fraction of drug is cleared from the body per unit of time. The compartmental pharmacokinetic model helps to explain the delay in recovery with high or multiple doses or constant infusions of barbiturates in which termination of effect becomes increasingly dependent on the redistribution from adipose tissue and elimination by hepatic metabolism. The nonlinear zero-order Michaelis–Menten kinetics is due to receptor saturation and results in a constant **amount** of drug being cleared per unit of time (Vuyk et al. 2020). The context-sensitive half-time (the time for the plasma concentration to decrease by 50%) after prolonged infusions of thiopental is long since reentry of the drug to the circulation from muscle and fat prevents plasma levels from decreasing (Rathmell and Rosow 2015).

The distribution of barbiturates is determined by their lipid solubility, degree of ionization and protein binding (Berry 2015). High-lipid solubility and a high degree of non-ionized drug results in rapid crossing of the blood–brain barrier and rapid onset of action. Thiopental and methohexital are more lipid soluble than pentobarbital and therefore, have a more rapid onset of action. Barbiturates, in general, are highly protein bound. Only unbound drug can cross the blood brain–barrier; therefore, the greater the amount of unbound drug, the more rapid and greater the CNS effect. Protein binding of barbiturates parallels the lipid solubility of the non-ionized form since the ionized molecule is poorly lipid soluble (Stoelting and Hillier 2006). Thiobarbiturates are more highly protein bound than oxybarbiturates due to the sulfur substitution increasing affinity for the hydrophobic portion of the protein. Hypoalbuminemia, displacement by other highly protein bound drugs such as aspirin or phenylbutazone or competitive binding inhibition in uremic patients all result in enhanced drug effect (Stoelting and Hillier 2006; Berry 2015). Neonates have also decreased protein binding which may be exacerbated by fetal acidosis during delivery. Elimination half-time is prolonged during pregnancy because of the increased protein binding of thiopental and greater volume of distribution (Stoelting and Hillier 2006).

The pKa (acid dissociation constant) and the pH of the environment determine the degree of ionization of barbiturates. The pKa is the pH at which barbiturates exist as

50% ionized and 50% non-ionized forms. Barbiturates penetrate cell lipid layers in the non-ionized form; as blood becomes more acidic, more barbiturate drug exists in the non-ionized form leading to an increase in CNS penetration of the drug and clinical effect (Berry 2015). Metabolic changes in blood pH produce more pronounced effects on drug distribution than do respiratory changes. During metabolic changes, the intracellular pH in the brain remains relatively unchanged due to the inability of hydrogen ions to cross the lipid barrier and drug movement across the blood–brain barrier is increased. In contrast, ventilation-induced changes in blood pH are associated with rapid diffusion of carbon dioxide and therefore, similar changes in intracellular and extracellular pH, resulting in less net movement of drug (Stoelting and Hillier 2006).

Thiopental and methohexital have a rapid effect-site equilibration with maximal brain uptake within 30 seconds, resulting in CNS depression (Stoelting and Hillier 2006). This is followed by a decrease to ½ the peak concentration by redistribution from the brain to other tissues and causes rapid awakening from a single IV dose (Stoelting and Hillier 2006). By 30 minutes, only about 10% remains in the brain (Stoelting and Hillier 2006). Disappearance from plasma is divided into a rapid redistribution phase, a slow metabolic phase and a second redistribution phase (Reves et al. 2009). Termination of effects is determined by the same factors that determine the rate of onset of action. Distribution from the CNS to plasma is determined by lipid solubility, protein binding and degree of ionization but lipid solubility is the most important (Stoelting and Hillier 2006). The initial high uptake of lipid-soluble drug into the brain and other highly perfused tissues causes the plasma concentration of barbiturate to decrease. This causes a reversal of the concentration gradient for the movement of drug between blood and tissues and results in rapid redistribution and awakening. The drug is redistributed from highly perfused CNS to well-perfused skeletal muscles which are the primary sites for initial redistribution. Equilibrium with skeletal muscles is reached in about 15 minutes after IV injection (Stoelting and Hillier 2006). Doses should be lowered in conditions of decreased skeletal muscle perfusion such as shock or decreased muscle mass (Stoelting and Hillier 2006). Tissue blood flow is also a major determinant of drug delivery to tissues and their ultimate distribution in the body and may be affected by changes in blood volume or distribution of blood flow to tissues (Stoelting and Hillier 2006). Hypovolemia or shock may decrease blood flow to skeletal muscles, whereas blood flow to the brain and heart are maintained resulting in increased cerebral and cardiac depression (Stoelting and Hillier 2006).

Barbiturate concentration continues to increase into the fat compartment 30 minutes after injection (Stoelting and

Hillier 2006). Despite a high fat: blood partition coefficient (~11) for thiopental, the initial uptake into adipose tissue is slow due to low blood flow limiting delivery of drug to the tissue (Stoelting and Hillier 2006). Thus, redistribution to fat does not significantly affect early awakening. The elimination half-time is prolonged in obese patients compared with non-obese patients, due to an increased volume of distribution from excess fat storage sites. Large or repeated doses will result in a cumulative effect where adipose tissue becomes a reservoir for maintaining plasma concentrations. Therefore, thiopental should be dosed according to lean body mass and repeated doses should be avoided to prevent overdose and/or prolonged recovery (Stoelting and Hillier 2006). Repeated dosing or constant infusion results in a prolonged context-sensitive half time due to saturation of tissues. The reservoir of drug in skeletal muscle and fat re-enters the circulation, preventing the plasma concentration from decreasing. Termination of effect depends on the elimination of the drug from blood which becomes more dependent on metabolism (Reves et al. 2009). Sighthounds such as the whippet and irish wolfhound have small fat stores and are known to have very prolonged and rough recoveries from thiobarbiturates. Greyhounds are classified as sighthounds and are also deficient in the CYP450 oxidative enzymes required for metabolism of thiobarbiturates (Robinson et al. 1986). Greyhounds can have extremely prolonged recoveries thus thiopental is not recommended for use in greyhounds. Greyhounds recover significantly quicker from methohexital (Sams et al. 1985).

Metabolism

Redistribution from the brain to inactive tissues rather than hepatic metabolism is the most important determinant of awakening following a single IV injection of barbiturates. Metabolism of thiopental is slow, with only 10–24% metabolized per hour. Although hepatic clearance of methohexital is 3–4 times faster than thiopental, early awakening from a single IV dose is still due to redistribution away from the brain to inactive tissue sites (Stoelting and Hillier 2006). With the exception of phenobarbital, barbiturates are metabolized in the liver. Metabolites are mostly inactive, water-soluble and excreted in the urine. Barbiturates are metabolized via four processes: (i) Oxidation of the aryl, alkyl or phenyl groups at C5; (ii) N-dealkylation; (iii) Desulfuration of thiobarbiturates at C2 and (iv) Hydrolytic disruption of the barbituric acid ring (Stoelting and Hillier 2006; Vuyk et al. 2020). Oxidation of the C5 side chain is the most important step in terminating the pharmacologic activity of barbiturates and occurs in the hepatocyte endoplasmic reticulum (Stoelting and

Hillier 2006). Drugs that induce oxidative microsomes enhance the metabolism of barbiturates. Oxybarbiturates are only metabolized in hepatocytes, whereas thiobarbiturates have a small amount of extra-hepatic metabolism in the kidney and CNS (Stoelting and Hillier 2006; Rathmell and Rosow 2015). Thiopental is metabolized to hydroxythiopental and carboxylic acid derivatives in the liver which are more water soluble and have little CNS activity (Stoelting and Hillier 2006). Metabolism of thiopental is 99% complete, with only ~1% excreted unchanged in the urine (Stoelting and Hillier 2006; Rathmell and Rosow 2015). Clearance of thiopental is characterized by a low hepatic extraction ratio (0.15) and capacity-dependent elimination, making metabolism more dependent on hepatic enzyme activity rather than hepatic blood flow (Stoelting and Hillier 2006; Rathmell and Rosow 2015).

Methohexital is less lipid soluble than thiopental, therefore, more of the drug remains in the plasma and available for metabolism. Methohexital has a similar distribution half-life, volume of distribution and protein binding as thiopental, however, the elimination half-life is markedly different (4 hours for methohexital and 12 hours for thiopental) (Vuyk et al. 2020). This difference is due to the more rapid hepatic clearance rate which is three times that of thiopental (Stoelting and Hillier 2006; Vuyk et al. 2020). Methohexital has a hepatic extraction ratio (clearance to hepatic blood flow) of 0.5 indicating that the liver extracts 50% of the drug presented to it in the circulation as compared to thiopental which is 0.15 (Vuyk et al. 2020). This also means that clearance of methohexital is more dependent on changes in cardiac output and hepatic blood flow than the clearance of thiopental (Stoelting and Hillier 2006; Reves et al. 2009). Methohexital is metabolized by oxidation in the liver to an alcohol and N-dealkylation to form the inactive metabolite 4-hydroxymethohexital (Stoelting and Hillier 2006; Reves et al. 2009; Vuyk et al. 2020).

Most barbiturates are filtered by the renal glomeruli, but the high degree of protein binding limits filtration and high lipid solubility favors reabsorption of any filtered drug back into the circulation, accounting for the low amount (<1%) excreted unchanged in urine. In contrast, phenobarbital is less lipid soluble and less protein bound and renal excretion accounts for 60–90% of drug elimination in the unchanged form (Stoelting and Hillier 2006; Reves et al. 2009; Vuyk et al. 2020).

Mechanism of Action

Barbiturate effects on the CNS include enhancement of synaptic action of inhibitory neurotransmitters and inhibition of synaptic actions of excitatory neurotransmitters. Gamma aminobutyric acid (GABA) is the major inhibitory neurotransmitter in the mammalian CNS and the $GABA_A$ receptor is the only site proven to be involved in barbiturate-induced anesthesia (Vuyk et al. 2020). The $GABA_A$ receptor is a chloride ion channel composed of at least five subunits with specific sites of action for GABA, barbiturates, benzodiazepines, and other molecules (Vuyk et al. 2020). At lower concentrations, interaction of barbiturates at the $GABA_A$ receptor increases the affinity of GABA for its binding site and decreases the rate of dissociation of GABA from the receptor. Both of these result in increased duration of the $GABA_A$-activated opening of chloride channels and hyperpolarization, which increases the threshold of excitability of the post-synaptic cell membrane and neuron (Vuyk et al. 2020). This enhancement of the action of GABA is considered responsible for the sedative-hypnotic effects. At higher drug concentrations, barbiturates can directly activate the chloride-ion channel associated with the $GABA_A$ receptor, acting as an agonist itself and is thought to be responsible for the anesthetic effects of barbiturates (Rathmell and Rosow 2015; Vuyk et al. 2020).

The second mechanism of action involves the inhibition of synaptic transmission of excitatory neurotransmitters such as glutamate and acetylcholine and are specific for synaptic ion channels (Rathmell and Rosow 2015; Vuyk et al. 2020). Thiopental may also exert effects on the N-methyl-D-aspartate (NMDA)-glutaminergic system by decreasing extracellular glutamate levels in the CNS and inhibiting excitatory activities through inhibition of NMDA receptors (Reves et al. 2009; Vuyk et al. 2020).

Pharmacodynamics

Barbiturates, at appropriate doses, cause loss of consciousness, amnesia and cardiovascular and respiratory depression. The amnesic effects are less pronounced compared to benzodiazepines. Studies indicate that barbiturates may lower the pain threshold, especially at lower plasma levels (Vuyk et al. 2020).

Effects on Cerebral Metabolism

Barbiturates cause a dose-related decrease in cerebral metabolic oxygen consumption rate (CMRO2), decreases adenosine triphosphate (ATP) consumption and protects during partial cerebral ischemia (Vuyk et al. 2020). The electroencephalogram (EEG) shows progressive slowing until it becomes isoelectric and CMRO2 is ~50% of baseline. This decrease in CMRO2 parallels the portion of metabolic activity related to neuronal signaling and impulse traffic, particularly in cortical areas. This portion does not include basal metabolic function which can only be suppressed through hypothermia. Therefore, the effect of barbiturates on cerebral metabolism is maximized at a 50% reduction in CMRO2 which leaves the rest of metabolic energy for the maintenance of cellular integrity. Along with reduced CMRO2, there is an increase in cerebral vascular resistance and cerebral blood flow (CBF) and intra-cranial pressure (ICP) both decrease. However, the ratio of CBF to CMRO2 remains unchanged since ICP decreases more than mean arterial pressure (MAP) and therefore, cerebral perfusion pressure (CPP) is preserved (Reves et al. 2009; Berry 2015; Vuyk et al. 2020). This increase in perfusion-to-metabolism ratio makes thiobarbiturates an appropriate drug choice for patients with intracranial disease, head trauma or a history of seizures (Stoelting and Hillier 2006; Berry 2015; Rathmell and Rosow 2015). In contrast, methohexital is associated with generalized excitement, activation of epileptic foci and seizures and should be avoided in patients with seizures.

Barbiturates can be used to treat patients with high ICP that are refractory to hyperventilation and drug-induced diuresis to lower ICP. However, significant hypotension occurs and improved outcome in head trauma has not been demonstrated (Stoelting and Hillier 2006; Rathmell and Rosow 2015). Effectiveness in metabolic suppression only occurs when the EEG is active, therefore, brain survival is not improved after global cerebral ischemia due to cardiac arrest with a flat EEG. Metabolic suppression by barbiturates is more likely to improve outcome with incomplete or focal cerebral ischemia since the decrease in CMRO2 exceeds that of CBF and provides protection to ischemic areas of the brain (Stoelting and Hillier 2006; Rathmell and Rosow 2015). However, these patients also have an increased requirement for inotropic support and moderate hypothermia may provide superior neuroprotection without prolonging recovery.

Effects on Cardiovascular System

Cardiovascular effects of induction with barbiturates result from both central and peripheral effects. The mechanisms for the decrease in cardiac output associated with barbiturate induction include direct negative inotropic effects due to a decrease in calcium influx into cells, decreased ventricular filling caused by increased capacitance and a decrease in sympathetic outflow from the CNS (Vuyk et al. 2020). However, the primary effect is peripheral vasodilation through depression of the medullary vasomotor center and decreased CNS sympathetic nervous system (SNS) outflow. This results in increased capacitance, decreased venous return and ventricular filling, causing decreased cardiac output and blood pressure. Dose-related direct negative inotropic effects that are less pronounced than that

caused by volatile anesthetics may be seen to be due to decreased calcium influx at sarcolemma sites (Reves et al. 2009; Vuyk et al. 2020). A baroreceptor-mediated increase in SNS activity causes a compensatory increase in heart rate and myocardial contractility to compensate for the decrease in cardiac output and blood pressure. The cardiac index and MAP are unchanged or slightly reduced in healthy patients (Vuyk et al. 2020). Hemodynamic changes are related to the infusion rate. Hypovolemic patients are less able to compensate for the peripheral vasodilation caused by barbiturates and may experience sustained decreases in venous return, cardiac output, and systemic blood pressure (Stoelting and Hillier 2006; Reves et al. 2009; Vuyk et al. 2015).

Healthy dogs exhibit similar cardiovascular responses with hypotension, decreased stroke volume and contractility which are compensated for by an increase in heart rate. Dogs and pigs require a smaller dose following significant hemorrhage, therefore, caution should be used in patients with dehydration, hypovolemia, anemia or cardiac disease. Cardiac dysrhythmias, particularly ventricular arrhythmias, including bigeminy may be seen after induction of anesthesia with barbiturates. These may be due to the reflex SNS stimulation and/or hypercapnia or hypoxemia from respiratory depression and apnea (Berry 2015). Caution should be used when administering thiopental to patients with high sympathetic tone or pre-existing cardiac arrhythmias. Adequate premedication, preoxygenation and administration of lidocaine (2.0 mg/kg IV slowly over two minutes) can be administered as an adjunct prior to thiopental to reduce the thiopental dosage and incidence of ventricular arrhythmias. Vasodilation contributes to heat loss in anesthetized patients and also leads to splenic sequestration of red blood cells and decreased packed cell volume (Berry 2015; Posner 2018).

Effects on the Respiratory System

Barbiturates cause dose-dependent depression of the medullary and pontine respiratory centers by decreasing sensitivity to carbon dioxide. The correlation between EEG suppression and decreased minute ventilation provides evidence for this mechanism of central depression (Vuyk et al. 2020). A high incidence of apnea can be seen, especially when used with other depressant drugs. After an induction dose of thiopental, peak respiratory depression occurs 1–1.5 minutes after administration (Vuyk et al. 2020). Apnea is usually short-lived (~30 seconds) and resumption of spontaneous ventilation is characterized by decreased frequency, tidal volume and minute ventilation. The ventilatory pattern with thiopental has been described as "double apnea" which is a period of initial apnea upon drug administration, followed by a few breaths with adequate tidal volume and then followed by a longer period of apnea (Vuyk et al. 2020). Patients should be intubated and ventilation assisted or controlled if necessary. Laryngeal and cough reflexes are depressed only at high doses, therefore, stimulation of the upper airway by laryngoscopy or intubation may result in laryngospasm in prone species (Stoelting and Hillier 2006; Reves et al. 2009; Rathmell and Rosow 2015). Induction doses of methohexital also cause central respiratory depression and significantly decrease the slope of the ventilatory response to carbon dioxide. Maximal reduction in tidal volume occurs approximately one minute after administration. Although patients awaken within about five minutes, respiratory variables may take up to 15 minutes to return to baseline (Vuyk et al. 2020). Therefore, patient oxygenation should be monitored and supplementation of oxygen provided where indicated.

Other Effects

Barbiturates produce minimal decreases in hepatic blood flow and do not affect post-operative hepatic or gastrointestinal (GI) function, however, thiopental will decrease lower esophageal sphincter tone (Stoelting and Hillier 2006; Berry 2015). Barbiturates stimulate liver microsomal enzyme induction after 2–7 days of sustained administration (Stoelting and Hillier 2006; Rathmell and Rosow 2015; Berry 2015). Phenobarbital is the most potent hepatic enzyme inducer, causing a 20–40% increase in microsomal enzymes and doubling metabolism for up to 30 days. Phenobarbital is also used experimentally as an inducer of cytochrome p450 (CYP) enzyme systems in rodents, especially CYP2B. Phenobarbital is an inducer of CYP2B6, CYP2C9, CYP2C19 and CYP3A in human hepatocyte cultures (Rathmell and Rosow 2015). Enzyme induction increases metabolism of barbiturates themselves, contributing to tolerance. It also increases the metabolism of other drugs such as anticoagulants, phenytoin and tricyclic antidepressants, as well as endogenous substances including corticosteroids, bile salts and vitamin K (Stoelting and Hillier 2006; Rathmell and Rosow 2015; Vuyk et al. 2020). Barbiturates cause modest decreases in renal blood flow and glomerular filtration rate (GFR) due to decreased cardiac output and systemic blood pressure.

Barbiturates readily cross the placenta and a dynamic equilibrium exists between fetal and maternal plasma levels. Peak umbilical vein concentrations occur within one minute after administration. Fetal plasma concentrations are significantly less than maternal plasma levels and the fetal brain is exposed to lower concentrations than are measured in the umbilical vein due to dilution and clearance by the fetal liver (Stoelting and Hillier 2006). Thiopental results in more profound depression of neurologic reflexes in puppies born via cesarean section

compared to propofol (Berry 2015). Thiopental impairs neutrophil function and nuclear transcription factor kB which is a central regulator of the immune response. Long-term use of high doses may be associated with bone-marrow suppression, leukopenia and increased nosocomial infections (Stoelting and Hillier 2006).

Acute tolerance to barbiturates occurs more rapidly and of higher magnitude than can be attributed to induction of microsomal enzymes. Effective doses can be increased sixfold which is twice that which can be accounted for by enzyme induction. Tolerance develops more for the sedative effects than anticonvulsant and lethal effects, therefore, the therapeutic index decreases. Acute tolerance also develops to the effects on CMRO2. The degree of tolerance is directly related to physical dependence and the severity of withdrawal; abrupt discontinuation can cause compensatory CNS excitation (Stoelting and Hillier 2006).

Inadvertent arterial injection of thiopental results in intense vasoconstriction, pain and blanching of the skin along the distribution of the artery. Arteritis and microembolism causing occlusion of arterial circulation is most likely due to precipitation of barbiturate crystals and can lead to gangrene and permanent nerve damage. The risk of vascular injury rises with increasing concentrations. Treatment includes dilution of the drug with saline, vasodilators such as lidocaine or phenoxybenzamine to prevent arterial spasm and heparinization to prevent thrombosis (Stoelting and Hillier 2006; Reves et al. 2009; Rathmell and Rosow 2015; Vuyk et al. 2020). Barbiturate crystal deposition can also lead to venous thrombosis. The incidence is again related to the concentration of solution but is less of a concern than in arteries due to the increasing diameter of veins (Stoelting and Hillier 2006).

A transient urticarial rash has been reported in human patients and develops on the head, neck, and trunk. More severe reactions, such as facial edema, hives, bronchospasm, and anaphylaxis, can occur. Anaphylaxis (antigen-antibody interaction) occurs in patients with prior exposure but in the absence of prior exposure, the anaphylactoid reactions are thought to be caused by histamine release from mast cells (Stoelting and Hillier 2006; Reves et al. 2009; Rathmell and Rosow 2015; Vuyk et al. 2020).

Clinical Use in Veterinary Medicine

Thiopental

Thiopental is no longer commercially available in the US and Canada. Where it is still available, it comes as a powder that can be reconstituted with sterile water, normal saline or 5% dextrose in water to a 2–2.5% (20 or 25 mg/ml) solution for small animals and a 2.5–5.0% solution in large animals (Posner 2018; Plumb 2018c). It is incompatible with most drugs however, it is chemically stable as a 1:1 volume mixture with propofol for one week at room temperature and is bacteriocidal against *Staphylococcus aureus*, *Escherichia coli* and *Pseudomonas aeruginosa* and bacteriostatic against *Candida albicans* (Crowther et al. 1996; Lazar et al. 1998; Joubert et al. 2005). Anesthetic induction quality is similar to either drug alone but recovery time and quality are similar to propofol and superior to thiopental alone (Ko et al. 1999).

The volume of distribution of thiopental in rabbits, sheep and dogs is 38.6±10 ml/kg, 44.5±9.1 ml/kg and 38.1±18.4 ml/kg, respectively (Ilkiw et al. 1991). The elimination half-life is shortest in rabbits (43.1±3.4 minutes), longest in sheep (251.9±107.8 minutes) and intermediate in dogs (182.4±57.9 minutes) (Ilkiw et al. 1991). In horses, thiopental has a rapid distribution phase with a half-life of 1.4±1.2 minutes in horses and 1.3±0.7 minutes in ponies (Abass et al. 1994). Horses have a slightly shorter elimination half-life than ponies (147±21 minutes vs. 222±44 minutes), and there was no significant difference in clearance (Abass et al. 1994).

The induction dose in pre-medicated dogs and cats is 6–10 mg/kg IV. Since a subinduction dose of thiopental tends to cause excitement, especially in non-premedicated patients, one quarter to one half of the calculated dose should be administered rapidly as a bolus to carry the patient through the excitement phase (Ko 2019). Additional amounts can be titrated to effect for endotracheal intubation (ET). The onset of action is approximately 20–30 seconds. Patients that are premedicated or have a compromised physical status such as hypovolemia, hypoproteinemia, acidosis or uremia will require a lower induction dose; slower administration over one minute may decrease cardiopulmonary depression. Thiopental can be used for short-term immobilization; the duration of action is ~5–8 minutes or up to 15 minutes in premedicated dogs and cats (Ko 2019). Appropriate analgesia should be provided as barbiturates do not provide analgesia. Repeated dosing is not recommended as this can result in prolonged rough recoveries (Ko 2019). Thiopental can also be used for laryngeal function examination since it has minimal effect on laryngeal function (Ko 2019). Perivascular injection can result in necrosis and sloughing of tissue in skin, therefore IV administration should always be via a meticulously placed IV catheter. Ventricular arrhythmias or bigeminy can occur with thiopental, therefore, avoid use in patients with cardiac disease or arrhythmias. Electrocardiogram (ECG) should be placed prior to induction. Should arrhythmias occur, the patient should be intubated and ventilated with 100% oxygen; lidocaine (2.0 mg/kg IV slowly over two minutes) can be administered if the arrhythmia persists (Ko 2019). Co-induction with lidocaine may decrease the

incidence of ventricular arrhythmias and the induction dose of thiopental (Rawlings and Kolata 1983). Use of thiopental should be avoided in sighthound breeds of dogs due to their relative deficiency in hepatic microsomal enzymes and their low body fat resulting in prolonged and rough recoveries (>8 hours) (Berry 2015; Posner 2018; Ko 2019). Thiopental can be administered as a 1:1 mixture with propofol (propofol 2 mg/kg, 10 mg/ml and thiopental 5 mg/kg, 25 mg/ml). Clinical experience with this mixture allows for more titration of induction doses and decreases the requirement of an initial bolus of induction agent to avoid excitement. A study comparing propofol or thiopental alone with a 1:1 mixture of propofol and thiopental found a similar quality of induction to propofol or thiopental alone but the recovery times and quality were similar to those of propofol and superior to those of thiopental (Ko et al. 1999).

Although the administration of barbiturates for anesthesia in horses has drastically decreased, they may still be used where available for induction, short-term maintenance and as an adjunct to inhalant anesthesia (Muir 2009). Methohexital and pentobarbital are not used for induction of anesthesia in horses. Thiopental can be administered as a bolus at 5–8 mg/kg in premedicated horses or 1–3 g of thiopental may be added to 1 l of 5% guaifenesin and administered rapidly to effect. Both induction and recovery can be associated with excitement, therefore, appropriate sedation and well-trained staff should be available to assist during induction and recovery. Hypoventilation and apnea are common, therefore, intubation along with oxygen supplementation and a demand valve for intermittent positive pressure ventilation should be available. Recovery to standing may be uncoordinated and sedation with acepromazine and/or an α-2 agonist facilitates a smoother recovery. A recent study compared induction with alphaxalone, ketamine or thiopental after premedication with medetomidine and midazolam in thoroughbred horses (Wakuno et al. 2017). Induction and recovery quality was not significantly different between protocols, however, alfaxalone and thiopental resulted in a significantly longer recovery time compared to ketamine (Wakuno et al. 2017).

Thiopental in 5% guaifenesin may also be used for induction in adult cattle. Six to 10 mg/kg IV given to unsedated patients will provide approximately 10–15 minutes of anesthesia (Riebold 2015). Use in swine is limited by the ability to procure IV access in larger individuals of this species.

Methohexital

Methohexital, although still available in the US, has been superseded by propofol for most indications. Where it is still available, it may be a useful agent for anesthetic induction, especially in sighthounds. It is associated with very rough recoveries when used as a sole agent, therefore, premedication and continuation with gas anesthesia is recommended. The dose for premedicated dogs and cats is 5.0 mg/kg IV with ~1/2 of the dose administered rapidly to avoid excitement, then to effect after ~30 seconds (Plumb 2018a). Profound respiratory depression may occur and the lethal dose is only 2–3 times the anesthetic induction dose. The human label contains a black box warning as a reminder of the importance of continuous monitoring of respiratory and cardiac function and availability of emergency resuscitative equipment and drugs (Plumb 2018a).

Pentobarbital Sodium

The duration of action pentobarbital (4–8 times thiopental) and its low therapeutic index has led to it being replaced with newer injectable anesthetics and inhalants in veterinary medicine. It is no longer used in North America for anesthesia in dogs and cats, cattle, small ruminants and horses. It may still be used as an anesthetic in laboratory animals especially for non-survival procedures, as a sedative for animals on mechanical ventilation and as a major component of euthanasia solutions (Berry 2015; Plumb 2018b). Pentobarbital is less lipid soluble than thiopental and methohexital, therefore, it does not cross the blood–brain barrier as rapidly and anesthetic induction is slower (30–60 seconds vs. 20–30 seconds for thiopental).

The constant rate infusion (CRI) dose for sedation in mechanically ventilated dogs and cats is 1–3 mg/kg/hour. It is recommended to change to a propofol CRI ~12 hours prior to weaning from the ventilator to avoid seizures and to allow pentobarbital plasma levels to decrease (Plumb 2018b). Pentobarbital may be used in patients with seizures intractable to benzodiazepines. Ruminants, especially sheep and goats, are reported to metabolize pentobarbital very rapidly; goats have a half-life of about one hour compared to eight hours in dogs (Berry 2015; Plumb 2018b). Pentobarbital can be used for chemical restraint in small rodents/mammals administered either intraperitoneally or IV (Plumb 2018b).

References

Abass, B.T., Weaver, B.M., Staddon, G.E. et al. (1994). Pharmacokinetics of thiopentone in the horse. *J. Vet. Pharmacol. Ther.* 17 (5): 331–338.

Berry, S.H. (2015). Injectable anesthetics. In: *Veterinary Anesthesia and Analgesia, the Fifth Edition of Lumb and Jones*, vol. 5 (ed. K.A. Grimm, L.A. Lamont, W.J. Tranquilli, et al.), Ames, IA, Wiley: 277–280.

Crowther, J., Hrazdil, J., Jolly, D.J. et al. (1996). Growth of microorganisms in propofol, thiopental, and a 1:1 mixture of propofol and thiopental. *Anesth. Analg.* 82: 475–478.

Ilkiw, J.E., Benthuysen, J.A., Ebling, W.F. et al. (1991). A comparative study of the pharmacokinetics of thiopental in the rabbit, sheep and dog. *J. Vet. Pharmacol. Ther.* 14 (2): 134–140.

Joubert, K.E., Picard, J., and Sethusa, M. (2005). Inhibition of bacterial growth by different mixtures of propofol and thiopentone. *J. S. Afr. Vet. Assoc.* 76 (2): 85–89.

Ko, J.C. (2019). Chapter 4: Intravenous injection techniques and intravenous anesthetic agents. In: *Small Animal Anesthesia and Pain Management* (ed. J.C. Ko), 81–82. Boca Raton, FL: CRC Press, Taylor and Francis Group.

Ko, J.C., Golder, F.J., Mandsager, R.E. et al. (1999). Anesthetic and cardiorespiratory effects of a 1:1 mixture of propofol and thiopental sodium in dogs. *J. Am. Vet. Med. Assoc.* 215 (9): 1292–1296.

Lazar, E.R., Jolly, D.T., Tam, Y.K. et al. (1998). Propofol and thiopental in a 1:1 volume mixture is chemically stable. *Anesth. Analg.* 86: 422–426.

Michic, S.J. and Harris, R.A. (2011). Hypnotics and sedatives. In: *Goodman and Gilman's the Pharmacological Basis of Therapeutics*, vol. 12 (ed. L.L. Brunton), 469–474. New York, USA: McGraw Medical.

Muir, W.W. (2009). Intravenous anesthetic drugs. In: *Equine Anesthesia: Monitoring and Emergency Therapy* (ed. W.W. Muir and J.A.E. Hubbell), 244–248. St. Louis, MO: Saunders Elsevier.

Plumb, D.C. (2018a). Methohexital sodium. In: *Plumb's Veterinary Drug Handbook*, vol. 9 (ed. D.C. Plumb), 776–777. Hoboken, NJ: Wiley-Blackwell.

Plumb, D.C. (2018b). Pentobarbital sodium. In: *Plumb's Veterinary Drug Handbook*, 9e (ed. D.C. Plumb), 922–925. Hoboken, NJ: Wiley-Blackwell.

Plumb, D.C. (2018c). Thiopental sodium. In: *Plumb's Veterinary Drug Handbook*, vol. 9 (ed. D.C. Plumb), 1132–1134. Hoboken, NJ: Wiley-Blackwell.

Posner, L.P. (2018). Injectable anesthetic agents. In: *Veterinary Pharmacology & Therapeutics*, vol. 9 (ed. J.E. Riviere and M.G. Papich), 248–255. Wiley-Blackwell: Hoboken, NJ.

Rathmell, J.P. and Rosow, C.E. (2015). Intravenous sedatives and hypnotics. In: *Stoelting's Pharmacology and Physiology in Anesthetic Practice* (ed. P. Flood, J.P. Rathmell and

S. Shafer) 5 pp, 183–186. Philadelphia, PA: Wolters Kluwer Health.

Rawlings, C.A. and Kolata, R.J. (1983). Cardiopulmonary effects of thiopental/lidocaine combination during anesthetic induction in the dog. *Am. J. Vet. Res.* 44: 144–149.

Reves, J.G., Glass, P.S.A., Lubarsky, D.A. et al. (2009). Intravenous anesthetics. In: *Miller's Anesthesia*, vol. 7 (ed. R.D. Miller), 1191–1200. Churchill Livingston.

Robinson, E.P., Sams, R.A., and Muir, W.W. (1986). Barbiturate anesthesia in greyhound and mixed-breed dogs: comparative cardiopulmonary effect, anesthetic effects and recovery rates. *Am. J. Vet. Res.* 47: 2105–2112.

Riebold T. (2015). Ruminants. In: *Veterinary Anesthesia and Analgesia, the Fifth Edition of Lumb and Jones*, vol. 5 (ed. K.A. Grimm, L.A. Lamont, W.J. Tranquilli, et al.), 912–925. Ames, IA: Wiley.

Sams, R.A., Muir, W.W., Detra, R.L. et al. (1985). Comparative pharmacokinetics and anesthetic effects of methohexital, pentobarbital, thiamylal, and thiopental in greyhound dogs and non-greyhound, mixed-breed dogs. *Am. J. Vet. Res.* 46: 1677–1683.

Stoelting, R.K. and Hillier, S.C. (2006). Barbiturates. In: *Pharmacology and Physiology in Anesthetic Practice* (ed. R.K. Stoelting and S.C. Hillier) 4 pp, 127–138. Philadelphia, PA: Lippincott Williams & Wilkins.

Vuyk, J., Sitsen, E., and Reekers, M. (2015). Intravenous anesthetics. In: *Miller's Anesthesia*, vol. 8 (ed. R.D. Miller), 835. Philadelphia, PA: Elsevier.

Vuyk, J., Sitsen, E., and Reekers, M. (2020). Intravenous anesthetics. In: *Miller's Anesthesia*, vol. 9 (ed. M.A. Gropper), 638–653. Philadelphia, PA: Elsevier.

Wakuno, A., Aoki, M., Kushiro, A., et al. (2017). Comparison of alfaxalone, ketamine and thiopental for anaesthetic induction and recovery in Thoroughbred horses premedicated with medetomidine and midazolam. *Equine Vet. J.* 49(1): 94–98.

Woolston, C. (2013). Death row incurs drug penalty. *Nature* 502: 417–418.

9

Induction Drugs

Jennifer E. Carter

Introduction

Induction of anesthesia of most small and large animal species in veterinary medicine is typically carried out by intravenous (IV) injection of one or more agents that induce central nervous system (CNS) depression and facilitate orotracheal intubation. Ideal agents facilitate rapid loss of consciousness while maintaining acceptable cardiorespiratory function and are rapidly redistributed from the CNS to facilitate timely emergence. In pocket pets and laboratory rodents, IV injection is not always possible or practical, so agents that facilitate loss of consciousness via other routes of administration are used.

Propofol

Propofol is available commercially in three formulations: a 1% aqueous lipid emulsion with no added preservatives, a 1% aqueous lipid emulsion with 2% benzyl alcohol added to prolong shelf life, and a 1% microemulsion formulation with added surfactants designed to reduce potential side effects associated with the original lipid emulsion.

Mechanism of Action

Propofol is a non-barbiturate phenolic IV induction agent that is used widely in veterinary medicine. Its mechanism of action is via interaction with the gamma aminobutyric acid (GABAA) receptor, the binding site of the inhibitory neurotransmitter GABA (Ying and Goldstein 2005). When propofol interacts with the $GABA_A$ receptor, it appears to promote the continued binding of the GABA neurotransmitter and, therefore, a hyperpolarization of the membrane (Concas et al. 1991). While GABA receptors are located in both the brain and spinal cord, research in humans suggests that the anesthetic effects of propofol are limited to a brain site of action (Kerz et al. 2001).

Pharmacokinetics

The pharmacokinetics of propofol have been described in dogs using a two-compartment model (Zoran et al. 1993). In the dog, it has a rapid uptake into the CNS and is quickly redistributed to other tissues allowing for a quick recovery (Zoran et al. 1993). As it is a highly lipophilic drug, it has a large volume of distribution, however, one study found that the volume of distribution was significantly smaller in the greyhound, owing likely to their relative lack of body fat (Zoran et al. 1993). Interestingly, greyhounds have a much lower clearance of propofol (54 ± 10 ml/kg/min) when compared to mixed-breed dogs (114.8 ± 46 ml/kg/min) (Zoran et al. 1993). In a smaller study using beagles and a non-compartmental analysis, the clearance time fell compared with the rates published in the other study (76 ± 4 ml/minute/kg) (Cockshott et al. 1992). In cats, propofol has been described with both a non-compartmental model and two-compartment model (Cleale et al. 2009; Griffenhagen et al. 2014). In one study, cats appeared to have a similar volume of distribution for propofol compared to dogs, however, their clearance appears to be much slower than dogs (1148 ± 228 ml/kg/hour for the macroemulsion formulation) (Cleale et al., 2009). A second study showed a slightly smaller volume of distribution but was in agreement with a slower clearance rate. This is likely owing to the inefficient nature of hepatic conjugation in the cat. Pigs and rabbits both followed a two-compartment pharmacokinetic model with a rapid redistribution of propofol from the central compartment and relatively large volumes of distribution (Cockshott et al. 1992). The total body clearance of propofol from the pig was similar to the beagle dog. However, rabbits displayed extremely rapid clearance rates (337 ± 35 ml/minute/kg) (Cockshott et al. 1992). Although the authors call into question whether that is an over representation of the actual value, clearance appears to be very fast in the rabbit. Lastly, the rat has been studied using a three-compartment open model which showed a rapid uptake and redistribution of the drug with a longer elimination phase not unlike the dog and cat (Cockshott et al. 1992).

Metabolism

In humans, it has been established that propofol is metabolized by both hepatic and extrahepatic routes and metabolism in the dog is likely similar. Hepatic biotransformation of propofol in the dog is largely mediated by glucuronidation to inactive metabolites. However, cytochrome P450-mediated hydroxylation also appears to play a significant role in the dog (Simons et al. 1991; Court et al. 1999). It has been proposed that a relative deficiency in the cytochrome P450 enzymes (CYP2B11) responsible for this hydroxylation may explain the decreased clearance of propofol in greyhounds when compared to other dogs (Court et al. 1999; Hay Kraus et al. 2000). In addition to hepatic biotransformation, uptake and elimination at the lung has been described in the cat (Matot et al. 1993). The rat and rabbit also appear to rely on conjugation and elimination of inactive metabolites in urine for the major route of propofol metabolism but there are definite species differences in the extent and enzymes involved (Simons et al. 1991).

Clinical Uses

Propofol is used in many species as a single IV injection for the induction of general anesthesia. Table 9.1 summarizes the species differences in dose recommendations for anesthetic induction. However, propofol inductions are recommended in most species as "to effect". Repeated doses have also been reported as the use of propofol in continuous rate infusion (CRI) or target-controlled infusion for maintenance of general anesthesia or long-term sedation.

Effects on Organ Systems

Cardiovascular
Propofol administration can result in transient systemic hypotension due to systemic vasodilation and, to a lesser extent, reduction in myocardial contractility (Ilkiw et al. 1992; Wouters et al. 1995). Despite changes in systemic vascular resistance, heart rate remains largely unchanged by propofol in dogs and horses (Whitwam et al. 2000; Muir et al. 2009b).

Respiratory
Post-induction apnea is the most reported respiratory consequence with administration of propofol. The rate of

Table 9.1 Suggested induction drug doses for Propofol in various species.

Species	IV dose	References
Dog	4.7–6.9 mg/kg[a]	Watkins et al. (1987), Morgan and Legge (1989), Weaver and Raptopoulos (1990), Watney and Pablo (1992), Geel (1991)
	2.1–4.5 mg/kg[b]	Weaver and Raptopoulos (1990), Morgan and Legge (1989), Watney and Pablo (1992), Geel (1991)
	1.1–3.58 mg/kg[c]	Covey-Crump and Murison (2008), Robinson and Borer-Weir (2013), Sanchez et al. (2013)
	2.9 mg/kg[d]	Covey-Crump and Murison (2008)
Cat	5–8.03 mg/kg[a]	Geel (1991), Morgan and Legge (1989)
	2.3–5.97 mg/kg[b]	Geel (1991), Morgan and Legge (1989), Slingsby et al. (2014)
	2.5–2.7 mg/kg[c]	Robinson and Borer-Weir (2015)
Horses	0.4[b,e]–2 mg/kg[b]	Frias et al. (2003), Mama et al. (1996), Posner et al. (2013), Jarrett et al. (2018)
Sheep	3–6 mg/kg	Lin et al. (1997), Waterman (1988)
Swine	2–5 mg/kg	Tendillo et al. (1996)
Rabbit	2–10 mg/kg	Cockshott et al. (1992)
Rat	3–10 mg/kg	Glen (1980)
Mouse	3–25 mg/kg	Glen (1980)

[a] Unpremedicated.
[b] Premedicated.
[c] Midazolam/benzodiazepine co-induction.
[d] Fentanyl co-induction.
[e] Ketamine co-induction.

administration is the most important factor in avoiding apnea, however, it can occur despite appropriate precautions and provisions for endotracheal intubation (ET), and ventilation should always be available with propofol use. Hypercapnia and bradypnea have been reported in dogs breathing 100% oxygen after induction and maintenance with propofol while significant hypoxemia is reported in horses breathing room air (Robertson et al. 1992; Muir et al. 2009b).

Central Nervous System
Propofol produces dose-dependent depression of the CNS. It is considered to be neuroprotective due to its ability to decrease intracranial pressure (ICP), cerebral metabolic oxygen demand, and cerebral perfusion pressure (CPP) in man and in dogs (Pinaud et al. 1990; Artru et al. 1992). At low to moderate doses, propofol preserves cerebral autoregulation. However, at high doses, this can be impaired due

to significant decreases in CPP (Artru et al. 1992). Due to the decrease in electroencephalogram (EEG) activity seen with propofol administration it has been used as an anticonvulsant agent in dogs (see Chapter 25) (Gommeren et al. 2010; Heldmann et al. 1999b).

Other Effects

Myoclonus has been reported with propofol administration in dogs and goats, however, its underlying mechanism is not understood (Cattai et al. 2015; Pablo et al. 1997). Although it is not well described in the literature, transient myoclonus is not an unusual phenomenon when propofol is administered to dogs. Propofol has been evaluated for suitability in canine cesarean section surgery and, despite transplacental drug transfer, results in viable puppies with appropriate cardiovascular variables and neurologic vigor (Luna et al. 2004). Although propofol is reported to decrease intraocular pressure in people, induction doses of propofol cause transient increases in intraocular pressure when administered to dogs with normal intraocular pressure (Costa et al. 2015; Hasiuk et al. 2014).

Prolonged infusions of propofol in humans can result in the development of Propofol Infusion Syndrome (PRIS). PRIS manifests as bradycardia, metabolic acidosis, rhabdomyolysis, hyperlipidemia, and an enlarged or fatty liver. The exact mechanism of this condition is not fully understood but is believed to be related to impaired or inhibited mitochondrial function. PRIS has not been described in veterinary patients. However, organ toxicity and mitochondrial dysfunction has been described in rabbits after prolonged propofol infusion (Campos et al. 2016; Ypsilantis et al. 2011; Ypsilantis et al. 2007).

Contraindications

Due to the potential for post-induction apnea, propofol use may be contraindicated in patients where ET may be difficult or contraindicated. There are conflicting reports surrounding the suitability of propofol for repeated or continuous administration in cats due to the potential to cause red blood cell oxidative injury which results in the formation of Heinz bodies (Andress et al. 1995; Baetge et al. 2020; Bley et al. 2007). Many current recommendations still state to avoid consecutive day dosing of propofol. However, a recent study highlighted the use of propofol CRIs for 24 hours to maintain manual ventilation in cats and reported a full recovery with no untoward effects (Boudreau et al. 2012). Propofol use has also been associated with an increased rate of wound infections in clean wounds in dogs potentially caused by injection of microbial-contaminated propofol (Heldmann et al. 1999a).

There are some suggestions that propofol use should be avoided in patients with pancreatitis due to reports in the human literature of the development of pancreatitis after propofol use. However, no such report exists in the veterinary literature.

Drug Interactions

Propofol (without benzyl alcohol) is physically compatible with 5% dextrose and thiopental, however, does not appear to have any adverse effects when mixed with saline, lactated Ringer's solution, midazolam, diazepam, fentanyl, or ketamine as its administration concurrently with these solutions have all been reported.

Alfaxalone

Alfaxalone is commercially available as a 1% cyclodextrin solution.

Mechanism of Action

Alfaxalone's mechanism of action is comparable to that of propofol. Alfaxalone binds to the $GABA_A$ receptor which promotes the binding of the inhibitory neurotransmitter GABA and leads to inhibition of the post-synaptic neuron and, therefore, CNS depression (Weir et al. 2004).

Pharmacokinetics

The pharmacokinetics of the current formulation of alfaxalone have been described in the dog, cat, horse, and rat using a non-compartmental model (Ferre et al. 2006; Whittem et al. 2008; Pasloske et al. 2009; Goodwin et al. 2011; Goodwin et al. 2012; Lau et al. 2013). In dogs, horses, and rats, it has a large volume of distribution due to lipid solubility and rapid clearance (Ferre et al. 2006; Goodwin et al. 2011; Lau et al. 2013; Pasloske et al. 2009). In dogs and horses, the $t_{1/2}$ is approximately 30 minutes while it is about 17–19 minutes in the rat (Goodwin et al. 2011; Lau et al. 2013; Pasloske et al. 2009; Ferre et al. 2006). A study comparing greyhounds to beagles failed to demonstrate a meaningful difference in alfaxalone pharmacokinetics in the greyhound (Pasloske et al. 2009). Foals have a smaller V_d than the horse, likely due to a lower fat to water ratio in the foal compared to the adult horse as well as a reduced clearance likely due to decreased hepatic metabolic capabilities (Goodwin et al. 2012). The pharmacokinetics of alfaxalone in the cat demonstrate nonlinearity making their metabolism dose dependent. Alfaxalone has a large V_d in the cat with a $t_{1/2}$ of approximately 45 minutes and rapid clearance at clinically relevant doses (5 mg/kg). The $t_{1/2}$ and clearance of this clinically relevant dose are slower than doses of 2 mg/kg or 10 mg/kg in the dog. In addition, when cats are given a supraclinical dose of alfaxalone (25 mg/kg), the $t_{1/2}$ increases considerably while the clearance decreases significantly. This pattern suggests that alfaxalone may accumulate in the cat at higher doses or with continuous infusions (Whittem et al. 2008).

Metabolism

The metabolism of alfaxalone has been described in the dog and rat and is expected to be similar in other mammalian species (Ferre et al. 2006; Celotti et al. 1997; Nicholas et al. 1981; Sear and McGivan 1981; Sear 1996). The alfaxalone molecule is primarily metabolized via phase I and II hepatic biotransformation with inactive metabolites primarily excreted in urine. The rapid hepatic metabolism has been suggested as the reason behind the short clinical duration of the anesthetic effect. Some additional metabolism may occur via renal, pulmonary and cerebral routes and excretion in bile may be a secondary, less significant, mechanism of elimination.

Clinical Uses

Alfaxalone is used in many species as a single IV injection for the induction of general anesthesia. Table 9.2

Table 9.2 Suggested induction doses for Alfaxalone for various species.

Species	IV dose	References
Dog	2–2.6 mg/kg[a]	Keates and Whittem (2012), Maney et al. (2013)
	0.8–1.7 mg/kg[b]	Pinelas et al. (2014), O'Hagan et al. (2012b), Amengual et al. (2013), Maddern et al. (2010)
Cat	4.2–5 mg/kg[a]	Zaki et al. (2009), Kalchofner Guerrero et al. (2014)
	2–2.7 mg/kg[a]	Bortolami et al. (2013), Zaki et al. (2009)
Horses	1 mg/kg[b]	Kloppel and Leece (2011), Keates et al. (2012)
Sheep	2 mg/kg[a,b]	Andaluz et al. (2013), Walsh et al. (2012)
Swine	5 mg/kg (IM)	Santos Gonzalez et al. (2013)
Rabbit	2–10 mg/kg[b]	Navarrete-Calvo et al. (2014), Grint et al. (2008)

[a] Unpremedicated.
[b] Premedicated.

summarizes the species differences in dose recommendations for anesthetic induction. However, alfaxalone inductions are recommended in most species as "to effect". Repeated doses have also been reported as the use of alfaxalone in CRI or target-controlled infusion for maintenance of general anesthesia or long-term sedation. Alfaxalone has also been described for use in koi, red-eared sliders, goats, bullfrogs, marmosets, tortoises, iguanas, axolotl, as well as anecdotal reports of its use in kangaroos, wallabies, and wombats.

Effects on Organ Systems

Cardiovascular

Alfaxalone produces dose-dependent decreases in arterial blood pressure and increases in heart rate in dogs and cats (Muir et al. 2008; Muir et al. 2009a). A study comparing propofol and alfaxalone induction demonstrated no significant difference in the cardiovascular effects of the two drugs in dogs (Maney et al. 2013). The cardiovascular effects of alfaxalone were found to be acceptable when used as an induction agent for dogs that have moderate to severe systemic disease (Psatha et al. 2011). In two studies on alfaxalone induction in dogs and cats less than 12 weeks of age, all cardiopulmonary parameters were maintained from baseline making it an acceptable induction agent in these juvenile patients (O'Hagan et al. 2012b; O'Hagan et al. 2012a). Alfaxalone also appears to maintain cardiopulmonary parameters within an acceptable limit in horses (Keates et al. 2012; Goodwin et al. 2011). IM alfaxalone, in combination with butorphanol, provided good sedation with minimal effects on echocardiogram (ECG) measurements in cats (Ribas et al. 2014).

Respiratory

Alfaxalone produces mild respiratory depressant effects with dose-dependent post-induction apnea being the most common effect in dogs and cats (Muir et al. 2008; Muir et al. 2009a). In unpremedicated dogs, alfaxalone appears to be less likely than propofol to cause post-induction apnea. However, studies with premedicated dogs demonstrated no difference between the two drugs with regard to the incidence of apnea (Keates and Whittem 2012; Amengual et al. 2013; Bigby et al. 2017a, b).

Central Nervous System

Alfaxalone produces dose-dependent depression of CNS activity. It is considered to be neuroprotective due to its ability to decrease cerebral metabolic oxygen demand, cerebral blood flow, and therefore, ICP (Rasmussen et al. 1978). In addition, it preserves the sensitivity of the cerebral autoregulatory functions to changes in carbon dioxide partial pressure in the blood (Sari et al. 1976). When compared to propofol for induction of dogs undergoing magnetic resonance imaging (MRI) of neurological conditions following a methadone premedication, alfaxalone resulted in a poorer quality of recovery (Jimenez et al. 2012).

Other Effects

Myoclonus and tremors on recovery have been reported in dogs and cats with alfaxalone administration (Maney et al. 2013; Mathis et al. 2012). In addition, tremors during induction have been reported in horses (Keates et al. 2012). Alfaxalone causes a transient increase in intraocular pressure followed by a decrease as well as a decrease in tear production (Costa et al. 2015). Alfaxalone has been evaluated for suitability in canine cesarean section surgery and results in better neonatal vitality in the first 60 minutes than propofol (Doebeli et al. 2013). When compared to propofol in the dog, recovery from anesthesia is prolonged with alfaxalone (Maney et al. 2013).

Contraindications

Due to the potential for post-induction apnea, alfaxalone use may be contraindicated in patients where ET may be difficult or contraindicated. The earlier formulation of alfaxalone (Saffan™) resulted in facial edema in cats and histamine release in dogs. However, these problems were later attributed to the cremophor carrier molecule of the formulation which is not present in the current alfaxalone formulation. Although not a specific contraindication, the use of alfaxalone as an IM induction agent in cats is not recommended due to poor quality of recovery (Grubb et al. 2013).

Drug Interactions

There are clinical reports of alfaxalone administration with acepromazine, atropine, diazepam, midazolam, xylazine, dexmedetomidine, as well as most opioids and non-steroidal anti-inflammatory drugs (NSAIDs). Alfaxalone is also routinely administered with isotonic crystalloid fluids.

Dissociative Anesthetics (Ketamine and Tiletamine)

Ketamine is commercially available as a 10% racemic mixture in the US. Tiletamine is available in combination with zolazepam (a benzodiazepine) and is supplied as a dehydrated powder reconstituted to a 100 mg/ml solution under the trade names of Telazol® or Zoletil® depending on the country of registration.

Mechanism of Action

Dissociative anesthetics exert their mechanism of action by non-competitively antagonizing the N-methyl-D-aspartate (NMDA) receptor at the phencyclidine binding site which prevents glutamate binding and results in CNS depression in the limbic, thalamocortical, and reticular activating systems. In addition, they appear to have some opioid receptor agonism and monoaminergic and cholinergic receptor antagonism.

Pharmacokinetics

Both ketamine and tiletamine are highly lipophilic molecules that rapidly cross the blood–brain barrier which results in rapid establishment of therapeutic CNS concentrations. Racemic ketamine pharmacokinetics have been described in the dog, cat, horse, and calves using a two-compartment model characterized by a rapid distribution phase (1.95–6.9 minutes) and a longer elimination phase (42–78.7 minutes) after IV injection (Kaka and Hayton 1980; Hanna et al. 1988; Baggot and Blake 1976; Waterman 1984; Waterman et al. 1987; Kaka et al. 1979). IM injection in the cat resulted in peak plasma concentrations after approximately 10 minutes (Baggot and Blake 1976). The clearance of S-ketamine has been reported as higher than the racemic mixture in humans resulting in faster elimination and more rapid recovery (Engelhardt 1997; Ihmsen et al. 2001). These findings have also been supported in Shetland Ponies (Larenza et al. 2008b; Larenza et al. 2007).

As tiletamine is only available in combination with zolazepam, its pharmacokinetics have not been widely studied due to the difficulty of assaying both drugs. In pigs, tiletamine has been described using a two-compartment model with zolazepam modeled with a one-compartment model (Kumar et al. 2014). When delivered IM, the plasma half-life of the parent drugs was 1.97 and 2.76 hours and the apparent clearance was 6.63 and 0.54 l/hour/kg respectively for tiletamine and zolazepam indicating that tiletamine was cleared much faster than zolazepam in this species (Kumar et al. 2014). This agrees with a previously published review that indicated a more rapid clearance of tiletamine in dogs, cats, monkeys, and rats (Lin et al. 1993). However, according to the manufacturer package insert (Zoetis 2014), the duration of effect of tiletamine exceeds that of zolazepam in dogs while the reverse is true in cats. This is most likely explained by the presence of active metabolites which may have different species-specific clearance rates.

Metabolism

Ketamine is metabolized to the active metabolite norketamine via hepatic demethylation. Norketamine is approximately 10–30% as active as ketamine in rats and had an elimination half-life of nearly 10× that of the parent drug in calves (Leung and Baillie 1986; Waterman 1984). In most species, norketamine is further biotransformed then conjugated to glucuronide metabolites for excretion in urine (White et al. 1982). Potentially owing to deficiencies in glucuronidation in the cat, norketamine is excreted unchanged in urine (Hanna et al. 1988).

In pigs, tiletamine is biotransformed to desethyl tiletamine and zolazepam is metabolized to 8-desmethyl zolazepam, 6-hydroxy zolazepam, and 1-desmethyl zolazepam (Kumar et al. 2014). Desethyl tiletamine is eliminated via urine and is cleared from the plasma more quickly than the parent tiletamine molecule. Although the activity of the three zolazepam metabolites is unknown, they are eliminated very slowly compared to the parent molecule and based on the known activity of other benzodiazepine metabolites, it is assumed that they are likely to be active (Kumar et al. 2014).

Clinical Uses

Ketamine is registered for IM use in cats and non-human primates in the US. However, it is used extensively off label in multiple species via multiple routes of administration including IV, IM, subcutaneous, and oral. It is most commonly used as a single IV injection along with a muscle relaxant such as a benzodiazepine for induction of general anesthesia. However, it can be used for chemical restraint via other routes of administration and is often used as part of a total IV anesthesia maintenance protocol in horses.

More recently, S-ketamine use has been described in dogs, cats (domestic and Oncilla), horses, ponies, goats, pigs, and marmosets (Larenza et al. 2008a; Larenza et al. 2009a; Larenza et al. 2009b; Casoni et al. 2015a; Casoni et al. 2015b; Rossetti et al. 2008; Furtado et al. 2010; Jud et al. 2010; Bettschart-Wolfensberger et al. 2013; Lima et al. 2016). Clinical impression has generally been positive with smooth induction and more rapid recovery when compared to the racemic mixture although caution is given that specific recommendations regarding dosing are not available at this time. A recent study evaluating the relative potency of S-ketamine in comparison to the racemic drug found their potency to be equivalent in dogs (Casoni et al. 2015a). This is of particular interest given that many of the clinical studies comparing S-ketamine to racemic ketamine were designed on the premise that S-ketamine was more potent and, as such, lower doses were used. This discrepancy may provide explanation in some of the studies where inadequate anesthesia was achieved.

Telazol is registered for IM administration in dogs and cats in the US. However, it is also used extensively off label in multiple species via multiple routes of administration. It is most commonly given as a single injection for chemical restraint or induction of anesthesia (dose dependent) (Table 9.3).

As dissociative anesthetics are so commonly used in veterinary medicine, suggested dosages and combinations for all species are well described in other literature and will not be covered extensively here.

Effects on Organ Systems

Cardiovascular

Dissociative anesthetics indirectly stimulate the cardiovascular system under normal conditions via increases in central sympathetic tone as well as norepinephrine reuptake inhibition (Wong and Jenkins 1974; Baraka et al. 1973). This results in increases in cardiac output, systemic blood pressure, pulmonary arterial pressure, and myocardial oxygen

Table 9.3 Suggested induction doses for Ketamine and Telazol for various species.

Species	Ketamine	Telazol
Dog	5–10 mg/kg IV	6 mg/kg IV
	5–20 mg/kg IM	6–13 mg/kg IM
Cat	5–10 mg/kg IV	
	11–33 mg/kg IM	3–16 mg/kg IM
Horse	2–3 mg/kg IV	1–3 mg/kg IV
Cattle	2–4 mg/kg IV	2–4 mg/kg IV
Sheep	2–4 mg/kg IV	
	22 mg/kg IM	
Swine	2–4 mg/kg IV	
	10–20 mg/kg IM	6 mg/kg IM
Rabbits	10–60 mg/kg IV	
	20–80 mg/kg IM	30–60 mg/kg IM[a]
Rats	40–50 mg/kg IV	
	40–100 mg/kg IM or IP	20–60 mg/kg IM
Mice	50 mg/kg IV	
	50–200 mg/kg IM or IP	80–100 mg/kg IM

[a] Do not use in New Zealand White rabbits (see contraindications). When drugs are given with other sedative agents, lower doses may be used.

demand in dogs (Haskins et al. 1985). Dissociative anesthetic use should be avoided in patients with pathologic increases in sympathetic tone such as pheochromocytoma or hyperthyroidism. The direct effect of ketamine on the heart is negative inotropy which can become evident in patients with relative adrenal insufficiency or reduced sympathetic reserves due to illness (Diaz et al. 1976; Waxman et al. 1980).

Respiratory

Dissociative anesthetics have minimal effects on respiratory function under normal conditions and chemoreceptor responses to changes in plasma carbon dioxide and oxygen tension are maintained when ketamine is used as a solo agent (Soliman et al. 1975). However, when dissociative agents are used with other CNS depressants, respiratory depression can occur. Administration of ketamine has been associated with a transient apneustic respiratory pattern of inspiratory breath holding but this pattern does not generally result in a change in minute ventilation (Jaspar et al. 1983).

Ketamine maintains laryngeal and pharyngeal reflexes. However, they may not be fully coordinated and, as ketamine also increases salivation, ET should be performed to provide a protected airway (Taylor and Towey 1971).

Finally, dissociative anesthetics cause bronchial smooth muscle relaxation and decrease resistance to breathing (Hirshman et al. 1979). Patients with obstructive lower airway diseases may benefit from dissociative anesthetic induction.

Central Nervous System

Dissociative anesthetics antagonize the NMDA receptors in the CNS to produce dissociation of the thalamocortical and limbic systems which results in altered consciousness but not unconsciousness (Reich and Silvay 1989).

Cerebral blood flow is increased with dissociative anesthesia due to vasodilation of cerebral blood vessels as well as increases in systemic blood pressure. The increase in cerebral blood flow leads to an increase in ICP which could be detrimental for individuals with intracranial lesions or traumatic brain injury (TBI). However, control of ventilation appears to provide some degree of attenuation of this response (Pfenninger et al. 1985). Dissociative anesthetics also cause an increase in cerebral metabolic oxygen demand and should be avoided in patients with significant oxygen delivery compromise.

EEG tracings following administration of dissociative anesthetics demonstrate epileptiform patterns. However, there is also evidence that ketamine possesses anticonvulsive properties (Kayama 1982; Reder et al. 1980). In addition, recent work has demonstrated that the NMDA receptor plays a role in the pathophysiology of TBI and that antagonism of that receptor actually reduces neuronal degeneration and apoptosis after TBI (Han et al. 2009). At this time, the use of dissociatives in epileptic patients or patients with brain injuries remains controversial.

Emergency delirium can be seen with recovery from dissociative anesthetics and can result in uncoordinated movements, thrashing, and vocalizing. These side effects can be minimized by administration of sedatives or other CNS depressant agents (White et al. 1982).

Other Effects

Muscle rigidity and myoclonus characterize dissociative anesthesia unless the agents are given concurrently with a muscle relaxant.

Dissociative anesthesia has traditionally been regarded as increasing intraocular pressure and suggestions have been made to avoid the administration of these agents in glaucoma patients or ocular trauma cases (Hahnenberger 1976; Ferreira et al. 2013; Kovalcuka et al. 2013). However, some recent work in children failed to demonstrate an increase in intraocular pressure when ketamine was used at clinical doses (≤4 mg/kg) (Drayna et al. 2012). In addition, no increase in intraocular pressure has been reported when Telazol was evaluated in both dogs and cats (Hahnenberger 1976; Jang et al. 2015).

Dissociative anesthetics provide analgesia and antihyperalgesia through antagonism of the NMDA receptor and likely through interactions with mu and kappa opioid receptors within the CNS and the periphery. Ketamine has been shown to provide excellent analgesia in acute surgical pain situations when administered at sub-anesthetic dosages (Annetta et al. 2005). The NMDA receptor plays an important role in the phenomenon of central sensitization or wind-up and NMDA antagonists have been shown to minimize this effect when given pre-emptively and to attenuate the effects when given after central sensitization has occurred (Aida et al. 2000; Castel et al. 2013). Lastly, ketamine and other NMDA antagonists have been shown to be beneficial in the treatment of neuropathic pain in humans and rodent models (Guirimand et al. 2000; Kang et al. 2010; Chen et al. 2009).

Contraindications

Tiletamine has been reported to cause severe renal tubular necrosis in New Zealand White rabbits when administered at anesthetic doses (Brammer et al. 1991; Doerning et al. 1992). The suggestion to avoid Telazol in all rabbits is extrapolated from these studies.

Table 9.4 summarizes the relative contraindications for administration of dissociative anesthetics classified by organ system.

Table 9.4 Relative contraindications to the use of dissociative agents for anesthetic induction.

Organ system	Disease or condition
CNS	Increased intracranial pressure ±Traumatic Brain Injury
Cardiovascular	Hypertrophic Cardiomyopathy Cardiac Failure Systemic Hypertension Tachyarrhythmias Dysrhythmias
Genitourinary	Oliguric or Anuric Renal Disease (especially in cats) Urethral Obstruction Cesarean Section in Dogs
Endocrine	Phaeochromocytoma Hyperthyroidism
Ocular	Glaucoma (or other causes of IOP) Ocular Trauma Deep Cornea Ulcers

Drug Interactions

Administration of concurrent CNS depressants and sedatives can result in cardiovascular and respiratory depression. Concurrent use of chloramphenicol can prolong recovery from ketamine (Amouzadeh et al. 1989).

Etomidate

Although both the R(+) and S(−) enantiomers of etomidate exist, the R(+) form is considerably more potent and is the component of the commercially available product (Tomlin et al. 1998). Etomidate is available in a 2 mg/mL solution with a propylene glycol carrier molecule. Etomidate is supplied by a human anesthesia drug manufacturer and not labeled for use in veterinary species.

Mechanism of Action

Etomidate enhances the binding of the inhibitory neurotransmitter GABA at its receptor leading to hyperpolarization of post-synaptic neurons in the CNS (Olsen and Li 2011).

Pharmacokinetics

The pharmacokinetics of etomidate have been described in the cat using an open three-compartment model. The drug is rapidly redistributed from the brain (0.05 hours) and has an elimination half-life of 2.89 hours. Etomidate has a large volume of distribution at steady state (4.88 l/kg) with a clearance rate of 2.47 l/kg/hour (Wertz et al. 1990). The rapid redistribution phase from the CNS into body tissues is responsible for a quick anesthetic recovery. In dogs, a two-compartment model has been used to describe etomidate with a fairly small volume of distribution (0.69 l/kg), slow clearance (0.0061 l/minute/kg), but short elimination half-life (0.56 hours) when a 50 mg dose (roughly 1.5 mg/kg) was administered IV (Zhang et al. 1998). Etomidate is approximately 75% bound to plasma proteins in the dog (Meuldermans and Heykants 1976). In rats, etomidate is also modeled using a three-compartment open model with rapid equilibration with brain tissue and rapid redistribution from the brain with a first phase half-life of 1.19 minutes (Lewi et al., 1976).

Metabolism

Etomidate is metabolized by ester hydrolysis in both the plasma and the liver. Plasma elimination is linear whereas hepatic metabolism appears to be non-linear and capacity limited (Lewi et al. 1976; Heykants et al. 1975). Hydrolysis is nearly complete and results in the formation of pharmacologically inactive metabolites which are largely excreted via urine (~85%) with the remainder excreted in bile. Less than 3% of etomidate is excreted unchanged.

Clinical Uses

Etomidate is not registered for use in veterinary patients in the US or abroad. It is most commonly used for its favorable lack of cardiovascular effects. It is generally titrated to effect and allows for rapid ET. Myoclonus is common with etomidate administration and dosing should be preceded by administration of muscle relaxant agents. Table 9.5 provides a summary of suggested dosage ranges for etomidate in several small animal and laboratory species.

Effects on Organ Systems

Cardiovascular

Etomidate exerts little to no meaningful effects on the cardiovascular system. In unpremedicated dogs receiving approximately 2.9 mg/kg IV there were no significant changes from baseline for heart rate, direct arterial blood pressures, systemic vascular resistance index, stroke volume index, cardiac index, contractility, and central venous pressure (Rodriguez et al. 2012). In another study, dogs receiving midazolam followed by approximately 2 mg/kg of etomidate experienced no significant changes in heart rate or Doppler blood pressure from baseline values (Gunderson et al. 2013). A study on humans with documented left ventricular dysfunction did show a significant

Table 9.5 Suggested dosages for Etomidate in various species.

Species	IV dose	References
Dog	2–2.91 mg/kg[a]	Moon (1997), Clutton et al. (1997)
	2–4 mg/kg[b]	Suresh and Nelson (1985), Dominguez et al. (2013)
	0.5–4 mg/kg	*Unreferenced range in many sources*
Cat	2–3 mg/kg[a]	Moon (1997), Wertz et al. (1990)
	0.5–4 mg/kg	*Unreferenced range in many sources*
Pig	0.2–0.9 mg/kg[b]	Clutton et al. (1997), Suresh and Nelson (1985)
	2–4 mg/kg	*Unreferenced range in many sources*
Sheep	1 mg/kg[a]	Dominguez et al. (2013), Fresno et al. (2008)
Mice	23.7 mg/kg (IP)	Gomwalk and Healing (1981)

[a] Unpremedicated.
[b] Premedicated.

decrease in heart rate and blood pressure immediately following administration of etomidate. However, these values returned to baseline after intubation and were deemed clinically acceptable (Aghdaii et al. 2015).

Respiratory

Etomidate has minimal effects on respiratory function. In unpremedicated dogs, there were no significant changes from baseline in respiratory rate or end-tidal carbon dioxide measurements after IV etomidate administration (Rodriguez et al. 2012). In people, post-induction apnea was reported in one study, however, it was also suggested that etomidate stimulated ventilation independently of carbon dioxide tensions and would be a suitable choice for induction of patients where maintenance of spontaneous ventilation was required (Choi et al. 1985).

Central Nervous System

Etomidate exerts its CNS depressant effects by promoting the binding of the inhibitory neurotransmitter GABA to the $GABA_A$ receptor (O'Meara et al. 2004). Etomidate administration results in cerebral vasoconstriction causing decreases in cerebral blood flow and cerebral metabolic oxygen demand but maintains the cerebrovascular response to carbon dioxide (Renou et al. 1978; Cold et al. 1985). As there are no meaningful changes in mean arterial pressure, this results in maintenance of CPP (Cold et al. 1985). In study of brain trauma in people, etomidate use resulted in a significant decrease in ICP (Bramwell et al. 2006).

Controversy surrounds the use of etomidate in seizure patients. A study comparing etomidate and thiopental in humans demonstrated similar EEG patterns with both drugs. However, seizures have been reported following use of etomidate (Ghoneim and Yamada 1977; Ebrahim et al. 1986). A recent human study demonstrated that etomidate administration resulted in epileptic high frequency oscillations and EEG spikes (Rampp et al. 2014).

Other Effects

Etomidate inhibits the enzyme 11-beta-hydroxylase which is an important step in the adrenal cortical pathway that converts cholesterol into cortisol and aldosterone (Wagner et al. 1984). Inhibition is transient and has been reported to persist up to 6 hours in the dog and 5 hours in the cat (Dodam et al. 1990; Moon 1997). Adrenocortical suppression of greater than 24 hours has been reported in critically ill people and has been correlated with increased duration of mechanical ventilation and prolonged hospitalization (Absalom et al. 1999; Hildreth et al. 2008). While the adrenocortical suppression is of minor clinical relevance in most patients, the use of etomidate in patients with known adrenocortical dysfunction or relative adrenal insufficiency should be avoided. Etomidate may be used, however, in controlled Addison's disease patients receiving cortisol supplementation as it does not interfere with the action of cortisol.

Etomidate does not provide any muscle relaxation and development of myoclonus on induction and recovery of anesthesia is well documented in both veterinary patients and humans. It is recommended that a muscle relaxant be administered either in the premedication or as a co-induction agent when etomidate is used.

Early reports indicated that etomidate decreased intraocular pressure in normal eyes. However, a recent report in normal dogs indicated that the co-induction of midazolam and etomidate resulted in clinically significant increased intraocular pressure as well as miosis (Calla et al. 1987; Gunderson et al. 2013).

Lastly, pain has been reported on injection of etomidate in veterinary and human patients. This is likely due to the propylene glycol carrier vehicle and administration of analgesics such as opioids or α-2 agonists as well as administration into a large vein or with IV fluids minimizes this effect. Pain on injection has been studied in humans where it was found that replacement of the propylene glycol carrier with a lipid emulsion greatly reduced the incidence of pain on injection (Doenicke et al. 1999).

Contraindications

While there are no specific contraindications for the use of etomidate in veterinary patients, as stated previously, use in epileptics and patients with adrenal insufficiency should be with caution. In addition, several sources recommend caution in cats due to the potential for intravascular hemolysis. However, no peer-reviewed literature appears to exist regarding this issue.

Drug Interactions

Administration with other CNS depressants can potentiate the effects of etomidate and, as such, it should always be administered "to effect".

Miscellaneous Induction Agents

The agents listed below are mostly used in laboratory animal medicine although some also have historical significance within the broader realm of veterinary anesthesia.

Chloral Hydrate

Chloral hydrate appears to exert its effects by binding to the GABA receptor. However, its exact mechanism of action remains unknown. IV injection in rats provides approximately 1–2 hours of stable anesthesia albeit at a light plane, but intraperitoneal injections have been reported to cause cardiovascular and respiratory depression as well as peritonitis and ileus (Sisson and Siegel 1989; Field et al. 1993; Fleischman et al. 1977). In addition, differing dosage requirements between strains have been reported (Sisson et al. 1991).

Historically, chloral hydrate was used for sedation and anesthesia of horses and cattle. However, it has a very narrow safety margin and doses necessary to produce anesthesia resulted in significant cardiorespiratory depression.

Chloral hydrate is available in combination with magnesium sulfate (a CNS depressant and muscle relaxant) and pentobarbital (a barbiturate anesthetic). This combination is not only used to maintain the benefits of both chloral hydrate and pentobarbital but also to reduce some of the unwanted side-effects. However, ileus has still been reported with this combination.

Alpha-Chloralose

Although the exact mechanism of action of alpha-chloralose remains unknown, it is suspected to bind to the GABA receptor in the CNS. It produces prolonged anesthesia at a light plane and provides no meaningful analgesia. It does not appear to affect baroreceptor or chemoreceptor reflexes which make it an ideal agent for long-term cardiopulmonary studies (Holzgrefe et al. 1987).

The onset of action after IV administration can be up to 15 minutes so it is generally suggested to induce anesthesia with an alternative agent and administer alpha-chloralose for the maintenance stage where 8–10 hours of light anesthesia can be achieved. Generally, alpha-chloralose is only given for non-recovery procedures owing to very prolonged recovery times and the potential for seizure-like activity.

Intraperitoneal injection is not recommended due to pain and inflammation on injection.

Urethane

Urethane's mechanism of action is not fully understood. However, a recent study in rats showed that it affected potassium channels to decrease neuron firing and did not exert any effect on GABA receptors (Sceniak and Maciver 2006). It produces long-acting anesthesia and maintains stable cardiovascular variables by stimulation of the sympathetic nervous system (Buelke-Sam et al. 1978; Janssen et al. 2004; Carruba et al. 1987). Respiratory function is generally good however, ventilation may be required in small mammals (Moldestad et al. 2009).

Urethane is no longer recommended for use as it has been shown to be mutagenic and carcinogenic and is listed on the National Institute of Health list of drugs that are anticipated to be human carcinogens (Field and Lang 1988). Personnel exposure can be via both direct and indirect (i.e. inhaled, etc.) contact.

References

Absalom, A., Pledger, D., and Kong, A. (1999). Adrenocortical function in critically ill patients 24 h after a single dose of etomidate. *Anaesthesia* 54 (9): 861–867.

Aghdaii, N., Ziyaeifard, M., Faritus, S.Z., and Azarfarin, R. (2015). Hemodynamic responses to two different anesthesia regimens in compromised left ventricular function patients undergoing coronary artery bypass graft surgery: etomidate-midazolam versus propofol-ketamine. *Anesth. Pain Med.* 5 (3): e27966.

Aida, S., Yamakura, T., Baba, H. et al. (2000). Preemptive analgesia by intravenous low-dose ketamine and epidural morphine in gastrectomy: a randomized double-blind study. *Anesthesiol.* 92 (6): 1624–1630.

Amengual, M., Flaherty, D., Auckburally, A. et al. (2013). An evaluation of anaesthetic induction in healthy dogs using rapid intravenous injection of propofol or alfaxalone. *Vet. Anaesth. Analg.* 40 (2): 115–123.

Amouzadeh, H.R., Sangiah, S., and Qualls, C.W. Jr. (1989). Effects of some hepatic microsomal enzyme inducers and inhibitors on xylazine-ketamine anesthesia. *Vet. Hum. Toxicol.* 31 (6): 532–534.

Andaluz, A., Santos, L., Garcia, F. et al. (2013). Maternal and foetal cardiovascular effects of the anaesthetic alfaxalone in 2-hydroxypropyl-beta-cyclodextrin in the pregnant ewe. *Sci. World J.* 2013: 189843.

Andress, J.L., Day, T.K., and Day, D. (1995). The effects of consecutive day propofol anesthesia on feline red blood cells. *Vet. Surg.* 24 (3): 277–282.

Annetta, M.G., Iemma, D., Garisto, C. et al. (2005). Ketamine: new indications for an old drug. *Curr. Drug Targets* 6 (7): 789–794.

Artru, A.A., Shapira, Y., and Bowdle, T.A. (1992). Electroencephalogram, cerebral metabolic, and vascular responses to propofol anesthesia in dogs. *J. Neurosurg. Anesthesiol.* 4 (2): 99–109.

Baetge, C.L., Smith, L.C., and Azevedo, C.P. (2020). Clinical Heinz body anemia in a cat after repeat propofol administration case report. *Front. Vet. Sci.* 26 (7): 591556.

Baggot, J.D. and Blake, J.W. (1976). Disposition kinetics of ketamine in the domestic cat. *Arch. Int. Pharmacodyn. Ther.* 220 (1): 115–124.

Baraka, A., Harrison, T., and Kachachi, T. (1973). Catecholamine levels after ketamine anesthesia in man. *Anesth. Analg.* 52 (2): 198–200.

Bettschart-Wolfensberger, R., Stauffer, S., Hassig, M. et al. (2013). Racemic ketamine in comparison to S-ketamine in combination with azaperone and butorphanol for castration of pigs. *Schweiz. Arch. Tierheilkd* 155 (12): 669–675.

Bigby, S.E., Beths, T., Bauquier, S., and Carter, J.E. (2017a). Postinduction apnoea in dogs premedicated with acepromazine or dexmedetomidine and anaesthetized with alfaxalone or propofol. *Vet. Anaesth. Analg.* 44 (5): 1007–1015.

Bigby, S.E., Beths, T., Bauquier, S., and Carter, J.E. (2017b). Effect of rate of administration of propofol or alfaxalone on induction requirements and occurrence of apnea in dogs. *Vet. Anaesth. Analg.* 44 (6): 1267–1275.

Bley, C.R., Roos, M., Price, J. et al. (2007). Clinical assessment of repeated propofol-associated anesthesia in cats. *J. Am. Vet. Med. Assoc.* 231 (9): 1347–1353.

Bortolami, E., Murrell, J.C., and Slingsby, L.S. (2013). Methadone in combination with acepromazine as premedication prior to neutering in the cat. *Vet. Anaesth. Analg.* 40 (2): 181–193.

Boudreau, A.E., Bersenas, A.M., Kerr, C.L. et al. (2012). A comparison of 3 anesthetic protocols for 24 hours of mechanical ventilation in cats. *J. Vet. Emerg. Crit. Care (San Antonio)* 22 (2): 239–252.

Brammer, D.W., Doerning, B.J., Chrisp, C.E., and Rush, H.G. (1991). Anesthetic and nephrotoxic effects of Telazol in New Zealand white rabbits. *Lab. Anim. Sci.* 41 (5): 432–435.

Bramwell, K.J., Haizlip, J., Pribble, C. et al. (2006). The effect of etomidate on intracranial pressure and systemic blood pressure in pediatric patients with severe traumatic brain injury. *Pediatr. Emerg. Care* 22 (2): 90–93.

Buelke-Sam, J., Holson, J.F., Bazare, J.J., and Young, J.F. (1978). Comparative stability of physiological parameters during sustained anesthesia in rats. *Lab. Anim. Sci.* 28 (2): 157–162.

Calla, S., Gupta, A., Sen, N., and Garg, I.P. (1987). Comparison of the effects of etomidate and thiopentone on intraocular pressure. *Br. J. Anaesth.* 59 (4): 437–439.

Campos, S., Felix, L., Venancio, C. et al. (2016). In vivo study of hepatic oxidative stress and mitochondrial function in rabbits with severe hypotension after propofol prolonged infusion. *Springerplus* 5 (1): 1349.

Carruba, M.O., Bondiolotti, G., Picotti, G.B. et al. (1987). Effects of diethyl ether, halothane, ketamine and urethane on sympathetic activity in the rat. *Eur. J. Pharmacol.* 134 (1): 15–24.

Casoni, D., Spadavecchia, C., and Adami, C. (2015a). S-ketamine versus racemic ketamine in dogs: their relative potency as induction agents. *Vet. Anaesth. Analg.* 42 (3): 250–259.

Casoni, D., Spadavecchia, C., Wampfler, B. et al. (2015b). Clinical and pharmacokinetic evaluation of S-ketamine for intravenous general anaesthesia in horses undergoing field castration. *Acta Vet. Scand.* 57 (1): 21.

Castel, A., Helie, P., Beaudry, F., and Vachon, P. (2013). Bilateral central pain sensitization in rats following a unilateral thalamic lesion may be treated with high doses of ketamine. *BMC Vet. Res.* 9: 59.

Cattai, A., Rabozzi, R., Natale, V., and Franci, P. (2015). The incidence of spontaneous movements (myoclonus) in dogs undergoing total intravenous anaesthesia with propofol. *Vet. Anaesth. Analg.* 42 (1): 93–98.

Celotti, F., Negri-Cesi, P., and Poletti, A. (1997). Steroid metabolism in the mammalian brain: 5alpha-reduction and aromatization. *Brain Res. Bull.* 44 (4): 365–375.

Chen, S.R., Samoriski, G., and Pan, H.L. (2009). Antinociceptive effects of chronic administration of uncompetitive NMDA receptor antagonists in a rat model of diabetic neuropathic pain. *Neuropharmacol.* 57 (2): 121–126.

Choi, S.D., Spaulding, B.C., Gross, J.B., and Apfelbaum, J.L. (1985). Comparison of the ventilatory effects of etomidate and methohexital. *Anesthesiol.* 62 (4): 442–447.

Cleale, R.M., Muir, W.W., Waselau, A.C. et al. (2009). Pharmacokinetic and pharmacodynamic evaluation of propofol administered to cats in a novel, aqueous, nano-droplet formulation or as an oil-in-water macroemulsion. *J. Vet. Pharmacol. Ther.* 32 (5): 436–445.

Clutton, R.E., Blissitt, K.J., Bradley, A.A., and Camburn, M.A. (1997). Comparison of three injectable anaesthetic techniques in pigs. *Vet. Rec.* 141 (6): 140–146.

Cockshott, I.D., Douglas, E.J., Plummer, G.F., and Simons, P.J. (1992). The pharmacokinetics of propofol in laboratory animals. *Xenobiotica* 22 (3): 369–375.

Cold, G.E., Eskesen, V., Eriksen, H. et al. (1985). CBF and CMRO2 during continuous etomidate infusion supplemented with N_2O and fentanyl in patients with supratentorial cerebral tumour. A dose–response study. *Acta Anaesthesiol. Scand.* 29 (5): 490–494.

Concas, A., Santoro, G., Serra, M. et al. (1991). Neurochemical action of the general anaesthetic propofol on the chloride ion channel coupled with GABAA receptors. *Brain Res.* 542 (2): 225–232.

Costa, D., Leiva, M., Moll, X. et al. (2015). Alfaxalone versus propofol in dogs: a randomised trial to assess effects on peri-induction tear production, intraocular pressure and globe position. *Vet. Rec.* 176 (3): 73.

Court, M.H., Hay-Kraus, B.L., Hill, D.W. et al. (1999). Propofol hydroxylation by dog liver microsomes: assay development and dog breed differences. *Drug Metab. Dispos.* 27 (11): 1293–1299.

Covey-Crump, G.L. and Murison, P.J. (2008). Fentanyl or midazolam for co-induction of anaesthesia with propofol in dogs. *Vet. Anaesth. Analg.* 35 (6): 463–472.

Diaz, F.A., Bianco, J.A., Bello, A. et al. (1976). Effects of ketamine on canine cardiovascular function. *Br. J. Anaesth.* 48 (10): 941–946.

Dodam, J.R., Kruse-Elliott, K.T., Aucoin, D.P., and Swanson, C.R. (1990). Duration of etomidate-induced adrenocortical suppression during surgery in dogs. *Am. J. Vet. Res.* 51 (5): 786–788.

Doebeli, A., Michel, E., Bettschart, R. et al. (2013). Apgar score after induction of anesthesia for canine cesarean section with alfaxalone versus propofol. *Theriogenology* 80 (8): 850–854.

Doenicke, A.W., Roizen, M.F., Hoernecke, R. et al. (1999). Solvent for etomidate may cause pain and adverse effects. *Br. J. Anaesth.* 83 (3): 464–466.

Doerning, B.J., Brammer, D.W., Chrisp, C.E., and Rush, H.G. (1992). Nephrotoxicity of tiletamine in New Zealand white rabbits. *Lab. Anim. Sci.* 42 (3): 267–269.

Dominguez, E., Rivera Del Alamo, M.M., Novellas, R. et al. (2013). Doppler evaluation of the effects of propofol, etomidate and alphaxalone on fetoplacental circulation hemodynamics in the pregnant ewe. *Placenta* 34 (9): 738–744.

Drayna, P.C., Estrada, C., Wang, W. et al. (2012). Ketamine sedation is not associated with clinically meaningful elevation of intraocular pressure. *Am. J. Emerg. Med.* 30 (7): 1215–1218.

Ebrahim, Z.Y., DeBoer, G.E., Luders, H. et al. (1986). Effect of etomidate on the electroencephalogram of patients with epilepsy. *Anesth. Analg.* 65 (10): 1004–1006.

Engelhardt, W. (1997). Recovery and psychomimetic reactions following S-(+)-ketamine. *Anaesthesist* 46 (Suppl 1): S38–S42.

Ferre, P.J., Pasloske, K., Whittem, T. et al. (2006). Plasma pharmacokinetics of alfaxalone in dogs after an intravenous bolus of Alfaxan-CD RTU. *Vet. Anaesth. Analg.* 33 (4): 229–236.

Ferreira, T.H., Brosnan, R.J., Shilo-Benjamini, Y. et al. (2013). Effects of ketamine, propofol, or thiopental administration on intraocular pressure and qualities of induction of and recovery from anesthesia in horses. *Am. J. Vet. Res.* 74 (8): 1070–1077.

Field, K.J. and Lang, C.M. (1988). Hazards of urethane (ethyl carbamate): a review of the literature. *Lab. Anim.* 22 (3): 255–262.

Field, K.J., White, W.J., and Lang, C.M. (1993). Anaesthetic effects of chloral hydrate, pentobarbitone and urethane in adult male rats. *Lab. Anim.* 27 (3): 258–269.

Fleischman, R.W., McCracken, D., and Forbes, W. (1977). Adynamic ileus in the rat induced by chloral hydrate. *Lab. Anim. Sci.* 27 (2): 238–243.

Fresno, L., Andaluz, A., Moll, X., and Garcia, F. (2008). The effects on maternal and fetal cardiovascular and acid–base variables after the administration of etomidate in the pregnant ewe. *Vet. J.* 177 (1): 94–103.

Frias, A.F., Marsico, F., Gomez de Segura, I.A. et al. (2003). Evaluation of different doses of propofol in xylazine pre-medicated horses. *Vet. Anaesth. Analg.* 30 (4): 193–201.

Furtado, M.M., Nunes, A.L., Intelizano, T.R. et al. (2010). Comparison of racemic ketamine versus (S+) ketamine when combined with midazolam for anesthesia of *Callithrix jacchus* and *Callithrix penicillata*. *J. Zoo Wildl. Med.* 41 (3): 389–394.

Geel, J.K. (1991). The effect of premedication on the induction dose of propofol in dogs and cats. *J. S. Afr. Vet. Assoc.* 62 (3): 118–123.

Ghoneim, M.M. and Yamada, T. (1977). Etomidate: a clinical and electroencephalographic comparison with thiopental. *Anesth. Analg.* 56 (4): 479–485.

Glen, J.B. (1980). Animal studies of the anaesthetic activity of ICI 35 868. *Br. J. Anaesth.* 52 (8): 731–742.

Gommeren, K., Claeys, S., de Rooster, H. et al. (2010). Outcome from status epilepticus after portosystemic shunt attenuation in 3 dogs treated with propofol and phenobarbital. *J. Vet. Emerg. Crit. Care (San Antonio)* 20 (3): 346–351.

Gomwalk, N.E. and Healing, T.D. (1981). Etomidate: a valuable anaesthetic for mice. *Lab. Anim.* 15 (2): 151–152.

Goodwin, W.A., Keates, H.L., Pasloske, K. et al. (2011). The pharmacokinetics and pharmacodynamics of the injectable anaesthetic alfaxalone in the horse. *Vet. Anaesth. Analg.* 38 (5): 431–438.

Goodwin, W., Keates, H., Pasloske, K. et al. (2012). Plasma pharmacokinetics and pharmacodynamics of alfaxalone in neonatal foals after an intravenous bolus of alfaxalone following premedication with butorphanol tartrate. *Vet. Anaesth. Analg.* 39 (5): 503–510.

Griffenhagen, G.M., Rezende, M.L., Gustafson, D.L. et al. (2014). Pharmacokinetics and pharmacodynamics of propofol with or without 2% benzyl alcohol following a single induction dose administered intravenously in cats. *Vet. Anaesth. Analg.*.

Grint, N.J., Smith, H.E., and Senior, J.M. (2008). Clinical evaluation of alfaxalone in cyclodextrin for the induction of anaesthesia in rabbits. *Vet. Rec.* 163 (13): 395–396.

Grubb, T.L., Greene, S.A., and Perez, T.E. (2013). Cardiovascular and respiratory effects, and quality of anesthesia produced by alfaxalone administered intramuscularly to cats sedated with dexmedetomidine and hydromorphone. *J. Feline Med. Surg.* 15 (10): 858–865.

Guirimand, F., Dupont, X., Brasseur, L. et al. (2000). The effects of ketamine on the temporal summation (wind-up) of the R(III) nociceptive flexion reflex and pain in humans. *Anesth. Analg.* 90 (2): 408–414.

Gunderson, E.G., Lukasik, V.M., Ashton, M.M. et al. (2013). Effects of anesthetic induction with midazolam-propofol and midazolam-etomidate on selected ocular and cardiorespiratory variables in clinically normal dogs. *Am. J. Vet. Res.* 74 (4): 629–635.

Hahnenberger, R. (1976). Influence of various anesthetic drugs on the intraocular pressure of cats. *Albrecht Von Graefes Arch. Klin. Exp. Ophthalmol.* 199 (2): 179–186.

Han, R.Z., Hu, J.J., Weng, Y.C. et al. (2009). NMDA receptor antagonist MK-801 reduces neuronal damage and preserves learning and memory in a rat model of traumatic brain injury. *Neurosci. Bull.* 25 (6): 367–375.

Hanna, R.M., Borchard, R.E., and Schmidt, S.L. (1988). Pharmacokinetics of ketamine HCl and metabolite I in the cat: a comparison of i.v., i.m., and rectal administration. *J. Vet. Pharmacol. Ther.* 11 (1): 84–93.

Hasiuk, M.M., Forde, N., Cooke, A. et al. (2014). A comparison of alfaxalone and propofol on intraocular pressure in healthy dogs. *Vet. Ophthalmol.* 17 (416): 411–416.

Haskins, S.C., Farver, T.B., and Patz, J.D. (1985). Ketamine in dogs. *Am. J. Vet. Res.* 46 (9): 1855–1860.

Hay Kraus, B.L., Greenblatt, D.J., Venkatakrishnan, K., and Court, M.H. (2000). Evidence for propofol hydroxylation by cytochrome P4502B11 in canine liver microsomes: breed and gender differences. *Xenobiotica* 30 (6): 575–588.

Heldmann, E., Brown, D.C., and Shofer, F. (1999a). The association of propofol usage with postoperative wound infection rate in clean wounds: a retrospective study. *Vet. Surg.* 28 (4): 256–259.

Heldmann, E., Holt, D.E., Brockman, D.J. et al. (1999b). Use of propofol to manage seizure activity after surgical treatment of portosystemic shunts. *J. Small Anim. Pract.* 40 (12): 590–594.

Heykants, J.J., Meuldermans, W.E., Michiels, L.J. et al. (1975). Distribution, metabolism and excretion of etomidate, a short-acting hypnotic drug, in the rat. Comparative study of (R)-(+)-(−)-Etomidate. *Arch. Int. Pharmacodyn. Ther.* 216 (1): 113–129.

Hildreth, A.N., Mejia, V.A., Maxwell, R.A. et al. (2008). Adrenal suppression following a single dose of etomidate for rapid sequence induction: a prospective randomized study. *J. Trauma* 65 (3): 573–579.

Hirshman, C.A., Downes, H., Farbood, A., and Bergman, N.A. (1979). Ketamine block of bronchospasm in experimental canine asthma. *Br. J. Anaesth.* 51 (8): 713–718.

Holzgrefe, H.H., Everitt, J.M., and Wright, E.M. (1987). Alpha-chloralose as a canine anesthetic. *Lab. Anim. Sci.* 37 (5): 587–595.

Ihmsen, H., Geisslinger, G., and Schuttler, J. (2001). Stereoselective pharmacokinetics of ketamine: R(−)-ketamine inhibits the elimination of S(+)-ketamine. *Clin. Pharmacol. Ther.* 70 (5): 431–438.

Ilkiw, J.E., Pascoe, P.J., Haskins, S.C., and Patz, J.D. (1992). Cardiovascular and respiratory effects of propofol administration in hypovolemic dogs. *Am. J. Vet. Res.* 53 (12): 2323–2327.

Jang, M., Park, S., Son, W.G. et al. (2015). Effect of tiletamine-zolazepam on the intraocular pressure of the dog. *Vet. Ophthalmol.* 18 (6): 481–484.

Janssen, B.J., De Celle, T., Debets, J.J. et al. (2004). Effects of anesthetics on systemic hemodynamics in mice. *Am. J. Physiol. Heart Circ. Physiol.* 287 (4): H1618–H1624.

Jarrett, M.A., Bailey, K.M., Messenger, K.M. et al. (2018). Recovery of horses from general anesthesia after induction with propofol and ketamine versus midazolam and ketamine. *J. Am. Vet. Med. Assoc.* 253 (1): 101–107.

Jaspar, N., Mazzarelli, M., Tessier, C., and Milic-Emili, J. (1983). Effect of ketamine on control of breathing in cats. *J. Appl. Physiol. Respir. Environ. Exerc. Physiol.* 55 (3): 851–859.

Jimenez, C.P., Mathis, A., Mora, S.S. et al. (2012). Evaluation of the quality of the recovery after administration of propofol or alfaxalone for induction of anaesthesia in dogs anaesthetized for magnetic resonance imaging. *Vet. Anaesth. Analg.* 39 (2): 151–159.

Jud, R., Picek, S., Makara, M.A. et al. (2010). Comparison of racemic ketamine and S-ketamine as agents for the induction of anaesthesia in goats. *Vet. Anaesth. Analg.* 37 (6): 511–518.

Kaka, J.S. and Hayton, W.L. (1980). Pharmacokinetics of ketamine and two metabolites in the dog. *J. Pharmacokinet. Biopharm.* 8 (2): 193–202.

Kaka, J.S., Klavano, P.A., and Hayton, W.L. (1979). Pharmacokinetics of ketamine in the horse. *Am. J. Vet. Res.* 40 (7): 978–981.

Kalchofner Guerrero, K.S., Reichler, I.M., Schwarz, A. et al. (2014). Alfaxalone or ketamine-medetomidine in cats undergoing ovariohysterectomy: a comparison of intra-operative parameters and post-operative pain. *Vet. Anaesth. Analg.* 41 (6): 644–653.

Kang, J.G., Lee, C.J., Kim, T.H. et al. (2010). Analgesic effects of ketamine infusion therapy in korean patients with neuropathic pain: a 2-week, open-label, uncontrolled study. *Curr. Ther. Res. Clin. Exp.* 71 (2): 93–104.

Kayama, Y. (1982). Ketamine and e.e.g. seizure waves: interaction with anti-epileptic drugs. *Br. J. Anaesth.* 54 (8): 879–883.

Keates, H. and Whittem, T. (2012). Effect of intravenous dose escalation with alfaxalone and propofol on occurrence of apnoea in the dog. *Res. Vet. Sci.* 93 (2): 904–906.

Keates, H.L., van Eps, A.W., and Pearson, M.R. (2012). Alfaxalone compared with ketamine for induction of anaesthesia in horses following xylazine and guaifenesin. *Vet. Anaesth. Analg.* 39 (6): 591–598.

Kerz, T., Hennes, H.J., Feve, A. et al. (2001). Effects of propofol on H-reflex in humans. *Anesthesiology* 94 (1): 32–37.

Kloppel, H. and Leece, E.A. (2011). Comparison of ketamine and alfaxalone for induction and maintenance of anaesthesia in ponies undergoing castration. *Vet. Anaesth. Analg.* 38 (1): 37–43.

Kovalcuka, L., Birgele, E., Bandere, D., and Williams, D.L. (2013). The effects of ketamine hydrochloride and diazepam on the intraocular pressure and pupil diameter of the dog's eye. *Vet. Ophthalmol.* 16 (1): 29–34.

Kumar, A., Mann, H.J., Remmel, R.P. et al. (2014). Pharmacokinetic study in pigs and in vitro metabolic characterization in pig- and human-liver microsomes reveal marked differences in disposition and metabolism of tiletamine and zolazepam (Telazol). *Xenobiotica* 44 (4): 379–390.

Larenza, M.P., Landoni, M.F., Levionnois, O.L. et al. (2007). Stereoselective pharmacokinetics of ketamine and norketamine after racemic ketamine or S-ketamine administration during isoflurane anaesthesia in Shetland ponies. *Br. J. Anaesth.* 98 (2): 204–212.

Larenza, M.P., Althaus, H., Conrot, A. et al. (2008a). Anaesthesia recovery quality after racemic ketamine or S-ketamine administration to male cats undergoing neutering surgery. *Schweiz. Arch. Tierheilkd.* 150 (12): 599–607.

Larenza, M.P., Knobloch, M., Landoni, M.F. et al. (2008b). Stereoselective pharmacokinetics of ketamine and norketamine after racemic ketamine or S-ketamine administration in Shetland ponies sedated with xylazine. *Vet. J.* 177 (3): 432–435.

Larenza, M.P., Peterbauer, C., Landoni, M.F. et al. (2009a). Stereoselective pharmacokinetics of ketamine and norketamine after constant rate infusion of a subanesthetic dose of racemic ketamine or S-ketamine in Shetland ponies. *Am. J. Vet. Res.* 70 (7): 831–839.

Larenza, M.P., Ringer, S.K., Kutter, A.P. et al. (2009b). Evaluation of anesthesia recovery quality after low-dose racemic or S-ketamine infusions during anesthesia with isoflurane in horses. *Am. J. Vet. Res.* 70 (6): 710–718.

Lau, C., Ranasinghe, M.G., Shiels, I. et al. (2013). Plasma pharmacokinetics of alfalaxone after a single intraperitoneal or intravenous injection of Alfaxan((R)) in rats. *J. Vet. Pharmacol. Ther.* 36 (5): 516–520.

Leung, L.Y. and Baillie, T.A. (1986). Comparative pharmacology in the rat of ketamine and its two principal metabolites, norketamine and (Z)-6-hydroxynorketamine. *J. Med. Chem.* 29 (11): 2396–2399.

Lewi, P.J., Heykants, J.J., and Janssen, P.A. (1976). Intravenous pharmacokinetic profile in rats of etomidate, a short-acting hypnotic drug. *Arch. Int. Pharmacodyn. Ther.* 220 (1): 72–85.

Lima, C.F., Cortopassi, S.R., de Moura, C.A. et al. (2016). Comparison between dexmedetomidine-S-ketamine and midazolam-S-ketamine in immobilization of Oncilla (*Leopardus tigrinus*). *J. Zoo Wildl. Med.* 47 (1): 17–24.

Lin, H.C., Thurmon, J.C., Benson, G.J., and Tranquilli, W.J. (1993). Telazol – a review of its pharmacology and use in veterinary medicine. *J. Vet. Pharmacol. Ther.* 16 (4): 383–418.

Lin, H.C., Purohit, R.C., and Powe, T.A. (1997). Anesthesia in sheep with propofol or with xylazine-ketamine followed by halothane. *Vet. Surg.* 26 (3): 247–252.

Luna, S.P., Cassu, R.N., Castro, G.B. et al. (2004). Effects of four anaesthetic protocols on the neurological and cardiorespiratory variables of puppies born by caesarean section. *Vet. Rec.* 154 (13): 387–389.

Maddern, K., Adams, V.J., Hill, N.A., and Leece, E.A. (2010). Alfaxalone induction dose following administration of medetomidine and butorphanol in the dog. *Vet. Anaesth. Analg.* 37 (1): 7–13.

Mama, K.R., Steffey, E.P., and Pascoe, P.J. (1996). Evaluation of propofol for general anesthesia in premedicated horses. *Am. J. Vet. Res.* 57 (4): 512–516.

Maney, J.K., Shepard, M.K., Braun, C. et al. (2013). A comparison of cardiopulmonary and anesthetic effects of an induction dose of alfaxalone or propofol in dogs. *Vet. Anaesth. Analg.* 40 (3): 237–244.

Mathis, A., Pinelas, R., Brodbelt, D.C., and Alibhai, H.I. (2012). Comparison of quality of recovery from anaesthesia in cats induced with propofol or alfaxalone. *Vet. Anaesth. Analg.* 39 (3): 282–290.

Matot, I., Neely, C.F., Katz, R.Y., and Neufeld, G.R. (1993). Pulmonary uptake of propofol in cats. Effect of fentanyl and halothane. *Anesthesiology* 78 (6): 1157–1165.

Meuldermans, W.E. and Heykants, J.J. (1976). The plasma protein binding and distribution of etomidate in dog, rat and human blood. *Arch. Int. Pharmacodyn. Ther.* 221 (1): 150–162.

Moldestad, O., Karlsen, P., Molden, S., and Storm, J.F. (2009). Tracheotomy improves experiment success rate in mice during urethane anesthesia and stereotaxic surgery. *J. Neurosci. Methods* 176 (2): 57–62.

Moon, P.F. (1997). Cortisol suppression in cats after induction of anesthesia with etomidate, compared with ketamine-diazepam combination. *Am. J. Vet. Res.* 58 (8): 868–871.

Morgan, D.W. and Legge, K. (1989). Clinical evaluation of propofol as an intravenous anaesthetic agent in cats and dogs. *Vet. Rec.* 124 (2): 31–33.

Muir, W., Lerche, P., Wiese, A. et al. (2008). Cardiorespiratory and anesthetic effects of clinical and supraclinical doses of alfaxalone in dogs. *Vet. Anaesth. Analg.* 35 (6): 451–462.

Muir, W., Lerche, P., Wiese, A. et al. (2009a). The cardiorespiratory and anesthetic effects of clinical and supraclinical doses of alfaxalone in cats. *Vet. Anaesth. Analg.* 36 (1): 42–54.

Muir, W.W., Lerche, P., and Erichson, D. (2009b). Anaesthetic and cardiorespiratory effects of propofol at 10% for induction and 1% for maintenance of anaesthesia in horses. *Equine Vet. J.* 41 (6): 578–585.

Navarrete-Calvo, R., Gomez-Villamandos, R.J., Morgaz, J. et al. (2014). Cardiorespiratory, anaesthetic and recovery effects of morphine combined with medetomidine and alfaxalone in rabbits. *Vet. Rec.* 174 (4): 95.

Nicholas, T.E., Jones, M.E., Johnson, D.W., and Phillipou, G. (1981). Metabolism of the steroid anaesthetic alphaxalone by the isolated perfused rat lung. *J. Steroid Biochem.* 14 (1): 45–51.

O'Hagan, B., Pasloske, K., McKinnon, C. et al. (2012a). Clinical evaluation of alfaxalone as an anaesthetic induction agent in dogs less than 12 weeks of age. *Aust. Vet. J.* 90 (9): 346–350.

O'Hagan, B.J., Pasloske, K., McKinnon, C. et al. (2012b). Clinical evaluation of alfaxalone as an anaesthetic induction agent in cats less than 12 weeks of age. *Aust. Vet. J.* 90 (10): 395–401.

Olsen, R.W. and Li, G.D. (2011). GABA(A) receptors as molecular targets of general anesthetics: identification of binding sites provides clues to allosteric modulation. *Can. J. Anaesth.* 58 (2): 206–215.

O'Meara, G.F., Newman, R.J., Fradley, R.L. et al. (2004). The GABA-A beta3 subunit mediates anaesthesia induced by etomidate. *Neuroreport* 15 (10): 1653–1656.

Pablo, L.S., Bailey, J.E., and Ko, J.C. (1997). Median effective dose of propofol required for induction of anaesthesia in goats. *J. Am. Vet. Med. Assoc.* 211 (1): 86–88.

Pasloske, K., Sauer, B., Perkins, N., and Whittem, T. (2009). Plasma pharmacokinetics of alfaxalone in both premedicated and unpremedicated Greyhound dogs after single, intravenous administration of Alfaxan at a clinical dose. *J. Vet. Pharmacol. Ther.* 32 (5): 510–513.

Pfenninger, E., Dick, W., and Ahnefeld, F.W. (1985). The influence of ketamine on both normal and raised intracranial pressure of artificially ventilated animals. *Eur. J. Anaesthesiol.* 2 (3): 297–307.

Pinaud, M., Lelausque, J.N., Chetanneau, A. et al. (1990). Effects of propofol on cerebral hemodynamics and metabolism in patients with brain trauma. *Anesthesiology* 73 (3): 404–409.

Pinelas, R., Alibhai, H.I., Mathis, A. et al. (2014). Effects of different doses of dexmedetomidine on anaesthetic induction with alfaxalone – a clinical trial. *Vet. Anaesth. Analg.* 41 (4): 378–385.

Posner, L.P., Kasten, J.I., and Kata, C. (2013). Propofol with ketamine following sedation with xylazine for routine induction of general anaesthesia in horses. *Vet. Rec.* 173 (22): 550.

Psatha, E., Alibhai, H.I., Jimenez-Lozano, A. et al. (2011). Clinical efficacy and cardiorespiratory effects of alfaxalone, or diazepam/fentanyl for induction of anaesthesia in dogs that are a poor anaesthetic risk. *Vet. Anaesth. Analg.* 38 (1): 24–36.

Rampp, S., Schmitt, H.J., Heers, M. et al. (2014). Etomidate activates epileptic high frequency oscillations. *Clin. Neurophysiol.* 125 (2): 223–230.

Rasmussen, N.J., Rosendal, T., and Overgaard, J. (1978). Althesin in neurosurgical patients: effects on cerebral hemodynamics and metabolism. *Acta Anaesthesiol. Scand.* 22 (3): 257–269.

Reder, B.S., Trapp, L.D., and Troutman, K.C. (1980). Ketamine suppression of chemically induced convulsions in the two-day-old white leghorn cockerel. *Anesth. Analg.* 59 (6): 406–409.

Reich, D.L. and Silvay, G. (1989). Ketamine: an update on the first twenty-five years of clinical experience. *Can. J. Anaesth.* 36 (2): 186–197.

Renou, A.M., Vernhiet, J., Macrez, P. et al. (1978). Cerebral blood flow and metabolism during etomidate anaesthesia in man. *Br. J. Anaesth.* 50 (10): 1047–1051.

Ribas, T., Bublot, I., Junot, S. et al. (2014). Effects of intramuscular sedation with alfaxalone and butorphanol on echocardiographic measurements in healthy cats. *J. Feline Med. Surg.* 530–536.

Robertson, S.A., Johnston, S., and Beemsterboer, J. (1992). Cardiopulmonary, anesthetic, and postanesthetic effects of intravenous infusions of propofol in greyhounds and non-Greyhounds. *Am. J. Vet. Res.* 53 (6): 1027–1032.

Robinson, R. and Borer-Weir, K. (2013). A dose titration study into the effects of diazepam or midazolam on the propofol dose requirements for induction of general anaesthesia in client owned dogs, premedicated with methadone and acepromazine. *Vet. Anaesth. Analg.* 42 (5): 493–501.

Robinson, R. and Borer-Weir, K. (2015). The effects of diazepam or midazolam on the dose of propofol required to induce anaesthesia in cats. *Vet. Anaesth. Analg.* 493–501.

Rodriguez, J.M., Munoz-Rascon, P., Navarrete-Calvo, R. et al. (2012). Comparison of the cardiopulmonary parameters after induction of anaesthesia with alphaxalone or etomidate in dogs. *Vet. Anaesth. Analg.* 39 (4): 357–365.

Rossetti, R.B., Gaido Cortopassi, S.R., Intelizano, T. et al. (2008). Comparison of ketamine and S(+)-ketamine, with romifidine and diazepam, for total intravenous anesthesia in horses. *Vet. Anaesth. Analg.* 35 (1): 30–37.

Sanchez, A., Belda, E., Escobar, M. et al. (2013). Effects of altering the sequence of midazolam and propofol during co-induction of anaesthesia. *Vet. Anaesth. Analg.* 40 (4): 359–366.

Santos Gonzalez, M., Bertran de Lis, B.T., and Tendillo Cortijo, F.J. (2013). Effects of intramuscular alfaxalone alone or in combination with diazepam in swine. *Vet. Anaesth. Analg.* 40 (4): 399–402.

Sari, A., Maekawa, T., Tohjo, M. et al. (1976). Effects of Althesin on cerebral blood flow and oxygen consumption in man. *Br. J. Anaesth.* 48 (6): 545–550.

Sceniak, M.P. and Maciver, M.B. (2006). Cellular actions of urethane on rat visual cortical neurons in vitro. *J. Neurophysiol.* 95 (6): 3865–3874.

Sear, J.W. (1996). Steroid anesthetics: old compounds, new drugs. *J. Clin. Anesth.* 8 (3 Suppl): 91S–98S.

Sear, J.W. and McGivan, J.D. (1981). Metabolism of alphaxalone in the rat: evidence for the limitation of the anaesthetic effect by the rate of degradation through the hepatic mixed function oxygenase system. *Br. J. Anaesth.* 53 (4): 417–424.

Simons, P.J., Cockshott, I.D., Douglas, E.J. et al. (1991). Species differences in blood profiles, metabolism and excretion of 14C-propofol after intravenous dosing to rat, dog and rabbit. *Xenobiotica* 21 (10): 1243–1256.

Sisson, D.F. and Siegel, J. (1989). Chloral hydrate anesthesia: EEG power spectrum analysis and effects on VEPs in the rat. *Neurotoxicol. Teratol.* 11 (1): 51–56.

Sisson, D.F., Siegel, J., and Westenberg, I.S. (1991). Are the differential effects of chloral hydrate on hooded rats vs. albino rats due to pigmentation or strain differences? *Pharmacol. Biochem. Behav.* 39 (3): 665–670.

Slingsby, L.S., Bortolami, E., and Murrell, J.C. (2015). Methadone in combination with medetomidine as premedication prior to ovariohysterectomy and castration in the cat. *J. Feline Med. Surg.* 17 (10): 864–872.

Soliman, M.G., Brindle, G.F., and Kuster, G. (1975). Response to hypercapnia under ketamine anaesthesia. *Can. Anaesth. Soc. J.* 22 (4): 486–494.

Suresh, M.S. and Nelson, T.E. (1985). Malignant hyperthermia: is etomidate safe? *Anesth. Analg.* 64 (4): 420–424.

Taylor, P.A. and Towey, R.M. (1971). Ketamine anaesthesia. *Br. Med. J.* 3 (5771): 432.

Tendillo, F.J., Mascias, A., Santos, M. et al. (1996). Cardiorespiratory and analgesic effects of continuous infusion of propofol in swine as experimental animals. *Rev. Esp. Anestesiol. Reanim.* 43 (4): 126–129.

Tomlin, S.L., Jenkins, A., Lieb, W.R., and Franks, N.P. (1998). Stereoselective effects of etomidate optical isomers on gamma-aminobutyric acid type A receptors and animals. *Anesthesiol.* 88 (3): 708–717.

Wagner, R.L., White, P.F., Kan, P.B. et al. (1984). Inhibition of adrenal steroidogenesis by the anesthetic etomidate. *N. Engl. J. Med.* 310 (22): 1415–1421.

Walsh, V.P., Gieseg, M., Singh, P.M. et al. (2012). A comparison of two different ketamine and diazepam combinations with an alphaxalone and medetomidine combination for induction of anaesthesia in sheep. *N. Z. Vet. J.* 60 (2): 136–141.

Waterman, A.E. (1984). The pharmacokinetics of ketamine administered intravenously in calves and the modifying effect of premedication with xylazine hydrochloride. *J. Vet. Pharmacol. Ther.* 7 (2): 125–130.

Waterman, A.E. (1988). Use of propofol in sheep. *Vet. Rec.* 122 (11): 260.

Waterman, A.E., Robertson, S.A., and Lane, J.G. (1987). Pharmacokinetics of intravenously administered ketamine in the horse. *Res. Vet. Sci.* 42 (2): 162–166.

Watkins, S.B., Hall, L.W., and Clarke, K.W. (1987). Propofol as an intravenous anaesthetic agent in dogs. *Vet. Rec.* 120 (14): 326–329.

Watney, G.C. and Pablo, L.S. (1992). Median effective dosage of propofol for induction of anesthesia in dogs. *Am. J. Vet. Res.* 53 (12): 2320–2322.

Waxman, K., Shoemaker, W.C., and Lippmann, M. (1980). Cardiovascular effects of anesthetic induction with ketamine. *Anesth. Analg.* 59 (5): 355–358.

Weaver, B.M. and Raptopoulos, D. (1990). Induction of anaesthesia in dogs and cats with propofol. *Vet. Rec.* 126 (25): 617–620.

Weir, C.J., Ling, A.T., Belelli, D. et al. (2004). The interaction of anaesthetic steroids with recombinant glycine and GABAA receptors. *Br. J. Anaesth.* 92 (5): 704–711.

Wertz, E.M., Benson, G.J., Thurmon, J.C. et al. (1990). Pharmacokinetics of etomidate in cats. *Am. J. Vet. Res.* 51 (2): 281–285.

White, P.F., Way, W.L., and Trevor, A.J. (1982). Ketamine – its pharmacology and therapeutic uses. *Anesthesiology* 56 (2): 119–136.

Whittem, T., Pasloske, K.S., Heit, M.C., and Ranasinghe, M.G. (2008). The pharmacokinetics and pharmacodynamics of alfaxalone in cats after single and multiple intravenous administration of Alfaxan at clinical and supraclinical doses. *J. Vet. Pharmacol. Ther.* 31 (6): 571–579.

Whitwam, J.G., Galletly, D.C., Ma, D., and Chakrabarti, M.K. (2000). The effects of propofol on heart rate, arterial pressure and adelta and C somatosympathetic reflexes in anaesthetized dogs. *Eur. J. Anaesthesiol.* 17 (1): 57–63.

Wong, D.H. and Jenkins, L.C. (1974). An experimental study of the mechanism of action of ketamine on the central nervous system. *Can. Anaesth. Soc. J.* 21 (1): 57–67.

Wouters, P.F., Van de Velde, M.A., Marcus, M.A. et al. (1995). Hemodynamic changes during induction of anesthesia with eltanolone and propofol in dogs. *Anesth. Analg.* 81 (1): 125–131.

Ying, S.W. and Goldstein, P.A. (2005). Propofol suppresses synaptic responsiveness of somatosensory relay neurons to excitatory input by potentiating GABA(A) receptor chloride channels. *Mol. Pain* 1 (2).

Ypsilantis, P., Politou, M., Mikroulis, D. et al. (2007). Organ toxicity and mortality in propofol-sedated rabbits under prolonged mechanical ventilation. *Anesth. Analg.* 105 (1): 155–166.

Ypsilantis, P., Politou, M., Mikroulis, D. et al. (2011). Attenuation of propofol tolerance conferred by remifentanil co-administration does not reduce propofol toxicity in rabbits under prolonged mechanical ventilation. *J. Surg. Res.* 168 (2): 253–261.

Zaki, S., Ticehurst, K.E., and Miyaki, Y. (2009). Clinical evaluation of Alfaxan-CD (R) as an intravenous anaesthetic in young cats. *Aust. Vet. J.* 87 (3): 82–87.

Zhang, J., Maland, L., Hague, B. et al. (1998). Buccal absorption of etomidate from a solid formulation in dogs. *Anesth. Analg.* 86 (5): 1116–1122.

Zoran, D.L., Riedesel, D.H., and Dyer, D.C. (1993). Pharmacokinetics of propofol in mixed-breed dogs and greyhounds. *Am. J. Vet. Res.* 54 (5): 755–760.

10

Inhalant Anesthetic Agents

Phillip Lerche and Linda Barter

Introduction

The advent of the use of inhalant anesthetic agents in the mid-1800s changed the medical profession profoundly, as these volatile agents were able to produce unconsciousness and immobility, allowing procedures to be performed on patients without them experiencing acute pain or moving in response to surgery. Despite this breakthrough, the early inhalants were not without their drawbacks, including flammability and toxicity, leading to the search for agents that were safer for patients, and safer for medical personnel to administer.

Addition of a halogen molecule to aliphatic hydrocarbons and ethers proved to render compounds of interest nonflammable, and in the 1950s halothane, a halogenated hydrocarbon derived from alkane, was introduced into clinical medical practice. Despite its favorable chemical profile as a general anesthetic, halothane was shown to decrease the dose of epinephrine required to produce cardiac arrhythmias, leading to continued investigation of compounds that might prove useful as inhalant anesthetic agents. Compounds with an ether linkage, i.e., having the general structure R-O-R′, either do not sensitize the myocardium to epinephrine, or have a vastly reduced sensitivity not clinically relevant. Inhalants classified as aliphatic ethers currently used in the practice of veterinary anesthesia include isoflurane, desflurane, and sevoflurane. Despite once being the most commonly used inhalant in the world, halothane is no longer available in the United States of America, however it is still in use in other countries. Several halogenated compounds used clinically in the past but withdrawn from general use for various reasons, most often due to toxicity, e.g. methoxyflurane, enflurane, will not be discussed.

Nitrous oxide (N_2O) a gas discovered in the 1800s, is not commonly used in veterinary anesthesia outside of specialty anesthetic practice but is sometimes used as an adjunct for its analgesic properties so will be discussed later in the chapter. The modern inhalant anesthetic agents halothane, isoflurane, sevoflurane and, to a much lesser extent, desflurane form the mainstay of maintenance of general anesthesia in animals undergoing surgery and medical procedures. They are manufactured as volatile liquids, which are delivered to the patient via the breathing circuit of an anesthetic machine using precision, inhalant-specific vaporizers in oxygen with or without other carrier gases (e.g. nitrogen, N_2O, medical air). Coupled with endotracheal intubation, this method of delivery allows for precise concentrations to be delivered easily and adjusted relatively quickly in response to changes in patient status.

Chemical Structure

Chemical structures of the commonly used halogenated inhalant anesthetics are shown in Figure 10.1. In general, the presence of fluorine decreases flammability and increases molecular stability. Halothane is classified as a halogenated alkane derivative. In the ether group, isoflurane is classified as a halogenated methyl ether, desflurane is a fluorinated methyl ethyl ether, and sevoflurane is a fluorinated methyl isopropyl ether. The chemical structure of the gas N_2O is also given.

Physical and Chemical Properties of Inhalant Anesthetics

Several physical and chemical properties of inhalant anesthetics are summarized in Table 10.1.

Boiling point – The volatile anesthetic agents halothane, isoflurane and sevoflurane exist as liquids at room temperature. Desflurane has a relatively low boiling point compared to the other volatile agents, and it requires a different type of vaporizer that is pressurized to prevent it from boiling at typical working temperatures. N_2O exists as a gas at

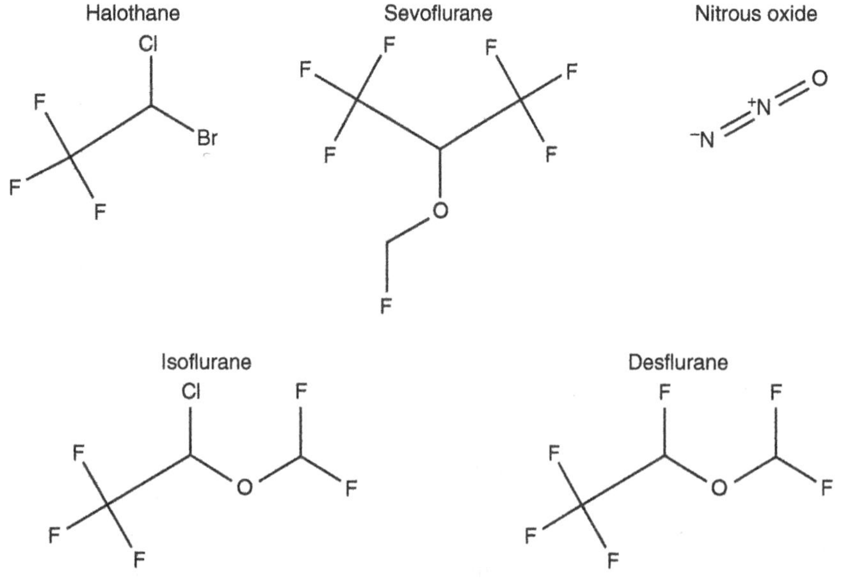

Figure 10.1 Chemical structures of inhalant anesthetics. Chemical structures of the gas N_2O and the volatile anesthetics halothane, isoflurane, sevoflurane and desflurane. *Source:* Redrawn from images downloaded from National Center for Biotechnology Information (2023). PubChem Compound Summary for CID 948, Nitrous Oxide. Retrieved August 1, 2023 from https://pubchem.ncbi.nlm.nih.gov/compound/Nitrous-Oxide. PubChem Compound Summary for CID 3562, Halothane. Retrieved August 1, 2023 from https://pubchem.ncbi.nlm.nih.gov/compound/Halothane. PubChem Compound Summary for CID 3763, Isoflurane. Retrieved August 1, 2023 from https://pubchem.ncbi.nlm.nih.gov/compound/Isoflurane. PubChem Compound Summary for CID 5206, Sevoflurane. Retrieved August 1, 2023 from https://pubchem.ncbi.nlm.nih.gov/compound/Sevoflurane. PubChem Compound Summary for CID 42113, Desflurane. Retrieved August 1, 2023 from https://pubchem.ncbi.nlm.nih.gov/compound/Desflurane.

Table 10.1 Selected physicochemical properties of halothane, isoflurane, sevoflurane, desflurane, and nitrous oxide.

	Halothane	Isoflurane	Sevoflurane	Desflurane	Nitrous oxide
Molecular weight (g/mol)	197	185	200	168	44
Boiling point (°C)	50	49	59	23	−89
Vapor pressure at 20 °C (mmHg)	244	240	170	669	Exists as a gas
mL vapor per mL liquid at 20 °C	227	195	183	210	N/A

N/A, not applicable.

room temperature and is therefore supplied in pressurized gas cylinders.

Vapor pressure – The term 'vapor' is used to describe the gas phase of a compound that is liquid at standard temperature (20 °C) and pressure (1 atm or 760 mmHg). Within a closed container, i.e. the bottle the manufacturer supplies the inhalant in, or the vaporization chamber of an anesthetic vaporizer, and at a constant temperature, an equilibrium will be reached between the molecules in the gas phase (i.e. above the liquid) and the liquid phase. This equilibrium is termed the saturated vapor pressure, commonly referred to as the vapor pressure. Vapor pressure can be used to determine the maximum concentration that can be reached for the given compound. For example, the vapor pressure of isoflurane is 240 mmHg.

The maximum concentration of isoflurane vapor in a closed space under standard conditions is therefore 240/760 mmHg, or 31.5%. This is far in excess of concentrations required to produce clinical anesthesia, hence the necessity to use precision vaporizers that allow delivery of lower concentrations, typically up to 5% for isoflurane. As each volatile anesthetic has its own specific vapor pressure, each agent requires a specific vaporizer calibrated for that specific agent. The vapor pressures of halothane and isoflurane are relatively close to each other and halothane vaporizers have been modified and relabeled for isoflurane use. Using isoflurane in a halothane vaporizer without professional modification is not recommended, although isoflurane output was only increased by a factor of between 1.08 and 1.15 compared to the output of halothane at low carrier gas flow rates and was lower than halothane at high gas flow rates (Steffey et al. 1983).

Vapor pressure is affected by ambient temperature. As temperature rises, the number of molecules having enough energy to move from the liquid phase to the gas phase increases, and vapor pressure rises. The opposite is true as temperature decreases. Agent specific vaporizers incorporate mechanisms to account for changes in ambient temperature that are within typical working conditions.

During vaporization, it is the molecules with higher energy that leave the liquid phase. In doing so, the liquid becomes cooler. A significant amount of vaporization may cool the liquid enough to noticeably decrease vaporization. This is the case with desflurane, which requires use of a vaporizer that, in addition to being pressurized, is heated to overcome the evaporative cooling of the liquid that occurs due to vaporization.

Note that, since N_2O exists as a gas at ambient temperatures, its concentration can be 100% if it is inadvertently used as the sole carrier gas (see below for hazards of N_2O use).

Degradation – The halogenated agents are generally very stable, and do not require preservatives. The exception is halothane, which may undergo spontaneous degradation to bromine, hydrobromic acid, chloride, hydrochloric acid, and phosgene. Halothane is therefore stored in opaque, amber-colored bottles and contains the preservative thymol to prevent this. Thymol accumulates in vaporizers, which can make vaporizer output inaccurate and also interfere with movement of the dial. Thymol accumulation can be decreased by draining vaporizers of halothane weekly and by maintaining regular servicing of vaporizers (Rosenberg and Alila 1984).

Stability in soda lime – Sevoflurane undergoes degradation to several compounds (compound A through compound E) (Wallin et al. 1975). Compound A – fluoromethy 1-2,2-difluoro-L-(trifluoromethyl) vinyl ether – is nephrotoxic to rats when administered via inhalation or peritoneal injection and occurs via metabolism to nephrotoxic haloalkenes (Kharasch et al. 2005). Levels of compound A present in the breathing circuit during sevoflurane anesthesia in studies in people (O'Keeffe and Healy 1999) and dogs (Muir and Gadawski 1998) were found to be below toxic levels, even when relatively low flow rates of oxygen were used. In a study where pigs were anesthetized with sevoflurane and dessicated Baralyme® was used as the carbon dioxide absorbent, compound A rose to levels that would be considered toxic in people and rats, yet produced minimal renal injury based on kidney histology after two to four hours of anesthesia (Steffey et al. 1997). Rats appear to be unique in their susceptibility to compound A; nephrotoxicity due to compound A anesthesia has not been definitively reported in other animal species.

Carbon monoxide production can occur when desflurane or isoflurane passes through dry absorbent that contains potassium or sodium hydroxide. The most likely clinical scenario for this to occur is when dry fresh gases are inadvertently left turned on, and flow though the absorbent for long periods of time (e.g. over a weekend when anesthesia machines are less likely to be in use) (Pearson et al. 2001). In horses, carbon monoxide increased with both halothane and isoflurane within the anesthetic circle breathing system, however levels were not clinically significant (Dodam et al. 1999). In a study in pigs, desflurane and isoflurane delivered via a circle system with purposely dried soda lime resulted in carbon monoxide levels of 5500 ppm (desflurane) and 800 ppm (isoflurane), despite using low-flow of carrier gases. Arterial carboxyhemoglobin was markedly elevated, with pigs of smaller size having higher concentrations (Bonome et al. 1999).

Mechanism of Action

Despite being discovered in the 1840s, and having been the subject of much research, the mechanism, or mechanisms, of action as to exactly how the inhalant anesthetics produce unconsciousness and immobility have not been fully elucidated. In terms of the general site of action, it has been demonstrated in a preferentially anesthetized goat brain model that immobility in response to painful stimuli is primarily mediated in the spinal cord, with unconsciousness being mediated in the brain (Antognini and Schwartz 1993). Traditional theories (the Meyer-Overton theory/critical volume hypothesis) hypothesized that all inhalant anesthetics work by the same mechanism. The proposed non-specific action on hydrophobic lipid components of cells, given the presence of sufficient molecules at the cell membrane, is that distortion of the cell membrane would occur, and alter cellular function. With the advent in the 1960s of the concept of MAC, the observed linear relationship between the MAC and oil:gas partition coefficients of the inhalants and their oil:gas partition coefficients (Tables 10.2 and 10.3) favored the theory of a lipid-based mechanism of action common to all inhalant anesthetics. Evidence against this theory includes the fact that effects of inhalants on the lipid bilayer of the cell membrane are small, and unlikely to result in interference with production of action potentials by cells (Franks and Lieb 1994). Additionally, inhalant anesthetics exist as stereoisomers, and potency of the enantiomers has been shown to be different, despite the fact that their lipid solubility is the same (Lysko et al. 1994). In the past several decades, researchers have generally moved away from the idea that multiple agents with diverse chemical structures share a non-specific, lipid-based cellular mechanism, and have focused

Table 10.2 Selected partition coefficients for inhaled anesthetics in people.

Partition coefficient	Halothane	Isoflurane	Sevoflurane	Desflurane	Nitrous oxide
Blood:gas	2.54	1.46	0.69	0.42	0.46
Brain:blood	1.9	1.46	1.7	1.3	1.1
Muscle:blood	3.4	2.9	3.1	2.0	1.2
Fat:blood	51.1	44.9	47.5	27.2	2.3
Oil:gas	224	98	55	18.7	1.4

on anesthetic-binding sites on specific receptor or ion channel proteins, as well as the likelihood that different aspects of anesthesia may be mediated by different mechanisms (Campagna et al. 2003).

In simple terms, neurotransmission can be decreased either by increasing inhibitory mediators or decreasing excitatory mediators. The impact of inhalant anesthetics on several receptors that affect neurotransmission has been studied.

Enhancement of receptors that mediate inhibition of neurotransmission – GABA and glycine are the most common inhibitory neurotransmitters in the brain and spinal cord respectively. Halogenated anesthetics have been shown to enhance the G-protein coupled $GABA_A$ and glycine receptors, leading to an increase in inhibition of neurotransmission. In contrast, N_2O has no effect on these receptors (Harrison et al. 1993; Mascia et al. 1996).

Reduction of excitatory neurotransmission – Glutamate is the most common excitatory neurotransmitter in the CNS. The ligand-gated glutamate receptors NMDA, AMPA, and kainite are all inhibited by the halogenated anesthetics, thus reducing excitatory neurotransmission. N_2O inhibits NMDA receptors, but not AMPA or kainite (Yamakura and Harris 2000; Kendig 2002). Inhalant anesthetics also inhibit some subtypes of voltage-gated Na^+ channels, decreasing release of glutamate (Shiraishi and Harris 2004).

Inhibition of neuronal nicotinic acetylcholine receptors by inhalant anesthetics is thought to contribute to amnesia and memory changes in people but does not result in immobility (Violet et al. 1997; Flood et al. 1997).

Two-pore-domain potassium (K_{2P}) receptors/ion channels regulate resting potential of the cell. Some of the K_{2P} channels within this group are potentiated by inhalant anesthetics, including the TASK-3 receptor associated with regulating natural sleep (Franks 2006; Pang et al. 2009).

Solubility

Inhalant anesthetic solubility has been thoroughly examined, and solubilities for the inhalants are typically expressed as partition coefficients (see Table 10.2, adapted from Steffey et al. 2015 and Flood 2022). Partition coefficients represent the ratio of the concentration at equilibrium in the two substances being compared. If the partition coefficient is 1, then the anesthetic is equally soluble in both substances. If the partition coefficient is 2, then the anesthetic is twice as soluble in the first substance, and if the partition coefficient is 0.5, then the anesthetic is twice as soluble in the second substance. As a general rule, the partition coefficients for all comparative pairings decrease in the following order: halothane > isoflurane > sevoflurane > desflurane > N_2O. Partition coefficients differ among different species, and have been reported in cats, dogs, ruminants, horses, rats and rabbits, with goats having values most similar to those reported in people (Soares et al. 2012). Species differences in hemoglobin, red blood cell membrane structure, albumin structure, and concentration of plasma triglycerides are possible causes for these differences.

Potency

The concept of minimal alveolar concentration (MAC) has been used to assess and compare the potency of inhalant anesthetics since its introduction in the 1960s. MAC is defined as the minimum alveolar anesthetic concentration at which 50% of subjects respond to a supramaximal noxious stimulus (Merkel and Eger 1963). MAC studies are performed with no other drugs present, so the MAC of an inhalant is therefore equivalent to a 50% effective dose (ED_{50}). ED_{95} is approximately 1.3 x MAC. MAC has been determined in many species (Steffey et al. 2015). Ranges of MAC values reported for the commonly anesthetized domestic species are given in Table 10.3. In general, MAC for a specific inhalant, with the exception of N_2O in people, is similar regardless of species. Differences in reported MAC values for a given inhalant in the same species are likely due to differences in methodology and the small numbers of animals used in each study given that, within a species, individual MAC can vary. MAC is additive, i.e. delivering 0.5 MAC of isoflurane and 0.5 MAC of sevoflurane is equivalent to delivering 1 MAC of either agent. This concept is used to extrapolate the MAC of N_2O.

Table 10.3 Range of MAC values (%) reported in the commonly anesthetized domestic species for halothane, isoflurane, sevoflurane, desflurane and nitrous oxide.

Species	Halothane	Isoflurane	Sevoflurane	Desflurane	Nitrous oxide
Dog	0.86–0.93[1,2]	0.9–1.5[3,4]	2.10–2.36[5,6]	7.2–10.3[7,8]	188–297[9,10]
Cat	0.99–1.19[11,12]	1.28–2.21[13,14]	2.58–3.41[15,16]	9.79–10.27[17,16]	255[18]
Horse	0.88–1.05[19,20]	1.31–1.64[19,21]	2.31–2.84[22,23]	7.02–8.02[24,25]	205[26]
Cattle	0.76[27]	1.14[28]	2.12[29]	–	223[27]
Sheep	0.97[30]	1.58[30]	2.74[31]	8.60–9.81[32,33]	–
Goat	1.30[34]	1.20–1.50[35,34]	2.33[36]	–	–
Pig	0.9–1.25[37,38]	1.45–2.04[39,40]	1.97–2.66[37,41]	10.00[40]	162–277[42,38]

[1] Eger et al. (1965b).
[2] Himes (1977)
[3] Johnson et al. (2019).
[4] Schwartz et al. (1989).
[5] Scheller et al. (1990).
[6] Kazama and Ikeda (1988).
[7] Doorley (1988).
[8] Hammond et al. (1994).
[9] Eger et al. (1965a).
[10] Young and Sawyer (1980).
[11] Webb and McMurphy (1987).
[12] Drummond et al. (1983).
[13] Ilkiw et al. (1997).
[14] Pypendop and Ilkiw (2005).
[15] Doi et al. (1998).
[16] Barter et al. (2004).
[17] McMurphy and Hodgson (1995).
[18] Steffey et al. (1974).
[19] Steffey et al. (1977).
[20] Bennett et al. (2004).
[21] Steffey et al. (2000).
[22] Aida et al. (1994).
[23] Steffey et al. (2005a).
[24] Tendillo et al. (1997).
[25] Steffey et al. (2005b).
[26] Steffey and Howland (1978b).
[27] Steffey and Howland (1979).
[28] Cantalapiedra et al. (2000).
[29] Araújo et al. (2017).
[30] Palahniuk et al. (1974).
[31] Columbano et al. (2018b).
[32] Sayre et al. (2015).
[33] Columbano et al. (2018a).
[34] Antognini and Eisele (1993).
[35] Antognini and Schwartz (1993).
[36] Hikasa et al. (1998).
[37] Lerman et al. (1990).
[38] Weiskopf and Bogetz (1984).
[39] Lundeen et al. (1983).
[40] Eger et al. (1988).
[41] Manohar and Parks (1984).
[42] Eisele et al. (1985).

The concept of MAC is used to determine derivatives of MAC with different end-points, for example, MAC-awake (the point at which a person responds to a verbal command) which is about 0.5 x MAC in people (Flood 2022). The MAC derivatives MAC-no movement (MAC-NM) and MAC-blunt adrenergic response (MAC-BAR) are useful in that they mimic the desired clinical result of inhalant anesthesia, i.e. a patient that does not move and has minimal autonomic response in response to a procedure. MAC-NM and MAC-BAR, in addition to MAC-extubation (MAC-EXT) have been evaluated in dogs anesthetized with isoflurane, and sevoflurane (Seddighi et al. 2023; Murahata et al. 2018; Ebner et al. 2013). MAC-EXT has also been evaluated for desflurane in dogs (Lopez et al. 2009). MAC-BAR has been determined in cats for halothane and isoflurane, and in sheep for sevoflurane (Schmeling et al. 1999; March and Muir 2023; Barletta et al. 2020). MAC-NM has been investigated in sevoflurane-anesthetized ponies receiving morphine and dexmedetomidine infusions (Gozalo-Marcilla et al. 2014). MAC-BAR is typically 20–40% higher than the MAC of a given inhalant, with marked variation among individuals, and MAC-NM is in the range of 10–20% higher than MAC. MAC-EXT in dogs occurs at 0.3–0.4 x MAC (Reed and Doherty 2018).

Due to MAC being determined in the absence of other drugs, MAC studies can be performed to determine the impact of drugs and physiologic conditions on inhalant requirement. Physiologic factors and pharmacologic agents which influence MAC are generally consistent regardless of species (Table 10.4). An exception is opioids in horses. Morphine given at 0.25 and 2 mg/kg IV increased MAC of isoflurane by 5% and 11% respectively, which was attributed to central nervous system (CNS) stimulation (Steffey et al. 2003). Within that study, the effect on MAC was inconsistent; MAC increased in three horses, decreased in one horse, and was unchanged in two horses given the

higher dose of morphine. In another study from the same research group, using the same conditions and methodology to determine MAC, morphine was given to halothane-anesthetized horses at 0.1 and 0.2 mg/kg IV immediately after xylazine at 0.5 mg/kg IV. Neither dose of morphine impacted MAC compared to xylazine alone, which decreased MAC by approximately 20% (Bennett et al. 2004). In contrast, isoflurane MAC was reduced by 49% when horses received a co-infusion of lidocaine and ketamine, and by 53% when morphine was added to the co-infusion at 0.1 mg/kg/h following a 0.15 mg/kg bolus (Villalba et al. 2011).

Pharmacokinetics

Inhalant anesthetic agents are administered via the lungs where they diffuse across a series of concentration gradients from the anesthetic vaporizer to the tissues. In the lung, inhalant anesthetics diffuse from the alveoli into pulmonary capillaries, and arterial blood then transports the anesthetic to the central nervous system (CNS) and other tissues, with the goal being to maintain a partial pressure in the CNS that maintains an adequate depth of anesthesia for the procedure the patient is undergoing. On cessation of administration of inhalant from the anesthetic machine, the process is reversed. Elimination occurs primarily via the lungs, although some agents do undergo metabolic biotransformation. The key partial pressure of an inhalant anesthetic is that in the alveoli (P_A). The brain

Table 10.4 Factors that influence MAC.

	Increases MAC	Decreases MAC	No effect on MAC
Patient		Increasing age Pregnancy	Gender
Physiologic	Hyperthermia Hypernatremia	Hypothermia Hyponatremia MAP <50 mmHg PaO_2 < 40 mmHg	Anesthetic metabolism Hyper- or hypokalemia MAP >50 mmHg PaO_2 > 40 mmHg $PaCO_2$ 15–95 mmHg
Pharmacologic	Ephedrine Morphine in horses Physostigmine	Acepromazine Alpha$_2$ agonists Opioids Benzodiazepines Ketamine Lidocaine Nitrous oxide Maropitant Gabapentin	Anticholinergics
Other			Duration of anesthesia

The impact of patient and physiologic factors, and pharmacologic drug classes on MAC.
MAP, mean arterial blood pressure; PaO_2, arterial partial pressure of oxygen; $PaCO_2$, arterial partial pressure of carbon dioxide.

is part of the vessel-rich group of organs, and the partial pressure at the brain rapidly equilibrates with the P_A. At steady state, the partial pressure at the brain (and other tissues) is in equilibrium with the P_A of the anesthetic, which can be measured in clinical practice using a gas analyzer. The partial pressure of an anesthetic gas is related to concentration (expressed in % volume) as follows: concentration = partial pressure / ambient pressure, where, for practical purposes, ambient pressure is considered to be 760 mmHg.

Anesthetic uptake – Several factors determine the P_A of inhalant anesthetics and fall into two main categories: increased delivery of anesthetic vapor to the alveoli, and decreased removal of anesthetic from the alveoli.

Increased delivery of anesthetic to the lungs can be achieved by increasing the inspired concentration, and by increasing alveolar ventilation. The inspired concentration is affected by the percentage selected on the vaporizer, the volume of the anesthetic breathing system, and the materials the breathing system and machine are made of, as the inhalants are soluble in rubber and plastic to some degree. Breathing system type is important – a non-rebreathing system has a relatively small total volume and delivers almost entirely fresh gases to the patient during inspiration, therefore, the concentration dialed on the vaporizer will be very close to the inspired concentration. Contrast this with a rebreathing system, which has a much larger volume, where oxygen (and other carrier gases) and inhalant anesthetics from expired gas are recirculated. Fresh gas flow rates at the start of inhalant anesthesia are considerably higher than those required for maintenance when using rebreathing systems. This ensures that the volume of gas in the anesthetic breathing system, which contains no inhalant at the start of anesthesia, is rapidly exchanged with gas that contains inhalant anesthetic in order for a rapid rise in the P_A to occur. The higher the inspired partial pressure, the faster the rate of rise of the P_A. This is known as the concentration effect (Eger 1963). This is demonstrated in Figure 10.2, where the rate of rise of N_2O in the alveoli is more rapid compared to desflurane. While desflurane has a lower blood:gas partition coefficient than desflurane, N_2O is delivered at much higher concentrations (up to 70% of the total carrier gas).

Increasing alveolar ventilation increases delivery of inhalant to the lungs leading to a rise in P_A. Conversely, decreases in alveolar ventilation will slow the rate of rise. Use of a mechanical ventilator typically increases alveolar ventilation, and therefore P_A. Hypoventilation is common following intravenous anesthetic induction, and as anesthetic depth increases.

Uptake of anesthetic vapor from the lungs in pulmonary arterial blood is determined by solubility of the anesthetic,

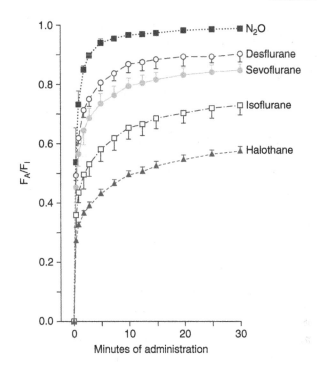

Figure 10.2 Time course of the rate of rise of inhalant anesthetics in the alveoli toward inspired concentration (F_A/F_I). The rate of rise of the alveolar concentration (F_A) toward the inspired concentration (F_I) expressed as the ratio F_A/F_I is determined by the solubility of the inhalant in blood, as well as the delivered concentration of the inhalant. *Source:* Redrawn from Yasuda et al. (1991).

cardiac output, and the difference between the P_A and the partial pressure in the pulmonary venous blood.

Inhalant anesthetics with low blood:gas solubility are associated with a more rapid equilibration in the tissues, as the low blood:gas solubility supports a rapid rate of rise of P_A, and therefore partial pressure in the CNS (Figure 10.2). Low blood:gas solubility is also advantageous during the maintenance phase of anesthesia as changes to inhaled partial pressures will be reflected quickly in the P_A, allowing for tighter control of anesthetic depth. When the administration of inhalant is terminated, anesthetic will be eliminated more quickly due to a rapid decrease in P_A compared to agents with higher blood:gas solubilities.

The rate of rise of the P_A of an inhalant increases as cardiac output decreases. Higher cardiac output removes inhalant from the lung faster, slows the rise of the P_A, and slows induction. Induction of anesthesia with inhalants in compromised patients, e.g. via nasotracheal intubation in foals, should therefore be done cautiously as the P_A can rise more rapidly than in healthy patients.

The alveolar-venous partial pressure difference is greatest when the anesthetic vaporizer is first turned on, as there is no inhalant in the blood. As inhalant anesthesia progresses, the difference will decrease due to the venous partial pressure rising. If, at any point, the venous partial pressure equals the P_A, then uptake will stop. The vessel-rich group of tissues, which includes the brain, receive the majority of cardiac output despite comprising approximately 10% of body mass. This tissue group therefore equilibrates more rapidly than the other tissue groups. The muscle group, which has an intermediate blood supply under anesthesia, receiving 10–15% of cardiac output, typically takes several hours to reach equilibrium. Fat receives a very small proportion of cardiac output, and inhalants are very soluble in this tissue, therefore it takes even longer for this vessel-poor tissue to equilibrate, and is unlikely to occur in clinical patients, even those anesthetized for more than a few hours.

Elimination – The inhalants are unique drugs in that they are largely eliminated via the lungs. Similar to the factors that determine anesthetic uptake, elimination is essentially the same process in reverse. Clearance of (and recovery from) inhalant anesthetic is directly proportional to alveolar ventilation, and inversely proportional to cardiac output and the blood:gas solubility. If the patient remains connected to the anesthetic breathing system clearance, as with uptake, may take longer. This can be overcome by increasing the oxygen flow rate to assist with wash out of the inhalant from the breathing system. Duration of anesthesia can impact elimination, as it may take longer to eliminate inhalant from adipose tissue (Eger and Saidman 2005). In the initial period of recovery, the arterial partial pressure will be higher than that in the muscle and fat groups, and they may take up additional anesthetic for a short time. This may be more noticeable during recovery from halothane and isoflurane anesthesia. The impact on recovery time from sevoflurane and desflurane, which have much lower blood:gas solubilities, has minimal clinical impact.

Context-sensitive half-time – The impact of anesthetic duration on the time it takes to make changes to the partial pressure of inhalant in the vessel-rich group can be modeled using computer simulation (Eger and Shafer 2005). In essence, the longer the duration of anesthesia, and the larger the decrease desired in partial pressure at the vessel-rich group, the longer it will take to reach the new concentration. Blood:gas solubility is an important factor; the longer the duration of anesthetic administration, the longer it will take for an anesthetic gas like isoflurane, with a higher blood:gas solubility, to reach target partial pressures compared to a gas like desflurane, which has the lowest blood:gas solubility. This type of modeling can be used to predict when a patient will wake up from inhalant anesthesia. At the time of writing, and to the best of the authors'

knowledge, modeling of this kind has not been investigated in animals.

Metabolism – While the majority of inhalant anesthetic delivered during anesthesia is removed via the lungs, tissue metabolism of halogenated inhalants does occur. Tissue metabolism of inhalants has mostly been studied in people. The liver is the main site of metabolism where inhalants initially undergo oxidation and/or hydrolysis via cytochrome P450 enzymes prior to conjugation. (Martin 2010) Metabolites are excreted in bile or urine. Halothane undergoes the most extensive metabolism (up to 46%) (Carpenter et al. 1986), followed by sevoflurane (up to 5%) (Holaday and Smith 1981), isoflurane (0.2%) (Holaday et al. 1975), and desflurane (0.02%) (Sutton et al. 1991). N_2O has not been shown to undergo tissue metabolism.

Pharmacodynamics of the Volatile Anesthetics

Central nervous system – Effects on cerebral metabolic rate – Volatile anesthetics cause a dose-dependent decrease in cerebral metabolic rate of oxygen consumption ($CMRO_2$) (Madsen et al. 1987; Scheller et al., 1988; Young 1992). Halothane has been shown to decrease $CMRO_2$ less when compared to isoflurane (Drummond et al. 1986; Todd and Drummond 1984) Isoflurane causes a marked decrease in $CMRO_2$ in dogs at 0.4 MAC (Eger 1981).

Effect on cranial blood flow and cerebral perfusion pressure – Inhalants cause a dose-dependent decrease in cerebrovascular resistance, resulting in increased CBF, although this may be somewhat counteracted as $CMRO_2$ is decreased. This increase in CBF results in an increase in the volume of blood within the cranium and, as a result, intracranial pressure (ICP) increases. Of the inhalants, halothane causes the greatest increase in CBF, likely as a result of its lesser impact on decreasing $CMRO_2$. Cerebral perfusion pressure (CPP) is defined as being equal to mean arterial blood pressure (MAP) minus ICP. Since inhalants decrease MAP in a dose-dependent fashion, and tend to increase ICP, CPP is generally decreased by inhalant anesthetics. Under normal physiologic conditions, i.e. in conscious patients, cerebrovascular autoregulation maintains a stable CBF despite changes in CPP, which can occur due to e.g. exercise or changes in ICP. This is achieved by either dilation or constriction of cerebral blood vessels. Inhalant anesthetics interfere with this mechanism as dose increases, and at 1.5 x MAC autoregulation is absent (Strebel et al. 1995).

Effect on intracranial pressure – Inhalant anesthesia decreases ventilation in a dose-dependent manner, resulting in hypercarbia, which causes vasodilation, thus contributing to increased ICP. This can effectively be counteracted by instituting hyperventilation to mild hypocapnia in small animals. In horses, however, ICP increased under isoflurane anesthesia and, despite initially being lower in ventilated horses, over time was not different regardless of mode of ventilation (Brosnan et al. 2003, Brosnan et al. 2008).

Effects on brain activity – The electroencephalogram (EEG) in conscious people is characterized by low-amplitude, high-frequency waves. Inhalant effects on the EEG in animals vary depending on the inhalant used, by species, and among individuals within a species. In people and dogs, the EEG progressively changes under isoflurane anesthesia as the delivered anesthetic concentration rises, with an initial increase in frequency, followed by a decrease in frequency. As concentration increases further (around 1.5 x MAC), a pattern of burst suppression is observed, where the waveform shows intermittent isoelectric periods. A completely isoelectric EEG ("flat line") is indicative of deep anesthesia. In another study in dogs, burst suppression with isoflurane and sevoflurane occurred at 2.17 x MAC and 2.14 x MAC respectively (Scheller et al. 1990). Increasing isoflurane concentration resulted in depressed activity on the EEG in cats, however, activity was variable in individuals, with burst suppression sometimes occurring at concentrations below MAC, and isoelectric EEG patterns seen in some cats at clinically relevant concentrations (1.8–2.5%) (March et al. 2003). In horses anesthetized with halothane or isoflurane, a high amount of individual variability can occur, burst suppression did not occur with halothane, and the presence of epileptiform-like discharges was noted with both inhalants (Williams et al. 2016).

Ocular effects – Intraocular pressure (IOP) can increase during inhalant anesthesia. This is not a direct effect on the eye; inhalants dose-dependently decrease ventilation, and the rise in the partial pressure of arterial carbon dioxide ($PaCO_2$) seen in spontaneously breathing animals can increase IOP (Duncalf and Weitzner 1963). Tear production is decreased during inhalant anesthesia, and in some, but not all, studies, lasted up to 24 hours after the anesthetic event (Herring et al. 2000; Shepard et al. 2011).

Cardiovascular system – Effects on cardiac output, heart rate and arterial blood pressure – Cardiac output (CO) can be decreased in a dose-dependent fashion by inhalant anesthetics due to a reduction in stroke volume (SV), although if there is a simultaneous decrease in systemic vascular resistance (SVR) then CO may be less affected (Klide 1976; Steffey and Howland 1978a; Merin et al. 1991). Of the four volatile inhalants discussed, halothane causes the greatest decrease in CO.

Heart rate tends to increase when an inhalant is the sole anesthetic agent compared to pre-anesthetic values in dogs (Pagel et al. 1991; Mutoh et al. 1997).

Arterial blood pressure decreases in a dose-dependent fashion. This is largely due to decreases in CO that result

from decreased SV but can also be due to decreased SVR as a result of vasodilation.

Halothane sensitizes the myocardium to epinephrine-induced ventricular arrhythmias. In contrast, the other volatile inhalants are much less arrhythmogenic (Joas and Stevens 1971; Weiskopf et al. 1989; Hikasa et al. 1996).

Respiratory system – As with most inhalant effects, ventilation is depressed in a dose-dependent manner. In spontaneously breathing animals, as the percentage inhalant delivered increases, tidal volume decreases. At the same time, respiration rate may increase, although this does not compensate enough to maintain normocapnia. If the percentage of inhalant delivered is further increased, respiratory arrest occurs. The point at which respiratory arrest occurs can be expressed as the apneic index (% inhalant where apnea occurs/MAC). The apneic index varies among species and inhalants (Table 10.5); (Steffey et al. 1977; Galloway et al. 2004; Regan and Eger 1967; Steffey and Howland 1977).

Hepatic effects – Since inhalant anesthetics decrease cardiac output, liver blood flow is also decreased. This can result in decreased clearance of drugs, and hepatic enzymes may increase after anesthesia. For example, clearance of lidocaine in anesthetized horses is decreased by approximately 50% compared to conscious horses (Feary et al. 2005). In cases of severe hypotension leading to decreased oxygen delivery to hepatocytes, necrosis can occur. Of the volatile agents discussed here, halothane has been associated with liver toxicity in animals (O'Brien et al. 1986; Gaunt et al. 1984).

Renal effects – Similar to the liver, reductions in cardiac output during inhalant anesthesia may decrease renal blood flow, glomerular filtration rate and urine production. Sevoflurane biotransformation in the kidneys can result in an increase in serum inorganic fluoride, however, this does not appear to lead to nephrotoxicity (Driessen et al. 2002).

Effect on insulin – Inhalant anesthetics have been shown to decrease insulin secretion in people and rabbits (Tanaka et al. 2005; Tanaka et al. 2009).

Musculoskeletal effects – Generally, inhalant anesthetics produce skeletal muscle relaxation. They have been shown to potentiate neuromuscular blockade (Nagahama et al. 2006). In susceptible individuals, inhalant anesthetics can trigger malignant hypothermia (MH), with halothane having a greater likelihood of doing so than the other inhalants discussed here. In veterinary medicine, MH is seen most commonly in pigs, but suspected cases of MH have been reported in other species (Brunson and Hogan 2004; Thomson et al. 2014; Hall et al. 1972; Aleman et al. 2005).

Pharmacodynamic considerations for clinical use of inhalants – Up to this point in the chapter, the pharmacodynamics of inhalants when used as sole anesthetic agents

Table 10.5 Apneic index in cats, dogs and pigs.

	Halothane	Isoflurane	Sevoflurane	Desflurane
Dog	2.9	2.5	3.5	2.4
Cat		2.4		
Horse	2.6	2.3		
Pig				1.6

Apneic index in commonly anesthetized domestic animals. Apneic index = % inhalant at which apnea occurs/MAC of the inhalant.

have been considered. In clinical veterinary anesthetic practice, it is rarely the case that inhalants are used alone. Sedatives, analgesics, injectable anesthetics and other adjuncts to anesthesia and analgesia are frequently used as part of anesthetic protocols, which often results in decreased concentrations of inhalant being required, referred to as MAC sparing. MAC sparing can result in decreased effects of the inhalant, as their effects are dose dependent, which can be beneficial (e.g. blood pressure effects may be lessened). Where a pharmacodynamic effect of a drug with MAC sparing properties is similar to that of inhalants, there may be no decrease in effect, or effects could be additive, e.g. hypotension with acepromazine, or decreased CO with alpha$_2$ agonists (Grasso et al. 2015).

The impact of mode of ventilation during inhalant anesthesia should also be factored in when considering the pharmacodynamic effects of inhalants. Inhalant anesthesia causes hypoventilation, which is characterized by increased PaCO$_2$. Elevated PaCO$_2$ can cause an increase in sympathetic tone, which could act to maintain higher blood pressure, although if PaCO$_2$ is above 95 mmHg, it causes CNS depression. In local tissue beds, elevated CO$_2$ causes vasodilation. Many anesthetized veterinary patients require ventilatory support and, in some species, this is routinely necessary (horses, ruminants). The main impact of controlled ventilation is to decrease CO, and therefore blood pressure, by reducing venous return as a result of positive intrathoracic pressure. Additionally, PaCO$_2$ will decrease, removing the effect on sympathetic tone.

Nitrous Oxide

N$_2$O differs from the volatile anesthetics in that it exists as a gas at 20 °C, therefore it does not need to be vaporized. N$_2$O is supplied in pressurized tanks and is administered as a percentage of fresh gas flow (FGF) to the anesthetic machine. As discussed earlier, N$_2$O has low potency as an inhaled anesthetic, and cannot produce general anesthesia on its own. It is used as a MAC sparing adjunct at concentrations no higher than 70% of the total FGF in order to

avoid delivering a gas mixture that could result in hypoxemia. N$_2$O has some unique pharmacokinetic and pharmacodynamic effects that impact its clinical use.

Second gas effect – When an anesthetic gas has significantly slower uptake than one of the carrier gases, a concentration effect occurs, known as the second gas effect. This is notable when N$_2$O, which has a very low blood:gas partition coefficient (0.46), is used with an inhalant like methoxyflurane, which has very slow uptake (blood: gas partition coefficient of 12). The first gas, N$_2$O, diffuses more rapidly into the bloodstream from the alveoli. The gases that are then drawn into the alveoli are in proportion to the original gases, and the P$_A$ of the second gas, methoxyflurane, (and oxygen) increases. Anesthetic gases with very low blood:gas solubility such as sevoflurane and desflurane render the second gas effect clinically insignificant.

Closed gas spaces – Any closed gas space in the body that contains air, 80% of which is nitrogen (N$_2$) will increase in size and/or pressure when N$_2$O is administered. N$_2$O is carried to the closed air space and diffuses from a region of high to a region of low partial pressure (i.e. from outside the closed air space to inside it). N$_2$ is transferred out of that space more slowly than N$_2$O enters as N$_2$ is much less soluble in blood than N$_2$O (blood:gas partition coefficients at 37°C for N$_2$O and N$_2$ 0.47 and 0.015 respectively). The increase in volume and/or pressure of the air space will increase with N$_2$O concentration and duration of exposure, and can have serious consequences, e.g. rapid expansion in the size of a pneumothorax.

For that reason, N$_2$O is contraindicated for use in patients with closed gas spaces in the body, e.g. pneumothorax, gastric dilation/volvulus, gas-filled intestines. Endotracheal tube cuffs inflated with air will also increase in volume and pressure.

Diffusion hypoxia – N$_2$O has a very low blood:gas solubility, therefore at the end of an anesthetic episode where it has been in use, it diffuses very rapidly out of the body into the alveoli. If this occurs in a large enough volume, N$_2$O will displace other gases, including oxygen, in the lung. If the patient is breathing room air at this stage of recovery, displacement will lead to a drastic decrease in the alveolar partial pressure of oxygen and result in hypoxia. This phenomenon is known as diffusion hypoxia and can be avoided by leaving the patient connected to oxygen for the first 5–10 minutes of recovery (Sheffer et al. 1972).

Analgesia – N$_2$O has analgesic properties. The exact mechanism for analgesia has not been fully elucidated. There is evidence that N$_2$O acts as a partial inhibitor at the N-methyl-D-aspartate receptor, inhibits low-voltage calcium channels, and is a weak opioid agonist, all of which may contribute to its analgesic action (Kalmoe et al. 2020).

Cardiorespiratory effects – The impact of N$_2$O on cardiorespiratory function is low compared to the volatile inhalants. N$_2$O has a direct depressant effect on the myocardium, and a stimulating effect on the sympathetic nervous system (Fukunaga and Epstein 1973). Clinically, this may result in minimal change to, or an increase in, blood pressure. An increase in sympathetic tone could predispose to development of arrhythmias.

N$_2$O does not cause significant depression of ventilation. It should be used cautiously or not at all in patients with impaired oxygenation.

The Future of Inhalant Anesthetics

All volatile inhalants are greenhouse gases, as they persist in the atmosphere for several years, and in the case of desflurane, decades. European Union legislation proposes to ban or restrict desflurane use by 2026, so the future of this inhalant is uncertain (Hendrickx et al. 2022). While total injectable anesthesia has a lower calculated carbon footprint than inhalant anesthesia, it is likely that isoflurane and sevoflurane will remain the mainstay of general anesthesia for the foreseeable future (Sherman et al. 2012).

References

Aida, H., Mizuno, Y., Hobo, S. et al. (1994). Determination of the minimum alveolar concentration (MAC) and physical response to sevoflurane inhalation in horses. *J. Vet. Med. Sci.* 56 (6): 1161–1165.

Aleman, M., Brosnan, R.J., Williams, D.C. et al. (2005). Malignant hyperthermia in a horse anesthetized with halothane. *J. Vet. Intern. Med.* 19 (3): 363–366.

Antognini, J.F. and Eisele, P.H. (1993). Anesthetic potency and cardiopulmonary effects of enflurane, halothane, and isoflurane in goats. *Lab. Anim. Sci.* 43 (6): 607–610.

Antognini, J.F. and Schwartz, K. (1993). Hypothesis: inhaled anesthetics produce immobility and amnesia by different mechanisms at different sites. *Anesthesiol.* 79 (6): 1244–1249.

Araújo, M.A., Deschk, M., Wagatsuma, J.T. et al. (2017). Cardiopulmonary effects of reverse Trendelenburg position at 5° and 10° in sevoflurane-anesthetized steers. *Vet. Anaesth. Analg.* 44 (4): 854–864.

Barletta, M., Quandt, J.E., Reed, R.A. et al. (2020). Determination of the minimum alveolar concentration of sevoflurane that blunts adrenergic responses and the effect of a constant rate infusion of ketamine in sheep. *Res. Vet. Sci.* 128: 230–235.

Barter, L.S., Ilkiw, J.E., Steffey, E.P. et al. (2004). Animal dependence of inhaled anesthetic requirements in cats. *Br. J. Anaesth.* 92 (2): 275–277.

Bennett, R.C., Steffey, E.P., Kollias-Baker, C., and Sams, R. (2004). Influence of morphine sulfate on the halothane sparing effect of xylazine hydrochloride in horses. *Am. J. Vet. Res.* 65 (4): 519–526.

Bonome, C., Belda, J., Alvarez-Refojo, F. et al. (1999). Low-flow anesthesia and reduced animal size increase carboxyhemoglobin levels in swine during desflurane and isoflurane breakdown in dried soda lime. *Anesth. Analg.* 89 (4): 909–916.

Brosnan, R.J., Steffey, E.P., LeCouteur, R.A. et al. (2003). Effects of duration of isoflurane anesthesia and mode of ventilation on intracranial and cerebral perfusion pressures in horses. *Am. J. Vet. Res.* 64 (11): 1444–1448.

Brosnan, R.J., Esteller-Vico, A., Steffey, E.P. et al. (2008). Effects of head-down positioning on regional central nervous system perfusion in isoflurane-anesthetized horses. *Am. J. Vet. Res.* 69 (6): 737–743.

Brunson, D.B. and Hogan, K.J. (2004). Malignant hyperthermia: a syndrome not a disease. *Vet. Clin. North Am. Small Anim. Pract.* 34 (6): 1419–1433.

Campagna, J.A., Miller, K.W., and Forman, S.A. (2003). Mechanisms of actions of inhaled anesthetics. *N. Engl. J. Med.* 348: 2110–2124.

Cantalapiedra, A.G., Villanueva, B., and Pereira, J.L. (2000). Anaesthetic potency of isoflurane in cattle: determination of the minimum alveolar concentration. *Vet. Anaesth. Analg.* 27 (1): 22–26.

Carpenter, R.L., Eger, E.I. 2nd, Johnson, B.H. et al. (1986). The extent of metabolism of inhaled anesthetics in humans. *Anesthesiol.* 65: 201–205.

Columbano, N., Duffee, L.R., Melosu, V. et al. (2018a). Determination of minimum alveolar concentration and cardiovascular effects of desflurane in positive-pressure ventilated sheep. *Am. J. Vet. Res.* 79 (7): 727–732.

Columbano, N., Scanu, A., Duffee, L. et al. (2018b). Determination of the minimum alveolar concentration (MAC) and cardiopulmonary effects of sevoflurane in sheep. *Vet. Anaesth. Analg.* 45 (4): 487–495.

Dodam, J.R., Branson, K.R., Gross, M.E., and Petroski, G.F. (1999). Inhaled carbon monoxide concentration during halothane or isoflurane anesthesia in horses. *Vet. Surg.* 28 (6): 506–512.

Doi, M., Yunoki, H., and Ikeda, K. (1998). The minimum alveolar concentration of sevoflurane in cats. *J. Anesth.* 2 (1): 113-4.

Doorley, B.M. (1988). MAC of I-653 in beagle dogs and New Zealand white rabbits. *Anesthesiol.* 69 (1): 89–91.

Driessen, B., Zarucco, L., Steffey, E.P. et al. (2002). Serum fluoride concentrations, biochemical and histopathological changes associated with prolonged sevoflurane anaesthesia in horses. *Vet. Med. A Physiol. Pathol. Clin. Med.* 49 (7): 337–347.

Drummond, J.C., Todd, M.M., and Shapiro, H.M. (1983). Minimal alveolar concentrations for halothane, enflurane, and isoflurane in the cat. *J. Am. Vet. Med. Assoc.* 182 (10): 1099–1101.

Drummond, J.C., Todd, M.M., Scheller, M.S., and Shapiro, H.M. (1986). A comparison of the direct cerebral vasodilating potencies of halothane and isoflurane in the New Zealand white rabbit. *Anesthesiol.* 65: 462–467.

Duncalf, D. and Weitzner, S.W. (1963). The influence of ventilation and hypercapnea on intraocular pressure. *Anesth. Analg.* 42 (2): 232–237.

Ebner, S.E., Lerche, P., Bednarski R.M., and Hubbell J.A.E. (2013). Effect of dexmedetomidine, morphine-lidocaine-ketamine, and dexmedetomidine-morphine-lidocaine-ketamine constant rate infusions on the minimum alveolar concentration of isoflurane and bispectral index in dogs. *Am. J. Vet. Res.* 74: 963–970.

Eger, E. (1963). Effect of inspired anesthetic concentration on the rate of rise of alveolar concentration. *Anesthesiol.* 24: 153–157.

Eger, E. 2nd (1981). Isoflurane: a review. *Anesthesiol.* 55 (5): 559–576.

Eger, E.I. 2nd, Brandstater, B., Saidman, L.J. et al. (1965a). Equipotent alveolar concentrations of methoxyflurane, halothane, diethyl ether, fluroxene, cyclopropane, xenon and nitrous oxide in the dog. *Anesthesiol.* 26 (6): 771–777.

Eger, E.I. 2nd, Saidman, L.J., and Brandstater, B. (1965b). Temperature dependence of halothane and cyclopropane anesthesia in dogs: correlation with some theories of anesthetic action. *Anesthesiol.* 26 (6): 764–770.

Eger, E.I. 2nd, Johnson, B.H., Weiskopf, R.B. et al. (1988). Minimum alveolar concentration of I-653 and isoflurane in pigs: definition of a supramaximal stimulus. *Anesth. Analg.* 67 (12): 1174–1176.

Eger, E.I. and Saidman, L.J. (2005). Illustrations of inhaled anesthetic uptake, including intertissue diffusion to and from fat. *Anesth. Analg.* 100 (4): 1020–1033.

Eger, E.I. and Shafer, S.L. (2005). Tutorial: context-sensitive decrement times for inhaled anesthetics. *Anesth. Analg.* 101 (3): 688–696.

Eisele, P.H., Talken, L., and Eisele, J.H. Jr. (1985). Potency of isoflurane and nitrous oxide in conventional swine. *Lab. Anim. Sci.* 35 (1): 76–78.

Feary, D.J., Mama, K.R., Wagner, A.E., and Thomasy, S.M. (2005). Influence of general anesthesia on pharmacokinetics of intravenous lidocaine infusion in horses. *Am. J. Vet. Res.* 66 (4): 574–580.

Flood, P. (2022). Inhaled anesthetics. In: *Stoelting's Pharmacology & Physiology in Anesthetic Practice*, 6e (ed. P. Flood, J.P. Rathmell, and R.D. Urman), 95–149. Philadelphia, PA: Wolters Kluwer.

Flood, P., Ramirez-Latorre, J., and Role, L. (1997). Alpha 4 beta 2 neuronal nicotinic acetylcholine receptors in the central nervous system are inhibited by isoflurane and propofol, but alpha 7-type nicotinic acetylcholine receptors are unaffected. *Anesthesiol.* 86: 859–865.

Franks, N.P. (2006). Molecular targets underlying general anesthesia. *Br. J. Pharmacol.* 147: S72–S81.

Franks, N.P. and Lieb, W.R. (1994). Molecular and cellular mechanisms of general anesthesia. *Nature*, 367 (6464): 607–614.

Fukunaga, A.F. and Epstein, R.M. (1973). Sympathetic excitation during nitrous-oxide-halothane anesthesia in the cat. *Anesthesiol.* 39 (1): 23–36.

Galloway, D.S., Ko, J.C.H., Reaugh, H.F. et al. (2004). Anesthetic indices of sevoflurane and isoflurane in unpremedicated dogs. *J. Am. Vet. Med. Assoc.* 225 (5): 700–704.

Gaunt, P.S., Meuten, D.J., and Pecquet-Goad, M.E. (1984). Hepatic necrosis associated with use of halothane in a dog. *J. Am. Vet. Med. Assoc.* 184 (4): 478–480.

Gozalo-Marcilla, M., Hopster, K., Gasthuys, F. et al. (2014). Minimum end-tidal sevoflurane concentration necessary to prevent movement during a constant rate infusion of morphine, or morphine plus dexmedetomidine in ponies. *Vet. Anaesth. Analg.* 41 (2): 212–219.

Grasso, S.C., Ko, J.C., Weil, A.B. et al. (2015). Hemodynamic influence of acepromazine or dexmedetomidine premedication in isoflurane-anesthetized dogs. *J. Am. Vet. Med. Assoc.* 246 (7): 754–764.

Hall, L.W., Trim, C.M., and Woolf, N. (1972). Further studies of porcine malignant hyperthermia. *Br. Med. J.* 2 (5806): 145–148.

Hammond, R.A., Alibhai, H.I.K., Walsh, K.P. et al. (1994). Desflurane in the dog; minimum alveolar concentration (MAC) alone and in combination with nitrous oxide. *Vet. Anaesth. Analg.* 21 (1): 21–23.

Harrison, N.L., Kugler, J.L., Jones, M.V. et al. (1993). Positive modulation of human gamma-aminobutyric acid type A and glycine receptors by the inhalation anesthetic isoflurane. *Mol. Pharmacol.* 44 (3): 628–632.

Hendrickx, J.F.A., Nielsen, O.J., De Hert, S., and De Wolf, A.M. (2022). The science behind banning desflurane: a narrative review. *Eur. J. Anaesthesiol.* 39 (10): 818–824.

Herring, I.P., Pickett, J.P., Champagne, E.S., and Marini, M. (2000). Evaluation of aqueous tear production in dogs following general anesthesia. *J. Am. Anim. Hosp. Assoc.* 36 (5): 427–430.

Hikasa, Y., Okabe, C., Takase, K., and Ogasawara, S. (1996). Ventricular arrhythmogenic dose of adrenaline during sevoflurane, isoflurane, and halothane anesthesia either with or without ketamine or thiopentone in cats. *Res. Vet. Sci.* 60 (2): 134–137.

Hikasa, Y., Okuyama, K., Kakuta, T. et al. (1998). Anesthetic potency and cardiopulmonary effects of sevoflurane in goats: comparison with isoflurane and halothane. *Can. J. Vet. Res.* 62 (4): 299–306.

Himes, R.S. (1977). Effects of lidocaine on the anesthetic requirements for nitrous oxide and halothane. *Anesthesiol.* 47 (5): 437–440.

Holaday, D.A. and Smith, F.R. (1981). Clinical characteristics and biotransformation of sevoflurane in healthy human volunteers. *Anesthesiol.* 54: 100–106.

Holaday, D.A., Fiserova-Bergerova, V., Latto, I.P., and Zumbiel, M.A. (1975). Resistance of isoflurane to biotransformation in man. *Anesthesiol.* 43: 325–332.

Ilkiw, J.E., Pascoe, P.J., and Fisher, L.D. (1997). Effect of alfentanil on the minimum alveolar concentration of isoflurane in cats. *Am. J. Vet. Res.* 58 (11): 1274–1279.

Joas, T.A. and Stevens, W.C. (1971). Comparison of the arrhythmic doses of epinephrine during forane, halothane, and fluroxene anesthesia in dogs. *Anesthesiol.* 35 (1): 48–53.

Johnson, B.A., Aarnes, T.K., Wanstrath, A.W. et al. (2019). Effect of oral administration of gabapentin on the minimum alveolar concentration of isoflurane in dogs. *Am. J. Vet. Res.* 80 (11): 1007–1009.

Kalmoe, M.C., Janski, A.M., Zorumski, C.F. et al. (2020). Ketamine and nitrous oxide: the evolution of NMDA receptor antagonists as antidepressant agents. *J. Neurol. Sci.* 15 (412): 116778.

Kazama, T. and Ikeda, K. (1988). Comparison of MAC and the rate of rise of alveolar concentration of sevoflurane with halothane and isoflurane in the dog. *Anesthesiol.* 68 (3): 435–437.

Kendig, J.J. (2002). *In vitro* networks: subcortical mechanisms of anesthetic action. *Br. J. Anaesth.* 89: 91–101.

Kharasch, E.D., Schroeder, J.L., Sheffels, P., and Liggitt, H.D. (2005). Influence of sevoflurane on the metabolism and renal effects of compound A in rats. *Anesthesiol.* 103 (6): 1183–1188.

Klide, A.M. (1976). Cardiopulmonary effects of enflurane and isoflurane in the dog. *Am. J. Vet. Res.* 37 (2): 127–131.

Lerman, J., Oyston, J.P., Gallagher, T.M. et al. (1990). The minimum alveolar concentration (MAC) and hemodynamic effects of halothane, isoflurane, and sevoflurane in newborn swine. *Anesthesiol.* 73 (4): 717–721.

Lopez, L.A., Hofmeister, E.H., Pavez, J.C., and Brainard, B.M. (2009). Comparison of recovery from anesthesia with isoflurane, sevoflurane, or desflurane in healthy dogs. *Am. J. Vet. Res.* 70 (11): 1339–1344.

Lundeen, G., Manohar, M., and Parks, C. (1983). Systemic distribution of blood flow in swine while awake and during 1.0 and 1.5 MAC isoflurane anesthesia with or without 50% nitrous oxide. *Anesth. Analg.* 62 (5): 499–512.

Lysko, G.S., Robinson, J.L., Casto, R., and Ferrone, R.A. (1994). The stereospecific effects of isoflurane isomers *in vivo. Eur. J. Pharmacol.* 263 (1-2): 25–29.

Madsen, J.B., Cold, G.E., Hansen, E.S., and Bardrum, B. (1987). Cerebral blood flow, cerebral metabolic rate of oxygen and relative CO2-reactivity during craniotomy for supratentorial cerebral tumors in halothane anesthesia. A dose–response study. *Acta Anaesthesiol. Scand.* 31 (5): 454–457.

Manohar, M. and Parks, C.M. (1984). Porcine systemic and regional organ blood flow during 1.0 and 1.5 minimum alveolar concentrations of sevoflurane anesthesia without and with 50% nitrous oxide. *J. Pharmacol. Exp. Ther.* 231 (3): 640–648.

March, P.A. and Muir, W.W. 3rd (2003). Minimum alveolar concentration measures of central nervous system activation in cats anesthetized with isoflurane. *Am. J. Vet. Res.* 64 (12): 1528–1533.

March, P.A., Teixeira Neto, F.J., Monteiro, E.R. et al. (2003). Use of the bispectral index as a monitor of anesthetic depth in cats anesthetized with isoflurane. *Am. J. Vet. Res.* 64 (12): 1534–1541.

Martin, J.L. (2010). Inhaled anesthetics: metabolism and toxicity. In: *Miller's Anesthesia*, 7e (ed. R.D. Miller), 633–666. Philadelphia PA: Churchill Livingstone Elsevier.

Mascia, M.P., Machu, T.K., and Harris, R.A. (1996). Enhancement of homomeric glycine receptor function by long-chain alcohols and anesthetics. *Br. J. Pharmacol.* 119 (7): 1331–1336.

McMurphy, R.M. and Hodgson, D.S. (1995). The minimum alveolar concentration of desflurane in cats. *Vet. Surg.* 24 (5): 453–455.

Merin, R.G., Bernard, J.M., Doursout, M.F. et al. (1991). Comparison of the effects of isoflurane and desflurane on cardiovascular dynamics and regional blood flow in the chronically instrumented dog. *Anesthesiol.* 74 (3): 568–574.

Merkel, G. and Eger, E.I. 2nd (1963). A comparative study of halothane and halopropane anesthesia including method for determining equipotency. *Anesthesiol.* 24: 346–357.

Muir, W.W. and Gadawski, J. (1998). Cardiorespiratory effects of low-flow and closed circuit inhalation anesthesia, using sevoflurane delivered with an in-circuit vaporizer and concentrations of compound A. *Am. J. Vet. Res.* 59 (5): 603–608.

Murahata, Y., Hikasa, Y., Hayashi, S. et al. (2018). The effect of remifentanil on the minimum alveolar concentration (MAC) and MAC derivatives of sevoflurane in dogs. *J. Vet. Med. Sci.* 80 (7): 1086–1093.

Mutoh, T., Nishimura, R., Kim, H.Y. et al. (1997). Cardiopulmonary effects of sevoflurane, compared with halothane, enflurane, and isoflurane, in dogs. *Am. J. Vet. Res.* 58 (8): 885–890.

Nagahama, S., Nishimura, R., Mochizuki, M., and Sasaki, N. (2006). The effects of propofol, isoflurane and sevoflurane on vecuronium infusion rates for surgical muscle relaxation in dogs. *Vet. Anaesth. Analg.* 33 (3): 169–174.

O'Brien, T.D., Raffe, M.R., Cox, V.S. et al. (1986). Hepatic necrosis following halothane anesthesia in goats. *J. Am. Vet. Med. Assoc.* 189 (12): 1591–1595.

O'Keeffe, N.J. and Healy, T.E. (1999). The role of new anesthetic agents. *Pharmacol. Ther.* 84: 233–248.

Pagel, P.S., Kampine, J.P., Schmeling, W.T., and Warltier, D.C. (1991). Comparison of the systemic and coronary hemodynamic actions of desflurane, isoflurane, halothane, and enflurane in the chronically instrumented dog. *Anesthesiol.* 74 (3): 539–551.

Palahniuk, R.J., Shnider, S.M., and Eger, E.I. 2nd (1974). Pregnancy decreases the requirement for inhaled anesthetic agents. *Anesthesiol.* 41 (1): 82–83.

Pang, D.S., Robledo, C.J., Carr, D.R. et al. (2009). An unexpected role for TASK-3 potassium channels in network oscillations with implications for sleep mechanisms and anesthetic action. *PNAS* 106 (41): 17546–17551.

Pearson, M.L., Levine, W.C., Finton, R.J. et al. (2001). Anesthesia-associated carbon monoxide exposures among surgical patients. *Infect. Cont. Hosp. Epidemiol.* 22 (6): 352–356.

Pypendop, B.H. and Ilkiw, J.E. (2005). The effects of intravenous lidocaine administration on the minimum alveolar concentration of isoflurane in cats. *Anaesth. Anlag.* 100 (1): 97–101.

Reed, R. and Doherty, T. (2018). Minimum alveolar concentration: key concepts and a review of its pharmacological reduction in dogs. Part 1. *Res. Vet. Sci.* 117: 266–270.

Regan, M.J. and Eger, E.I. 2nd (1967). Effect of hypothermia in dogs on anesthetizing and apneic doses of inhalation agents. Determination of the anesthetic index (apnea/MAC). *Anesthesiol.* 28 (4): 689–700.

Rosenberg, P.H. and Alila, A. (1984). Accumulation of thymol in halothane vaporizers. *Anesthesia.* 39 (6): 581–583.

Sayre, R.S., Lepiz, M.A., Horsley, K.T. et al. (2015). Effects of oxymorphone hydrochloride or hydromorphone hydrochloride on minimal alveolar concentration of desflurane in sheep. *Am. J. Vet. Res.* 76 (7): 583–590.

Scheller, M.S., Tateishi, A., Drummond, J.C., and Zornow, M.H. (1988). The effects of sevoflurane on cerebral blood flow, cerebral metabolic rate for oxygen, intracranial pressure, and the electroencephalogram are similar to those of isoflurane in the rabbit. *Anesthesiol.* 68 (4): 548–551.

Scheller, M.S., Nakakimura, K., Fleischer, J.E., and Zornow, M.H. (1990). Cerebral effects of sevoflurane in the dog: comparison with isoflurane and enflurane. *Br. J. Anaesth.* 65 (3): 388–392.

Schmeling, W.T., Ganjoo, P., Staunton, M. et al. (1999). Pretreatment with dexmedetomidine: altered indices of anesthetic depth for halothane in the neuraxis of cats. *Anesth. Analg.* 88 (3): 625–632.

Schwartz, A.E., Maneksha, F.R., Kanchuger, M.S. et al. (1989). Flumazenil decreases the minimum alveolar concentration isoflurane in dogs. *Anesthesiol.* 71 (1): 174.

Seddighi, R., Egger, C.M., Rohrbach, B.W. et al. (2012). Effect of nitrous oxide on the minimum alveolar concentration for sevoflurane and the minimum alveolar concentration derivatives that prevent motor movement and autonomic responses in dogs. *Am. J. Vet. Res.* 73 (3): 341–345.

Seddighi, R., Geist, A., Knych, H., and Sun, X. (2023). The effect of remifentanil infusion on sevoflurane minimum alveolar concentration-no movement (MACNM) and bispectral index in dogs. *Vet. Anaesth. Analg.* 50: 121–128.

Sheffer, L., Steffenson, J.L., and Birch, A.A. (1972). Nitrous-oxide-induced diffusion hypoxia in patients breathing spontaneously. *Anesthesiol.* 37 (4): 436–439.

Shepard, M.K., Accola, P.J., Lopez, L.A. et al. (2011). Effect of duration and type of anesthetic on tear production in dogs. *Am. J. Vet. Res.* 72 (5): 608–612.

Sherman, J., Le, C., Lamers, V., and Eckelman, M. (2012). Life cycle greenhouse gas emissions of anesthetic drugs. *Anesth. Analg.* 114 (5): 1086–1090.

Shiraishi, M. and Harris, R.A. (2004). Effects of alcohols and anesthetics on recombinant voltage-gated Na^+ channels. *J. Pharmacol. Exp. Ther.* 309 (3): 987–994.

Soares, J.H.N., Brosnan, R.J., Fukushima, F.B. et al. (2012). Solubility of haloether anesthetics in human and animal blood. *Anesthesiol.* 117 (1): 48–55.

Steffey, E.P. and Howland, D. Jr. (1977). Isoflurane potency in the dog and cat. *Am. J. Vet. Res.* 38 (11): 1833–1836.

Steffey, E.P. and Howland, D. Jr. (1978a). Potency of enflurane in dogs: comparison with halothane and isoflurane. *Am. J. Vet. Res.* 39 (4): 573–577.

Steffey, E.P. and Howland, D. Jr. (1978b). Potency of halothane-N20 in the horse. *Am. J. Vet. Res.* 39 (7): 1141–1146.

Steffey, E.P. and Howland, D. Jr. (1979). Halothane anesthesia in calves. *Am. J. Vet. Res.* 40 (3): 372–376.

Steffey, E.P., Gillespie, J.R., Berry, J.D. et al. (1974). Anesthetic potency (MAC) of nitrous oxide in the dog, cat, and stump-tail monkey. *J. Appl. Physiol.* 36 (5): 530–532.

Steffey, E.P., Howland, D. Jr., Giri, S., and Eger, E.I. 2nd (1977). Enflurane, halothane, and isoflurane potency in horses. *Am. J. Vet. Res.* 38 (7): 1037–1039.

Steffey, E.P., Woliner, M.J., and Howland, D. (1983). Accuracy of isoflurane delivery by halothane-specific vaporizers. *Am. J. Vet. Res.* 44 (6): 1072–1078.

Steffey, E.P., Laster, M.J., and Ionescu, P. (1997). Dehydration of baralyme(R) increases compound A resulting from sevoflurane degradation in a standard anesthetic circuit used to anesthetize swine. *Anesth. Analg.* 85 (6): 1382–1386.

Steffey, E.P., Pascoe, P.J., Woliner, M.J., and Berryman, E.R. (2000). Effects of xylazine hydrochloride during isoflurane-induced anesthesia in horses. *Am. J. Vet. Res.* 61 (10): 1225–1231.

Steffey, E.P., Eisele, J.H., and Baggot, J.D. (2003). Interactions of morphine and isoflurane in horses. *Am. J. Vet. Res.* 64 (2): 166–175.

Steffey, E.P., Mama, K.R., Galey, F.D. et al. (2005a). Effects of sevoflurane dose and mode of ventilation on cardiopulmonary function and blood biochemical variables in horses. *Am. J. Vet. Res.* 66 (4): 606–614.

Steffey, E.P., Woliner, M.J., Puschner, B., and Galey, F.D. (2005b). Effects of desflurane and mode of ventilation on cardiovascular and respiratory functions and clinicopathologic variables in horses. *Am. J. Vet. Res.* 66 (4): 669–677.

Steffey, E.P., Mama, K.R., and Brosnan, R.J. (2015). Inhalation anesthetics. In: *Veterinary Anesthesia and Analgesia*, 5e (ed. L.L. Grimm), 297–331. Ames, IA: Wiley.

Strebel, S., Lam, A.M., Matta, B. et al. (1995). Dynamic and static cerebral autoregulation during isoflurane, desflurane, and propofol anesthesia. *Anesthesiol.* 83 (1): 66–76.

Sutton, T.S., Koblin, D.D., and Gruenke, L.D. (1991). Fluoride metabolites after prolonged exposure of volunteers and patients to desflurane. *Anesth. Analg.* 73: 180–185.

Tanaka, T., Nabatame, H., and Tanifuji, Y. (2005). Insulin secretion and glucose utilization are impaired under general anesthesia with sevoflurane as well as isoflurane in a concentration-independent manner. *J. Anesth.* 277–281.

Tanaka, K., Kawano, T., Tomino, T. et al. (2009). Mechanisms of impaired glucose tolerance and insulin secretion during isoflurane anesthesia. *Anesthesiol.* 1044–1051.

Tendillo, F.J., Mascías, A., and Santos, M. (1997). Anesthetic potency of desflurane in the horse: determination of the minimum alveolar concentration. *Vet. Surg.* 26 (4): 354–357.

Thomson, S.M., Burton, C.A., and Armitage-Chan, E.A. (2014). Intra-operative hyperthermia in a cat with a fatal outcome. *Vet. Anaesth. Analg.* 41 (3): 290–296.

Todd, M.M. and Drummond, J.C. (1984). A comparison of the cerebrovascular and metabolic effects of halothane and isoflurane in the cat. *Anesthesiol.* 60 (4): 276–282.

Villalba, M., Santiago, I., and Gomez de Segura, I.A. (2011). Effects of constant rate infusion of lidocaine and ketamine, with or without morphine, on isoflurane MAC in horses. *Equine Vet. J.* 43 (6): 721–726.

Violet, J.M., Downie, D.L., Nakisa, R.C. et al. (1997). Differential sensitivities of mammalian neuronal and muscle nicotinic acetylcholine receptors to general anesthetics. *Anesthesiol.* 86 (4): 866–874.

Wallin, R.F., Regan, B.M., Napoli, M.D., and Stern, I.J. (1975). Sevoflurane: a new inhalational anesthetic agent. *Anesth. Analg.* 54: 758–767.

Webb, A.I. and McMurphy, R.M. (1987). Effect of anticholinergic preanesthetic medicaments on the requirements of halothane for anesthesia in the cat. *Am. J. Vet. Res.* 48 (12): 1733–1735.

Weiskopf, R.B. and Bogetz, M.S. (1984). Minimum alveolar concentrations (MAC) of halothane and nitrous oxide in swine. *Anesth. Analg.* 63 (5): 529–532.

Weiskopf, R.B., Eger, E.I. 2nd, and Holmes, M.A. (1989). Epinephrine-induced premature ventricular contractions and changes in arterial blood pressure and heart rate during I-653, isoflurane, and halothane anesthesia in swine. *Anesthesiol.* 70 (2): 293–298.

Williams, D.C., Aleman, M.R., Brosnan, R.J. et al. (2016). Electroencephalogram of healthy horses during inhaled anesthesia. *J. Vet. Intern. Med.* 30 (1): 304–308.

Yamakura, T. and Harris, R.A. (2000). Effects of gaseous anesthetics nitrous oxide and xenon on ligand-gated ion channels: comparison with isoflurane and ethanol. *Anesthesiol.* 93: 1095–1101.

Yasuda, N., Lockhart, S.H., Eger, E.I. 2nd, et al. (1991). Comparison of kinetics of sevoflurane and isoflurane in humans. *Anesth. Analg.* 72 (3): 316–324.

Young, W.L. (1992). Effects of desflurane on the central nervous system. *Anesth. Analg.* 75 (4 Suppl): S32–S37.

Young, D.J. and Sawyer, D.C. (1980). Anesthetic potency of nitrous oxide during halothane anesthesia in the dog. *J. Am. Anim. Hosp. Assoc.* 16 (1): 125–128.

11

Non-Steroidal Anti-Inflammatory Drugs

Craig Willette

Introduction

Non-steroidal anti-inflammatory drugs (NSAIDs) are drugs other than steroids that are widely used in both human and veterinary medicine to treat fever, inflammation, and pain. Many veterinary NSAIDs are approved in companion animals specifically for the management of pain and inflammation associated with osteoarthritis and perioperative pain. In horses, NSAIDs are a staple of in-hospital and ambulatory management. In food and fiber animals, the use of NSAIDs can be beneficial but the regulations set out by the US Food and Drug Administration (FDA) must be strictly adhered to. Veterinarians assume legal responsibility when using NSAIDs off-label in these animals. Importantly, ketoprofen was recently approved for use in certain beef and dairy cattle in the US, thus expanding the available approved analgesics in this species. Off-label use has also been investigated and is common in veterinary species.

NSAIDs specifically affect the synthesis of prostaglandins (PGs) from arachidonic acid (AA) by targeting cyclooxygenase (COX) enzymes. Synthesis of PGs is widespread throughout the body and is essential to maintaining homeostasis in addition to contributing to the inflammatory process. The potential for accidental ingestion due to widespread use and the possibility of adverse effects even at labeled doses mean that it is important for veterinarians to understand the basic mechanisms of action, labeled and off-label uses, and expected side effect profiles of these drugs.

Pharmacology

In veterinary species, NSAIDs are commonly administered orally, intravenously (IV), intramuscularly (IM), and, in some cases, subcutaneously or transdermally. Absorption after oral administration is variable among species and individuals but is often high compared to other orally administered medications. As a result, oral bioavailability is typically high (90%+), with peak plasma concentrations often achieved one to four hours after ingestion. Most NSAIDs are weak acids, leading to absorption in the stomach and upper gastrointestinal (GI) tract. The acidic pH of the stomach results in the majority of the drug being unionized and lipophilic, leading to effective absorption through the lipid membrane of gastric cells. Consumption of food or concurrent administration of gastroprotectants may prolong absorption, leading to lower peak plasma concentrations but little change in bioavailability. In the presence of food or gastroprotectants, more drug is absorbed in the small or large intestine. As administered dose increases, there is potential for more drug to remain in the hydrophilic, ionized form in the stomach, resulting in prolonged absorption and a smaller increase in peak plasma concentrations than expected.

NSAIDs are typically highly bound to plasma proteins, primarily albumin. Such high affinity for protein binding results in a relatively low volume of distribution. This is an important factor when considering coadministration with other drugs that are protein-bound, which may be displaced by the NSAID, as well as therapeutic dosing regimens in patients with hypoalbuminemia. Either scenario may result in an unintentionally high plasma concentration of a prescribed drug. Despite a limited volume of distribution, NSAIDs are typically effective at specific sites (such as synovial structures) after systemic administration. As weak organic acids, NSAIDs easily lose a hydrogen ion in plasma and become lipophilic, in which form they efficiently cross into the CNS and exhibit effects on the brain and spinal cord (Lees et al. 2004). The acidic nature of NSAIDs means that they tend to accumulate in sites where pH is lowered by inflammation, an advantageous characteristic given that such sites are often the therapeutic target of administration.

Pharmacology in Veterinary Anesthesia and Analgesia, First Edition. Edited by Turi Aarnes and Phillip Lerche.
© 2024 John Wiley & Sons, Inc. Published 2024 by John Wiley & Sons, Inc.

Metabolism of NSAIDs occurs primarily via hepatic biotransformation and renal excretion. Some NSAIDs first undergo hydroxylation or oxidation in the liver, and many are conjugated in the liver with glucuronic acid in a process called glucuronidation. It is of note that cats and other felidae have a significantly lower capacity for glucuronidation than other veterinary species (Van Beusekom et al. 2013). As a result, NSAID half-life can be significantly prolonged and plasma concentrations will reach higher levels than an equivalent dosage in other species. This can make cats especially susceptible to NSAID toxicity from accidental ingestion, or as a result of overdose from a well-intentioned owner. Following breakdown of the primary drug, metabolite elimination is primarily via excretion by the kidneys or GI tract in the bile, with a fraction of parent drug excreted prior to metabolism. In some cases, primary metabolites are further broken down prior to elimination. Elimination half-life varies greatly among NSAIDs, from as little as one hour (e.g. ketoprofen) to as long as one to two days (e.g. piroxicam). A short time-to-peak plasma concentration, combined with a short half-life, is optimal for treatment of acute pain. NSAIDs with longer half-lives are more well-suited to the treatment of chronic pain. The significant role played by both the liver and kidneys in the elimination of NSAIDs warrants careful consideration in patients with renal or liver disease.

Mechanism of Action

NSAIDs inhibit the activity of COX enzymes which bind AA to produce prostaglandins. COX enzymes include the isoforms COX-1 and COX-2, and the more recently described COX-3. COX-1 and COX-2 metabolize AA released from membrane phospholipids to produce the cyclic endoperoxides PGG_2 and PGH_2. The end-products of PGG_2 and PGH_2 are tissue-specific, including thromboxane $(TX)A_2$, PGE_2, and PGI_2. Leukotrienes are also a product of AA metabolism via lipoxygenase (LOX); LOX activity is not directly affected by NSAID administration. Leukotrienes and the end products of PGG_2 and PGH_2 are collectively known as eicosanoids. TX is produced in platelets and contributes to platelet aggregation and clot formation. PGs predominantly act locally (autocrine, paracrine) for a short period of time. Elimination within minutes of production means that eicosanoid activity requires constant production. COX-1 is constitutively expressed and is essential for many homeostatic mechanisms including maintenance of cardiovascular function, hemostasis, and blood flow to the GI mucosa and kidneys. COX-2 is significantly upregulated in response to inflammation and shear stress, although it also serves some homeostatic functions.

It is a significant factor in the maintenance of chronic inflammation and the development of central sensitization (Chen et al. 2013). Less is known about the specific functions of COX-3, but evidence suggests it may be an important binding target for the therapeutic effects of acetaminophen in veterinary species (Chandrasekharan et al. 2002).

Classification

NSAIDs can be classified by chemical structure or COX isoform selectivity. The chemical structure of most NSAIDs is comprised of an acidic moiety with an aromatic functional group, resulting in the relatively predictable absorption and distribution characteristic of weak acids. When grouped by chemical structure, NSAIDs can be separated into carboxylic acids or enolic acids, with the remaining COX-2 selective NSAIDs being grouped by a similar mechanism of action. Carboxylic acids include aspirin, carprofen, and etodolac. Enolic acids include meloxicam and phenylbutazone. COX-2 selective NSAIDs include coxibs, such as firocoxib and robenacoxib. NSAIDs are commonly distinguished clinically by their inhibition of COX isoforms and plasma half-life (duration of effectiveness). They primarily function either as isoform selective COX-2 inhibitors, or as isoform non-selective inhibitors of both COX-1 and COX-2. This inhibition is further classified as competitive, non-competitive, or mixed reversible. Aspirin, a salicylic acid derivative, differs from other commonly used NSAIDs in that it is a non-competitive irreversible COX inhibitor. Acetaminophen is often considered along with the NSAIDs, but its lack of anti-inflammatory properties despite analgesic and anti-pyretic effects means that it is not.

Adverse Effects

Gastrointestinal

The most reported side effects after NSAID administration are gastrointestinal (GI) in nature. Vomiting, soft stool or diarrhea, and loss of appetite are possible manifestations seen in companion animals. Gastric and intestinal ulceration and, in the case of horses, right dorsal ulcerative colitis (RDUC) are more serious manifestations. Gastric ulceration is thought to be a result of impairment of the constitutive expression of COX-1 in gastric epithelial cells, which produces PGI_2 and PGE_2. These prostaglandins maintain mucosal blood flow, inhibit gastric acid secretion, and promote secretion of the intestinal mucus layer. Without the mucoid layer, the acidic nature of the stomach may break down gastric epithelial cells. Further, blood flow to the GI tract may be altered by COX-1 inhibition, impairing the ability of the intestine to heal the developed lesions. COX-2 also contributes to the production of PGI_2 and PGE_2, and it may be necessary for healing of mucosal cells affected by ulceration. Ulcerative colitis in horses is most often associated with the administration of phenylbutazone, but its occurrence is also possible after treatment with other NSAIDs. RDUC is presumed to occur through a similar process as in other species, but it is only theorized as to why these lesions localize to the right dorsal colon (Karcher et al. 1990). Despite the widespread use of phenylbutazone in horses, the clinical manifestation of ulcerative colitis is rare. Upper GI endoscopy may often reveal some level of ulcerative gastritis in patients chronically administered NSAIDs, or in patients experiencing acute toxicity. Complications include discomfort and inappetence, ranging to diarrhea, anemia, and potentially death if significant hemorrhage or sepsis/endotoxemia develop.

Kidney

Blood flow to the renal cortex and medulla is locally mediated in part by COX enzymatic activity. COX-2 derived PGE_2 and PGI_2 both increase renal medullary blood flow and act to increase glomerular filtration rate (GFR) through local vasodilation (Hao and Breyer 2007). Prostaglandins derived from COX-1 contribute to sodium excretion in the collecting ducts, while increased medullary blood flow from products of COX-2 promote pressure diuresis and reduced Na^+ retention. Many other factors contribute to maintenance of renal perfusion, providing redundancy in a healthy animal. When these systems are compromised, prostaglandins become more important for maintaining renal perfusion and preventing cellular damage. Healthy patients administered a course of NSAIDs at clinically appropriate doses rarely show renal side effects. However, chronic NSAID use, NSAID toxicity, or NSAID use in the face of renal compromise can cause significant kidney damage. When a patient has developed azotemia as a result of renal damage, the benefits and disadvantages of NSAID administration are apparent. There remains much debate on NSAID administration to patients with conditions that may cause azotemia in the future, such as the challenges to renal blood flow encountered under general anesthesia, or when there is a question of subclinical renal compromise.

Coagulation

TXA_2, a major product of COX-1 activity in platelets, contributes to platelet aggregation and clot formation.

COX-1 inhibitors impair TXA_2 production, thus impairing coagulation. Aspirin, an acetylated salicylic acid, binds COX-1 irreversibly, leading to impairment of platelet function for the duration of the life of the platelet (Patrono et al. 2001). Other COX-1 inhibitors have less impact on coagulation due to the reversible nature of their binding. Impairment of coagulation is a major contributing factor in the hemorrhage that may follow severe GI ulceration. The discontinuation of aspirin prior to elective surgery to avoid complications related to hemorrhage is common practice. COX-2 selective drugs, such as the coxibs, do not significantly inhibit the production of TxA_2, but they do inhibit the production of PGI_2 and PGE_2. PGI_2 is important in the inhibition of platelet aggregation, and both PGI_2 and PGE_2 contribute to renal maintenance of blood pressure. Thus, the overall effect of COX-2 selective NSAID administration is to promote coagulation. This is less of a concern in veterinary species but is the primary reason COX-2 selective NSAIDs are often avoided in human patients who are at higher risk for infarction.

Liver

NSAID toxicity may lead to elevated liver enzymes as a result of cellular damage, and potentially altered hepatic function in severe cases; however, this is relatively rare at recommended doses. Carprofen has been reported to cause hepatocellular toxicity in a case series of 21 dogs (MacPhail et al. 1998). An investigation of long-term carprofen administration in dogs demonstrated no adverse effects when compared with a placebo (Raekallio et al. 2006). As with other adverse effects, dosage likely plays a significant role in hepatotoxicity. Acetaminophen is not an NSAID but is often considered along with them when discussing analgesic management. NAQPI, a reactive metabolic byproduct of acetaminophen, is normally produced in low enough numbers that conjugation with reduced glutathione (GSH) is sufficient to eliminate it safely. When GSH becomes saturated, as in acute overdose or chronic liver failure, NAQPI then reacts with local hepatocellular tissue which can lead to hepatocellular necrosis (Graham et al. 2005). Recently, a two-week course of acetaminophen was demonstrated to produce no elevation in liver enzymes at clinical doses in horses (Mercer et al. 2020). Hepatotoxicity due to acetaminophen is more likely in cats and other felidae which have a limited ability to metabolize drugs via glucuronidation, leading to more NAQPI production; there is no clinically safe dose of acetaminophen in cats. If a patient survives a hepatotoxic event, discontinuation of NSAIDs, combined with supportive care, is expected to ultimately reverse associated liver damage.

Interaction with Steroids

Corticosteroids are administered clinically as replacements for adrenal dysfunction in Addison's disease or, most commonly, for their significant anti-inflammatory and immunosuppressive activity. Like NSAIDs, corticosteroids are metabolized by the liver and excreted by the kidneys. Corticosteroids affect multiple enzymatic pathways, include COX and LOX. The shared activity, metabolism and excretion between corticosteroids and NSAIDs can amplify therapeutic effects. Correspondingly, the adverse effects may also be amplified by concurrent administration. Thus, administration of NSAIDs and corticosteroids to the same patient warrants careful consideration. Patients administered both steroids and NSAIDs are at significant risk for GI irritation and ulceration. Ultimately, GI perforation and hemorrhage are possible serious outcomes. While there may be therapeutic benefit to the combination of these two drug classes in the treatment of specific conditions, it is prudent to monitor appetite and for other signs of GI upset.

Acetaminophen

Acetaminophen is a phenol that has anti-pyretic and analgesic properties, but its minimal anti-inflammatory activity means that it is not classified as an NSAID. Nonetheless, acetaminophen is routinely considered when discussing NSAIDs. Acetaminophen may often be considered when developing an analgesic regimen for a patient already on an NSAID, or in a patient in which the renal and GI side effects of traditional NSAIDs wish to be avoided. Its low cost, availability, and typically minimal-to-mild side effect profile can be advantageous in clinical use.

Acetaminophen can be administered orally or, less often in veterinary medicine, IV. After oral administration, acetaminophen is primarily absorbed in the proximal small intestine. As a result, time to reach peak plasma levels can be affected by gastric emptying time. In horses, this characteristic has been used to measure gastric emptying time (Doherty et al. 1998). Absorption after oral absorption is not significantly different between fasted and fed dogs (Sartini et al. 2021). Bioavailability after IM administration averages 71% in goats (10 mg/kg) and a $t_{1/2}$-corrected 105% in dromedary camels (5 mg/kg) (Ali et al. 1996). More recently, San et al. (2019) demonstrated much lower peak plasma concentrations (0.96 μg/ml) after a similar dose of 4 mg/kg IM to Bactrian camels (compared with 4.05 μg/ml demonstrated by Ali et al. in dromedaries). Presumably this equates with a lower bioavailability in Bactrian camels, although an IV dose was not administered for comparison

by San et al. (2019). Following absorption, a large amount of acetaminophen remains unbound in plasma, with very little bound to protein. As a weak acid, it easily crosses into cells via passive diffusion, and can cross the blood–brain-barrier. Half-life of elimination is relatively short, typically less than two hours, the exception being horses, in which a half-life of elimination of over four hours has been demonstrated (Neirinckx et al. 2010; Mercer et al. 2020; Sartini et al. 2021). After one single IV administration of 20 mg/kg in adult female labrador dogs, plasma concentrations were detectable up to eight hours after administration (Sartini et al. 2021). Similarly, detectable plasma levels approached eight hours in beagles and galgo Español (Spanish greyhound) dogs after 20 mg/kg administered IV (Serrano-Rodríguez et al. 2019); detectable plasma concentrations lasted closer to six hours after 10 mg/kg IV in this study. The results of Serrano-Rodríguez et al. (2019) indicate some breed differences in acetaminophen metabolism in dogs. After IV administration in dromedary camels, acetaminophen is detectable for up to three hours, compared with less than an hour in goats (Ali et al. 1996). This can be attributed to a more rapid clearance in goats than in camels. In Bactrian camels, a more advanced liquid chromatography system combined with a slower clearance (9.9 ml/kg/min vs. 21.9 ml/kg/min in dromedaries) resulted in detectable plasma concentrations for up to 24 hours (San et al. 2019). This dramatic difference is a clear example of how species pharmacokinetics can affect dosing requirements. Metabolism occurs in the liver, where acetaminophen primarily undergoes conjugation with glucuronic acid and sulfuric acid, forming acetaminophen glucuronide and acetaminophen sulfate, respectively. Several peroxidases and cytochromes in the liver metabolize acetaminophen to a lesser extent via oxidation, the products of which (primarily NAPQI) can cause toxicity. At clinical doses in small animals, the oxidative metabolites of acetaminophen are produced in low enough numbers that hepatotoxicity is rare. A small amount is excreted unchanged in the urine.

Acetaminophen produces its clinical effects by binding and inhibition of multiple receptors. Its targets include the COX enzymes 1 and 2, where it non-selectively acts at the peroxide site. There is debate over its effects on a more recently discovered COX enzyme, COX-3, but this interaction may play a significant role in its effects in veterinary species (Chandrasekharan et al. 2002). COX-3 expression has been demonstrated in canine brain tissue. As peroxide concentrations increase with inflammation, the COX inhibitory activity of acetaminophen is reduced, which results in minimal anti-inflammatory effects. Inhibition of 5-HT-3 and PgE_2 receptors centrally, as well as its effects on PGE_2 and substance P peripherally, are likely the reason for the primary analgesic and antipyretic effects of the drug (Graham et al. 2013).

Use of acetaminophen in veterinary species is extra-label in the US. It may be prescribed by veterinarians for the treatment of mild pain or fever, or as an adjunct to other, more effective analgesics. Its effectiveness has been demonstrated in the treatment of post-surgical pain in dogs (Hernandez-Avalos et al. 2020). It may also be used in the clinical treatment of osteoarthritis in dogs, but no clinical studies have been performed on its effectiveness for this indication. In horses, there is some evidence that acetaminophen is an effective adjunct analgesic for orthopedic pain when combined with other medications (Tavanaeimanesh et al. 2018).

In contrast to traditional NSAIDs, the adverse effects of acetaminophen rarely involve the kidneys or GI tract. Accidental ingestion or overdose by well-intentioned owners is common in companion animals. In dogs, acetaminophen toxicity primarily involves hepatic damage. Less likely is some degree of hemolytic anemia and depressed bone marrow function (Salem et al. 2010). At clinical doses, hepatotoxicity is rare and idiosyncratic. In cats, acetaminophen is contraindicated due to their reduced ability to metabolize acetaminophen via glucuronidation; as a result, more of the highly reactive oxidative metabolite NAQPI is produced, which can cause significant hepatotoxicity. Little is known about the adverse effects of acetaminophen in pregnant or lactating veterinary species. In people, only a very small amount of acetaminophen is present in lactating mothers' milk (National Library of Medicine (US) 2022). Due to its limited anti-inflammatory effects, acetaminophen is unlikely to perpetuate the adverse effects of steroids.

Aspirin

Aspirin (acetylsalicylic acid, ASA) is a derivative of salicylic acid. ASA was first used by Mering in 1893. Soon thereafter it was being tested by the pharmaceutical company Bayer for widespread use. Willow bark, which contains salicylic acid, had been used for centuries to relieve fevers and pain. After investigations prompted by the irritating nature of salicylic acid, aspirin was the first salicylic acid derivative developed for human use. Aspirin is a nonselective inhibitor of COX-1 and COX-2, exhibiting its effects by irreversibly acetylating the catalytic subunits of these enzymes.

Aspirin is administered orally in veterinary species. It is available as a tablet or capsule for companion animals, and as a paste, bolus or liquid concentrate for horses, cattle and poultry. Like other NSAIDs, aspirin is absorbed in the stomach and proximal GI tract with relatively high bioavailability. Coatings, buffers or prolonged-release formulations that can be found in human aspirin products may alter oral bioavailability. Absorption is slightly prolonged in horses and cattle relative to cats and dogs. The acidic nature of aspirin means that it is relatively well-absorbed in the stomach and proximal small intestine, where local activity may potentiate adverse effects. Aspirin primarily reaches systemic circulation in its unmetabolized form, but a portion is hydrolyzed by esterases in the gastric mucosa and hepatic portal circulation (first-pass effect) to reach the systemic circulation as salicylic acid, the primary active metabolite of aspirin. Upon reaching systemic circulation, aspirin may also be converted to salicylic acid or two other primary salicylates via deacetylation by esterases in red blood cells, or by spontaneous hydrolysis in the plasma. Aspirin and the primary salicylates produced by aspirin metabolism are widely distributed throughout the body, including crossing the placental barrier and into the CSF. Protein binding of salicylic acid is high, giving the metabolites of aspirin the potential to compete with other medications for protein binding sites in the plasma, including other NSAIDs. Salicylic acid is metabolized via glucuronidation in the liver and excreted in the urine. Half-life of aspirin is very short (<1 hour in most species), and half-life of its metabolites is also relatively short at clinical doses (four to six hours). The glucuronide deficiency present in cats and other Felidae produces a significantly longer half-life of up to 37.5 hours (Gupta 2018). In an investigation of aspirin resistance in healthy dogs, Haines et al. (2019) sampled plasma concentrations up to three hours after administration of 4 mg/kg orally. Plasma concentrations were nearing the lower levels of detection at three hours after administration, although a variation in aspirin esterase activity of up to 15-fold. This is consistent with evidence of aspirin tolerance in horses (Roscher et al. 2017). First recognized in humans, aspirin resistance is likely affected by individual genetics, with clinical doses failing to produce inhibition of platelet function, although the complete mechanisms are still poorly understood.

Aspirin differs from its metabolites in its COX selectivity and reversibility of binding. Prior to its metabolism, aspirin binds COX-1 and COX-2 irreversibly, inhibiting their production of prostaglandins and, importantly, TxA_2. Due to the short half-life of aspirin, many cells in which COX enzyme activity is inhibited by aspirin can produce more COX enzymes following aspirin metabolism that are then unaffected. Platelets differ from most cells in that they have little ability to synthesize new proteins; they are thus significantly affected by aspirin binding in the portal circulation, where its concentrations are high prior to exposure to systemic circulation. Aspirin binding ultimately results in irreversible inhibition of platelet function with demonstrable prolongation of hemostasis; new platelets must be formed to recover hemostatic function. This inhibition may be cumulative as aspirin continues to affect newly formed platelets. Discontinuation requires time for hemostatic function to recover as platelet turnover occurs. Salicylic acid, in contrast to aspirin, is a reversible inhibitor of COX that may also interfere with upregulation of COX-2 during inflammation. The metabolites of aspirin have very limited effects on platelet function. Accordingly, the antithrombotic effects of aspirin are of longer duration than its effects on inflammation and pain.

Veterinary aspirin is labeled for anti-pyretic and mild analgesic use in cattle, horses, sheep, swine, dogs, and poultry. A major indication that is not on the label is for its antithrombotic activity in conditions that can promote thromboembolism (e.g. immune-mediated hemolytic anemia, protein-losing nephropathy) (Lunsford and Mackin 2007; Robinson and Sprayberry 2009). In dogs, the use of low-dose aspirin has been shown to correlate with improved outcome in the treatment of immune-mediated hemolytic anemia (Weinkle et al. 2005).

Aspirin has a high margin of safety in most species, with cats and other Felidae being the notable exception. The prolonged half-life of aspirin in cats means that accumulation can occur if dosed too often; a typical dosing regimen is 10–25 mg/kg every two to three days (Gupta 2018). The adverse effect profile of aspirin is relatively predictable between species, with gastric and intestinal ulceration being by far the most common. Emesis, hyporexia, and melena may accompany these lesions. Depression, restlessness, seizures, and coma due to salicylate toxicity have been reported in severe cases in dogs and cats, likely a result of hypoventilation, hypoglycemia, and acidosis (Gupta 2018). As with most NSAIDs, there is limited data on the toxicity of aspirin during pregnancy and lactation, although several studies suggest that very high doses can cause birth defects in rats (Cook et al. 2003). Further, aspirin crosses easily into milk, and it is known that animals metabolize aspirin more slowly in the first month of life (Gupta 2018). It is reasonable, then, to exercise caution when considering aspirin administration to pregnant or lactating animals. Aspirin is not approved for use in animals by the FDA, therefore its use is extra-label in all veterinary species in the US.

Carprofen

Carprofen is a propionic acid derivative available in both oral and subcutaneous injectable formulations for dogs. In the US, carprofen is one of the archetypal NSAIDs for management of pain and inflammation in dogs.

After oral administration, carprofen is absorbed in the stomach and proximal GI tract with bioavailability >90% (McKellar et al. 1990). After subcutaneous administration, peak plasma concentration is lower and half-life prolonged compared to oral administration, but ultimately drug exposure is bioequivalent (Clark et al. 2003). At clinical doses, peak plasma concentrations are achieved one to three hours after administration, and half-life is approximately eight hours. A single oral dose of carprofen in dogs at 4 mg/kg resulted in detectable plasma concentrations for up to 24 hours (Mckellar et al. 1994). As with most other NSAIDs, carprofen is highly protein-bound (99%+), with a low volume of distribution (Carprofen Package Insert 2020). Concurrent administration with other protein-bound medications or administration to patients with hypoalbuminemia warrants careful consideration. Metabolism occurs primarily in the liver via glucuronidation, with 70–80% eliminated in the feces and 10–20% excreted renally.

Carprofen inhibits COX-1 and COX-2 activity, with *in vitro* evidence of higher affinity for COX-2, although this selectivity was lower in canine whole blood than in canine cell lines (Brideau et al. 2001; Ricketts et al. 1998). The clinical relevance of this *in vitro* affinity is unknown. The accepted mechanism of action of carprofen is its inhibition of prostaglandin synthesis secondary to COX inhibition, leading to anti-pyretic, anti-inflammatory, and analgesic effects. There is evidence that COX inhibition is not the only mechanism of action of carprofen in some species (Delatour et al. 1996).

In the US, carprofen is labeled for the treatment of inflammation and pain associated with osteoarthritis and for postoperative analgesia following soft-tissue and orthopedic surgery in dogs. The labeled dosage is 4.4 mg/kg once per day or 2.2 mg/kg twice per day.

Long-term administration of carprofen is well-tolerated in dogs (Raekallio et al. 2006). The adverse effects of carprofen administration are most commonly GI, including mucosal ulceration, vomiting, and diarrhea. Altered GI permeability with subsequent protein loss is possible. Carprofen is often co-administered with gastroprotectants to protect against ulceration, but recent evidence suggests that co-administration with omeprazole may not be beneficial, with the potential to promote dysbiosis (Jones et al. 2020). Adverse effects associated with greater drug exposure include hepatocellular toxicity (MacPhail et al. 1998) and renal damage. Altered renal blood flow due to COX inhibition must always be considered in compromised patients. A single report of dermatitis and immune-mediated hematologic disorders in a Neapolitan mastiff associated with carprofen has been published (Mellor et al. 2005). The safety of carprofen in pregnant or lactating dogs has not been established, although there is evidence in dairy cattle that it does not affect pregnancy and is poorly excreted in milk (Ludwig et al. 1989, Heuweiser et al. 2010). Carprofen is only FDA approved for use in dogs in the US. Its use in all other species is extra-label.

Deracoxib

Deracoxib is a coxib-class NSAID available for oral administration to dogs in the US. It is available both as a tablet and a powder. It was the first coxib approved for use in dogs and is still routinely used today.

Deracoxib is absorbed in the stomach and proximal small intestine. It exhibits >90% bioavailability with a volume of distribution of 1.5 l/kg. Bioavailability is highest when administered with food. In plasma, deracoxib is >90% bound to plasma protein. Time-to-peak concentration in dogs is approximately two hours, with a dose-dependent elimination half-life approximating three hours at clinical doses (Deracoxib Package Insert 2021). The longest duration of detectable plasma concentrations in dogs is not published. In cats, after a single oral dose of 1 mg/kg, plasma concentrations of deracoxib were detectable for up to 60 hours (Gassel et al. 2006). Metabolism in dogs is primarily via hepatic biotransformation, with the majority of metabolites and parent drug excreted in feces. Some metabolites are excreted renally. No parent drug is excreted in urine. Deracoxib is a selective COX inhibitor, with significantly higher affinity for COX-2 than COX-1. COX-1 activity was not inhibited *in vitro* at clinical dosages of 2–4 mg/kg/day (Deracoxib Package Insert 2021). Selective inhibition of COX-2 decreases production of inflammatory prostaglandins primarily upregulated by COX-2 while maintaining constitutive production of gastroprotective and pro-thrombotic prostaglandins produced by COX-1. This is thought to produce the desired analgesic and anti-inflammatory effects of NSAIDs without the adverse GI effects commonly seen with non-selective COX inhibitors.

Deracoxib is labeled for the treatment of postoperative inflammation and pain after orthopedic surgery or dental procedures, and for the treatment of inflammation and pain due to osteoarthritis in dogs. Its effectiveness in providing analgesia has been demonstrated in dogs undergoing both soft-tissue surgery and dental procedures, as well as in an experimentally induced synovitis model (Bienhoff et al. 2011; Bienhoff et al. 2012; Millis et al. 2002). The product label specifically designates that it should not be used in cats. A significant extra-label use of deracoxib in dogs is for the treatment of cancer. Deracoxib has been shown to have anti-tumor effects *in vivo* in the treatment of canine transitional cell carcinoma (McMillan et al. 2011), as well as synergistic anti-proliferative effects when combined with doxorubicin to treat canine mammary tumor cell lines *in vitro* (Bakirel et al. 2016).

Deracoxib is typically well tolerated in systemically healthy dogs. The adverse effects of deracoxib are primarily GI at clinical doses. Vomiting, melena, weight loss, GI edema, and ulceration were observed in dogs administered 25–100 mg/kg/d for 10–11 days (6 to 25× labeled dosage), without evidence of renal damage. No dogs died in that study (Deracoxib Package Insert 2021). In healthy dogs at 1.5 mg/kg/day (in the dose range for treatment of osteoarthritis), deracoxib was demonstrated to have no difference in vomiting or gastric lesions when compared to a placebo, and significantly less gastric mucosal damage and vomiting when compared to aspirin at 25 mg/kg every eight hours (Sennello and Leib 2006). A case report series of three dogs developing proximal duodenal perforation after initiation of 2–3 mg/kg per day deracoxib for postoperative pain after orthopedic surgery has been published (Case et al. 2010). Altered renal blood flow due to COX inhibition must always be considered in azotemic or compromised patients. Safety of deracoxib in pregnant or lactating dogs has not been evaluated. Use of deracoxib in any species other than dogs is considered extra-label.

Etodolac

Etodolac is an acetic acid derivative developed for human use. It is available as a capsule and in various forms of extended-release tablets. Etodolac is manufactured for canine use in 150–500 mg tablets.

Data on the pharmacokinetics of etodolac in dogs is limited; until recently, veterinarians had to rely on bioavailability studies meant to validate use in humans (Kraml et al. 1984). In overnight fasted dogs, etodolac at 15–22 mg/kg reaches maximum plasma concentrations in less than an hour (Baek 2019). Kraml et al. (1984) demonstrated that administration of etodolac with food prolongs absorption in dogs but does not alter bioavailability of the drug. Coadministration with sucralfate prolonged absorption and reduced C_{max} but bioavailability was not affected. Unpublished data from studies performed for FDA approval of EtoGesic® indicate that etodolac exhibits nearly 100% bioavailability (EtoGesic® Freedom of Information Summary 1998). In plasma, etodolac is highly bound to plasma proteins (>99%), primarily albumin, resulting in a relatively low volume of distribution. It is metabolized in the liver; metabolites of glucuronidation and hydroxylation have been identified. The specific enzymes responsible for metabolism of etodolac are not yet known. Following metabolism, etodolac is primarily excreted via bile into the feces. Some primary drug is renally excreted, although glucuronide metabolites of etodolac have not been detected in urine (Cayen et al. 1981). Recent data has demonstrated a long half-life of elimination of almost 40 hours (Baek 2019). Cayen et al. (1981), in contrast, described a half-life of 10 hours in dogs. The difference may be attributable to differences in technology and/or duration of monitoring of plasma drug levels; Baek (2019) was able to detect plasma levels for up to 24 hours after a single oral dose. Sampling was not continued beyond this point. Etodolac exerts its clinical effects primarily by inhibition of the COX isoenzymes. There is some disparity in published literature as to the COX selectivity of etodolac in dogs, ranging from non-selective (Streppa et al. 2002) to COX-2 selective (Wilson et al. 2004). It has been demonstrated to be COX-2 selective in humans and is widely thought of as a COX-2 selective NSAID. It may also influence inflammation via inhibition of macrophage chemotaxis (Budsberg et al. 1999).

Etodolac is FDA approved for the treatment of pain and inflammation associated with osteoarthritis in dogs. Dogs with hip-joint osteoarthritis, treated with etodolac for eight days displayed improved ground reaction forces in a dose-dependent manner (Budsberg et al. 1999). It has also been shown to limit the progression of experimentally induced temporomandibular joint osteoarthritis in dogs, when compared with a placebo (Miyamoto et al. 2007). Despite its widespread clinical use, further studies on the efficacy of etodolac in managing pain and inflammation in dogs are warranted. Etodolac has also been demonstrated to reduce pain associated with navicular syndrome as evaluated by force-plate analysis, when administered once per day to chronically lame horses (Symonds et al. 2006).

The adverse effects of etodolac are primarily GI in nature, with vomiting, weight loss, hypoproteinemia, and fecal abnormalities reported. GI ulceration is evident in some dogs at clinical doses (15 mg/kg per day) following six months of administration. As dosage increases to three to five times the clinical dosage (40–80 mg/kg) adverse effects become more severe, and chronic administration at the highest doses resulted in the death of some dogs (EtoGesic® Freedom of Information Summary 1998). Etodolac has also been reported to be associated with keratoconjunctivitis sicca (KCS) in dogs, with an incidence rate of about 1 in every 2000 dogs treated (Klauss et al. 2007). KCS is a minor safety concern in any dog administered an anti-inflammatory agent. As with all NSAIDs, renal and hepatotoxicity must be considered in compromised animals. There is no information on the efficacy or safety of etodolac in pregnant or lactating dogs. The use of etodolac in horses and other species is extra-label.

Firocoxib

Firocoxib is a second-generation member of the coxib NSAIDs available specifically for veterinary use. It is the first coxib approved for use in horses and the second in dogs. It is available as an oral paste and tablet and IV solution in horses, and as an oral tablet in dogs.

The pharmacokinetics of firocoxib have been studied more in the horse than in the dog. In fasted dogs, the time-to-peak plasma concentration is one hour, which is prolonged to five hours when administered with food, without affecting bioavailability. In fasted horses administered the paste formulation, time-to-peak plasma concentration is four hours (Kvaternick et al. 2007). In fed horses, time-to-peak plasma concentration was six hours for the tablet and 9–10 hours when administered paste (Knych et al. 2014). Manufacturer data comparing the paste and tablet formulation in horses determined a T_{max} of 0.25–4 hours for the paste and 0.25–12 hours for the tablet formulation, with significant individual variability. The relatively short T_{max} for both species indicates absorption in the proximal GI tract. Upon absorption, bioavailability is approximately 38% in dogs and 79% in horses. Firocoxib is highly protein-bound (96%+), with a relatively high volume of distribution of 1.7 l/kg in horses, 2.3 l/kg in dromedary camels (Wasfi et al. 2015), and 4.6 l/kg in dogs. Firocoxib undergoes hepatic metabolism with elimination of metabolites primarily via the feces in the dog and via urine in the horse. The parent drug does not undergo significant excretion prior to metabolism. Dromedary camels metabolize firocoxib relatively quickly, with a terminal half-life of 5.75 hours. A terminal half-life of eight hours has been demonstrated in dogs, compared to a relatively slow 30–45 hours in horses. The long terminal half-life in horses means that bioaccumulation can occur, with steady state concentrations achievable after oral administration after 6 to 10 consecutive days of treatment (Letendre et al. 2008; Knych et al. 2014). There is no evidence of bioaccumulation in the dog, with detectable plasma concentrations approaching zero 24 hours after a single IV administration (McCann et al. 2004). While bioaccumulation seems unlikely, Wasfi et al. (2015) recommend a withdrawal period of seven days prior to racing to ensure zero detectable plasma levels in dromedary camels.

Firocoxib is a selective COX-2 inhibitor, with high selectivity for COX-2 over COX-1 demonstrated *in vitro* in both canine and equine whole blood (Kvaternick et al. 2007). Theoretically, COX-2 selectivity inhibits prostaglandin production in response to inflammation, without significantly affecting constitutively produced prostaglandins necessary for normal GI, cardiovascular, and renal function. The result should be an NSAID with fewer adverse effects at doses that produce clinical analgesic, antipyretic, and anti-inflammatory activity. It is labeled for the control of pain and inflammation associated with osteoarthritis in horses, and for the control of pain and inflammation associated with osteoarthritis, orthopedic, and soft-tissue surgery in dogs. In both species, dosing is labeled at once daily. Specifically, it is labeled once daily as needed for osteoarthritis, and once daily for three days for postoperative pain in dogs. In horses, administration of any formulation should not exceed once daily for 14 consecutive days. The efficacy of firocoxib has been demonstrated in both dogs and horses. Specifically, it has been demonstrated to have analgesic efficacy in the treatment of osteoarthritis in horses equivalent to that of phenylbutazone (Doucet et al. 2008; Orsini et al. 2012). In dogs, its analgesic efficacy has been demonstrated in dogs clinically affected by arthritis and following soft-tissue and orthopedic surgery (Pollmeier et al. 2006; Kondo et al. 2012; Davila et al. 2013).

The adverse effects of firocoxib in dogs are relatively uncommon when used as labeled. When they occur, adverse effects are primarily GI (vomiting, anorexia, diarrhea). Azotemia is possible in a small percentage of dogs after chronic administration, with more serious renal damage or hepatic damage less likely. A clinical study evaluating the long-term safety of firocoxib in dogs demonstrated very few side effects over the course of one year at the labeled dose of 5 mg/kg once daily; one dog died of duodenal perforation after administration of twice the recommended dose (Autefage et al. 2011). When administered for 14 or fewer days in horses at the labeled dose of 0.1 mg/kg per day, adverse effects are rare in systemically healthy horses. In manufacturer safety studies, as dosage or duration of treatment increased beyond label recommendations, horses developed oral ulceration, renal damage, and elevation of hepatic enzymes. Even at 12.5× the labeled dose (1.25 mg/kg/day) for 92 days, death did not occur in these safety studies (DailyMed 2020a). The safety and efficacy of firocoxib in pregnant or lactating horses and dogs has not been investigated.

Flunixin Meglumine

Flunixin Meglumine is an NSAID widely used across multiple veterinary species, particularly in food and fiber animals. It is available in the US in multiple formulations for transdermal, subcutaneous, intramuscular, oral, and IV administration. In accordance with the popularity of flunixin, a relatively high number of publications investigating its pharmacokinetics and pharmacodynamics in veterinary species are available.

As with other NSAIDs, the bioavailability of flunixin varies widely by species and route of administration. Transdermal administration typically results in the lowest bioavailability of the various routes. In Holstein calves, bioavailability reached 48% after transdermal administration (Kleinhenz et al. 2016). In Boer goats and Huacaya alpacas, transdermal flunixin bioavailability was closer to 25% (Reppert et al. 2019a,b) while, in mature sows, administration of a pour-over (transdermal) formulation of flunixin resulted in only about 1.5% bioavailability (Cramer et al. 2019). Reppert et al. (2019a,b) advised against transdermal administration in alpacas after demonstrating lower C_{max}, longer T_{max} a lower volume of distribution and more rapid clearance than after transdermal administration to goats or calves. Transdermal administration of flunixin has been investigated in horses, but bioavailability was not determined, and a transdermal formulation is not currently available for use in horses (Knych et al. 2021). Subcutaneous administration has been investigated in cattle (Kissell et al. 2012) and goats (Smith et al. 2020), with high bioavailability (89%+) in both species. IM administration results in relatively high bioavailability of approximately 85% in cattle (Kissell et al. 2012), >99% in piglets (Kittrell et al. 2020), 76% in mature swine (Pairis-Garcia et al. 2013), 70% in sheep (Welsh et al. 1993), 79% in dairy goats (Königsson et al. 2003), and likely close to 100% in horses (Dyke et al. 1997). After oral administration, flunixin is absorbed in the proximal GI tract. Bioavailability after oral administration ranges from 22% in mature swine (Kissell et al. 2012) to as high as 86% in horses (Soma et al. 1988). There is evidence that administration to fed versus fasted horses prolongs absorption, resulting in lower peak plasma concentrations without altering bioavailability (Welsh et al. 1992).

Upon reaching the blood, flunixin is highly protein-bound (99%) in plasma, with a relatively high volume of distribution. It is a lipid-soluble weak acid, so it readily leaves plasma to enter peripheral tissues, and it concentrates in areas of inflammation (Lees and Higgins 1984). After a single IV administration, plasma levels of flunixin were detectable for up 48 hours in greyhounds (1 mg/kg, Morris et al. 2019) and alpacas (2.2 mg/kg, Reppert et al. 2019a,b). Following a single oral administration, and regardless of dose, plasma concentrations were detected up to 24 hours after administration in beagles (McKellar et al. 1989). Flunixin administered at 2.2 mg/kg IV to horses produced alpha, beta, and lambda half-lives of 0.61, 1.5, and 6.0 hours, respectively (Soma et al. 1988). In cattle, a harmonic mean elimination half-life after 1.1 mg/kg IV approached 3.5 hours (Kissell et al. 2012). In llamas, a single IV dose at 2.2 mg/kg IV resulted in a rapid half-life of elimination of 1.47 hours, with a lower clearance and lower volume of distribution than had been demonstrated in other large animal species (Navarre et al. 2001). At the same IV dose, terminal $t_{1/2}$ was 4.5 hours in alpacas (Reppert et al. 2019a,b). Regardless of the method of half-life description, there is a consistency in the area under the curve (AUC) representing metabolism of flunixin among species in that there is an acute, rapid phase followed by a prolonged phase in which plasma levels drop more slowly. Presumably, this is attributable to rapid redistribution. Accordingly, plasma half-life and total body clearance can vary significantly by species and individual, and, due to its concentration at sites of activity, use of pharmacokinetic parameters to estimate dosing intervals may result in underestimation of its duration of effectiveness. While plasma concentration-over-time curves are available for most investigated species, species specifics of organ metabolism largely remain undetermined. Metabolism, as with other NSAIDs, is primarily via hepatic biotransformation, with elimination of metabolites in the bile and urine. In cattle, elimination of metabolites is primarily in bile (Kopcha and Ahl 1989). In horses, the majority of metabolite is excreted via the urine (Soma et al. 1988). A small fraction of parent drug is excreted primarily in the bile or kidneys.

Flunixin is a non-selective NSAID, with similar levels of inhibition of COX-1 and COX-2 *in vitro* (Beretta et al. 2005). As a result, it has anti-inflammatory, analgesic, and antipyretic properties. Its effects have been demonstrated in a wide range of species. Flunixin is labeled for the treatment of visceral pain associated with colic disorders and the treatment of inflammation and pain associated with musculoskeletal disorders in horses. In beef and dairy cattle, it is labeled for the control of pyrexia respiratory disease, endotoxemia, and mastitis, and for the control of inflammation in endotoxemia. In swine, flunixin is specifically labeled for the treatment of pyrexia associated with swine respiratory disease. Flunixin is widely used for its effectiveness in the suppression of the adverse effects of endotoxemia (Shuster et al. 1997). Recent evidence suggests that firocoxib may provide similar levels of analgesia with superior control of endotoxemia in horses undergoing postoperative treatment for small intestinal strangulating obstruction (Ziegler et al. 2019). The efficacy of flunixin in the treatment of pain and/or inflammation has been demonstrated in multiple species, including chickens (Hocking et al. 2005), sheep (Paull et al. 2007), cattle (Currah et al. 2009), horses (Gobbi et al. 2020) and pigs (Pairis-Garcia et al. 2015).

The adverse effects of flunixin administration are similar to those of other NSAIDs. A comparative study in horses in 1993 demonstrated that flunixin administration can cause gastric ulceration, specifically in the glandular region, as well as renal medullary necrosis (MacAllister et al. 1993). Neonatal foals treated with 0.55– 6.6 mg/kg IV daily for six days developed GI ulcerations and diarrhea, with no clinically significant hematologic or biochemical abnormalities detected (Carrick et al. 1989). At 3.3–5.5 mg/kg IV (3–5× the clinical dose) for nine days (3× the maximum duration) in cattle, some cattle developed hematuria or blood in the feces. No adverse effects were seen at 1.1 mg/kg for nine days Prevail® Package Insert 2021. A rare, but significant adverse effect is the possibility of development of bacterial (often clostridial) myositis in horses. In a case series of 37 horses with clostridial myonecrosis over 15 years at two university veterinary hospitals, 17 of the cases were attributable to the IM or perivascular (one case) administration of flunixin (Peek et al. 2003). For this reason, most clinicians do not recommend the IM use of flunixin in horses, despite its labeling.

The adverse effects of flunixin during the periparturient period and lactation have been heavily investigated in cattle. Flunixin metabolites are detectable in the milk of dairy cattle after systemic administration; the labeled withdrawal time is 36 hours after last administration. In cows with mastitis, however, violative residues were detected in the milk of 8 of 10 cattle 36 hours after administration and in 3 of 10 cattle after 60 hours (Kissell et al. 2015). In the periparturient period, a study of 1265 cattle demonstrated increased risk of stillbirth in cattle treated before calving, and increased risk of retained placenta and the accompanying adverse effects in cattle treated with flunixin immediately after calving. As a result, the authors recommend against the use of flunixin within 24 hours of parturition in dairy cattle (Newby et al. 2017). In early pregnancy mares, flunixin alters embryo motility, presumably by altering uterine prostaglandin production, which may affect maternal recognition of the conceptus (Okada et al. 2019). The safety of administration of flunixin in pregnant mares has not specifically been investigated.

The flunixin label specifically states that it is not intended for use in dry dairy cows or in veal calves. The use of flunixin in cats and dogs in the US is off label and, given the availability of other NSAIDs specifically labeled for use in these animals, would be difficult for a veterinarian to justify.

Grapiprant

Grapiprant is one of the most recently available NSAIDs on the market. Unlike traditional NSAIDs, grapiprant targets a specific prostanoid receptor rather than inhibiting the COX enzymes. It is available as an oral tablet for administration in dogs.

After oral administration, grapiprant is quickly absorbed, reaching maximum plasma concentrations in dogs in approximately two hours. In fasted cats, T_{max} was approximately one to two hours, with bioavailability approaching 40% (Lebkowska-Wieruszewska et al. 2017), while in exercised thoroughbreds T_{max} was 1.5 hours (Knych et al. 2018). In dogs, bioavailability is estimated to be at least 80% (DailyMed 2018). Administration of grapiprant with food reduces oral bioavailability in dogs, with reduction in peak plasma concentrations by a factor of 4, and a roughly 50% reduction in total AUC (representative of total drug exposure). After absorption, grapiprant is roughly 95% bound to protein. A single IV or oral dose of 0.5 or 2 mg/kg produces detectable plasma levels in labrador dogs for 24 and 36 hours, respectively (Lebkowska-Wieruszewska et al. 2017). Importantly, in collies, detectable plasma concentrations appear to be similar after a single oral dose of 2 mg/kg grapiprant, but exposure (maximum plasma concentrations) reached more than three times that observed in labradors after administration of the same oral dose (Heit et al. 2021). Elimination is via hepatic metabolism and excretion in the bile, urine, and feces, with the majority eliminated in the bile. Plasma half-life is roughly 4.6–5.7 hours in dogs, 4–5 hours in cats, and 5.8 hours in horses, with the majority of the dose excreted by dogs in the first three days. At the recommended once-daily dosing in dogs, little to no accumulation is expected (DailyMed 2018). Four grapiprant metabolites have been identified; their activity is unknown.

The activity of grapiprant is different from the prototypical COX inhibition effected by most NSAIDs. Grapiprant is a member of the priprant class of NSAIDs, drugs that specifically target specific prostanoid activity by antagonizing their receptors. PGE_2 is a prostanoid that exhibits its physiologic effects by binding four different receptors: EP1, EP2, EP3, and EP4. Grapiprant specifically antagonizes the EP4 receptor that is bound by PGE_2. The EP4 receptor mediates mucus secretion in the stomach and small intestine, acid secretion in the stomach, inhibition of small intestinal motility, inhibition of large intestinal cytokine expression (Takeuchi et al. 2010), and the antinatriuretic effect of PGE_2 in the kidney (Nasrallah et al. 2014). Gastric ulcer healing is also mediated by PGE_2 binding to EP4 (Hatazawa et al. 2007). The desirable clinical effects of EP4 receptor antagonism are likely due to its role as the primary mediator of sensory neuron sensitization and inflammation promoted by PGE_2 (Nakao et al. 2007; Murase et al. 2008). Thus, grapiprant has the potential for anti-inflammatory and analgesic effects. It is worth noting that EP4 receptors are present in canine cardiac tissue (Castleberry et al. 2001), although cardiovascular side effects of grapiprant administration have not been demonstrated.

Publications evaluating the clinical efficacy of grapiprant indicate that it may provide analgesia to dogs affected by osteoarthritis. A multisite clinical study in which owners evaluated pain at home with a pain scale demonstrated improvement in outcomes when compared to a placebo (Rausch-Derra et al. 2016). Dogs had been previously diagnosed with osteoarthritis and were treated with grapiprant once daily at 2 mg/kg. In a model of induced osteoarthritis in dogs, a single dose of firocoxib provided superior analgesia to a single dose of grapiprant, which did not differ from untreated controls (de Salazar Alcalá et al. 2019). Both drugs were administered at labeled doses; analgesia was evaluated by visual scale and weight-bearing analysis. In another induced synovitis study, dogs were administered four total doses of carprofen, grapiprant, or another EP4 antagonist. Two doses were administered before induction of synovitis and two after. Improvement in lameness was evaluated in the same way as Salazar Alcalá et al. Grapiprant provided inferior analgesia to the other two drugs; there was no control group (Budsberg et al. 2019). In an early rat study, an ED_{50} of 4.7 mg/kg was determined in the treatment of inflammatory pain (Murase et al. 2008). Similarly, in a rabbit model of inflammatory pain, a single IV dose of 2 mg/kg grapiprant provided an analgesic effect (De Vito et al. 2017). It is possible that superior analgesia could be provided to dogs at dosages higher than 2 mg/kg/day PO.

Grapiprant is labeled in the US for the control of pain and inflammation associated with osteoarthritis in dogs. It does not currently have any other clinical indications. Long-term safety has been evaluated in both dogs and cats. In a study of 24 healthy cats over 28 days, daily administration of up to 15 mg/kg PO resulted in no gross, histologic or clinical adverse effects (Rausch-Derra and Rhodes 2016). In dogs, daily administration of up to 50 mg/kg PO for nine months resulted in a higher rate of soft or mucoid feces than a control group, with mild changes in serum total protein and albumin that resolved within 30 days of discontinuation. One dog developed mild ileal mucosal regeneration after 50 mg/kg PO for nine months, with no other gross or histologic lesions found in any dogs (Rausch-Derra et al. 2015). In the multisite clinical study of dogs treated for osteoarthritis, dogs administered grapiprant were more likely than controls to develop occasional vomiting (17.5% vs. 6.25%; Rausch-Derra et al. 2016). In dogs, homozygous for the *MDR1* gene mutation, which alters brain penetration and biliary excretion of some drugs, grapiprant administered at 2 mg/kg PO for 28 days resulted in greater drug exposure but was otherwise well-tolerated, with similar occurrence of vomiting in treated dogs (Heit et al. 2021). The safety of grapiprant in pregnant, nursing or breeding animals has not been evaluated. Grapiprant is labeled only for use in dogs; it is not currently recommended for use in other species.

Ketoprofen

Ketoprofen is a non-selective COX-inhibiting NSAID available as an injectable solution for the treatment of cattle and horses in the US. In other countries, ketoprofen is also marketed for the treatment of acute (perioperative) pain in dogs and cats. It is provided as a racemic mixture of S(+) and R(−) stereoisomers.

Ketoprofen is labeled for IV injection but other routes have been investigated in multiple species. Ketoprofen exists in two enantiomeric forms, and the specific enantiomer can have a significant effect on the pharmacokinetics of the drug in different species. Commercially, veterinary ketoprofen is only available as a racemic mixture. Oral bioavailability has been investigated in a range of species and is typically reported as almost completely bioavailable in cats (Lees et al. 2003), dogs (Schmitt and Guentert 1990), and pigs (Raekallio et al. 2008). In horses, in contrast, oral bioavailability ranges from 50% (Landoni and Lees 1995) to 88% (Knych et al. 2016) depending on the formulation administered, and likely the fed/fasted state of the horse. The subcutaneous absolute bioavailability has not been investigated in cattle. Absorption after oral, subcutaneous, and IM administration is typically rapid: T_{max} ranges from 0.34 hours in horses administered the injectable solution orally (Knych et al. 2016) to one hour in pigs administered the solution IM or an oral powder PO (Raekallio et al. 2008). After absorption, ketoprofen is eliminated via hepatic biotransformation, with first-pass metabolism likely for specific enantiomers (Neirinckx et al. 2011). Elimination half-life varies from minutes in sheep (Arifah et al. 2001), goats (Arifah et al. 2003), and horses (Knych et al. 2016) to one to three hours in cats (Lees et al. 2003), dogs (Serrano-Rodríguez et al. 2014), pigs (Raekallio et al. 2008) and cattle (De Koster et al. 2021). In llamas, half-life after a single 4.4 mg/kg IV administration is approximately 5.4 hours (Navarre et al. 2001b), like that of camels which approaches 4.2 hours (Alkatheeri et al. 1999). Half-life can vary significantly by specific enantiomer. The S(+) enantiomer half-life is longer than or equivalent to that of the R(−) enantiomer in most species (Navarre et al. 2001a; Neirinckx et al. 2011). It is likely advantageous that the (S)(+) enantiomer is a more potent COX-inhibitor, with the R(−) enantiomer often irreversibly inverting to S(+) to some degree (Landoni et al. 1997). A single IV administration of ketoprofen to beagle dogs produced detectable plasma concentrations of S(+) for up to 12 hours at both 1 and 3 mg/kg (Serrano-Rodríguez et al. 2014). Significant inversion of the R(−) enantiomer to S(+) does not appear to occur in llamas (Navarre et al. 2001a). A predominance of R(−) was demonstrated in dromedary camels; the authors also demonstrated significant effects of gender (male vs. female

camels) on pharmacokinetics (Al Katheeri et al. 2000). A similar predominance of R(−) was demonstrated in sheep (Delatour et al. 1993). Renal elimination accounts for the majority of metabolite excretion in most species, with a small amount of parent drug also detectable in urine (Sams et al. 1995, Neirinckx et al. 2011).

The clinical effects of ketoprofen are due to non-selective inhibition of the COX enzymes. The resulting decrease in prostaglandin production leads to its anti-inflammatory, anti-pyretic, and analgesic effects. In the US, ketoprofen is labeled for the treatment of inflammation and pain associated with musculoskeletal disorders in horses, and for the treatment of pyrexia associated with Bovine Respiratory Disease (BRD) in beef heifers, beef steers, beef calves two months of age and older, beef bulls, replacement dairy heifers, and dairy bulls (DailyMed 2021). The effectiveness of ketoprofen in the treatment of pyrexia has been demonstrated in cattle (De Koster et al. 2021; DailyMed 2021) and in cats (Glew et al. 1996). Its effectiveness in the treatment of musculoskeletal disease has been demonstrated in horses (Owens et al. 1995), pigs (Mustonen et al. 2011), cattle (Alsaaod et al. 2019), and dogs (Grisneaux et al. 1999). Other indications in which the effectiveness of ketoprofen has been demonstrated include the treatment of platelet activating factor-induced lung injury in calves (Van De Weerdt et al. 1999), pain associated with soft-tissue surgery in cats (Slingsby and Waterman-Pearson 1998), chronic mastitis in cattle (Zecconi et al. 2018) and dehorning in calves (Mills et al. 2020; Duffield et al. 2010). There is indication that ketoprofen can improve recovery from left displaced abomasum (LDA) (Newby et al. 2013a) and parturition (Kovacevic et al. 2019) in cattle.

The adverse effects of ketoprofen administration are similar to those of other non-selective COX-inhibiting NSAIDs. Animal safety studies were performed prior to the marketing of ketoprofen in the US. Cattle were administered 3–15 mg/kg per day for nine days. At the labeled dose of 3 mg/kg, a small degree of renal tubular damage was noted after nine days, three times longer than the labeled duration. No other clinical or hematologic abnormalities were noted. A dose-dependent development of abomasal ulcers was seen as the dose was increased to 15 mg/kg. At up to 11 mg/kg (five times the labeled dosage) for 15 days (three times labeled duration) horses developed no clinical adverse effects. Renal, GI, and hepatic adverse effects developed in a dose-dependent manner as 15- and 25-fold overdoses were administered (DailyMed 2021). Horses administered 2.2 mg/kg every eight hours for a total of 12 days developed lesions of the glandular portion of the stomach, with no evidence of renal damage (MacAllister et al. 1993). Dogs administered ketoprofen for 28 days at the labeled dose for the treatment of osteoarthritis developed prolonged (although still clinically normal) buccal mucosal bleeding times, decreased GFR, and evidence of gastric lesions (Monteiro et al. 2019). The effects of ketoprofen on pregnancy, fertility, lactation, or fetal health have not been investigated in horses or cattle. It is specifically labeled as not for use in reproducing animals over one year of age, dairy calves, or veal calves, lactating dairy cattle or calves less than two months of age. The use of ketoprofen in species other than cattle or horses in the US is extra-label.

Meloxicam

Meloxicam is a COX-2 selective NSAID available as an injectable solution for dogs and cats and as an oral solution for dogs in the US. It should be administered only as a single dose in cats.

Meloxicam has approximately 100% bioavailability after oral and subcutaneous administration to dogs and cats (DailyMed 2020c). In other species, bioavailability ranges from 76% after oral administration to the llama (Kreuder et al. 2012) to 100% in pre-ruminant calves (Coetzee et al. 2009). Other species investigated include rabbits (Fredholm et al. 2013), goats (Wani et al. 2013), horses (Vander Werf et al. 2012; Mendoza et al. 2019), camels (Wasfi et al. 2012) and miniature pigs (Busch et al. 1998). Upon absorption, meloxicam protein binding reaches 97%+ (DailyMed 2020c; Mendoza et al. 2019). Hepatic biotransformation is the most important route of elimination for meloxicam, with very little parent drug excreted in any species (Busch et al. 1998). Volume of distribution at steady-state is relatively low due to high protein-binding and is lowest in dromedary camels (Wasfi et al. 2012). Half-life of elimination is relatively long in companion animals compared to many other NSAIDs, approaching 15 hours in the cat and 24 hours in the dog (DailyMed 2020c). After a single oral administration of 0.31 mg/kg to beagle dogs, plasma concentrations were detectable for up to four days, although they appeared to fall below estimated effective levels of 100 ng/ml between 48 and 72 hours after administration (Yuan et al. 2009). Llamas demonstrate a similar half-life of elimination to companion animals, at 22 and 17 hours after oral and IV administration, respectively (Kreuder et al. 2012). The authors concluded that a single dose of 1 mg/kg meloxicam IV administered to llamas could potentially produce therapeutic plasma concentrations for up to three days. An even longer terminal $t_{1/2}$ has been reported in dromedary camels of 40.2 hours (Wasfi et al. 2012); clearance in this species was extremely low at less than 2 ml/kg/hr. Half-life is shorter in other investigated species, ranging from five to eight hours in goats, pigs, horses, and rabbits in the

aforementioned studies. As can be inferred, the availability of different formulations for oral administration and species differences can affect rate of absorption as well as rate of elimination. Both the kidneys and biliary tract play a significant role in excretion of meloxicam metabolites in most species.

Meloxicam has significant selectivity for the inhibition of COX-2 over COX-1. As a result, it preferentially inhibits upregulation of inflammatory prostanoids over those necessary for homeostasis, theoretically providing a greater safety profile than COX non-selective NSAIDs. This inhibition is what leads to the anti-inflammatory, antipyretic, and analgesic effects of meloxicam. In the US, meloxicam is labeled for the control of pain and inflammation associated with osteoarthritis in dogs and the control of postoperative pain and inflammation associated with soft-tissue and orthopedic surgery in cats. Extra-label indications include the treatment of pain and inflammation associated with soft-tissue and orthopedic surgery in dogs, and in food and fiber animals and horses, for which it is used in other countries around the world.

The efficacy of meloxicam in the treatment of canine osteoarthritis has been demonstrated (Doig et al. 2000). Likewise, perioperative analgesia following soft-tissue (Gassel et al. 2005; Carroll et al. 2005) and orthopedic (Speranza et al. 2015) surgery in cats is evident after meloxicam administration. Extra-label indications in food and fiber animals, as well as horses, are many. In horses, meloxicam was demonstrated to be comparable to phenylbutazone for the treatment of musculoskeletal disease (Olson et al. 2016b), and effective in the treatment of post-castration pain (Olson et al. 2015), and perioperative pain associated with orthopedic surgery (Walliser et al. 2015). There is some evidence that meloxicam is superior to phenylbutazone for the treatment of inflammatory pain, while phenylbutazone is superior for the treatment of mechanical pain in horses (UCVM Class of 2016 et al. 2017). The efficacy of meloxicam has also been demonstrated in calves (Theurer et al. 2012; Olson et al. 2016a), adult cattle (Newby et al. 2013b; Swartz et al. 2018), goats (Ingvast-Larsson et al. 2011), and sheep (Colditz et al. 2019). IM administration of meloxicam to piglets at similar doses, however, does not appear to alleviate pain due to surgical castration (Viscardi and Turner 2018).

The adverse effects of meloxicam are of greatest concern in cats. The veterinary meloxicam label contains a black box warning that reads: "Warning: Repeated use of meloxicam in cats has been associated with acute renal failure and death. Do not administer additional injectable or oral meloxicam to cats." (DailyMed 2020c). The most likely adverse effects in cats include azotemia and renal failure, followed by anorexia, vomiting, and diarrhea (GI), lethargy and depression, and anemia. Target safety and repeated oral dosing studies performed prior to meloxicam approval led to GI and renal side effects, and death in two of nine cats subject to repeated dosing. GI signs and renal adverse effects were also seen in safety studies in dogs when meloxicam was administered at 1, 3, and 5 times the labeled dose (DailyMed 2020c). There appears to be good clinical safety of meloxicam when administered to horses and foals at clinical doses (D'Arcy-Moskwa et al. 2012; Raidal et al. 2013; Vander Werf et al. 2012), although as the dose increases, renal and GI side effects become apparent (Noble et al. 2012). Meloxicam does not appear to increase the risk of fetal membrane retention in cows (Newby et al. 2014). Tissue residues have been investigated in beef calves; a 21-day withholding period appears to be appropriate after repeated administration (Coetzee et al. 2015). The safety of meloxicam in pregnant, breeding, or lactating dogs or cats has not been evaluated. Due to a small safe therapeutic window, administration of meloxicam only at labeled or previously published doses is recommended.

Phenylbutazone

Phenylbutazone is a pyrazolone derivative available for use in horses and dogs in the US. It is supplied as a powder, paste, and tablets for oral administration, and as a solution for IV administration. It was originally developed in 1948, well before purification of the COX enzyme in 1976. Due to the nature of pharmacology knowledge at the time of its development, the use of phenylbutazone became widespread in human and veterinary medicine without significant information regarding its pharmacokinetics and pharmacodynamics. Phenylbutazone is no longer approved for use in human medicine.

The absorption of phenylbutazone after oral administration to horses is significantly affected by the presence of feed, as well as by inter- and within-individual variability. After oral administration to horses, bioavailability ranges from 69% to 91%. When administered to fasted horses, an expected single peak plasma concentration occurs four to six hours after administration. When administered with feed, an initial small peak occurs within the first two hours, followed by a larger maximum peak concentration 10–12 hours after administration. This is thought to be due to phenylbutazone binding to the fibrous component of the equine diet, which is later released for absorption by digestion in the large colon (Maitho et al. 1986; Lees et al. 1986a; Lees and Toutain 2013). Absorption in the large colon in the horse is thought to be a primary cause for one of phenylbutazone's most concerning side effects; RDUC (Karcher et al. 1990). Bioavailability in cattle varies greatly

from 41 to 95% after oral administration (De Backer et al. 1980), and in llamas oral bioavailability approaches 70% (Navarre et al. 2001). Upon absorption, phenylbutazone is ≥98% bound to plasma protein, resulting in a relatively small volume of distribution (Lees et al. 1986b). Metabolism of phenylbutazone is primarily via hepatic biotransformation, with excretion of metabolites in the urinary and biliary tracts. The primary metabolite of phenylbutazone is oxyphenbutazone, which also has anti-inflammatory and analgesic activity (Lees et al. 1986b); although the relative significance of phenylbutazone metabolite activity is unknown, their presence likely prolongs the clinical activity of the drug. Little is known about the plasma disposition of phenylbutazone in dogs, however, a single IV administration of 30 mg/kg IV to racing greyhounds produced detectable plasma concentrations of phenylbutazone at 24 hours, but not at 48 hours (Mills et al. 1995). Half-life of elimination varies greatly among treated species; it is less than two hours in the pig (Hvidberg and Rasmussen 1975), two and seven hours after IV and oral administration, respectively, in llamas (Navarre et al. 2001b), 12.5 hours in dromedary camels (Kadir et al. 1997), 50–60 hours in calves aged four to five months (Arifah and Lees 2002), and greater than 200 hours in neonatal calves (Semrad et al. 1993). Clearly, age can significantly affect phenylbutazone clearance (Eltom et al. 1993). While co-administration with gentamicin in horses does not affect phenylbutazone pharmacokinetics, it significantly alters the pharmacokinetics of gentamicin by decreasing half-life of elimination and volume of distribution (Whittem et al. 1996), an example of how concurrent administration of highly protein-bound drugs should be considered carefully.

The clinical effects of phenylbutazone as an anti-inflammatory, anti-pyretic, and analgesic agent are attributable to its inhibition of COX enzyme activity (Higgins et al. 1984; Lees and Higgins 1987; Beretta et al. 2005). Phenylbutazone is specifically labeled for the relief of inflammatory conditions associated with the musculoskeletal system in horses. Its long history of use in horses and the resulting knowledge of its clinical effects at specific doses and dosing intervals, as well as its relative safety when dosed according to labeling, make it one of the most widely prescribed anti-inflammatory medications in horses to this day. Phenylbutazone may also be used to treat pain and inflammation associated with musculoskeletal disease in dogs, although the availability of numerous other NSAIDs for dogs has made this practice relatively uncommon. The use of phenylbutazone in food-producing animals is controversial; the possibility of human exposure to phenylbutazone residues in treated animals is a significant concern. The anti-inflammatory activity of phenylbutazone in the horse has been demonstrated (Higgins et al. 1984; Lees and Higgins 1987). Phenylbutazone is an effective analgesic agent in the treatment of musculoskeletal disease in horses (Foreman et al. 2008). There does not seem to be a dose-dependent increase in its effectiveness beyond the labeled dose (Hu et al. 2005). In the treatment of specific musculoskeletal disorders, the effectiveness of phenylbutazone may be equivalent to flunixin meglumine (Erkert et al. 2005), despite a widespread belief that phenylbutazone provides superior activity in the treatment of musculoskeletal disorders while flunixin is thought to be superior for treatment of soft-tissue conditions. Phenylbutazone also provides comparable analgesia to that of butorphanol for castration of young horses (Sanz et al. 2009).

The adverse effects of phenylbutazone, like other NSAIDs, primarily involve the GI, renal, and, less often, hepatic systems. During peak phenylbutazone use in humans, some fatalities were reported in people despite appropriate clinical use. As concern for its adverse effects grew, the use of phenylbutazone in people declined, and along with its use in food-producing animals became far less common. In a toxicity study in horses, phenylbutazone administration at three times the daily dose for 12 days resulted in ulceration of the glandular portion of the stomach, edema of the small intestine and erosions and ulceration in the large colon. Renal crest necrosis was present in each of the three horses administered phenylbutazone (MacAllister et al. 1993). The pathogenesis underlying the development of glandular gastric lesions in horses does not appear to involve alterations in PGE_2 production (Pedersen et al. 2018). At 8.8 mg/kg/day (twice the current labeled dose rate) for 21 days, horses developed evidence of protein-losing nephropathy and alterations in volatile fatty acid production and blood flow to the right dorsal colon (McConnico et al. 2008). The safety of phenylbutazone administration to pregnant, lactating or breeding horses or dogs has not been evaluated.

The use of phenylbutazone in female dairy cattle 20 months of age or older is specifically prohibited by the US. FDA.

Piroxicam

Piroxicam is an oxicam derivative NSAID primarily used in the treatment of cancerous tumors in dogs and cats. It is available as generic capsules, chews, and liquid for oral administration in the US.

After oral administration, piroxicam reaches 100% bioavailability in dogs (Galbraith and McKellar 1991) and averages 80% bioavailability in cats (Heeb et al. 2003). In human

plasma, piroxicam is 99%+ bound to plasma protein (Piroxicam Package Insert 2019). The relatively low volume of distribution in dogs (0.29 l/kg) and cats (0.48 l/kg) suggest similarly high plasma protein binding in these species (Galbraith and McKellar 1991; Heeb et al. 2003). Metabolism of piroxicam occurs via hepatic biotransformation primarily through hydroxylation. A small amount of parent drug is excreted in urine, with metabolites found in both feces and urine. Evidence for enterohepatic recirculation has been demonstrated in dogs, cats, and people. This may explain the relatively long half-life of the drug, approaching 14 hours in cats (Heeb et al. 2005), and as high as 43 and 40 hours in dogs, respectively (Hobbs and Twomey 1981; Galbraith and McKellar 1991). After a single 0.3 mg/kg IV administration in the dog, plasma concentrations were equal to 50% of the initial plasma concentration 48 hours after administration. It remained detectable in plasma 72 hours after a single administration, with 47% of thromboxane B_2 inhibition demonstrated at this time. Similar results were demonstrated after oral administration (Galbraith and McKellar 1991). The authors suggested that daily dosing may lead to accumulation. Indeed, in people, piroxicam accumulates after daily dosing, typically reaching steady-state at 7–12 days (FDA 2021).

Piroxicam is a COX-2 selective NSAID. The anti-inflammatory, anti-pyretic, and analgesic effects of piroxicam are due to its COX inhibition. Piroxicam selectivity for COX-2 has been demonstrated in dogs. At concentrations that inhibit 50% (IC_{50}) of COX activity, the COX-2 selectivity of piroxicam is similar to that of meloxicam. At IC_{80}, meloxicam becomes more selective for COX-2 while piroxicam approaches equal COX-1 and COX-2 selectivity (Streppa et al. 2002). The pharmacodynamics behind the anti-tumor activity of piroxicam *in vivo* when combined with chemotherapeutic agents are not clearly understood.

The use of piroxicam in any veterinary species in the US is off label. While the clinical effects of piroxicam mean that it could be used as an anti-inflammatory, analgesic agent for the treatment of osteoarthritis, meloxicam has been demonstrated to have similar efficacy with a superior adverse effect profile (Dequeker et al. 1998). As a result, piroxicam is primarily used as an anti-neoplastic agent in combination with chemotherapeutics. The anti-tumor activity of piroxicam has been demonstrated in dogs with urinary bladder TCC (Mohammed et al. 2003), oral malignant melanoma and oral squamous cell carcinoma (Boria et al. 2004). There is evidence that piroxicam is also an effective anti-tumor agent in cats (DiBernardi et al. 2007; Spugnini et al. 2008). Feline lymphocytic-plasmacytic gingivitis stomatitis has also been effectively treated with piroxicam in combination with bovine lactoferrin (Hung et al. 2014).

The use of piroxicam as an anti-tumor agent means that it may be administered for a longer duration in veterinary patients than other NSAIDs used for the treatment of acute inflammation or pain. The longer an animal is exposed to a drug, at equivalent dose and dosing intervals, the more likely they are to develop toxicity. The adverse effect profile of dogs treated with piroxicam and cisplatin in one study included mild azotemia that resolved with discontinuation of cisplatin, mild GI toxicosis in two of 20 dogs, and severe GI toxicosis in one dog that resolved with treatment (Boria et al. 2004). Early investigation of piroxicam administered in combination with cisplatin for the treatment of canine bladder TCC led to a dose-dependent, clinically significant renal toxicity (Mohammed et al. 2003). In a retrospective study of 73 cats administered piroxicam at clinical doses for various neoplasms, 29% of cats were reported to experience adverse effects, the majority of which were mild and transient. In eight of the 73 cats, piroxicam was discontinued due to significant adverse effects, with azotemia being a significant concern (Bulman-Fleming et al. 2010). An investigation into the acute toxicity of piroxicam due to overdose in various monogastric animals demonstrated GI, hepatic, renal, and neurologic adverse effects culminating in death (Saganuwan and Orinya 2016). The pharmacology of piroxicam has not been investigated in breeding, pregnant or lactating dogs or cats. Use of piroxicam in all veterinary species is off label in the US.

Robenacoxib

Robenacoxib is a COX-2 selective NSAID available as a tablet, injectable solution, and powder for reconstitution for use in dogs and cats in the US. It is one of the more recently developed NSAIDs for use in companion animals.

The pharmacokinetics of robenacoxib have been investigated in both the dog and the cat. After subcutaneous administration, bioavailability of robenacoxib in cats averages 69%. The presence of food in the stomach significantly affects bioavailability of oral administration in cats; after 12 hours of fasting oral bioavailability approached 49%, whereas bioavailability when administered with food is only 10% (King et al. 2013). The authors recommended either subcutaneous administration, or administration with little to no food in cats. Bioavailability is somewhat higher in dogs, averaging 88% after subcutaneous administration, 62% with feed and 84% after fasting (Jung et al. 2009). Time--to-peak plasma concentration is short in both species indicating rapid absorption, ranging from 15 minutes after oral administration to fed dogs to 90 minutes after oral administration in cats. Protein-binding in plasma is ≥98%, coinciding with a low steady-state volume

of distribution of 0.24 l/kg in dogs. After IV administration of 1 mg/kg, robenacoxib was detectable for six hours in plasma; after oral and subcutaneous administration of the same dose, plasma concentrations were detected up to eight hours after administration in some dogs (Jung et al. 2009). Metabolism of robenacoxib occurs primarily via hepatic biotransformation, with minimal parent drug excretion. The majority of the metabolites are excreted via the fecal route, with some eliminated in the urine (DailyMed 2020b). Terminal half-life of elimination is ≤1 hour in dogs and one to two hours in cats.

The anti-inflammatory and analgesic effects for which robenacoxib is prescribed are due to COX inhibition and subsequent reduction in production of prostaglandins. Robenacoxib has been shown to have high selectivity for COX-2 in both cats (Giraudel et al. 2009; Pelligand et al. 2014) and dogs (King et al. 2010). King et al. (2010) compared the COX selectivity of robenacoxib to that of meloxicam, carprofen, deracoxib, and other NSAIDs in dogs. Of the NSAIDs investigated, robenacoxib was found to have the greatest selectivity for COX-2. Robenacoxib is specifically labeled for the treatment of postoperative pain and inflammation associated with orthopedic surgery, ovariohysterectomy, and castration in cats ≥4 months of age, and for the control of pain and inflammation associated with soft-tissue surgery in dogs ≥4 months of age (DailyMed 2020b). In cats administered three robenacoxib doses perioperatively, robenacoxib provided sufficient analgesia after ovariohysterectomy (Sattasathuchana et al. 2018). In a multisite study, 96 cats were administered either a single dose of meloxicam or robenacoxib before induction of anesthesia for soft-tissue or orthopedic surgery; robenacoxib was found to have superior analgesic efficacy (Kamata et al. 2012). It is noteworthy that the majority of surgeries in that study were ovariohysterectomies. A later multisite study of 147 cats demonstrated non-inferior efficacy of robenacoxib compared to meloxicam for the treatment of perioperative pain associated with orthopedic surgery (Speranza et al. 2015). Robenacoxib is also non-inferior in efficacy compared to ketoprofen in the treatment of musculoskeletal disorders (Giraudel et al. 2010; Sano et al. 2012), with Sano et al. (2012) reporting superior efficacy as compared to ketoprofen in owners' assessment of activity and the human/animal relationship. The efficacy of robenacoxib for its labeled indications was further confirmed with a large multi-center study of 349 cats (King et al. 2016[a]). In dogs, analgesic efficacy in a model of acute joint inflammation was non-inferior to meloxicam (Schmid et al. 2010). Robenacoxib is also effective in the treatment of canine osteoarthritis, with similar efficacy and tolerability when compared to carprofen over a three-month treatment period (Reymond et al. 2012).

Robenacoxib has been demonstrated to have relatively high safety margins in comparison to administration of other NSAIDs. In preclinical trials, the most common adverse effects were incisional infection, dehiscence or bleeding in cats, and mild GI signs in cats and dogs (DailyMed 2020b). Robenacoxib has been shown to have no effect on GFR in cats (King et al. 2016b) or dogs (Panteri et al. 2017) when administered orally at 2 mg/kg for seven days. King et al. (2011) demonstrated no adverse effects of robenacoxib on the kidney, liver or GI tract when administered at up to 5× (10 mg/kg) the clinical dose orally for six months to healthy young beagle dogs. Toutain et al. (2018) published similar results. In cats administered up to 10 mg/kg orally for up to 42 days, no adverse effects were demonstrated clinically or histologically (King et al. 2012). In the clinical efficacy trial comparing robenacoxib to carprofen for the treatment of canine osteoarthritis, some dogs developed mild GI signs when administered

2 mg/kg orally for 12 weeks (Reymond et al. 2012). It is unknown whether these adverse events are related to robenacoxib administration. Toutain et al. (2017) also demonstrated that the oral and subcutaneous formulations may be safely interchanged in healthy young dogs over a series of 20-day cycles. Preclinical trials demonstrated some subcutaneous tissue inflammation and necrosis when subcutaneous injections were repeatedly administered over periods longer than three days. Long-term administration of robenacoxib may prolong the QT interval; cardiovascular health should be monitored (DailyMed 2020b). A single IV dose of robenacoxib does not appear to have significant adverse cardiovascular effects in healthy adult dogs (Desevaux et al. 2017). The safety of robenacoxib has not been investigated in breeding, pregnant or lactating cats or dogs. Use of robenacoxib for more than three days, or in species other than cats and dogs is off label in the US.

References

Al Katheeri, N.A., Wasfi, I.A., Lambert, M. et al. (2000). Pharmacokinetics of ketoprofen enantiomers after intravenous administration of racemate in camels: effect of gender. *J. Vet. Pharmacol. Ther.* 3: 137–143.

Ali, B.H., Cheng, Z., el Hadrami, G. et al. (1996). Comparative pharmacokinetics of paracetamol (acetaminophen) and its sulphate and glucuronide metabolites in desert camels and goats. *J. Vet. Pharmacol. Ther.* 3: 238–244.

Alkatheeri, N.A., Wasfi, I.A., and Lambert, M. (1999). Pharmacokinetics and metabolism of ketoprofen after intravenous and intramuscular administration in camels. *J. Vet. Pharmacol. Ther.* 2: 127–135.

Alsaaod, M., Fadul, M., Deiss, R. et al. (2019). Use of validated objective methods of locomotion characteristics and weight distribution for evaluating the efficacy of ketoprofen for alleviating pain in cows with limb pathologies. *PLoS One* 6: e0218546.

Arifah, A.K. and Lees, P. (2002). Pharmacodynamics and pharmacokinetics of phenylbutazone in calves. *J. Vet. Pharmacol. Ther.* 4: 299–309.

Arifah, A.K., Landoni, M.F., Frean, S.P., and Lees, P. (2001). Pharmacodynamics and pharmacokinetics of ketoprofen enantiomers in sheep. *Am. J. Vet. Res.* 1: 77–86.

Arifah, A.K., Landoni, M.F., and Lees, P. (2003). Pharmacodynamics, chiral pharmacokinetics and PK-PD modelling of ketoprofen in the goat. *J. Vet. Pharmacol. Ther.* 2: 139–150.

Autefage, A., Palissier, F.M., Asimus, E., and Pepin-Richard, C. (2011). Long-term efficacy and safety of firocoxib in the treatment of dogs with osteoarthritis. *Vet. Rec.* 23: 617.

Baek, I. (2019). Pharmacokinetic modeling and simulation of etodolac following single oral administration in dogs. *Xenobiotica* 8: 981–986.

Bakirel, T., Alkan, F.U., Üstüner, O. et al. (2016). Synergistic growth inhibitory effect of deracoxib with doxorubicin against a canine mammary tumor cell line, CMT-U27. *J. Vet. Med. Sci.* 4: 657–668.

Beretta, C., Garavaglia, G., and Cavalli, M. (2005). COX-1 and COX-2 inhibition in horse blood by phenylbutazone, flunixin, carprofen and meloxicam: an in vitro analysis. *Pharmacol. Res.* 4: 302–306.

Bienhoff, S.E., Smith, E.S., Roycroft, L.M. et al. (2011). Efficacy and safety of deracoxib for the control of postoperative pain and inflammation associated with dental surgery in dogs. *ISRN Vet. Sci.* 2011: 593015.

Bienhoff, S.E., Smith, E.S., Roycroft, L.M., and Roberts, E.S. (2012). Efficacy and safety of Deracoxib for control of postoperative pain and inflammation associated with soft tissue surgery in dogs. *Vet. Surg.* 41: 336–344.

Boria, P.A., Murry, D.J., Bennett, P.F. et al. (2004). Evaluation of cisplatin combined with piroxicam for the treatment of oral malignant melanoma and oral squamous cell carcinoma in dogs. *J. Am. Vet. Med. Assoc.* 3: 388–394.

Brideau, C., Van Staden, C., and Chan, C.C. (2001). In vitro effects of cyclooxygenase inhibitors in whole blood of horses, dogs, and cats. *Am. J. Vet. Res.* 11: 1755–1760.

Budsberg, S.C., Johnston, S.A., Schwarz, P.D. et al. (1999). Efficacy of etodolac for the treatment of osteoarthritis of the hip joints in dogs. *J. Am. Vet. Med. Assoc.* 2: 206–210.

Budsberg, S.C., Kleine, S.A., Norton, M.M., and Sandberg, G.S. (2019). Comparison of two inhibitors of E-type prostanoid receptor four and carprofen in dogs with experimentally induced acute synovitis. *Am. J. Vet. Res.* 11: 1001–1006.

Bulman-Fleming, J.C., Turner, T.R., and Rosenberg, M.P. (2010). Evaluation of adverse events in cats receiving long-term piroxicam therapy for various neoplasms. *J. Feline Med. Surg.* 4: 262–268.

Busch, U., Schmid, J., Heinzel, G. et al. (1998). Pharmacokinetics of meloxicam in animals and the relevance to humans. *Drug Metab. Dispos.* 6: 576–584.

Carprofen Package Insert (2020). *Carprofen Caplets 75mg.* Dublin OH: Covetrus North America Available at: https://dailymed.nlm.nih.gov/dailymed/drugInfo.cfm?setid=1dbbfaa4-aff3-4dfc-895b-38d9f5dcdf87.

Carrick, J.B., Papich, M.G., Middleton, D.M. et al. (1989). Clinical and pathological effects of flunixin meglumine administration to neonatal foals. *Can. J. Vet. Res.* 2: 195–201.

Carroll, G.L., Howe, L.B., and Peterson, K.D. (2005). Analgesic efficacy of preoperative administration of meloxicam or butorphanol in onychectomized cats. *J. Am. Vet. Med. Assoc.* 6: 913–919.

Case, J.B., Fick, J.L., and Rooney, M.B. (2010). Proximal duodenal perforation in three dogs following deracoxib administration. *J. Am. Anim. Hosp. Assoc.* 46: 255–258.

Castleberry, T.A., Lu, B., Smock, S.L., and Owen, T.A. (2001). Molecular cloning and functional characterization of the canine prostaglandin E2 receptor EP4 subtype. *Prostaglandins Other Lipid Mediat.* 4: 167–187.

Cayen, M.N., Kraml, M., Ferdinandi, E.S. et al. (1981). The metabolic disposition of etodolac in rats, dogs, and man. *Drug Metab. Rev.* 2: 339–362.

Chandrasekharan, N.V., Dai, H., Turepu Roos, K.L. et al. (2002). COX-3, a cyclooxygenase-1 variant inhibited by acetaminophen and other analgesic/antipyretic drugs: cloning, structure, and expression. *Proc. Natl. Acad. Sci. U.S.A.* 21: 13926–13931.

Chen, L., Yang, G., and Grosser, T. (2013). Prostanoids and inflammatory pain. *Prostaglandins Other Lipid Mediat.* 104, 105: 58–66.

Clark, T.P., Chieffo, C., Huhn, J.C. et al. (2003). The steady-state pharmacokinetics and bioequivalence of carprofen administered orally and subcutaneously in dogs. *J. Vet. Pharmacol. Therap.* 26: 187–192.

Coetzee, J.F., KuKanich, B., Mosher, R., and Allen, P.S. (2009). Pharmacokinetics of intravenous and oral meloxicam in ruminant calves. *Vet. Ther.* 4: E1–E8.

Coetzee, J.F., Mosher, R.A., Griffith, G.R. et al. (2015). Pharmacokinetics and tissue disposition of meloxicam in beef calves after repeated oral administration. *J. Vet. Pharmacol. Ther.* 6: 556–562.

Colditz, I.G., Paull, D.R., Lloyd, J.B. et al. (2019). Efficacy of meloxicam in a pain model in sheep. *Aust. Vet. J.* 1, 2: 23–32.

Cook, J.C., Jacobson, C.F., Gao, F. et al. (2003). Analysis of the nonsteroidal anti-inflammatory drug literature for potential developmental toxicity in rats and rabbits. *Birth Defects Res.* 68: 5–26.

Cramer, M.C., Pairis-Garcia, M.D., Bowman, A.S. et al. (2019). Pharmacokinetics of transdermal flunixin in sows. *J. Vet. Pharmacol. Ther.* 4: 492–495.

Currah, J.M., Hendrick, S.H., and Stookey, J.M. (2009). The behavioral assessment and alleviation of pain associated with castration in beef calves treated with flunixin meglumine and caudal lidocaine epidural anesthesia with epinephrine. *Can. Vet. J.* 4: 375–382.

DailyMed (2018). Galliprant- grapiprant tablet. https://dailymed.nlm.nih.gov/dailymed/drugInfo.cfm?setid=a38cc5c6-93e8-4c90-aabc-33bc8423beab (accessed 30 June 2022).

DailyMed (2020a). Equioxx-firocoxib tablet, chewable. https://dailymed.nlm.nih.gov/dailymed/drugInfo.cfm?setid=3f891a61-ce58-4cc1-97e2-a161907ea8eb (accessed 30 June 2022).

DailyMed (2020b). Onsior- robenacoxib injection. https://dailymed.nlm.nih.gov/dailymed/drugInfo.cfm?setid=f4f307a0-88b5-4740-b198-35edef954bf1 (accessed 30 June 2022).

DailyMed (2020c). Ostilox- meloxicam injection, solution. https://dailymed.nlm.nih.gov/dailymed/drugInfo.cfm?setid=88df74f2-853c-433f-a398-a3bc60b3e984 (acessed 30 June 2022).

DailyMed (2021). Ketofen- ketoprofen injection, solution. https://dailymed.nlm.nih.gov/dailymed/drugInfo.cfm?setid=412cb3e9-53dc-4068-a1ab-00b771112f88 (accessed 30 June 2022).

D'Arcy-Moskwa, E., Noble, G.K., Weston, L.A. et al. (2012). Effects of meloxicam and phenylbutazone on equine gastric mucosal permeability. *J. Vet. Intern. Med.* 6: 1494–1499.

Davila, D., Keeshen, T.P., Evans, R.B., and Conzemius, M.G. (2013). Comparison of the analgesic efficacy of perioperative firocoxib and tramadol administration in dogs undergoing tibial plateau leveling osteotomy. *J. Am. Vet. Med. Assoc.* 2: 225–231.

De Backer, P., Braeckman, R., Belpaire, F., and Debackere, M. (1980). Bioavailability and pharmacokinetics of phenylbutazone in the cow. *J. Vet. Pharmacol. Therap.* 3: 29–33.

De Koster, J., Tena, J.K., and Stegemann, M.R. (2021). Treatment of bovine respiratory disease with a single administration of tulathromycin and ketoprofen. *Vet. Rec.* 2: e834.

De Vito, V., Salvadori, M., Poapolathep, A. et al. (2017). Pharmacokinetic/pharmacodynamic evaluation of grapiprant in a carrageenan-induced inflammatory pain model in the rabbit. *J. Vet. Pharmacol. Ther.* 5: 468–475.

Delatour, P., Benoit, E., Bourdin, M. et al. (1993). Enantiosélectivité comparée de la disposition de deux anti-inflammatoires non stéroïdiens, le kétoprofène et le carprofène, chez l'homme et l'animal [Comparative enantioselectivity of the disposition of two non-steroidal anti-inflammatory agents, ketoprofen and carprofen, in man and animals]. *Bull. Acad. Natl. Med.* 3: 515–526. discussion 526–527.

Delatour, P., Foot, R., Foster, A.P. et al. (1996). Pharmacodynamics and chiral pharmacokinetics of Carprofen in calves. *Br. Vet. J.* 153: 183–198.

Dequeker, J., Hawkey, C., Kahan, A. et al. (1998). Improvement in gastrointestinal tolerability of the selective cyclooxygenase (COX)-2 inhibitor, meloxicam, compared with piroxicam: results of the safety and efficacy large-scale evaluation of COX-inhibiting therapies (SELECT) trial in osteoarthritis. *Br. J. Rheumatol.* 37 (9): 946–951.

Deracoxib Package Insert (2021). *Deracoxib Chewable Tables 12mg*. North America, Dublin, OH: Covetrus Available at: https://dailymed.nlm.nih.gov/dailymed/drugInfo.cfm?seti d=c5f4096c-3a57-49da-9f0a-285d93ba9d1e.

Desevaux, C., Marotte-Weyn, A.A., Champeroux, P., and King, J.N. (2017). Evaluation of cardiovascular effects of intravenous robenacoxib in dogs. *J. Vet. Pharmacol. Ther.* 6: e62–e64.

DiBernardi, L., Doré, M., Davis, J.A. et al. (2007). Study of feline oral squamous cell carcinoma: potential target for cyclooxygenase inhibitor treatment. *Prostaglandins Leukot. Essent. Fatty Acids* 4: 245–250.

Doherty, T.J., Andrews, F.M., Provenza, M.K., and Frazier, D.L. (1998). Acetaminophen as a marker of gastric emptying in ponies. *Equine Vet. J.* 30: 349–351.

Doig, P.A., Purbrick, K.A., Hare, J.E., and McKeown, D.B. (2000). Clinical efficacy and tolerance of meloxicam in dogs with chronic osteoarthritis. *Can. Vet. J.* 4: 296–300.

Doucet, M.Y., Bertone, A.L., Hendrickson, D. et al. (2008). Comparison of efficacy and safety of paste formulations of firocoxib and phenylbutazone in horses with naturally occurring osteoarthritis. *J. Am. Vet. Med. Assoc.* 1: 91–97.

Duffield, T.F., Heinrich, A., Millman, S.T. et al. (2010). Reduction in pain response by combined use of local lidocaine anesthesia and systemic ketoprofen in dairy calves dehorned by heat cauterization. *Can. Vet. J.* 3: 283–288.

Dyke, T.M., Sams, R.A., and Cosgrove, S.B. (1997). Disposition of flunixin after intramuscular administration of flunixin meglumine to horses. *J. Vet. Pharmacol. Ther.* 4: 330–332.

Eltom, S.E., Guard, C.L., and Schwark, W.S. (1993). The effect of age on phenylbutazone pharmacokinetics, metabolism and plasma protein binding in goats. *J. Vet. Pharmacol. Ther.* 2: 141–151.

Erkert, R.S., MacAllister, C.G., Payton, M.E., and Clarke, C.R. (2005). Use of force plate analysis to compare the analgesic effects of intravenous administration of phenylbutazone and flunixin meglumine in horses with navicular syndrome. *Am. J. Vet. Res.* 2: 284–288.

EtoGesic® Freedom of Information Summary (1998). *Etogesic® Tablets*. MO USA: Boehringer Ingelheim Available at: https://animaldrugsatfda.fda.gov/adafda/app/ search/public/document/downloadFoi/2215.

FDA (2021). Feldene® Package Insert. https://www. accessdata.fda.gov/drugsatfda_docs/ label/2021/018147s050lbl.pdf (accessed 30 June 2022).

Foreman, J.H., Barange, A., Lawrence, L.M., and Hungerford, L.L. (2008). Effects of single-dose intravenous phenylbutazone on experimentally induced, reversible lameness in the horse. *J. Vet. Pharmacol. Ther.* 1: 39–44.

Fredholm, D.V., Carpenter, J.W., KuKanich, B., and Kohles, M. (2013). Pharmacokinetics of meloxicam in rabbits after oral administration of single and multiple doses. *Am. J. Vet. Res.* 4: 636–641.

Galbraith, E.A. and McKellar, Q.A. (1991). Pharmacokinetics and pharmacodynamics of piroxicam in dogs. *Vet. Rec.* 24: 561–565.

Gassel, A.D., Tobias, K.M., Egger, C.M., and Rohrbach, B.W. (2005). Comparison of oral and subcutaneous administration of buprenorphine and meloxicam for preemptive analgesia in cats undergoing ovariohysterectomy. *J. Am. Vet. Med. Assoc.* 12: 1937–1944.

Gassel, A.D., Tobias, K.M., and Cox, S.K. (2006). Disposition of deracoxib in cats after oral administration. *J. Am. Anim. Hosp. Assoc.* 3: 212–217.

Giraudel, J.M., Toutain, P.L., King, J.N., and Lees, P. (2009). Differential inhibition of cyclooxygenase isoenzymes in the cat by the NSAID robenacoxib. *J. Vet. Pharmacol. Ther.* 1: 31–40.

Giraudel, J.M., Gruet, P., Alexander, D.G. et al. (2010). Evaluation of orally administered robenacoxib versus ketoprofen for treatment of acute pain and inflammation associated with musculoskeletal disorders in cats. *Am. J. Vet. Res.* 7: 710–719.

Glew, A., Aviad, A.D., Keister, D.M., and Meo, N.J. (1996). Use of ketoprofen as an antipyretic in cats. *Can. Vet. J.* 4: 222–225.

Gobbi, F.P., Di Filippo, P.A., Mello, L.M. et al. (2020). Effects of flunixin meglumine, firocoxib, and meloxicam in equines after castration. *J. Equine Vet. Sci.* 94: 103229.

Graham, G., Scott, K.F., and Day, O.R. (2005). Tolerability of paracetamol. *Drug Saf.* 3: 227–240.

Graham, G.G., Davies, M.J., Day, R.O. et al. (2013). The modern pharmacology of paracetamol: therapeutic actions, mechanism of action, metabolism, toxicity and recent pharmacological findings. *Inflammopharmacology* 21: 201–232.

Grisneaux, E., Pibarot, P., Dupuis, J., and Blais, D. (1999). Comparison of ketoprofen and carprofen administered prior to orthopedic surgery for control of postoperative pain in dogs. *J. Am. Vet. Med. Assoc.* 8: 1105–1110.

Gupta, R. (2018). *Veterinary Toxicology: Basica and Clinical Principles*, 3e, 370–373. London, UK: Saunders Elsevier.

Haines, J.M., Lee, P.M., Hegedus, R.M. et al. (2019). Investigation into the causes of aspirin resistance in healthy dogs. *J. Vet. Pharmacol. Therap.* 42: 160–170.

Hao, C.M. and Breyer, M.D. (2007). Physiologic and pathophysiologic roles of lipid mediators in the kidney. *Kidney Int.* 71: 1105–1115.

Hatazawa, R., Tanaka, A., Tanigami, M. et al. (2007). Cyclooxygenase-2/prostaglandin E2 accelerates the healing of gastric ulcers via EP4 receptors. *Am. J. Physiol. Gastrointest. Liver Physiol.* 4: G788–G797.

Heeb, H.L., Chun, R., Koch, D.E. et al. (2003). Single dose pharmacokinetics of piroxicam in cats. *J. Vet. Pharmacol. Ther.* 26 (4): 259–263.

Heeb, H.L., Chun, R., Koch, D.E. et al. (2005). Multiple dose pharmacokinetics and acute safety of piroxicam and cimetidine in the cat. *J. Vet. Pharmacol. Ther.* 5: 447–452.

Heit, M.C., Mealey, K.L., and King, S.B. (2021). Tolerance and pharmacokinetics of Galliprant™ administered orally to collies homozygous for MDR1-1Δ. *J. Vet. Pharmacol. Ther.* 5: 705–713.

Hernandez-Avalos, I., Valverde, A., Ibancovichi-Camarillo, J.A. et al. (2020). Clinical evaluation of postoperative analgesia, cardiorespiratory parameters and changes in liver and renal function tests of paracetamol compared to meloxicam and carprofen in dogs undergoing ovariohysterectomy. *PLoS One* 15 (2): e0223697.

Heuweiser, W., Iwersen, M., and Goetze, L. (2010). Efficacy of carprofen on conception rates in lactating dairy cows after subcutaneous or intrauterine administration at the time of breeding. *J. Dairy Sci.* 94: 146–151.

Higgins, A.J., Lees, P., and Taylor, J.B. (1984). Influence of phenylbutazone on eicosanoid levels in equine acute inflammatory exudate. *Cornell Vet.* 3: 198–207.

Hobbs, D.C. and Twomey, T.M. (1981). Metabolism of piroxicam by laboratory animals. *Drug Metab. Dispos.* 9 (2): 114–118.

Hocking, P.M., Robertson, G.W., and Gentle, M.J. (2005). Effects of non-steroidal anti-inflammatory drugs on pain-related behaviour in a model of articular pain in the domestic fowl. *Res. Vet. Sci.* 1: 69–75.

Hu, H.H., MacAllister, C.G., Payton, M.E., and Erkert, R.S. (2005). Evaluation of the analgesic effects of phenylbutazone administered at a high or low dosage in horses with chronic lameness. *J. Am. Vet. Med. Assoc.* 3: 414–417.

Hung, Y.P., Yang, Y.P., Wang, H.C. et al. (2014). Bovine lactoferrin and piroxicam as an adjunct treatment for lymphocytic-plasmacytic gingivitis stomatitis in cats. *Vet. J.* 1: 76–82.

Hvidberg, E.F. and Rasmussen, F. (1975). Pharmacokinetics of phenylbutazone and oxyphenabutazone in the pig. *Can. J. Comp. Med.* 1: 80–88.

Ingvast-Larsson, C., Högberg, M., Mengistu, U. et al. (2011). Pharmacokinetics of meloxicam in adult goats and its analgesic effect in disbudded kids. *J. Vet. Pharmacol. Ther.* 1: 64–69.

Jones, S.M., Gaier, A., Enomoto, H. et al. (2020). The effect of combined carprofen and omeprazole administration on gastrointestinal permeability and inflammation in dogs. *J. Vet. Int. Med.* 34: 1886–1893.

Jung, M., Lees, P., Seewald, W., and King, J.N. (2009). Analytical determination and pharmacokinetics of robenacoxib in the dog. *J. Vet. Pharmacol. Ther.* 1: 41–48.

Kadir, A., Ali, B.H., al Hadrami, G. et al. (1997). Phenylbutazone pharmacokinetics and bioavailability in the dromedary camel (*Camelus dromedarius*). *J. Vet. Pharmacol. Ther.* 1: 54–60.

Kamata, M., King, J.N., Seewald, W. et al. (2012). Comparison of injectable robenacoxib versus meloxicam for peri-operative use in cats: results of a randomised clinical trial. *Vet. J.* 1: 114–118.

Karcher, L.F., Dill, S.G., Anderson, W.I., and King, J.M. (1990). Right dorsal colitis. *J. Vet. Int. Med.* 4: 247–253.

King, J.N., Rudaz, C., Borer, L. et al. (2010). In vitro and ex vivo inhibition of canine cyclooxygenase isoforms by robenacoxib: a comparative study. *Res. Vet. Sci.* 3: 497–506.

King, J.N., Arnaud, J.P., Goldenthal, E.I. et al. (2011). Robenacoxib in the dog: target species safety in relation to extent and duration of inhibition of COX-1 and COX-2. *J. Vet. Pharmacol. Ther.* 3: 298–311.

King, J.N., Hotz, R., Reagan, E.L. et al. (2012). Safety of oral robenacoxib in the cat. *J. Vet. Pharmacol. Ther.* 3: 290–300.

King, J.N., Jung, M., Maurer, M.P. et al. (2013). Effects of route of administration and feeding schedule on pharmacokinetics of robenacoxib in cats. *Am. J. Vet. Res.* 3: 465–472.

King, S., Roberts, E.S., and King, J.N. (2016a). Evaluation of injectable robenacoxib for the treatment of post-operative pain in cats: results of a randomized, masked, placebo-controlled clinical trial. *BMC Vet. Res.* 1: 215.

King, J.N., Panteri, A., Graille, M. et al. (2016b). Effect of benazepril, robenacoxib and their combination on glomerular filtration rate in cats. *BMC Vet. Res.* 1: 124.

Kissell, L.W., Smith, G.W., Leavens, T.L. et al. (2012). Plasma pharmacokinetics and milk residues of flunixin and

5-hydroxy flunixin following different routes of administration in dairy cattle. *J. Dairy Sci.* 12: 7151–7157.

Kissell, L.W., Leavens, T.L., Baynes, R.E. et al. (2015). Comparison of pharmacokinetics and milk elimination of flunixin in healthy cows and cows with mastitis. *J. Am. Vet. Med. Assoc.* 1: 118–125.

Kittrell, H.C., Mochel, J.P., Brown, J.T. et al. (2020). Pharmacokinetics of intravenous, intramuscular, oral, and transdermal administration of flunixin meglumine in pre-wean piglets. *Front. Vet. Sci.* 7: 586.

Klauss, G., Giuliano, E.A., Moore, C.P. et al. (2007). Keratoconjunctivitis sicca associated with administration of etodolac in dogs: 211 cases (1992–2002). *J. Am. Vet. Med. Assoc.* 4: 541–547.

Kleinhenz, M.D., Van Engen, N.K., Gorden, P.J. et al. (2016). The pharmacokinetics of transdermal flunixin meglumine in Holstein calves. *J. Vet. Pharmacol. Therap.* 39: 612–615.

Knych, H.K., Stanley, S.D., Arthur, R.M., and Mitchell, M.M. (2014). Detection and pharmacokinetics of three formulations of firocoxib following multiple administrations to horses. *Equine Vet. J.* 46: 734–738.

Knych, H.K., Arthur, R.M., Steinmetz, S., and McKemie, D.S. (2016). Pharmacokinetics of ketoprofen enantiomers following intravenous and oral administration to exercised thoroughbred horses. *Vet. J.* 207: 196–198.

Knych, H.K., Seminoff, K., and McKemie, D.S. (2018). Detection and pharmacokinetics of grapiprant following oral administration to exercised thoroughbred horses. *Drug Test. Anal.*.

Knych, H.K., Arthur, R.M., Gretler, S.R. et al. (2021). Pharmacokinetics of transdermal flunixin meglumine and effects on biomarkers of inflammation in horses. *J. Vet. Pharmacol. Ther.* 5: 745–753.

Kondo, Y., Takashima, K., Matsumoto, S. et al. (2012). Efficacy and safety of firocoxib for the treatment of pain associated with soft tissue surgery in dogs under field conditions in Japan. *J. Vet. Med. Sci.* 10: 1283–1289.

Königsson, K., Törneke, K., Engeland, I.V. et al. (2003). Pharmacokinetics and pharmacodynamic effects of flunixin after intravenous, intramuscular and oral administration to dairy goats. *Acta Vet. Scand.* 3-4: 153–159.

Kopcha, M. and Ahl, A.S. (1989). Experimental uses of flunixin meglumine and phenylbutazone in food-producing animals. *J. Am. Vet. Med. Assoc.* 1: 45–49.

Kovacevic, Z., Stojanovic, D., Cincovic, M. et al. (2019). Effect of postpartum administration of ketoprofen on proinflammatory cytokine concentration and their correlation with lipogenesis and ketogenesis in Holstein dairy cows. *Pol. J. Vet. Sci.* 3: 609–615.

Kraml, M., Cosyns, L., Hicks, D.R. et al. (1984). Bioavailability studies with etodolac in dogs and man. *Biopharm. Drug Dispos.* 5: 63–74.

Kreuder, A.J., Coetzee, J.F., Wulf, L.W. et al. (2012). Bioavailability and pharmacokinetics of oral meloxicam in llamas. *BMC Vet. Res.* 8: 85.

Kvaternick, V., Pollmeier, M., Fischer, J., and Hanson, P.D. (2007). Pharmacokinetics and metabolism of orally administered firocoxib, a novel second generation coxib, in horses. *J. Vet. Pharmacol. Therap.* 30: 208–217.

Landoni, M.F. and Lees, P. (1995). Influence of formulation on the pharmacokinetics and bioavailability of racemic ketoprofen in horses. *J. Vet. Pharmacol. Ther.* 6: 446–450.

Landoni, M.F., Soraci, A.L., Delatour, P., and Lees, P. (1997). Enantioselective behaviour of drugs used in domestic animals: a review. *J. Vet. Pharmacol. Ther.* 1: 1–16.

Lebkowska-Wieruszewska, B., De Vito, V., Owen, H. et al. (2017). Pharmacokinetics of grapiprant, a selective EP4 prostaglandin PGE2 receptor antagonist, after 2 mg/kg oral and i.v. administrations in cats. *J. Vet. Pharmacol. Ther.* 6: e11–e15.

Lees, P. and Higgins, A.J. (1984). Flunixin inhibits prostaglandin E2 production in equine inflammation. *Res. Vet. Sci.* 3: 347–349.

Lees, P. and Higgins, A.J. (1987). Physiological, biochemical and haematological effects on horses of a phenylbutazone paste. *Vet. Rec.* 3: 56–60.

Lees, P. and Toutain, P.L. (2013). Pharmacokinetics, pharmacodynamics, metabolism, toxicology and residues of phenylbutazone in humans and horses. *Vet. J.* 3: 294–303.

Lees, P., Higgins, A.J., Mawhinney, I.C., and Reid, D.S. (1986a). Absorption of phenylbutazone from a paste formulation administered orally to the horse. *Res. Vet. Sci.* 2: 200–206.

Lees, P., Taylor, J.B., Higgins, A.J., and Sharma, S.C. (1986b). Phenylbutazone and oxyphenbutazone distribution into tissue fluids in the horse. *J. Vet. Pharmacol. Ther.* 2: 204–212.

Lees, P., Taylor, P.M., Landoni, F.M. et al. (2003). Ketoprofen in the cat: pharmacodynamics and chiral pharmacokinetics. *Vet. J.* 1: 21–35.

Lees, P., Landoni, M.F., Giraudel, J., and Toutain, P.L. (2004). Pharmacodynamics and pharmacokinetics of nonsteroidal anti-inflammatory drugs in species of veterinary interest. *J. Vet. Pharmacol. Therap.* 27: 479–490.

Letendre, L.T., Tessman, R.K., McClure, S.R. et al. (2008). Pharmacokinetics of firocoxib after administration of multiple consecutive daily doses to horses. *Am. J. Vet. Res.* 11: 1399–1405.

Ludwig, B., Jordan, J.C., and Rehm, W.F. (1989). Carprofen in veterinary medicine: 1. Plasma disposition, milk excretion and tolerance in milk-producing cows. *Schweiz. Arch. Tierheilk.* 131: 99–106.

Lunsford, K.V. and Mackin, A.J. (2007). Thromboembolic therapies in dogs and cats: an evidence-based approach. *Vet. Clin. Small Anim.* 37: 579–609.

MacAllister, C.G., Morgan, S.J., Borne, A.T., and Pollet, R.A. (1993). Comparison of adverse effects of phenylbutazone, flunixin meglumine, and ketoprofen in horses. *J. Am. Vet. Med. Assoc.* 1: 71–77.

MacPhail, C.M., Lappin, M.R., Meyer, D.J. et al. (1998). Hepatocellular toxicosis associated with administration of carprofen in 21 dogs. *J. Am. Vet. Med. Assoc.* 12 (1): 895–901.

Maitho, T.E., Lees, P., and Taylor, J.B. (1986). Absorption and pharmacokinetics of phenylbutazone in Welsh Mountain ponies. *J. Vet. Pharmacol. Ther.* 1: 26–39.

McCann, M.E., Andersen, D.R., Zhang, D. et al. (2004). In vitro effects and in vivo efficacy of a novel cyclooxygenase-2 inhibitor in dogs with experimentally induced synovitis. *Am. J. Vet. Res.* 4: 503–512.

McConnico, R.S., Morgan, T.W., Williams, C.C. et al. (2008). Pathophysiologic effects of phenylbutazone on the right dorsal colon in horses. *Am. J. Vet. Res.* 11: 1496–1505.

McKellar, Q.A., Galbraith, E.A., Bogan, J.A. et al. (1989). Flunixin pharmacokinetics and serum thromboxane inhibition in the dog. *Vet. Rec.* 25: 651–654.

McKellar, Q.A., Pearson, T., Bogan, J.A. et al. (1990). Pharmacokinetics, tolerance and serum thromboxane inhibition of carprofen in the dog. *J. Small. Anim. Pract.* 9: 443–448.

McKellar, Q.A., Delatour, P., and Lees, P. (1994). Stereospecific pharmacodynamics and pharmacokinetics of carprofen in the dog. *J. Vet. Pharmacol. Ther.* 6: 447–454.

McMillan, S.K., Boria, P., Moore, G.E. et al. (2011). Antitumor effects of deracoxib treatment in 26 dogs with transitional cell carcinoma of the urinary bladder. *J. Am. Vet. Med. Assoc.* 8: 1084–1089.

Mellor, P.J., Roulois, A.J.A., Day, M.J. et al. (2005). Neutrophilic dermatitis and immune-mediated haematological disorders in a dog: suspected adverse reaction to carprofen. *J. Small Anim. Pract.* 5: 237–242.

Mendoza, F.J., Serrano-Rodriguez, J.M., and Perez-Ecija, A. (2019). Pharmacokinetics of meloxicam after oral administration of a granule formulation to healthy horses. *J. Vet. Intern. Med.* 2: 961–967.

Mercer, M.A., McKenzie, H.C., Davis, J.L. et al. (2020). Pharmacokinetics and safety of repeated oral dosing of acetaminophen in adult horses. *Equine Vet. J.* 52: 120–125.

Millis, D.L., Weigel, J.P., Moyers, T., and Buonomo, F.C. (2002). Effect of deracoxib, a new COX-2 inhibitor, on the prevention of lameness induced by chemical synovitis in dogs. *Vet. Ther.* 4: 453–464.

Mills, P.C., Ng, J.C., Skelton, K.V. et al. (1995). Phenylbutazone in racing greyhounds: plasma and urinary residues 24 and 48 hours after a single intravenous administration. *Aust. Vet. J.* 8: 304–308.

Mills, P.C., Ghodasara, P., Satake, N. et al. (2020). A novel transdermal ketoprofen formulation provides effective analgesia to calves undergoing amputation dehorning. *Animals (Basel)* 12: 2442.

Miyamoto, H., Onuma, H., Shigematsu, H. et al. (2007). The effect of etodolac on experimental temporomandibular joint osteoarthritis in dogs. *J. Cranio-Maxillofacial. Surg.* 35: 358–363.

Mohammed, S.I., Craig, B.A., Mutsaers, A.J. et al. (2003). Effects of the cyclooxygenase inhibitor, piroxicam, in combination with chemotherapy on tumor response, apoptosis, and angiogenesis in a canine model of human invasive urinary bladder cancer. *Mol. Cancer Ther.* 2 (2): 183–188.

Monteiro, B.P., Lambert, C., Bianchi, E. et al. (2019). Safety and efficacy of reduced dosage ketoprofen with or without tramadol for long-term treatment of osteoarthritis in dogs: a randomized clinical trial. *BMC Vet. Res.* 1: 213.

Morris, T., Paine, S.W., Zahra, P. et al. (2019). Plasma and urine pharmacokinetics of intravenously administered flunixin in greyhound dogs. *J. Vet. Pharmacol. Ther.* 5: 505–510.

Murase, A., Okumura, T., Sakakibara, A. et al. (2008). Effect of prostanoid EP4 receptor antagonist, CJ-042,794, in rat models of pain and inflammation. *Eur. J. Pharmacol.* 1, 2: 116–121.

Mustonen, K., Ala-Kurikka, E., Orro, T. et al. (2011). Oral ketoprofen is effective in the treatment of non-infectious lameness in sows. *Vet. J.* 1: 55–59.

Nakao, K., Murase, A., Ohshiro, H. et al. (2007). CJ-023,423, a novel, potent and selective prostaglandin EP4 receptor antagonist with antihyperalgesic properties. *J. Pharmacol. Exp. Ther.* 2: 686–694.

Nasrallah, R., Hassouneh, R., and Hébert, R.L. (2014). Chronic kidney disease: targeting prostaglandin E2 receptors. *Am. J. Physiol. Renal Physiol.* 3: F243–F250.

National Library of Medicine (US) (2022). Acetaminophen. In: *Drugs and Lactation Database (LactMed)*. Bethesda (MD): National Library of Medicine (US).

Navarre, C.B., Ravis, W.R., Nagilla, R. et al. (2001). Pharmacokinetics of phenylbutazone in llamas following single intravenous and oral doses. *J. Vet. Pharmacol. Ther.* 3: 227–231.

Navarre, C.B., Ravis, W.R., Campbell, J. et al. (2001a). Stereoselective pharmacokinetics of ketoprofen in llamas following intravenous administration. *J. Vet. Pharmacol. Ther.* 3: 223–226.

Navarre, C.B., Ravis, W.R., Nagilla, R. et al. (2001b). Pharmacokinetics of flunixin meglumine in llamas following a single intravenous dose. *J. Vet. Pharmacol. Ther.* 5: 361–364.

Neirinckx, E., Vervaet, C., De Boever, S. et al. (2010). Species comparison of oral bioavailability, first-pass metabolism and pharmacokinetics of acetaminophen. *Res. Vet. Sci.* 1: 113–119.

Neirinckx, E., Croubels, S., De Boever, S. et al. (2011). Species comparison of enantioselective oral bioavailability and pharmacokinetics of ketoprofen. *Res. Vet. Sci.* 3: 415–421.

Newby, N.C., Pearl, D.L., LeBlanc, S.J. et al. (2013a). The effect of administering ketoprofen on the physiology and behavior of dairy cows following surgery to correct a left displaced abomasum. *J. Dairy Sci.* 3: 1511–1520.

Newby, N.C., Pearl, D.L., Leblanc, S.J. et al. (2013b). Effects of meloxicam on milk production, behavior, and feed intake in dairy cows following assisted calving. *J. Dairy Sci.* 6: 3682–3688.

Newby, N.C., Renaud, D., Tremblay, R., and Duffield, T.F. (2014). Evaluation of the effects of treating dairy cows with meloxicam at calving on retained fetal membranes risk. *Can. Vet. J.* 12: 1196–1199.

Newby, N.C., Leslie, K.E., Dingwell, H.D.P. et al. (2017). The effects of periparturient administration of flunixin meglumine on the health and production of dairy cattle. *J. Dairy Sci.* 1: 582–587.

Noble, G., Edwards, S., Lievaart, J. et al. (2012). Pharmacokinetics and safety of single and multiple oral doses of meloxicam in adult horses. *J. Vet. Intern. Med.* 5: 1192–1201.

Okada, C.T.C., Andrade, V.P., Freitas-Dell'Aqua, C.P. et al. (2019). The effect of flunixin meglumine, firocoxib and meloxicam on the uterine mobility of equine embryos. *Theriogenology* 123: 132–138.

Olson, M.E., Fierheller, E., Burwash, L. et al. (2015). The efficacy of meloxicam oral suspension for controlling pain and inflammation after castration in horses. *J. Equine Vet. Sci.* 35: 724–730.

Olson, M.E., Ralston, B., Burwash, L. et al. (2016a). Efficacy of oral meloxicam suspension for prevention of pain and inflammation following band and surgical castration in calves. *BMC Vet. Res.* 1: 102.

Olson, M.E., Nagel, D., Custead, S. et al. (2016b). The palatability and comparative efficacy of meloxicam oral suspension for the treatment of chronic musculoskeletal disease in horses. *J. Equine Vet. Sci.* 44: 26–31.

Orsini, J.A., Ryan, W.G., Carithers, D.S., and Boston, R.C. (2012). Evaluation of oral administration of firocoxib for the management of musculoskeletal pain and lameness associated with osteoarthritis in horses. *Am. J. Vet. Res.* 5: 664–671.

Owens, J.G., Kamerling, S.G., Stanton, S.R., and Keowen, M.L. (1995). Effects of ketoprofen and phenylbutazone on chronic hoof pain and lameness in the horse. *Equine Vet. J.* 4: 296–300.

Pairis-Garcia, M.D., Karriker, L.A., Johnson, A.K. et al. (2013). Pharmacokinetics of flunixin meglumine in mature swine after intravenous, intramuscular and oral administration. *BMC Vet. Res.* 9: 165.

Pairis-Garcia, M.D., Johnson, A.K., Abell, C.A. et al. (2015). Measuring the efficacy of flunixin meglumine and meloxicam for lame sows using a GAITFour pressure mat and an embedded microcomputer-based force plate system. *J. Anim. Sci.* 5: 2100–2110.

Panteri, A., Kukk, A., Desevaux, C. et al. (2017). Effect of benazepril and robenacoxib and their combination on glomerular filtration rate in dogs. *J. Vet. Pharmacol. Ther.* 1: 44–56.

Patrono, C., Coller, B., Dalen, J.E. et al. (2001). Platelet-active drugs. The relationships among dose, effectiveness, and side effects. *Chest* 119: 39S–63S.

Paull, D.R., Lee, C., Colditz, I.G. et al. (2007). The effect of a topical anaesthetic formulation, systemic flunixin and carprofen, singly or in combination, on cortisol and behavioural responses of merino lambs to mulesing. *Aust. Vet. J.* 3: 98–106.

Pedersen, S.K., Cribb, A.E., Read, E.K. et al. (2018). Phenylbutazone induces equine glandular gastric disease without decreasing prostaglandin E2 concentrations. *J. Vet. Pharmacol. Ther.* 2: 239–245.

Peek, S.F., Semrad, S.D., and Perkins, G.A. (2003). Clostridial myonecrosis in horses (37 cases 1985-2000). *Equine Vet. J.* 1: 86–92.

Pelligand, L., King, J.N., Hormazabal, V. et al. (2014). Differential pharmacokinetics and pharmacokinetic/pharmacodynamic modelling of robenacoxib and ketoprofen in a feline model of inflammation. *J. Vet. Pharmacol. Ther.* 4: 354–366.

Piroxicam Package Insert (2019). *Piroxicam Capsules USP 20mg*. NJ USA: West-Ward Pharmaceuticals Corp Available at: https://dailymed.nlm.nih.gov/dailymed/drugInfo.cfm?setid=4eab0dcc-e134-45a3-b63b-9c06540bfa21.

Pollmeier, M., Toulemonde, C., Fleishman, C., and Hanson, P.D. (2006). Clinical evaluation of firocoxib and carprofen for the treatment of dogs with osteoarthritis. *Vet. Rec.* 159: 547–551.

Prevail ® Package Insert (2021). *Flunixin Meglumine Injectable Solution 50mg/mL*. Boise ID: MWI Veterinary Supply Available at: https://dailymed.nlm.nih.gov/dailymed/drugInfo.cfm?setid=9d09fe7d-569b-476c-88db-af31519c7491.

Raekallio, M.R., Hielm-Björkman, A.K., Kejonen, J. et al. (2006). Evaluation of adverse effects of long-term orally administered carprofen in dogs. *J. Am. Vet. Med. Assoc.* 6: 876–880.

Raekallio, M.R., Mustonen, K.M., Heinonen, M.L. et al. (2008). Evaluation of bioequivalence after oral, intramuscular, and intravenous administration of racemic ketoprofen in pigs. *Am. J. Vet. Res.* 1: 108–113.

Raidal, S.L., Edwards, S., Pippia, J. et al. (2013). Pharmacokinetics and safety of oral administration of meloxicam to foals. *J. Vet. Intern. Med.* 2: 300–307.

Rausch-Derra, L.C. and Rhodes, L. (2016). Safety and toxicokinetic profiles associated with daily oral administration of grapiprant, a selective antagonist of the prostaglandin E2 EP4 receptor, to cats. *Am. J. Vet. Res.* 7: 688–692.

Rausch-Derra, L.C., Huebner, M., and Rhodes, L. (2015). Evaluation of the safety of long-term, daily oral administration of grapiprant, a novel drug for treatment of osteoarthritic pain and inflammation, in healthy dogs. *Am. J. Vet. Res.* 10: 853–859.

Rausch-Derra, L., Huebner, M., Wofford, J., and Rhodes, L. (2016). A prospective, randomized, masked, placebo-controlled multisite clinical study of Grapiprant, an EP4 prostaglandin receptor antagonist (PRA), in dogs with osteoarthritis. *J. Vet. Intern. Med.* 3: 756–763.

Reppert, E.J., Kleinhenz, M.D., Montgomery, S.R. et al. (2019a). Pharmacokinetics and pharmacodynamics of intravenous and transdermal flunixin meglumine in meat goats. *J. Vet. Pharmacol. Ther.* 3 (1): 309–317.

Reppert, E.J. et al. (2019b). Pharmacokinetics and pharmacodynamics of intravenous and transdermal flunixin meglumine in alpacas. *J. Vet. Pharmacol. Therap.* 42 (5): 572–579. https://doi.org/10.1111/jvp.12800 (2).

Reymond, N., Speranza, C., Gruet, P. et al. (2012). Robenacoxib vs. carprofen for the treatment of canine osteoarthritis; a randomized, noninferiority clinical trial. *J. Vet. Pharmacol. Ther.* 2: 175–183.

Ricketts, A.P., Lundy, K.M., and Seibel, S.B. (1998). Evaluation of selective inhibition of canine cyclooxygenase 1 and 2 by carprofen and other nonsteroidal anti-inflammatory drugs. *Am. J. Vet. Res.* 11: 1441–1446.

Robinson, N.E. and Sprayberry, K.A. (2009). *Current Therapy in Equine Medicine*, 7e, 498. St. Louis, MO: Saunders Elsevier.

Roscher, K.A., Failing, K., Schenk, I., and Moritz, A. (2017). Suspected aspirin resistance in individual healthy adult warmblood horses. *J. Vet. Pharmacol. Therap.* 40: 16–22.

Saganuwan, S.A. and Orinya, O.A. (2016). Toxico-neurological effects of piroxicam in monogastric animals. *J. Exp. Neurosci.* 10: 121–128.

de Salazar Alcalá, A.G., Gioda, L., Dehman, A., and Beugnet, F. (2019). Assessment of the efficacy of firocoxib (Previcox®) and grapiprant (Galliprant®) in an induced model of acute arthritis in dogs. *BMC Vet. Res.* 1: 309.

Salem, S.I., Elgayed, S.S.A., El-Kelany, W.M., and Abd El-Baky, A.A. (2010). Diagnostic studies on acetaminophen toxicosis in dogs. *Glob. Vet.* 2: 72–83.

Sams, R., Gerken, D.F., and Ashcraft, S.M. (1995). Pharmacokinetics of ketoprofen after multiple intravenous doses to mares. *J. Vet. Pharmacol. Ther.* 2: 108–116.

San, R., Yue, W., and Hasi, S. (2019). Effects of CYP1A enzyme specific inhibitor on pharmacokinetics of Para-acetaminophen in Bactrian camel. *J. Vet. Sci.* 3: e12.

Sano, T., King, J.N., Seewald, W. et al. (2012). Comparison of oral robenacoxib and ketoprofen for the treatment of acute pain and inflammation associated with musculoskeletal disorders in cats: a randomised clinical trial. *Vet. J.* 2: 397–403.

Sanz, M.G., Sellon, D.C., Cary, J.A. et al. (2009). Analgesic effects of butorphanol tartrate and phenylbutazone administered alone and in combination in young horses undergoing routine castration. *J. Am. Vet. Med. Assoc.* 10: 1194–1203.

Sartini, I., Lebkowska-Wieruszewska, B., Lisowski, A. et al. (2021). Pharmacokinetics of acetaminophen after intravenous and oral administration in fasted and fed Labrador Retriever dogs. *J. Vet. Pharmacol. Therap.* 44: 28–35.

Sattasathuchana, P., Phuwapattanachart, P., and Thengchaisri, N. (2018). Comparison of post-operative analgesic efficacy of tolfenamic acid and robenacoxib in ovariohysterectomized cats. *J. Vet. Med. Sci.* 6: 989–996.

Schmid, V.B., Spreng, D.E., Seewald, W. et al. (2010). Analgesic and anti-inflammatory actions of robenacoxib in acute joint inflammation in dog. *J. Vet. Pharmacol. Ther.* 2: 118–131.

Schmitt, M. and Guentert, T.W. (1990). Biopharmaceutical evaluation of ketoprofen following intravenous, oral, and rectal administration in dogs. *J. Pharm. Sci.* 7: 614–616.

Semrad, S.D., McClure, J.T., Sams, R.A., and Kaminski, L.M. (1993). Pharmacokinetics and effects of repeated administration of phenylbutazone in neonatal calves. *Am. J. Vet. Res.* 11: 1906–1912.

Sennello, K.A. and Leib, M.S. (2006). Effects of deracoxib or buffered aspirin on the gastric mucosa of healthy dogs. *J. Vet. Intern. Med.* 20: 1291–1296.

Serrano-Rodríguez, J.M., Serrano, J.M., Rodríguez, J.M. et al. (2014). Pharmacokinetics of the individual enantiomer S-(+)-ketoprofen after intravenous and oral administration in dogs at two dose levels. *Res. Vet. Sci.* 3: 523–525.

Serrano-Rodríguez, J.M., Mengual, C., Quirós-Carmona, S. et al. (2019). Comparative pharmacokinetics and a clinical laboratory evaluation of intravenous acetaminophen in Beagle and Galgo Español dogs. *Vet. Anaesth. Analg.* 2: 226–235.

Shuster, R., Traub-Dargatz, J., and Baxter, G. (1997). Survey of diplomates of the American College of Veterinary Internal Medicine and the American College of Veterinary Surgeons regarding clinical aspects and treatment of endotoxemia in horses. *J. Am. Vet. Med. Assoc.* 1: 87–92.

Slingsby, L.S. and Waterman-Pearson, A.E. (1998). Comparison of pethidine, buprenorphine and ketoprofen for postoperative analgesia after ovariohysterectomy in the cat. *Vet. Rec.* 7: 185–189.

Smith, J.S., Marmulak, T.L., Angelos, J.A. et al. (2020). Pharmacokinetic parameters and estimated milk withdrawal intervals for domestic goats (*Capra aegagrus hircus*) after administration of single and multiple intravenous and subcutaneous doses of flunixin meglumine. *Front. Vet. Sci.* 7: 213.

Soma, L.R., Behrend, E., Rudy, J., and Sweeney, R.W. (1988). Disposition and excretion of flunixin meglumine in horses. *Am. J. Vet. Res.* 11: 1894–1898.

Speranza, C., Schmid, V., Giraudel, J.M. et al. (2015). Robenacoxib versus meloxicam for the control of peri-operative pain and inflammation associated with orthopaedic surgery in cats: a randomised clinical trial. *BMC Vet. Res.* 11: 79.

Spugnini, E.P., Crispi, S., Scarabello, A. et al. (2008). Piroxicam and intracavitary platinum-based chemotherapy for the treatment of advanced mesothelioma in pets: preliminary observations. *J. Exp. Clin. Cancer Res.* 1: 6.

Streppa, H.K., Jones, C.J., and Budsberg, S.C. (2002). Cyclooxygenase selectivity of nonsteroidal anti-inflammatory drugs in canine blood. *Am. J. Vet. Res.* 63: 91–94.

Swartz, T.H., Schramm, H.H., Bewley, J.M. et al. (2018). Meloxicam administration either prior to or after parturition: effects on behavior, health, and production in dairy cows. *J. Dairy Sci.* 11: 10151–10167.

Symonds, K.D., MacAllister, C.G., Erkert, R.S., and Payton, M.E. (2006). Use of force plate analysis to assess the analgesic effects of etodolac in horses with navicular syndrome. *Am. J. Vet. Res.* 4: 557–561.

Takeuchi, K., Kato, S., and Amagase, K. (2010). Prostaglandin EP receptors involved in modulating gastrointestinal mucosal integrity. *J. Pharmacol. Sci.* 3: 248–261.

Tavanaeimanesh, H., Azarnoosh, A., Ashar, F.S. et al. (2018). Comparison of analgesic effects of a constant rate infusion of both tramadol and acetaminophen versus those of infusions of each individual drug in horses. *J. Equine Vet. Sci.* 64: 101–106.

Theurer, M.E., White, B.J., Coetzee, J.F. et al. (2012). Assessment of behavioral changes associated with oral meloxicam administration at time of dehorning in calves using a remote triangulation device and accelerometers. *BMC Vet. Res.* 8: 48.

Toutain, C.E., Heit, M.C., King, S.B., and Helbig, R. (2017). Safety evaluation of the interchangeable use of robenacoxib (Onsior™) tablets and solution for injection in dogs. *BMC Vet. Res.* 1: 359.

Toutain, C.E., Brossard, P., King, S.B., and Helbig, R. (2018). Six-month safety evaluation of robenacoxib tablets (Onsior™) in dogs after daily oral administrations. *BMC Vet. Res.* 1: 242.

UCVM Class of 2016, Banse, H., and Cribb, A.E. (2017). Comparative efficacy of oral meloxicam and phenylbutazone in 2 experimental pain models in the horse. *Can. Vet. J.* 2: 157–167.

Van Beusekom, C.D., Fink-Gremmels, J., and Schrickx, J.A. (2013). Comparing the glucuronidation capacity of the feline liver with substratespecific glucuronidation in dogs. *J. Vet. Pharmacol. Therap.* 37: 18–24.

Van de Weerdt, M.L., Coghe, J., Uystepruyst, C. et al. (1999). Ketoprofen and phenylbutazone attenuation of PAF-induced lung inflammation in calves. *Vet. J.* 1: 39–49.

Vander Werf, K.A., Davis, E.G., and Kukanich, B. (2012). Pharmacokinetics and adverse effects of oral meloxicam tablets in healthy adult horses. *J. Vet. Pharmacol. Ther.* 4: 376–381.

Viscardi, A.V. and Turner, P.V. (2018). Use of meloxicam or ketoprofen for piglet pain control following surgical castration. *Front. Vet. Sci.* 5: 299.

Walliser, U., Fenner, A., Mohren, N. et al. (2015). Evaluation of the efficacy of meloxicam for post-operative management of pain and inflammation in horses after orthopaedic surgery in a placebo controlled clinical field trial. *BMC Vet. Res.* 11: 113.

Wani, A.R., Roy, R.K., Ashraf, A., and Roy, D.C. (2013, 2013). Pharmacokinetic studies of meloxicam after its intravenous administration in local goat (*Capra hircus*) of Assam. *Vet. World* 8: 516–552.

Wasfi, I.A., Al Ali, W.A., Agha, B.A. et al. (2012). The pharmacokinetics and metabolism of meloxicam in camels after intravenous administration. *J. Vet. Pharmacol. Ther.* 2: 155–162.

Wasfi, I.A., Saeed, H.M., Agha, B.A. et al. (2015). Pharmacokinetics and metabolism study of firocoxib in camels after intravenous administration by using high-resolution bench-top orbitrap mass spectrometry. *J. Chromatogr. B Analyt. Technol. Biomed. Life Sci.* 974: 17–23.

Weinkle, K.T., Center, S.A., Randolph, J.F. et al. (2005). Evaluation of prognostic factors, survival rates, and treatment protocols for immune-mediated hemolytic anemia in dogs: 151 cases (1993–2002). *J. Am. Vet. Med. Assoc.* 226: 1869–1880.

Welsh, J.C., Lees, P., Stodulski, G. et al. (1992). Influence of feeding schedule on the absorption of orally administered flunixin in the horse. *Equine Vet. J.* 11: 62–65.

Welsh, E.M., McKellar, Q.A., and Nolan, A.M. (1993). The pharmacokinetics of flunixin meglumine in the sheep. *J. Vet. Pharmacol. Ther.* 2: 181–188.

Whittem, T., Firth, E.C., Hodge, H., and Turner, K. (1996). Pharmacokinetic interactions between repeated dose phenylbutazone and gentamicin in the horse. *J. Vet. Pharmacol. Ther.* 6: 454–459.

Wilson, J.E., Chandrasekharan, N.V., Westover, K.D. et al. (2004). Determination of expression of cyclooxygenase-1 and -2 isozymes in canine tissues and their differential sensitivity to nonsteroidal anti-inflammatory drugs. *Am. J. Vet. Res.* 65: 810–818.

Yuan, Y., Chen, X.Y., Li, S.M. et al. (2009). Pharmacokinetic studies of meloxicam following oral and transdermal administration in Beagle dogs. *Acta Pharmacol. Sin.* 7: 1060–1064.

Zecconi, A., Frosi, S., Cipolla, M., and Gusmara, C. (2018). Effects of chronic mastitis and its treatment with ketoprofen on the milk ejection curve. *J. Dairy Res.* 1: 50–52.

Ziegler, A.L., Freeman, C.K., Fogle, C.A. et al. (2019). Multicentre, blinded, randomised clinical trial comparing the use of flunixin meglumine with firocoxib in horses with small intestinal strangulating obstruction. *Equine Vet. J.* 3: 329–335.

12

Local Anesthetics

Turi K. Aarnes

Pharmacology of Local Anesthetics

Local anesthetics are membrane-stabilizing agents. The resting membrane potential of most nerve cells is −60 to −90 mV. Nerve cells at rest are more permeable to potassium ions, and the potassium ion concentration inside the cell is approximately 30 times greater than the concentration outside the cell. When the nerve is active, sodium channels are triggered to open, and sodium permeability increases so the membrane potential becomes less negative. If the membrane potential increases enough, additional sodium channels open and a wave of depolarization is propagated along the length of the axon.

When local anesthetic drugs are injected near the site of desired action, they diffuse to nerve cells or nociceptors. They cross cell membranes and bind to sodium channels. Local anesthetics stabilize the membranes preventing the depolarization process and initiation or conduction of impulses.

Local anesthetic drugs are weak bases, which dissociate into ionized and un-ionized forms in water. The ionized form of the drug is more water-soluble than the unionized form. Local anesthetics are purchased as acidic solutions, so the majority of the drug is in the ionized form. Once injected into a milieu with a more neutral pH (7.4), the amount of the unionized (neutral) form increases. The un-ionized (neutral) form is lipid soluble and diffuses rapidly through cell membranes to reach the sodium channels (onset of action). Once the local anesthetic reaches the site of action (sodium channel), the ionized (charged) form is responsible for its activity. Thus, the non-ionized form of the drug crosses the cell membrane, and the ionized drugs blocks sodium channels. The ratio of ionized to un-ionized forms depends on the pKa of the drug and the pH of the environment. The pKa determines the degree of ionization and onset of action. As the pKa of the local anesthetic is increased, less free diffusible drug at tissue pH (7.4) is available, delaying the onset of action. For example, the pKa of bupivacaine is higher than that of lidocaine (8.1 vs. 7.6), making bupivacaine slower in onset of action.

The effectiveness of local anesthetics is also affected by the tissue pH. The local environment depends to some degree on the blood supply. Local anesthetics are less effective in an acidic environment, such as tissue with infection and swelling (pH = 3), because there is less uncharged drug present. Other factors that affect activity include protein binding and lipid solubility. As the protein binding of a drug is increased, the duration of the anesthetic effect is prolonged. For example, lidocaine is more protein bound than procaine (80% vs. 6%) so it has a longer duration of action. As the lipid solubility of a drug increases, its potency and toxicity are also increased. Bupivacaine is more lipid soluble than lidocaine, thus it is more potent and potentially more toxic.

Neural Blockade

In veterinary medicine, local anesthetics are most frequently injected near nerves in order to block conduction of impulses through the nerve. Local anesthetic blockade can affect sensory function, autonomic function, motor function or combinations of all three. Many nerves are mixed nerves, which contain fibers of varying diameters and amounts of myelin (e.g. trigeminal, facial, vagus). The fibers are positioned at various places within the nerve sheath.

Nerve Classification

Nerves fibers are classified as large or small, depending on their diameter. Myelin acts like insulation allowing the energy of the nerve impulse activity to be conserved so that the impulse travels farther and at greater speeds. The more myelin, the harder it is to block nerve conduction. Large nerve fibers have a myelin sheath and are not as easily blocked by local anesthetics, and small nerve fibers have little to no myelin and are readily blocked.

Peripheral nerves can be classified according to size. In general, the larger the nerve the more difficult it is to block.

Table 12.1 Nerve Classification based on size, ease of blockade, type of nerve, and primary function.

Size	Ease of block	Nerve	Primary function
Large	Resistant to block	A-alpha	motor
		A-beta	pressure
		A-gamma	proprioception
		A-delta	pain, temperature
		B	preganglionic, sympathetic
Small	Easily blocked	C	pain

Nerve Blockade

Pain and temperature are blocked before touch and motor function. A dog with regional anesthetic blockade (e.g. brachial plexus block, epidural block) can be pain free and still have movement of the limb (differential blockade). Human patients feel no pain in their paralyzed arms or legs after regional anesthetic blockade (e.g. brachial plexus blocks, epidural blocks). We assume that animals are adequately anesthetized if they don't move after a surgical stimulus.

Nerve fibers located on the outer side of the nerve (mantle fibers) supply the more proximal parts of the body (e.g. shoulder, pelvis). Nerve fibers located in the center of the nerve (core fibers) supply the more distal parts of the body (e.g. fingers and toes). Anesthetic blockade progresses from mantle to core. Shoulders and pelvis become anesthetized first, digits become anesthetized last. Spread of anesthesia may take up to 20 minutes. Recovery from blockade occurs from the mantle to the core, because of the larger blood supply around the nerve, so sensation returns first in the shoulder and pelvis. The patient is fully recovered if the sensation in the digits returns.

Other Factors that Influence Local Anesthetic Activity

Other factors that influence local anesthetic activity include the dose of the anesthetic agent (large volume of drug improves diffusion speeding up onset of action), additives, site of injection, and pregnancy.

Additives

Additives that influence local anesthetic activity include vasoconstrictors, hyaluronidase, sodium bicarbonate, and liposomes. Drugs such as epinephrine or the α-2 agonists cause vasoconstriction, which reduce vascular absorption thus prolonging the duration of the local anesthetic effect. Because vasoconstrictors decrease blood flow, they should be added with caution when utilizing in end-arterial areas such as tails or ears as tissue necrosis could occur. Addition of epinephrine to lidocaine decreased the chondrotoxicity of lidocaine following 30-minute exposure (Di Salvo et al. 2016).

Hyaluronidase is an enzyme that break down hyaluronic acid in tissues. Hyaluronidase facilitates the spread of local anesthetic, speeding up the onset of action and broadening the effect. Hyaluronidase also enhances systemic absorption reducing duration and potential increasing toxicity.

Sodium bicarbonate can be combined with some local anesthetic drugs, which will result in alkalinization of local anesthetic solution, which shortens the onset of neural blockade, enhances the depth of sensory and motor blockade, and increases the spread of epidural blockade. Alkalinization increases the percentage of local anesthetic existing in the lipid soluble form that is available to diffuse across lipid cellular barriers. Adding sodium bicarbonate will speed the onset of peripheral nerve block and epidural block by three to five minutes. However, the addition of sodium bicarbonate to some local anesthetics can result in precipitation.

Liposomes are vesicles consisting of bilayers of phospholipid surrounding an aqueous phase. The phospholipid can act as a barrier to drug diffusion from the liposome, effectively resulting in a slow-release preparation with a prolonged duration of action (Mashimo et al. 1992). Incorporation of local anesthetics into liposomes also decreases toxicity. Liposome formulations are available. A new liposome encapsulated bupivacaine has been approved for use in dogs and cats in which bupivacaine has been incorporated into biodegradable microcapsules to prolong the duration of action (see bupivacaine below).

Site of Injection

Intrathecal administration has the shortest activity. Peripheral nerve blocks have the longest activity.

Pregnancy

Duration of ester-linked local anesthetics may be prolonged due to decreased plasma cholinesterase activity. Increased spread and depth of an epidural or spinal (intrathecal) local anesthetic is also reported, due to mechanical factors and hormone changes.

Toxicity of Local Anesthetics

Toxicity of local anesthetic relates to the concentration of local anesthetic in the systemic circulation based on the dose, absorption rate, and metabolism. The clinical signs and order of appearance (from first to last) are seizures (or convulsions), apnea, hypotension, and death. The toxic effects of local anesthetic are typically related to their plasma concentration. Pharmacokinetics are altered (clearance is reduced) in animals following convulsions suggesting prolongation of a toxic effect (Arthur et al. 1988a; Copeland et al. 2008b). However, toxicity effects may be blunted by general anesthesia, resulting in differences in hemodynamic and CNS effects even at the same dosages (Copeland et al. 2008a). Chondrocyte toxicity has been reported with all of the local anesthetics and their intra-articular use has decreased in recent years while infiltration use remains a mainstay of veterinary practice.

Allergic reactions are rare, despite frequent use. It is estimated that less than 1% of all adverse reactions to local anesthetics are due to allergic reactions (humans). Most adverse responses that are attributed to allergic reactions are instead manifestations of excess plasma concentrations.

Chemical Structure of Local Anesthetics and Classification of Local Anesthetics

All clinically used local anesthetics have a similar chemical structure consisting of a lipophilic aromatic ring, and intermediate chain (with either ester or amide linkage), and a hydrophilic secondary chain (Figure 12.1). Lipophilicity may influence the pharmacokinetics of different local anesthetics based on the route of administration (e.g. epidural) and the octanol: water partition coefficient (Nava-Ocampo and Bello-Ramirez 2004).

Ester-Linked Local Anesthetics

Ester-linked local anesthetics are rapidly metabolized by enzymes in the blood (pseudocholinesterase, procaine esterase). The ester-linked local anesthetic drugs typically

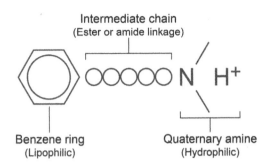

Figure 12.1 Chemical structure of local anesthetics.

have a short anesthetic duration (usually less than one hour), but allergic reactions have occurred (rare). Examples of ester-linked local anesthetics include cocaine, procaine, chloroprocaine, proparacaine, and benzocaine. The ester-linked local anesthetics are not commonly used in veterinary anesthesia.

Amide-Linked Local Anesthetics

Amide-linked local anesthetics are metabolized by the liver. The amide-linked local anesthetic drugs typically have an intermediate (2 hour) or longer (8 hour) anesthetic duration. Examples of amide-linked local anesthetics include lidocaine, mepivacaine, bupivacaine, and ropivacaine.

EMLA cream is a Eutectic Mixture of Local Anesthetics: lidocaine and prilocaine. A eutectic mixture is one in which the individual components are soluble in each other and the resulting compound has a lower melting point than the separate components. A 50:50 (weight: weight) mixture of lidocaine powder and prilocaine powder forms an oil that penetrates intact skin better than either drug alone. There is prolonged time to effect (approximately 60 minutes). There is also a potential for methemoglobinemia formation and so EMLA should not be used in cats. EMLA was as effective as infiltration of 2% lidocaine for episioplasty in mares (Erkert et al. 2005).

Table 12.2 Commonly used local anesthetic in veterinary medicine.

Drug	Onset	Duration	Suggested dose (infiltration)
Lidocaine	5–15 min	1–2 hr	<10 mg/kg
Mepivacaine	5–10 min	2–2.5 hr	<4 mg/kg
Ropivacaine	5–15 min	2.5–4 hr	<4 mg/kg
Bupivacaine	20–30 min	2.5–6 hr	<4 mg/kg

Lidocaine

Lidocaine has an intermediate potency and duration (approximately two hours). The pharmacokinetics of intravenous (IV) lidocaine are discussed in Chapter 20. Lidocaine is metabolized in the liver to two active metabolites in the horse: glycinexylidide and monoethylglycinexylidide as well as inactive metabolites, such as 3-hydroxylidocaine, 4-hydroxylidocaine, dimethylamine, and 4-hydroxydimethylalinine (Dirikolu et al. 2000). Elimination is via urinary excretion (Dirikolu et al. 2000; Dickey et al. 2008). The metabolites in cattle are unknown (Cox et al. 2011).

IV lidocaine has been demonstrated to cause a dose-dependent reduction in the MAC of sevoflurane and isoflurane in dogs (Matsubara et al. 2009; Muir et al. 2003; Wilson et al. 2008), horses (Dzikiti et al. 2003; Rezende et al. 2011; Villalba et al. 2011), and goats (Doherty et al. 2007). Pharmacokinetics of IV lidocaine demonstrated higher serum concentrations in sevoflurane-anesthetized horses compared with awake horses following administration of a 1.3 mg/kg IV loading dose and infusion of 50 mcg/kg/min, likely due to changes in volume of distribution and clearance (Freary et al. 2005). Lidocaine may increase intestinal motility following IV administration (Guschlbauer et al. 2011). Lidocaine has been found in milk following lidocaine infiltration for surgery in cows (Sellers et al. 2009; Puente and Josephy 2001). Significant placental transfer occurs in pregnant ewes and lidocaine should be administered with caution during pregnancy (Kennedy et al. 1990).

Lidocaine has long been the mainstay of local anesthetic techniques in veterinary medicine due to its ubiquity in practice, it is inexpensive, and complications are uncommon.

Topical patches containing 5% lidocaine are utilized to desensitize skin following surgical incisions. Following 72 hours of patch application, dogs and cats had lidocaine accumulation in the skin and low plasma lidocaine concentrations (Ko et al. 2007; Ko et al. 2008; Valverde et al. 2004; Weiland et al. 2006). Systemic lidocaine absorption was also low following 5% lidocaine patch placement in horses (Bidwell et al. 2007).

Mepivacaine

Mepivacaine has intermediate potency and prolonged duration (approximately 2.5 hours) compared to lidocaine. Mepivacaine is supplied as a racemic mixture of two enantiomers (R and S). The major metabolite of mepivacaine in the horse is 3-hydroxymepivacaine, which is excreted in urine (Harkins et al. 1999a).

Mepivacaine is more commonly used in a clinical setting in equine practice compared with small animal practice. It is used for tissue infiltration blocks (Crandall et al. 2020), intraarticular administration (Adler et al. 2020), and nerve blockade (Harcourt et al. 2021).

Ropivacaine

Ropivacaine has a higher potency and longer duration compared with lidocaine and a similar onset as lidocaine. Ropivacaine is supplied as a single enantiomer (S). Due to the potential for cardiac toxicity, ropivacaine should not be administered intravenously.

In comparison to bupivacaine, ropivacaine is less potent (approximately 60%) (Capogna et al. 1999). Ropivacaine has been associated with lower toxicity and less motor blockade than bupivacaine (Brockway et al. 1991), possible related to the formulation as the single S enantiomer. The major urinary metabolite in horses was determined to be 3-hydroxyropivacaine (Harkins et al. 2001).

Clinical use of ropivacaine in veterinary medicine includes for local blockade of nerves (Harkins et al. 2001), regional blockade (Skarda and Muir 2003; Ganidagli et al. 2004), epidural and spinal administration (Arujo et al. 2012), "splash" blockade and surgical site infiltration (Nicacio et al. 2020; de OL Carapeba et al. 2020), and tissue blockade (Cicirelli et al. 2022) in many veterinary species.

Short-term ropivacaine use may result in less chondrotoxicity in equine chondrocytes compared with mepivacaine (Silva et al. 2019) but, in a later study, viability of chondrocytes and fibroblast-like synoviocytes was decreased following ropivacaine exposure (Adler et al. 2021). Bovine chondrocyte viability was negatively affected following ropivacaine exposure (Lo et al. 2009) but there was little effect on bovine tenocytes following exposure to 0.5% ropivacaine (Piper et al. 2012). Ropivacaine may also be associated with decreased toxicity following accidental IV administration due to a more rapid decrease in plasma concentrations compared with bupivacaine (Arthur et al. 1988b).

Bupivacaine

Bupivacaine has a higher potency and longer duration compared with lidocaine, but time to onset tends to be prolonged. Bupivacaine is supplied as a racemic mixture for two enantiomers: D-bupivacaine [R(+)-bupivacaine] and L-bupivacaine [S(−)-bupivacaine] for clinical administration. While pharmacokinetic differences exist in the different racemates, only the racemic mixture of bupivacaine is available clinically (Derossi et al. 2005; Mather et al. 1994). In the horse, bupivacaine is metabolized to 3-hydroxybupivacaine which is excreted in urine (Harkins et al. 1999a, Harkins et al. 1999b).

Bupivacaine has been evaluated for intraarticular administration, and was associated with rapid dilution and a concomitant drop in synovial fluid concentrations suggesting that chondrocyte damage from intraarticular administration would be minimal (Barry et al. 2014). Intermittent infusion of bupivacaine into surgical wounds in dogs was associated with systemic absorption but not anesthesia of the wound (Hardie et al. 2011). Bupivacaine is most often used for infiltration blocks of nerves, for dentistry procedures, epidural and subarachnoid administration, and wound infiltration due to its prolonged duration of action.

A liposome encapsulated formulation of bupivacaine has been approved for use in people, and also recently for use in dogs and cats. The safety of the liposome encapsulated formulation has been evaluated in pre-clinical studies in dogs which determined that the safety of this formulation may be superior to that of the traditional bupivacaine formulation following IV, intraarterial, intrathecal, and epidural administration (Joshi et al. 2015). Incisional administration of the liposome encapsulated formulation dogs and rapids showed no adverse effects, although granulomatous inflammation was noted in one-third of the rabbits (Richard et al. 2011). Similarly, granulomatous inflammation was also associated with its use for peripheral nerve block (brachial plexus) in rabbits and dogs, with a lower maximum plasma concentration compared with bupivacaine solution (Richard et al. 2012). In horses, this formulation was evaluated for perineural injection and was not associated with prolonged analgesia (Le et al. 2020).

References

Adler, D.M.T., Serteyn, D., Franck, T. et al. (2020). Effects of intra-articular administration of lidocaine, mepivacaine, and the preservative methyl parahydroxybenzoate on synovial fluid biomarkers of horses. *Am. J. Vet. Res.* 81: 479–487.

Adler, D.M.T., Frellesen, J.F., Karlsen, C.V. et al. (2021). Evaluation of the in vistro effects of local anesthetics on equine chondrocytes and fibroblast-like synoviocytes. *Am. J. Vet. Res.* 82: 478–486.

Arthur, G.R., Feldman, H.S., and Covino, B.G. (1988a). Alterations in the pharmacokinetic properties of amide local anaesthetics following local anaesthetic induced convulsions. *Acta Anesthesiol. Scand.* 32: 522–529.

Arthur, G.R., Feldman, H.S., and Covino, B.G. (1988b). Comparative pharmacokinetics of bupivacaine and ropivacaine, a new amide local anesthetic. *Anesth. Analg.* 67: 1053–1058.

Arujo, M.A., Albuquergue, V.B., Deschk, M. et al. (2012). Cardiopulmonary and analgesic effects of caudal epidurally administered ropivacaine in cattle. *Vet. Anaesth. Analg.* 39: 409–413.

Barry, S.L., Martinez, S.A., Davies, N.M. et al. (2014). Synovial fluid bupivacaine concentration following single intra-articular injection in normal and osteoarthritic canine stifles. *J. Vet. Pharmacol. Therap.* 38: 97–100.

Bidwell, L.A., Wilson, D.V., and Caron, J.P. (2007). Lack of systemic absorption of lidocaine from 5% patches placed on horses. *Vet. Anaesth. Analg.* 34: 443–446.

Brockway, M.S., Bannister, J., McClure, J.H. et al. (1991). Comparison of extradural ropivacaine and bupivacaine. *Bri. J. Anaesth.* 66: 31–33.

Capogna, G., Celleno, D., Fusco, P. et al. (1999). Relative potencies of bupivacaine and ropivacaine for analgesia in labor. *Bri. J. Anaesth.* 82: 371–373.

Cicirelli, V., Matteo, B., Di Bella, C. et al. (2022). The ultrasound-guided funicular block in cats undergoing orchiectomy: a ropivacaine injection into the spermatic cord to improve intra and postoperative analgesia. *BMC Vet. Res.* 18: 169.

Copeland, S.E., Ladd, L.A., Gu, X. et al. (2008a). The effects of general anesthesia on the central nervous and cardiovascular system toxicity of local anesthetics. *Anesth. Analg.* 106: 1429–1439.

Copeland, S.E., Ladd, L.A., Gu, X. et al. (2008b). The effects of general anesthesia on whole body and regional pharmacokinetics of local anesthetics at toxic doses. *Anesth. Analg.* 106: 1440–1449.

Cox, S., Wilson, J., and Doherty, T. (2011). Pharmacokinetics of lidocaine after intravenous administration to cows. *J. Vet. Pharmacol. Therap.* 35: 305–308.

Crandall, A., Hopster, K., Grove, A. et al. (2020). Intratesticular mepivacaine versus lidocaine in anaesthetised horses undergoing Henderson castration. *Equine Vet. J.* 52: 805–810.

Derossi, R., Migel, G.L.S., Frazilio, F.O. et al. (2005). L-bupivacaine 0.5% vs. racemic 0.5% bupivacaine for caudal epidural analgesia in horses. *J. Vet. Pharmacol. Therap.* 28: 293–297.

Di Salvo, A., Chiaradia, E., Della Rocca, G. et al. (2016). Intra-articular administration of lidocaine plus adrenaline in dogs: pharmacokinetic profile and evaluation of toxicity in vivo and in vitro. *Vet. J.* 208: 70–75.

Dickey, E.J., McKenzie, H.C. III, Brown, J.A. et al. (2008). Serum concentrations of lidocaine and its metabolites after prolonged infusion in healthy horses. *Equine Vet. J.* 40: 348–352.

Dirikolu, L., Lehner, A.F., Karpiesiuk, W. et al. (2000). Identification of lidocaine and its metabolites in post-administration equine urine by ELISA and MS/MS. *J. Vet. Pharmacol. Therap.* 23: 215–222.

Doherty, T., Redua, M.A., Queiroz-Castro, P. et al. (2007). Effect of intravenous lidocaine and ketamine on the minimum alveolar concentration of isoflurane in goats. *Vet. Anaesth. Analg.* 34: 125–131.

Dzikiti, T.B., Hellebrekers, L.J., and van Dijk, P. (2003). Effects of intravenous lidocaine on isoflurane concentration, physiological parameters, metabolic parameters and stress-related hormones in horses undergoing surgery. *J. Vet. Med. A Physiol. Pathol. Clin. Med.* 50: 190–195.

Erkert, R.S., Macallister, C.G., Campbell, G. et al. (2005). Comparison of topical lidocaine/prilocaine anesthetic cream and local infiltration of 2% lidocaine for episioplasty in mares. *J. Vet. Pharmacol. Therap.* 28: 299–304.

Freary, D.J., Mama, K.R., Wagner, A.E. et al. (2005). Influence of general anesthesia on pharmacokinetics of intravenous lidocaine infusion in horses. *Am. J. Vet. Res.* 66: 574–580.

Ganidagli, S., Cetin, H., Biricik, H.S. et al. (2004). Comparison of ropivacaine with a combination of ropivacaine and fentanyl for the caudal epidural anaesthesia of mares. *Vet. Rec.* 154: 329–332.

Guschlbauer, M., Feige, K., Geburek, F. et al. (2011). Effects of in vivo lidocaine administration at the time of ischemia and reperfusion on in vitro contractility of equine jejunal smooth muscle. *Am. J. Vet. Res.* 72: 1449–1455.

Harcourt, M.M., Smith, R.L., and Hosgood, G. (2021). Duration of skin desensitization following palmar digital nerve blocks with lidocaine, bupivacaine, mepivacaine, and prilocaine. *Aust. Vet. J.* 99: 541–546.

Hardie, E.M., Lascelles, B.D.X., Meuten, T. et al. (2011). Evaluation of intermittent infusion of bupivacaine into surgical wounds of dogs postoperatively. *Vet. J.* 190: 287–289.

Harkins, J.D., Karpiesiuk, W., Woods, W.E. et al. (1999a). Mepivacaine: its pharmacological effects and their relationship to analytical findings in the horse. *J. Vet. Pharmacol. Therap.* 22: 107–121.

Harkins, J.D., Lehner, A., Karpiesiuk, W. et al. (1999b). Bupivacaine in the horse: relationship of local anaesthetic responses and urinary concentrations of 3-hydroxybupivacaine. *J. Vet. Pharmacol. Therap.* 22: 181–195.

Harkins, J.D., Karpiesiuk, W., Lehner, A. et al. (2001). Ropivacaine in the horse: its pharmacological responses, urinary detection and mass spectral confirmation. *J. Vet. Pharmacol. Therap.* 24: 89–98.

Joshi, G.P., Patou, G., and Kharitonov, V. (2015). The safety of liposome bupivacaine following various routes of administration in animals. *J. Pain Res.* 8: 781–789.

Kennedy, R.L., Bell, J.U., Miller, R.P. et al. (1990). Uptake and distribution of lidocaine in fetal lambs. *Anesthesiology* 72: 483–489.

Ko, J., Weil, A., Maxwell, L. et al. (2007). Plasma concentrations of lidocaine in dogs following lidocaine patch application. *J. Am. Anim. Hosp. Assoc.* 43: 280–283.

Ko, J.C.H., Maxwell, L.K., Abbo, L.A. et al. (2008). Pharmacokinetics of lidocaine following the application of 5% lidocaine patches to cats. *J. Vet. Pharmacol. Therap.* 31: 359–367.

Le, K.M., Caston, S.S., Hossetter, J.M. et al. (2020). Comparison of analgesic and tissue effects of subcutaneous perineural injection of liposomal bupivacaine and bupivacaine hydrochloride in horses with forelimb lameness induced via circumferential clamp. *Am. J. Vet. Res.* 81: 551–556.

Lo, I.K., Sciore, P., Chung, M. et al. (2009). Local anesthetics induce chondrocyte death in bovine articular cartilage disks in a dose- and duration-dependent manner. *Arthroscopy* 25: 707–715.

Mashimo, T., Uchida, I., Pak, M. et al. (1992). Prolongation of canine epidural anesthesia by liposome encapsulation of lidocaine. *Anesth. Analg.* 74: 827–834.

Mather, L.E., Rutten, A.J., and Plummer, J.L. (1994). Pharmacokinetics of bupivacaine enantiomers in sheep: influence of dosage regimen and study design. *J. Pharmacokinet. Biopharm.* 22: 481–498.

Matsubara, L.M., Olivia, V.N.L.S., Gabas, D.T. et al. (2009). Effect of lidocaine on the minimum alveolar concentration of sevoflurane in dogs. *Vet. Anaesth. Analg.* 36: 407–413.

Muir, W.W. III, Wiese, A.J., and March, P.A. (2003). Effects of morphine, lidocaine, ketamine, and morphine-lidocaine-ketamine drug combination on minimum alveolar concentration in dogs anesthetized with isoflurane. *Am. J. Vet. Res.* 64: 1155–1160.

Nava-Ocampo, A.A. and Bello-Ramirez, A.M. (2004). Lipophilicity affects the pharmacokinetics and toxicity of local anaesthetic agents administered by caudal block. *Clin. Exp. Pharmacol. Physiol.* 31: 116–118.

Nicacio, I.P., Stelle, A.B.F., Bruno, T.S. et al. (2020). Comparison of intraperitoneal ropivacaine and ropivacaine-dexmedetomidine for postoperative analgesia in cats undergoing ovariohysterectomy. *Vet. Anaesth. Analg.* 47: 396–404.

de OL Carapeba, G., IPGA, N., ABF, S. et al. (2020). Comparison of perioperative analgesia using the infiltration of the surgical site with ropivacaine alone and in combination with meloxicam in cats undergoing ovariohysterectomy. *BMC Vet. Res.* 16: 88.

Piper, S.L., Laron, D., Manzano, G. et al. (2012). A comparison of lidocaine, ropivacaine and dexamethasone toxicity on bovine tenocytes in culture. *J. Bone Joint Surg.* 94: 856–862.

Puente, N.W. and Josephy, P.D. (2001). Analysis of the lidocaine metabolite 2,6-dimethylaniline in bovine and human milk. *J. Anal. Toxicol.* 25: 711–715.

Rezende, M.L., Wagner, A.E., Mama, K.R. et al. (2011). Effects of intravenous administration of lidocaine on the minimum alveolar concentration of sevoflurane in horses. *Am. J. Vet. Res.* 72: 446–451.

Richard, B.M., Ott, L.R., Haan, D. et al. (2011). The safety and tolerability evaluation of DepoFoam bupivacaine (bupivacaine extended-release liposome injection) administered by incision wound infiltration in rabbits and dogs. *Exp. Opin. Investig. Drugs* 20: 10.

Richard, B.M., Newton, P., Ott, L.R. et al. (2012). The safety of EXPAREL (bupivacaine liposome injectable suspension) administered by peripheral nerve block in rabbits and dogs. *J. Drug Deliv.* 2012: 962101.

Sellers, G., Lin, H.C., Riddell, M.G. et al. (2009). Pharmacokinetics of lidocaine in serum and milk of mature Holstein cows. *J. Vet. Pharmacol. Therap.* 32: 446–450.

Silva, G., De La Corte, F.D., Brass, K.E. et al. (2019). Viability of equine chondrocytes after exposure to mepivacaine and ropivacaine in vitro. *J. Equine Vet. Sci.* 77: 80–85.

Skarda, R.T. and WWIII, M. (2003). Analgesic, behavioral, and hemodynamic and respiratory effects of midsacral subarachnoidally administered ropivacaine hydrochloride in mares. *Vet. Anaesth. Analag.* 30: 37–50.

Valverde, A., Doherty, T.J., Hernández, J. et al. (2004). Effect of lidocaine on the minimum alveolar concentration of isoflurane in dogs. *Vet. Anaesth. Analg.* 31: 264–271.

Villalba, M., Santiago, I., and Gomez de Segura, I.A. (2011). Effects of constant rate infusion of lidocaine and ketamine, with or without morphine, on isoflurane MAC in horses. *Equine Vet. J.* 43: 721–726.

Weiland, L., Croubels, S., Baert, K. et al. (2006). Pharmacokinetics of a lidocaine patch 5% in dogs. *J. Vet. Med. A Physiol. Pathol. Clin. Med.* 53: 34–39.

Wilson, J., Doherty, T.J., Egger, C.M. et al. (2008). Effects of intravenous lidocaine, ketamine, and the combination on the minimum alveolar concentration of sevoflurane in dogs. *Vet. Anaesth. Analg.* 35: 289–296.

13

Anticholinergics

Phillip Lerche

Introduction

Anticholinergics occur naturally in several plant species in high concentrations, including deadly nightshade (*Atropa belladonna*), henbane (*Hyoscyamus niger*), and *Datura* species. The tropane alkaloids from these plants (atropine, hyoscyamine, and scopolamine) are toxic to many species in relatively low concentrations (Lee 2007). The isolation of the atropine molecule in the 1830s was a landmark discovery for two reasons: first, it could then be used much more safely in clinical medicine, and second it was essential to performing research that identified the important parasympathetic neurotransmitter acetylcholine (Lee 2007). Glycopyrrolate, initially approved to treat gastric ulcers in people in 1961, was approved in injectable form for intraoperative use in 1975 (Chabicovsky et al. 2019). The anticholinergic drugs atropine and glycopyrrolate are frequently used in the perianesthetic period in veterinary medicine to prevent bradycardia, treat bradyarrhythmias, decrease airway secretions, prevent or diminish vagal reflexes, and for their parasympatholytic action when reversing neuromuscular blockade with drugs like neostigmine that have undesirable cholinergic effects (see Chapter 17).

Mechanism of Action

Anticholinergics competitively antagonize acetylcholine at postganglionic muscarinic cholinergic receptors in the parasympathetic nervous system. Five subtypes of muscarinic receptor are known to exist, and are classified as M1–M5 (Caulfield & Birdsall 1998). Muscarinic receptors are part of the family of G protein coupled receptors, and can activate multiple G proteins within the same cell (Karakiulakis and Roth 2012). The muscarinic receptors can be placed into two groups based on the primary G protein to which they couple. The odd-numbered receptors M1, M3, and M5 are excitatory. They couple with $G_{q/11}$-type proteins and generally activate cellular mechanisms via phospholipase C, which produces diacyl glycerol and inositol triphosphate; these second messengers result in an increased concentration of intracellular ionized calcium. The even-numbered M2 and M4 receptors are inhibitory. They couple with $G_{i/o}$-type proteins and result in inhibition of adenylyl cyclase, which decreases cyclic adenosine monophosphate (AMP) within cells (Caulfield and Birdsall 1998). M1, M2, and M3 receptors can also activate protein kinase (Rosenblum et al. 2000). Muscarinic receptors are present in virtually all tissues, with different receptor subtypes generally having a tissue-specific anatomic distribution, and physiologic response (Table 13.1) (Eglen 2012; Saternos et al. 2018; Cuevas and Adams 1997; Croy et al. 2016; Raffa 2009).

Chemical Structure and Pharmacokinetics

Atropine

Atropine, manufactured as atropine sulfate, is a racemic mixture of l- and d-hyoscyamine. The l-isomer is responsible for the majority of pharmacologic activity. The atropine molecule consists of a tropic acid ester-linked to an organic base, yielding a lipid-soluble tertiary amine (see Figure 13.1) (National Center for Biotechnology Information 2022a), which easily crosses the blood–brain and blood–placenta barriers (Proakis and Harris 1978).

Onset of action at the M2 receptor (increased heart rate) is rapid after intravenous (IV) and intramuscular (IM) atropine administration in dogs, with effects apparent at approximately one and five minutes after injection,

Table 13.1 Muscarinic receptor subtypes, predominant response, tissue location, and physiologic responses.

Receptor	Predominant response	Tissue location	Physiologic response
M₁	Stimulation	CNS	Modulates cognitive functioning (e.g. learning, memory)
			Analgesia
		Cardiovascular	↑ heart rate
			↑ inotropy
			Vascular tone modulation
		Gastrointestinal	↑ Gastric secretions
			↑ Salivation
M₂	Inhibition	Cardiovascular	↓ Heart rate
			↓ AV conduction (and associated AV block)
			↓ Inotropy
			Vasodilation
M₃	Stimulation	CNS	Insulin homeostasis
			Emesis
		Ocular	Mydriasis
		Gastrointestinal	↑ Gastric secretions
			↑ Salivation
			↑ Peristalsis
		Airway smooth muscle	Bronchoconstriction, ↑ secretions
		Cardiovascular	Vasodilation
M₄	inhibition	CNS	Modulates locomotion
			Dopamine regulation
		Heart	Modulates high-voltage-activated Ca²⁺ channels
			Modulates K⁺ channels
M₅	stimulation	CNS	Dopamine regulation

AV, atrioventricular; CNS, central nervous system; SA, sinoatrial.

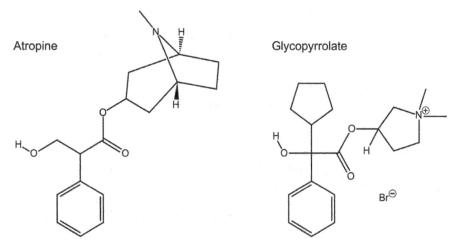

Figure 13.1 Chemical structure of atropine (left) and glycopyrrolate (right).

respectively, with a duration of 30 minutes (Hendrix and Robinson 1997). Other body systems are generally affected for one to several hours, although mydriasis after topical administration can persist for up to three days.

Hypovolemia induced by controlled hemorrhage decreased volume of distribution, but not other pharmacokinetic parameters, after IM administration of atropine when compared to normovolemic dogs (Smallridge et al. 1989). Compared to euthyroid dogs, the presence of hypothyroidism reduced clearance of atropine, and resulted in increased bioavailability and peak plasma concentrations after IM administration (Paret et al. 1911). The pharmacokinetics of atropine administered to dogs endotracheally and endobronchially have been reported (Paret et al. 1911). Times to peak plasma concentration were shorter than one minute in both cases. Peak plasma concentration was higher, half-life was longer (39 ± 5 vs. 28 ± 9 minutes), and clearance was slower after endobronchial administration when compared to endotracheal administration.

Atropine is hydrolyzed to tropic acid by atropine esterase activity in the plasma. Atropinase levels vary considerably among species. Rabbits have been shown to have high levels of atropinase, which may render typical clinical doses ineffective in this species, however, this enzyme is not present in high concentrations in all rabbits (Harrison et al. 2000). Tropic acid has been detected in the plasma of dogs, goats, pigs, and people in much smaller quantities than seen in rabbits after the addition of atropine *in vitro*, suggesting either very low levels of atropinase, or metabolism via other esterases (Harrison et al. 2000). In dogs, up to 90% of atropine is excreted by the kidney unchanged (Albanus et al. 1968). Cats and rats metabolize atropine via hepatic esterases (Godeaux and Tønnsen 1949).

Glycopyrrolate

Glycopyrrolate, also known as glycopyrronium bromide, is a synthetic quaternary ammonium compound consisting of a mandelic acid ester-linked to an organic base (Figure 13.1) (National Center for Biotechnology Information 2022b). As it has low lipid solubility, it does not cross the blood–brain or blood–placenta barriers (Proakis and Harris 1978).

The onset of action of glycopyrrolate is slightly slower than that of atropine, usually occurring within a few minutes. In awake dogs, the cardiovascular effects of glycopyrrolate have been shown to last for about 60 minutes, which is longer than those seen with atropine (Lemke 2001). Following IV injection, glycopyrrolate distributes rapidly to the vessel-rich group of tissues, except the brain. Glycopyrrolate undergoes hepatic metabolism in mice and rats, however, in dogs and people liver metabolism is more limited (Chabicovsky et al. 2019). Liver metabolism is likely a function of hydroxylation and hydrolysis, with the main metabolite being M9 (2(RS)-2-cyclopentyl-2-hydroxy-2-phenylacetic acid), which has not been shown to have muscarinic activity. In species where biotransformation is low, glycopyrrolate is mostly excreted unchanged in urine.

Pharmacodynamics

Both atropine and glycopyrrolate are relatively nonselective in their binding to muscarinic receptor subtypes. As a general rule, muscarinic receptors in salivary, cardiac, bronchial and ocular tissues are more sensitive to these drugs compared to responses seen other tissue groups. Atropine and glycopyrrolate differ in the response seen in a specific tissue type at clinically used doses. The degree of response is compared in Table 13.2 (Lerche 2015).

Central nervous system: Unlike glycopyrrolate, atropine crosses the blood–brain barrier. It is theoretically possible that atropine may cause sedation by blocking M1 receptors, however, the low doses used clinically do not produce noticeable sedation.

Cardiovascular system: M2 receptors in the sinoatrial node, the atrioventricular node, and the atrial myocardium mediate cardiac anticholinergic effects. Systemic administration of atropine and glycopyrrolate blocks M2 receptors, which usually leads to an increase in heart rate, acceleration of conduction through the electrical pathway of the heart, and increased contraction of the atria. Cardiac arrhythmias can occur following atropine administration (Muir 1978). At lower doses, bradycardia and second-degree atrioventricular block may be seen (Richards et al. 1989). This transient effect is likely caused by presynaptic M1 receptors being blocked, which results in an

Table 13.2 Effects of atropine and glycopyrrolate on saliva production, heart rate, smooth muscle, and the eye (Lerche, 2015).

Drug	Antisialagogue effects	Heart rate increase	Smooth muscle relaxation	Ocular effects
Atropine	+	+++	++	++
Glycopyrrolate	++	+	++	No effect

increase in acetylcholine release, leading to further slowing of heart rate (Wellstein and Pitschner 1988). This usually resolves spontaneously, and can also can be overcome by administering an additional dose of the anticholinergic drug. A relatively high dose of atropine in sheep (0.08 mg/kg) has been shown to cause bradycardia (Clutton and Glasby 2008).

Heart rate can sometimes exceed the normal range after anticholinergic administration, resulting in sinus tachycardia or other tachyarrhythmias. This is usually short-lived, typically resolving within 20–30 minutes. Drastic increases in heart rate can result in sudden increases in cardiac work and myocardial oxygen consumption, and a decrease in cardiac output. These effects may be undesirable in patients with cardiac disease.

Respiratory system: Antagonism of M2 and M3 receptors results in bronchodilation and decreased airway secretions. Bronchodilation decreases airway resistance, however, anatomic dead space ventilation increases, resulting in a decrease in alveolar ventilation if tidal ventilation stays the same (West and Luks 2021). This could potentially contribute to the development of hypoxemia, however, since most patients under anesthesia are intubated and breathing oxygen-enriched gases, it is unlikely to have any clinical impact.

Ocular effects: Topical application of atropine to the cornea blocks the action of acetylcholine in cholinergic fibers innervating the circular muscles of the iris, resulting in mydriasis, and the ciliary muscle, resulting in cycloplegia in sheep, goats, cats, and horses (Ribeiro et al. 2013; Whelan et al. 2011; Stadtbäumer et al. 2006; Davis et al. 2003; Mughannam et al. 1999). This is also the case with glycopyrrolate in rabbits (Varsanno et al. 1996). Intraocular pressure (IOP) increases in cats after topical application of anticholinergics due to drainage angle closure (Stadtbäumer et al. 2006), however, this does not occur in sheep and horses (Ribeiro et al. 2013; Mughannam et al. 1999). Atropine and glycopyrrolate both decrease tear production (Ludders and Heavner 1979; Arnett et al. 1984).

Topical glycopyrrolate induces mydriasis and cycloplegia in rabbits (Varsanno et al. 1996), while systemic administration to dogs had minimal effects (Frischmeyer et al. 1993).

Gastrointestinal tract: Acting by blocking M3 receptors, glycopyrrolate and atropine decrease saliva production in monogastrics. Anticholinergic administration for anti-sialagogue effects in ruminants is contra-indicated as saliva becomes viscous and thickens to the point where it may result in obstruction of the laryngopharynx. Blockade of M3 receptors in the gastrointestinal (GI) tract may lead to ileus. Motility was decreased for up to 30 minutes in dogs and more than six hours in horses following glycopyrrolate administration (Short et al. 1974;

Table 13.3 Doses of anticholinergics (Lerche, 2015; Flecknell, 2016).

Animal	Atropine	Glycopyrrolate
Cats and dogs	0.02–0.04 (IV or IM)	0.005–0.01 (IV or IM)
Horses	0.02–0.04	0.0025–0.005
Ruminants	0.04–0.08	0.0025–0.005
Pigs	0.04–0.08	0.0025–0.005
Rabbits	—	0.01 (IV) 0.1 (IM or SC)

Doses for anticholinergics in mg/kg. Route of administration is IV except where noted. IV, intravenous; IM, intramuscular; SC, subcutaneous.

Singh et al. 1997). Development of colic postoperatively in horses is multifactorial and antimuscarinic drug administration may be a contributing factor. Of 17 horses that received glycopyrrolate intraoperatively, one subsequently showed signs of colic (Gonçalves et al. 2002; Dyson et al. 1999). Anticholinergics are therefore not routinely used in horses (Ducharme and Fubini 1983), and, like in ruminants, are reserved for treating bradycardia. In monogastric animals, anticholinergics can decrease lower esophageal sphincter function, increasing the risk of gastroesophageal reflux and associated complications such as aspiration pneumonia, esophagitis, and esophageal stricture (Roush et al. 1990).

Role in cardiopulmonary–cerebral resuscitation (CPR): – CPR guidelines for cats and dogs published in 2012 state that atropine can be administrated after every second basic life support cycle, i.e. every four minutes, particularly when asystole or pulseless electrical activity is thought to have occurred as a result of high vagal tone (Fletcher et al. 2012). The longer onset time of action of glycopyrrolate precludes its use for CPR.

Dose ranges for anticholinergics are presented in Table 13.3.

Use with Other Drugs

In clinical veterinary anesthetic practice, anticholinergics are frequently mixed in the same syringe with other water-soluble drugs (e.g. acepromazine and opioids) in preanesthetic medication combinations for their ability to prevent and counteract parasympathetic effects encountered in the perianesthetic period. Bradycardia is a common side effect of general anesthesia, and may be due to direct drug effects (opioids, alpha$_2$ agonists), decreases in sympathetic tone (general anesthetics) or vagally-mediated reflexes. The use of anticholinergics to treat bradycardia associated with alpha$_2$ agonists should be considered in light of the underlying mechanism. If bradycardia occurs secondary to a baroreceptor response as a result of vasoconstriction and high blood pressure, increasing the heart rate in the face of this increased afterload has the potential to decrease cardiac output while simultaneously increasing myocardial oxygen consumption (Lemke et al. 1993). Cardiac output is usually not significantly improved when dogs are sedated with dexmedetomidine and atropine compared with dexmedetomidine alone. Use of atropine with alpha$_2$ agonists did not improve cardiac output and caused arrhythmias in dogs (Monteiro et al. 2009). No benefit was noted when cats were sedated with dexmedetomidine and atropine versus dexmedetomidine alone, however, cardiac output was not evaluated in that study (Monteiro et al. 2009).

Several groups of drugs commonly used in the perianesthetic period directly decrease GI activity (anticholinergics, opioids, alpha$_2$ agonists), and these effects may be additive.

Electing to use an anticholinergic as part of an anesthetic protocol should be done after weighing the overall impact on the patient.

References

Albanus, L., Sundwall, A., Vangbo, B., and Winbladh, B. (1968). The fate of atropine in the dog. *Acta Pharmacol. Toxicol.* 26: 571–582.

Arnett, B.D., Brightman, A.H., and Mussleman, E.E. (1984). Effect of atropine sulfate on tear production in the cat when used with ketamine hydrochloride and acetylpromazine maleate. *J. Am. Vet. Med. Assoc.* 185: 214–215.

Caulfield, M.P. and Birdsall, N.J.M. (1998). International Union of Pharmacology. XVII. Classification of muscarinic acetylcholine receptors. *Pharmacol. Rev.* 50: 279–290.

Chabicovsky, M., Winkler, S., Soeberdt, M. et al. (2019). Pharmacology, toxicology and clinical safety of glycopyrrolate. *Toxicol. Appl. Pharmacol.* 370: 154–169.

Clutton, R.E. and Glasby, M.A. (2008). Cardiovascular and autonomic nervous effects of edrophonium and atropine combinations during neuromuscular blockade antagonism in sheep. *Vet. Anaesth. Analg.* 35: 191–200.

Croy, C.H., Chan, W.Y., Castetter, A.M. et al. (2016). Characterization of PCS1055, a novel muscarinic M4 receptor antagonist. *Eur. J. Pharmacol.* 782: 70–76.

Cuevas, J. and Adams, D.J. (1997). M4 muscarinic receptor activation modulates calcium channel currents in rat intracardiac neurons. *J. Neurophysiol.* 78 (4): 1903–1912.

Davis, J.L., Stewart, T., Brazik, E. et al. (2003). The effect of topical administration of atropine sulfate on the normal equine pupil: influence of age, breed and gender. *Vet. Ophthalmol.* 6: 329–332.

Ducharme, N.G. and Fubini, S.L. (1983). Gastrointestinal complications associated with the use of atropine in horses. *J. Am. Vet. Med. Assoc.* 167: 200–202.

Dyson, D.H., Pascoe, P.J., and McDonell, W.N. (1999). Effects of intravenously administered glycopyrrolate in anesthetized horses. *Can. Vet. J.* 40: 29–32.

Eglen, R.M. (2012). Overview of muscarinic receptor subtypes. In: *Muscarinic Receptors*, Handbook of Experimental Pharmacology, vol. 208 (ed. A. Fryer, A. Christopoulos and N. Nathanson), 3–28. Berlin, Heidelberg: Springer.

Flecknell, P. (2016). Rodent and rabbit anesthesia. In: *Anesthesia and Analgesia for Veterinary Technicians*, 5e (ed. J. Thomas and P. Lerche), 2016. St. Louis, MO: Elsevier.

Fletcher, D., Boller, M., Brainard, B.M. et al. (2012). RECOVER evidence and knowledge gap analysis on veterinary CPR. Part 7: Clinical guidelines. *J. Vet. Emerg. Crit. Care* 22 (S): S102–S131.

Frischmeyer, K.J., Miller, P.E., Bellay, Y. et al. (1993). Parenteral anticholinergics in dogs with normal and elevated intraocular pressure. *Vet. Surg.* 22: 230–234.

Godeaux, J. and Tønnsen, M. (1949). Investigations into atropine metabolism in the animal organism. *Acta Pharm.* 5: 95–109.

Gonçalves, S., Julliand, V., and Leblond, A. (2002). Risk factors associated with colic in horses. *Vet. Res.* 33: 641–652.

Harrison, P.K., Tattersall, J.E., and Gosden, E. (2000). The presence of atropinesterase activity in animal plasma. *Naunyn Schmiedebergs Arch. Pharmacol.* 373: 230–236.

Hendrix, P.K. and Robinson, E.P. (1997). Effects of a selective and a nonselective muscarinic cholinergic antagonist on heart rate and intestinal motility in dogs. *J. Vet. Pharmacol. Ther.* 20: 387–395.

Karakiulakis, G. and Roth, M. (2012). Muscarinic receptors and their antagonists in COPD: anti-inflammatory and antiremodeling effects. *Mediators Inflamm.* 40: 95–80.

Lee, M.R. (2007). Solanaceae IV: *Atropa belladonna*, deadly nightshade. *J. R. Coll. Physic. Edinb.* 37: 77–84.

Lemke, K.A. (2001). Electrocardiographic and cardiopulmonary effects of intramuscular administration of glycopyrrolate and romifidine in conscious Beagle dogs. *Vet. Anaesth. Analg.* 28: 75–86.

Lemke, K.A., Tranquilli, W.J., Thurmon, J.C. et al. (1993). Hemodynamic effects of atropine and glycopyrrolate in isoflurane–xylazine-anesthetized dogs. *Vet. Surg.* 22: 163–169.

Lerche, P. (2015). Anticholinergics. In: *Veterinary Anesthesia and Analgesia*, 5e, 178–182. Ames IA: Blackwell Publishing.

Ludders, J.W. and Heavner, J.E. (1979). Effect of atropine on tear formation in anesthetized dogs. *J. Am. Vet. Med. Assoc.* 175: 585–586.

Monteiro, E.R., Campagnol, D., Parrilha, L.R., and Furlan, L.Z. (2009). Evaluation of cardiorespiratory effects of combinations of dexmedetomidine and atropine in cats. *J. Feline Med. Surg.* 11: 783–792.

Mughannam, A.J., Buyukmihci, N.C., and Kass, P.H. (1999). Effect of topical atropine on intraocular pressure and pupil diameter in the normal horse eye. *Vet. Ophthalmol.* 2: 213–215.

Muir, W.W. (1978). Effects of atropine on cardiac rate and rhythm in dogs. *J. Am. Vet. Med. Assoc.* 172: 917–921.

National Center for Biotechnology Information (2022a). PubChem Compound Summary for CID 174174, Atropine. https://pubchem.ncbi.nlm.nih.gov/compound/Glycopyrrolate#section=2D-Structure (accessed 1 May 2022).

National Center for Biotechnology Information (2022b). PubChem Compound Summary for CID 11693, Glycopyrrolate. https://pubchem.ncbi.nlm.nih.gov/compound/Glycopyrrolate#section=2D-Structure (accessed 1 May 2022).

Paret, G., Mazkereth, R., Sella, R. et al. (1911). Atropine pharmacokinetics and pharmacodynamics following endotracheal versus endobronchial administration in dogs. *Resuscitation* 41 (1): 57–62.

Proakis, A.G. and Harris, G.B. (1978). Comparative penetration of glycopyrrolate and atropine across the blood–brain and placental barriers in anesthetized dogs. *Anesthesiology* 48: 339–344.

Raffa, R.B. (2009). The M_5 muscarinic receptor as possible target for treatment of drug abuse. *J. Clin. Pharm. Ther.* 34: 623–629.

Ribeiro, A.P., Crivelaro, R.M., Teixeira, P.P. et al. (2013). Effects of different mydriatics on intraocular pressure, pupil diameter, and ruminal and intestinal motility in healthy sheep. *Vet. Ophthalmol.* 17: 297–402.

Richards, D.L., Clutton, R.E., and Boyd, C. (1989). Electrocardiographic findings following intravenous glycopyrrolate to sedated dogs: a comparison with atropine. *J. Assoc. Vet. Anaesth.* 16: 46–50.

Rosenblum, K., Futter, M., Jones, M. et al. (2000). ERKI/II regulation by the muscarinic acetylcholine receptors in neurons. *J. Neurosci.* 20: 977–985.

Roush, J.K., Keene, B.W., Eicker, S.W. et al. (1990). Effects of atropine and glycopyrrolate on esophageal, gastric and tracheal pH in anesthetized dogs. *Vet. Surg.* 19: 88–92.

Saternos, H.C., Almarghalani, D.A., Gibson, H.M. et al. (2018). Distribution and function of the muscarinic receptor subtypes in the cardiovascular system. *Physiol. Genom.* 50: 1–9.

Short, C.E., Paddleford, R.R., and Cloyd, G.D. (1974). Glycopyrrolate for prevention of pulmonary complications during anesthesia. *Mod. Vet. Pract.* 55: 194–196.

Singh, S., McDonell, W.N., Young, S.S. et al. (1997). The effect of glycopyrrolate on heart rate and intestinal motility in conscious horses. *J. Vet. Anaesth.* 24: 14–19.

Smallridge, R.C., Chernow, B., Teich, S. et al. (1989). Atropine pharmacokinetics are affected by moderate hemorrhage and hypothyroidism. *Crit. Care Med.* 17 (12): 1254–1257.

Stadtbäumer, K., Frommlet, F., and Nell, B. (2006). Effects of mydriatics on intracoluar pressure and pupil size in the normal feline eye. *Vet. Ophthalmol.* 9: 233–237.

Varsanno, D., Rothamn, S., Haas, K. et al. (1996). The mydriatic effect of topical glycopyrrolate. *Graefes Arch. Clin. Exp. Ophthalmol.* 234: 205–207.

Wellstein, A. and Pitschner, H.F. (1988). Complex dose-response curves of atropine in man explained by different functions of M1- and M2-cholinoceptors. *Naunyn Schmiedebergs Arch. Pharmacol.* 338: 19–27.

West, J.B. and Luks, A.M. (2021). Ventilation. In: *West's Respiratory Physiology*, 11e, 2–30. Philadelphia, PA: Wolters Kluwer.

Whelan, N.C., Castillo-Alcala, F.C., and Lizarraga, I. (2011). Efficacy of tropicamide, homatropine, cyclopentolate, atropine and hyoscine as mydriatics in Angora goats. *N. Z. Vet. J.* 59: 328–331.

14

CNS Stimulants

Caitlin Tearney

Introduction

Analeptic drugs stimulate the central nervous system. This is accomplished by blocking inhibition or enhancing excitation. Analeptic drugs used in veterinary medicine today include doxapram and the methylxanthines (caffeine, theophylline, and aminophylline). Their original use was to provide CNS stimulation in the face of CNS depression but this use has fallen out of favor due to their lack of specificity and side effects. Doxapram and methylxanthines are used to stimulate respirations especially in apnea of prematurity in human infants and foals. The most common clinical use of doxapram is to evaluate airway function by stimulation of the arytenoids following dose-dependent depression by anesthetic drugs.

Doxapram

Evidence exists that doxapram has action both peripherally and centrally with the ultimate effect being concentration dependent. The peripheral effect is to act on chemoreceptors to stimulate respirations. This is accomplished mainly by an increase in tidal volume but can also be accompanied by an increase in respiratory rate. This increase in minute ventilation is accompanied by an increase in oxygen consumption. Doxapram also acts centrally. It was discovered that animals anesthetized with phenobarbital became responsive following doxapram 5 mg/kg IV and awake animals given the same dose had seizures. Early clinical studies in humans noted increased respiratory rate and tidal volume in patients anesthetized with inhalants with a respiratory alkalosis noted on arterial blood gas and a mild increase in blood pressure. Centrally, faster awakening from inhalants was noted which led to its recommendation to be used with patients with central nervous system (CNS) or respiratory depression (Stephen and Talton 1964).

Early studies in dogs who underwent spinal cord transection at C2 found the effect of doxapram was abolished, yet effects persisted with cutting of the vagus nerve suggesting activity at the respiratory centers in the brainstem (Ward and Franko 1962). Increased brainstem inspiratory and expiratory neuronal activity has been observed in response to doxapram (Funderburk et al. 1966). Recent work found direct input on the brainstem, specifically a rhythm generating center called the pre-Bötzinger complex (Kruszynski et al. 2019), which is important in the generation of eupnea and gasping (Lieske et al. 2000). Numerous researchers have also found increased respirations through stimulatory action on the carotid and aortic chemoreceptors (Kato and Buckley 1964; Hirsh and Wang 1974; Mitchell and Herbert 1975). Research into the membrane currents of carotid glomus cells, the primary chemosensing cell in the carotid body, has revealed a role for TWIK-related acid sensitive K^+ channels (TASK) and big potassium (BK) channels (voltage dependent and calcium-activated) (Peers 1991), with both hypoxia and doxapram appearing to inhibit these potassium channels. This inhibition causes depolarization of the cell and an influx of calcium through voltage-gated calcium channels which lead to neurotransmitters generating action potentials on carotid sinus nerve afferents to increase ventilation (Peers et al. 2010). TASK channels were further investigated and doxapram was found to specifically inhibit TASK-1 and TASK-3 channels in a dose-dependent manner (Cotton et al. 2006).

The ventilation stimulus following doxapram 1 mg/kg IV is comparable to hypoxemia with a PaO_2 of 38 mmHg in humans (Stoelting's p. 360).

Adult horses receiving a 1.1 mg/kg IV doxapram bolus show a short duration of effect likely due to redistribution out of the brain and plasma and display an elimination half-life of two to three hours (Wernette et al. 1986; Sams et al. 1992). The drug has a high extraction ratio with

Pharmacology in Veterinary Anesthesia and Analgesia, First Edition. Edited by Turi Aarnes and Phillip Lerche.
© 2024 John Wiley & Sons, Inc. Published 2024 by John Wiley & Sons, Inc.

clearance dependent on liver blood flow (Sams et al. 1992). Mean serum concentrations of doxapram in anesthetized neonatal foals were 1127 ng/ml (low dose: 0.5 mg/kg, 0.03 mg/kg/min) and 3246 ng/ml (high dose: 0.5 mg/kg, 0.08 mg/kg/min) (Giguère et al. 2007) which are similar to the therapeutic range of concentrations in infants (1500–4000 ng/ml) (Huon et al. 1998). A short duration of action due to a short elimination half-life and a rapid biotransformation to keto-doxapram which has a faster elimination rate than doxapram was confirmed in newborn lambs (Bairam et al. 1990).

Metabolism

Doxapram is rapidly metabolized and blood levels decline rapidly after a bolus, and low concentrations are excreted unchanged in the urine in dogs and horses (Pitts et al. 1973; Sams et al. 1992). The major metabolite is keto-doxapram which is a less potent respiratory stimulant (Bairam et al. 1990).

Clinical Use

In humans, clinical uses are slim as newer techniques and safer options have replaced its use. Doxapram is given to patients with chronic obstructive pulmonary disorder to maintain ventilation during oxygen supplementation as they rely on a hypoxic drive to breathe. In the past, it has been used when weaning a patient from mechanical ventilation and has been proposed for humans with obstructive sleep apnea. During the post-operative period, it can counteract both respiratory and CNS depression of opioids without reversing analgesia although its action is short lived. Doxapram has been shown to arouse patients following barbiturates, volatile anesthetics, nitrous oxide, and benzodiazepines (Yost 2006). It has utility in decreasing postoperative shivering, although minor (Komatsu et al. 2005). Premature apneic neonates in the ICU given doxapram can avoid intubation and ventilation with efficacy similar to commonly used methylxanthines (Henderson-Smart and Steer 2004), although undesirable side effects similar to caffeine and an increase in blood pressure have also been noted. Doxapram has been recommended for infants unresponsive to methylxanthines alone.

Foals affected by hypoxic–ischemic encephalopathy lose chemoreceptor sensitivity in the respiratory center resulting in apnea and severe respiratory acidosis. Pharmacological stimulation of respiration has been attempted with both doxapram and methylxanthines (Giguère et al. 2007). In this study, healthy neonatal foals were deeply anesthetized with isoflurane to achieve hypercapnia ($ETCO_2$ 70–80 mmHg), treatment with both low- and high-dose doxapram (low dose: 0.5 mg/kg loading dose, 0.03 mg/kg/min for 20 minutes, high dose: 0.5 mg/kg loading dose, 0.08 mg/kg/min for 20 minutes) increased respiratory rate, minute ventilation, arterial blood pH, and PaO_2 and decreased $PaCO_2$ significantly compared to saline control and caffeine citrate treatments [(10 mg/kg [5 mg/kg caffeine base/kg] given once in the low-dose group and repeated for the high dose)]. Doxapram also significantly increased arterial blood pressure. The authors noted respiratory depression from inhalant anesthesia may differ from the respiratory sequala of ischemic CNS damage.

Findings on the effects of doxapram on respiration are similar in a study on awake, healthy neonatal calves (Bleul and Bylang 2012) where a dose of doxapram 40 mg (0.9 mg/kg) IV increased respiratory rate, minute ventilation, and PaO_2 and decreased $PaCO_2$ for 90 minutes although maximal effect was seen at one minute post treatment. Lambs exhibited a similar increase in minute ventilation after doxapram 2.5 mg/kg IV (Bairam et al. 1990). Cats anesthetized with pentobarbitone given doxapram 0.25 mg/kg/min for 15 minutes showed increased ventilation and decreased $ETCO_2$ (Bopp et al. 1979).

Infusions of doxapram to stimulate ventilation to overcome the respiratory depression of halothane anesthesia in ponies has been studied (Taylor 1990). A dose of 0.05 mg/kg/min was found to stimulate ventilation without causing arousal under anesthesia.

Laryngeal paralysis is a common pathology in dogs and one in which the diagnosis requires direct visualization of the larynx or laryngoscopy. This requires a light plane of anesthesia which itself can affect laryngeal function and cause respiratory depression in a dose dependent fashion. To offset these effects, doxapram has been used to increase intrinsic laryngeal motion and respiratory effort (Miller et al. 2002). The anesthetic protocol in this study consisted of glycopyrrolate, acepromazine, butorphanol, and propofol. Doxapram significantly increased the average area of the rima glottis during both inspiration and expiration. Doses of 1.1 and 2.2 mg/kg have been used to evaluate laryngeal function in dogs (Miller et al. 2002; Tobias et al. 2004). Numerous other studies have used a variety of anesthetic protocols, a recent review found 67% of studies evaluated used doxapram as a respiratory stimulant and it successfully increased laryngeal motion in 75% of these studies (Ranninger et al. 2020). Dogs with laryngeal paralysis given doxapram can exhibit paradoxical motion of their arytenoids secondary to the Bernoulli effect of increased negative airway pressure. This finding was also noted in normal dogs who had good laryngeal motion prior to receiving doxapram IV (Radkey et al. 2018).

The use of doxapram for neonatal resuscitation is controversial (Traas 2008). Use was initially advocated in a non-controlled study of puppies delivered via cesarean section given doxapram IV via the umbilical vein (Holladay 1971). Effects of doxapram have been shown to be diminished in hypoxic brains of lambs (Bamford et al. 1986) so it is unlikely to be beneficial in the apneic newborn. Resuscitation efforts should focus on warming, stimulating, reversal of anesthetic drugs, with a focus on supporting airway, breathing, and circulation before other emergency drugs are used.

Doxapram does have a wide margin of safety. In humans, a mild pressor effect exists suspected to be due to release of catecholamines (Abelson et al. 1996). An increase in blood pressure has been noted following doxapram given to hypotensive or hypovolemic patients (Kim et al. 1971). However, a second study noted no change in hemodynamics when given to patients following thoracic surgery (Laxenaire et al. 1986). Effects seem to vary based on volume state. In euvolemic conscious dogs given 1.5 mg/kg doxapram IV, cardiac output increased by 15% but following hemorrhage to produce hypovolemia, cardiac output increased by 72% mainly due to an increased stroke volume (Kim et al. 1971). Healthy dogs anesthetized with medetomidine, propofol, and remifentanil showed a mild increase in arterial blood pressure following bolus and constant rate infusion (CRI) of doxapram compared to control (2 mg/kg bolus, 67 mcg/kg/min) (Yun and Kwon 2015). Potential for arrhythmias and effects on QT interval seem to be greater in infants, especially if premature (Maillard et al. 2001). Attempts to induce ventricular arrhythmias in dogs were unsuccessful following doxapram 4 mg/kg IV despite conditions of hypercapnia, halothane or cyclopropane anesthesia, and epinephrine IV (Huffington and Craythorne 1966).

Awake humans given doxapram have reported dyspnea. The increase in minute ventilation via increases in tidal volume and respiratory rate is well documented across species and discussed above. More in-depth respiratory mechanics have been investigated in horses where 0.3 mg/kg IV doxapram decreased airway compliance and increased airway resistance in horses with both normal and abnormal lungs (Aguilera-Tejero et al. 1997).

CNS excitation, anxiety, and panic are reported in people. Seizures can occur when 20–40 times the dose that is required to stimulate respirations is given (Funderburk et al. 1966). Continuous infusions which are given to maintain respiratory stimulations can produce signs of CNS stimulation (hypertension, tachycardia, cardiac arrhythmias, vomiting, hyperthermia). To investigate the effect of doxapram on cerebral blood flow, doxapram was injected into the cerebral circulation in instrumented goats. This resulted in a reduction in cerebral blood flow independent of blood carbon dioxide levels (Miletich et al. 1976). However, this study conflicts with others, when doxapram

was administered at 1 mg/kg IV a reduction in cardiac output, heart rate, and blood pressure, although very briefly (30 seconds) was also recorded. Preterm infants treated with doxapram because they were unresponsive to caffeine showed an increase in cerebral oxygen requirement and decrease cerebral blood flow assessed using Doppler sonography (Roll and Horsch 2004; Dani et al. 2006).

Doxapram's effects as a non-selective CNS stimulant have been investigated in dogs sedated with acepromazine 0.05 mg/kg IM (Zapata and Hofmeister 2013). Doxapram 1.25 and 2.5 mg/kg IV 30 minutes after acepromazine decreased sedation scores for at least 30 minutes with no significant difference in sedation scores between the two groups suggesting it has a ceiling effect on CNS stimulation (Zapata and Hofmeister 2013). Panting was noted in male dogs receiving the higher dose of doxapram.

The ability of doxapram to speed elimination of inhaled anesthetics via increased minute ventilation and potentially improve recovery has recently been investigated in horses. A small, randomized, crossover, blinded, prospective study compared two doses of doxapram (0.1 and 0.2 mg/kg) plus xylazine 0.2 mg/kg IV at recovery following 90 minutes of isoflurane anesthesia and found no difference in time to sternal, time to standing, or quality of recovery between groups, or compared to xylazine alone, or to saline control (Midon et al. 2022).

The LD50 is 72 mg/kg IV in rats manifesting in hyperactivity, tremors, and seizures as well as salivation, diarrhea, vomiting, urination, and defecation (Ward et al. 1968).

The current formulation contains benzyl alcohol as a preservative so its use should be avoided in populations with known sensitivities (premature neonates, high doses in felines). In patients with thoracic disease due to a mechanical disorder (flail chest, pneumothorax) or restrictive lung disease (pulmonary fibrosis) doxapram could potentially worsen respiratory fatigue and not improve ventilation (Yost 2006).

Use caution in patients receiving sympathomimetics or monoamine oxidase inhibitors due to potential for compounding cardiovascular stimulation.

Methylxanthines

Methylxanthines improve ventilation by direct stimulation of the respiratory center increasing sensitivity to carbon dioxide, improvement of diaphragmatic contractility, and antagonism of actions of adenosine (neurotransmitter that causes respiratory depression) facilitating release of catecholamines (Comer et al. 2001; Stark 2004). Caffeine is the preferred agent for treatment of apnea in premature infants. IV caffeine to apneic infants, neonatal lambs, and cats resulted in significant increases in minute ventilation and tidal volume, without changing respiratory rate (Aranda et al. 1983; Mazzarelli et al. 1986; Bairam et al. 1992). Clinical use of caffeine in veterinary medicine is limited.

Pharmacokinetic studies of oral caffeine in adult horses have revealed a bioavailability of 39%, peak serum levels in 2 hours, and a half-life of 10–21 hours (Greene et al. 1983; Aramaki et al. 1991; Schumacher et al. 1994). Extrapolating from clinical experience in infants led to the common recommendation of caffeine 10 mg/kg orally then 2.5–3 mg/kg orally once daily in foals (Vaala and Palmer 1998). However, based on the foal study (Giguère et al. 2007) where caffeine did not affect hypercapnia in neonatal foals under inhalant anesthesia and PK data in horses, it is unlikely these recommendations are clinically effective. A follow-up retrospective analysis of foals affected with suspect hypoxic–ischemic encephalopathy showed treatment with doxapram to have a more significant decrease in $PaCO_2$ than in foals treated with caffeine despite higher dosing of caffeine, loading dose of 7.5–12 mg/kg PO then 2.5–5 mg/kg once daily (Giguère et al. 2008). However, in this retrospective study, foals in the doxapram group had significantly lower baseline arterial pH and HCO_3^-.

Side effects of methylxanthines in infants include tachycardia, GI dysfunction, agitation, and irritability (Comer et al. 2001). Methylxanthines primarily undergo liver metabolism by hepatic cytochrome P450. The major metabolite of caffeine is theophylline.

Theophylline is more active than caffeine as an adenosine receptor antagonist and, at high concentrations, inhibits phosphodiesterase. The drug also has anti-inflammatory properties including reducing chemical mediators in mast cells, decreasing cytokine expression in T-lymphocytes and macrophages, and reducing recruitment of neutrophils (Barnes 2013). The combinations of these actions result in smooth muscle relaxation and bronchodilation. This drug was once commonly used for treatment of asthma in people. The use of theophylline as a bronchodilator has largely been replaced by a more selective class of drugs with fewer adverse effects, the β 2 adrenergic agonists. Therapeutic plasma concentrations of theophylline are believed to be 5–20 mcg/ml (extrapolated from humans), although toxicity can be seen within these doses and includes arrhythmias, CNS excitement, seizures, and GI irritation. Dogs appear to be more resistant to adverse effects until higher plasma concentrations are reached (Shibata et al. 2000). Recent work suggests therapeutic plasma concentrations in dogs to be 5–30 mcg/ml (Reinhart et al. 2021). In a clinical study of dogs with collapsing trachea, mean plasma concentrations of theophylline were 11.67 mcg/ml with a dosage range of 7.5–30 mg/kg (Jeung et al. 2019). Adverse signs in this study consisted of diarrhea, dyspnea, tremor, and anorexia. Theophylline undergoes enterohepatic recirculation.

Clinical use today is mainly restricted to management of collapsing trachea in dogs and chronic bronchitis in dogs and cats. It is also used clinically to prevent diaphragmatic fatigue (Rozanski 2014), and as a positive chronotrope in patients with bradycardia such as sick sinus syndrome (Fox et al. 1999). Available formulations of theophylline have been limited due to decline of use in human medicine, but recent compounded products evaluated in dogs appear to be well absorbed and have shown favorable pharmacokinetic properties (half-life 8.85 hours) with a recommended dose of 10 mg/kg every 12 hours orally (Cavett et al. 2019; Reinhart et al. 2021). Some inter-individual variation did exist in the studies which may warrant therapeutic drug monitoring with clinical use.

References

Abelson, J.L., Weg, J.G., Nesse, R.M., and Curtis, G.C. (1996). Neuroendocrine responses to laboratory panic: cognitive intervention in the doxapram model. *Psychoneuroendocrinology* 21: 375–390.

Aguilera-Tejero, E., Pascoe, J.R., Smith, B.L., and Woliner, M.J. (1997). The effect of doxapram-induced hyperventilation on respiratory mechanics in horses. *Res. Vet. Sci.* 62: 143–146.

Aramaki, S., Suzuki, E., Ishidaka, O. et al. (1991). Pharmacokinetics of caffeine and its metabolites in horses after intravenous, intramuscular or oral administration. *Chem. Pharm. Bull.* 39: 2999–3002.

Aranda, J.V., Turmen, T., Davis, J. et al. (1983). Effect of caffeine on control of breathing in infantile apnea. *J. Pediatr.* 103: 975–978.

Bairam, A., Blanchard, P.W., Mullahoo, K. et al. (1990). Pharmacodynamic effects and pharmacokinetic profiles of keto-doxapram and doxapram in newborn lambs. *Pediatr. Res.* 28: 142–146.

Bairam, A., Blanchard, P.W., Bureau, M.A. et al. (1992). Interactive ventilatory effects of two respiratory stimulants, caffeine and doxapram, in newborn lambs. *Biol. Neonate* 61: 201–208.

Bamford, O.S., Dawes, G.S., Hanson, M.A., and Ward, R.A. (1986). The effects of doxapram on breathing, heart rate and blood pressure in fetal lambs. *Respir. Physiol.* 66: 387–396.

Barnes, P.J. (2013). Theophylline. *Am. J. Respir. Crit. Care Med.* 188: 901–906.

Bleul, U. and Bylang, T. (2012). Effects of doxapram, prethcamide and lobeline on spirometric, blood gas and acid–base variables in healthy new-born calves. *Vet. J.* 194: 240–246.

Bopp, P., Drummond, G., Fisher, J., and Milic-Emili, J. (1979). Effect of doxapram on control of breathing in cats. *Can. J. Anesth.* 26: 191–195.

Cavett, C., Li, Z., McKiernan, B.C., and Reinhart, J.M. (2019). Pharmacokinetics of a modified, compounded theophylline product in dogs. *Vet. Pharmacol. Therap.* 42: 593–601.

Comer, A.M., Perry, C.M., and Figgitt, D.P. (2001). Caffeine citrate: a review of its use in apnoea of prematurity. *Paediatr. Drugs* 3: 61–79.

Cotton, J.F., Keshavaprasad, B., Laster, M.J. et al. (2006). The ventilatory stimulant doxapram inhibits TASK tandem pore (K2P) potassium channel function but does not affect minimum alveolar anesthetic concentration. *Anesth. Analg.* 102: 779–785.

Dani, C., Bertini, G., Pezzati, M. et al. (2006). Brain hemodynamic effects of doxapram in preterm infants. *Biol. Neonate* 89: 69–74.

Fox, P.R., Sisson, D., and Moïse, N.S. (1999). *Textbook of Canine and Feline Cardiology: Principles and Clinical Practice*, 2e. Philadelphia, PA: Saunders.

Funderburk, W.H., Oliver, K.L., and Ward, J.W. (1966). Electrophysiologic analysis of the site of action of doxapram hydrochloride. *J. Pharmacol. Exp. Ther.* 151: 360–368.

Giguère, S., Sanchez, L.C., Shih, A. et al. (2007). Comparison of the effects of caffeine and doxapram on respiratory and cardiovascular function in foals with induced respiratory acidosis. *Am. J. Vet. Res.* 68: 1407–1416.

Giguère, S., Slade, J.K., and Sanchez, L.C. (2008). Retrospective comparison of caffeine and doxapram for the treatment of hypercapnia in foals with hypoxic-ischemic encephalopathy. *J. Vet. Intern. Med.* 22: 401–405.

Greene, E.W., Woods, W.E., and Tobin, T. (1983). Pharmacology, pharmacokinetics, and behavioral effects of caffeine in horses. *Am. J. Vet. Res.* 44: 57–63.

Henderson-Smart, D. and Steer, P. (2004). Doxapram treatment for apnea in preterm infants. *Cochrane Database Syst. Rev.* 4: CD000074.

Hirsh, K. and Wang, S.C. (1974). Selective respiratory stimulating action of doxapram compared to pentylenetetrazaol. *J. Pharmacol. Exp. Therap.* 189: 1–11.

Holladay, J.R. (1971). Routine use of doxapram hydrochloride in neonatal pups delivered by cesarean section. *Vet. Med. Small Anim. Clin.* 66: 28.

Huffington, P. and Craythorne, N.W. (1966). Effect of doxapram on heart rhythm during anesthesia in dog and man. *Anesth. Analg.* 45: 558–563.

Huon, C., Rey, E., Mussat, P. et al. (1998). Low-dose doxapram for treatment of apnoea following early weaning in very low birthweight infants: a randomized, double-blind study. *Acta Paediatr.* 87: 1180–1184.

Jeung, S., Sohn, S., An, J. et al. (2019). A retrospective study of theophylline-based therapy with tracheal collapse in small-breed dogs: 47 cases (2013-2017). *J. Vet. Sci.* 20: e57.

Kato, H. and Buckley, J.P. (1964). Possible sites of action of the respiratory stimulant effect of doxapram hydrochloride. *J. Pharmacol. Exp. Ther.* 144: 260–264.

Kim, S.I., Winnie, A.P., Collins, V.J., and Shoemaker, W.C. (1971). Hemodynamic responses to doxapram in normovolemic and hypovolemic dogs. *Anesth. Analg.* 50: 705–710.

Komatsu, R., Sengupta, P., Cherynak, G. et al. (2005). Doxapram only slightly reduces the shivering threshold in healthy volunteers. *Anesth. Analg.* 101: 1368–1373.

Kruszynski, S., Stanaitis, K., Brandes, J. et al. (2019). Doxapram stimulates respiratory activity through distinct activation of neurons in the nucleus hypoglossus and the pre-Bötzinger complex. *J. Neurophysiol.* 121: 1102–1110.

Laxenaire, M.C., Boileau, S., Dagrenat, P. et al. (1986). Haemodynamic and respiratory effects of post-operative doxapram and almitrine in patients following pneumonectomy. *Eur. J. Anaesthesiol.* 3: 259–271.

Lieske, S.P., Thoby-Brisson, M., Telgkamp, P., and Ramirez, J.M. (2000). Reconfiguration of the neural network controlling multiple breathing patterns: eupnea, sighs and gasps. *Nat. Neurosci.* 3: 600–607.

Maillard, C., Boutroy, M.J., Fresson, J. et al. (2001). QT interval lengthening in premature infants treated with doxapram. *Clin. Pharmacol. Therap.* 70: 540–545.

Mazzarelli, M., Jaspar, N., Zin, W.A. et al. (1986). Dose effect of caffeine on control of breathing and respiratory response to CO_2 in cats. *J. Appl. Phys.* 60: 52–59.

Midon, M., Yamada, D.I., Filho, D.Z. et al. (2022). Evaluation of the effects of doxapram in combination with xylazine on recovery of horses isoflurane-anesthetized. *J. Equine Vet. Sci.*, Jan Epub ahead of print 111: 103872.

Miletich, D.J., Ivankovich, A.D., Albrecht, R.F. et al. (1976). The effects of Doxapram on cerebral blood flow and peripheral hernodynamics in the anesthetized and unanesthetized goat. *Anesth. Analg.* 55: 279–285.

Miller, C.J., McKiernan, B.C., Pace, J., and Fettman, M.J. (2002). The effects of doxapram hydrochloride (dopram-V) on laryngeal function in healthy dogs. *J. Vet. Intern. Med.* 16: 524–528.

Mitchell, R.A. and Herbert, D.A. (1975). Potencies of doxapram and hypoxia in stimulating carotid-body chemoreceptors and ventilation in anesthetized cats. *Anesthesiology* 42: 559–566.

Peers, C. (1991). Effects of doxapram on ionic currents recorded in isolated type I cells of the neonatal rat carotid body. *Brain Res.* 568: 116–122.

Peers, C., Wyatt, C.N., and Evans, A.M. (2010). Mechanisms for acute oxygen sensing in the carotid body. *Respir. Physiol. Neurobiol.* 174: 292–298.

Pitts, J.E., Bruce, R.B., and Forehand, I.B. (1973). Identification of doxapram metabolites using high pressure ion exchange chromatography and mass spectroscopy. *Xenobiotica* 3: 73–83.

Radkey, D.I., Hardie, R.J., and Smith, L.J. (2018). Comparison of the effects of alfaxalone and propofol with acepromazine, butorphanol and/or doxapram on laryngeal motion and quality of examination in dogs. *Vet. Anaesth. Analg.* 45: 241–249.

Ranninger, E., Kantyka, M., and Bektas, R.N. (2020). The influence of anaesthetic drugs on the laryngeal motion in dogs: a systematic review. *Animals* 10: 530.

Reinhart, J.M., Perkowski, C., Lester, C. et al. (2021). Multidose pharmacokinetics and safety of a modified, compounded theophylline product in dogs. *J. Vet. Pharmacol. Therap.* 44: 902–909.

Roll, C. and Horsch, S. (2004). Effect of doxapram on cerebral blood flow velocity in preterm infants. *Neuropediatrics* 35: 126–129.

Rozanski, E. (2014). Canine chronic bronchitis. In the veterinary clinics of North America. *Small Anim. Pract.* 44: 107–116.

Sams, R.A., Detra, R.L., and Muir, W.W.I.I.I. (1992). Pharmacokinetics and metabolism of intravenous doxapram in horses. *Equine Vet. J.* 11: 45–51.

Schumacher, J., Spano, J.S., Wilson, R.C. et al. (1994). Caffeine clearance in the horse. *Vet. Res. Commun.* 18: 367–372.

Shibata, M., Wachi, M., Kagawa, M. et al. (2000). Acute and subacute toxicities of theophylline are directly reflected by its plasma concentration in dogs. *Method Find. Exp. Clin. Pharmacol.* 22: 173–178.

Stark, A.R. (2004). Apnea. In: *Manual of Neonatal Care* (ed. J.P. Cloherty, E.C. Eichenwald and A.R. Stark), 388–393. Philadelphia: Lippincott Williams & Wilkins.

Stephen, C.R. and Talton, I. (1964). Investigation of doxapram as a postanesthetic respiratory stimulant. *Anesth. Analg.* 43: 628–640.

Taylor, P.M. (1990). Doxapram infusion during halothane anaesthesia in ponies. *Equine Vet. J.* 22: 329–332.

Tobias, K.M., Jackson, A.M., and Harvey, R.C. (2004). Effects of doxapram HCl on laryngeal function of normal dogs and dogs with naturally occurring laryngeal paralysis. *Vet. Anaesth. Analg.* 31: 258–263.

Traas, A.M. (2008). Resuscitation of canine and feline neonates. *Theriogenology* 70: 343–348.

Vaala, W.E. and Palmer, J.E. (1998). Neonatology: foal cardiopulmonary resuscitation. In: *Manual of Equine Emergencies: Treatment and Procedures* (ed. J.A. Orsini and T.J. Divers), 473–537. Philadelphia: WB Saunders Co.

Ward, J.W. and Franko, B.V. (1962). A new centrally acting agent (AHR-619) with marked respiratory stimulating, pressor, and "awakening" effects. *Fed. Proc.* 21: 325.

Ward, J.W., Gilbert, D.L., Franko, B.V. et al. (1968). Toxicological studies of doxapram hydrochloride. *Toxicol. Appl. Pharmacol.* 13: 242–250.

Wernette, K.M., Hubbell, J.A., Muir, W.W. III et al. (1986). Doxapram: cardiopulmonary effects in the horse. *Am. J. Vet. Res.* 47: 1360–1362.

Yost, S. (2006). A new look at the respiratory stimulant doxapram. *CNS Drug Rev.* 12: 236–249.

Yun, S. and Kwon, Y. (2015). The effect of doxapram on cardiopulmonary function in dogs under total intravenous anesthesia with remifentanil and propofol. *J. Vet. Clin.* 32: 491–498.

Zapata, M. and Hofmeister, E.H. (2013). Refinement of the dose of doxapram to counteract the sedative effects of acepromazine in dogs. *J. Small Anim. Pract.* 54: 405–408.

15

Centrally Acting Muscle Relaxants

Bonnie L. Hay Kraus

Introduction and Physiology

Muscle relaxants affect skeletal muscle tone and function and include two major therapeutic groups: neuromuscular blockers and centrally acting muscle relaxants. Neuromuscular blockers interfere with transmission at the neuromuscular end plate and do not have central nervous system (CNS) activity. "Centrally acting" muscle relaxants act at the level of the cortex, brainstem, or spinal cord. The neuronal signals generated in motor neurons that cause muscle contraction are dependent on the balance of synaptic excitation and inhibition that the motor neuron receives. Central muscle relaxants work by either enhancing the level of inhibition or reducing the level of excitation. Inhibition is enhanced by increasing the actions of endogenous inhibitory substances such as gamma-aminobutyric acid (GABA). Higher brain centers, including the cerebrum, cerebellum, and medulla oblongata, control activity in the ventral horn cells of the spinal cord which stimulate motor neurons and cause contraction.

Centrally acting muscle relaxant drugs used in veterinary medicine, such as guaifenesin and benzodiazepines, produce muscle relaxation by selectively depressing transmission of impulses at the internuncial or inter-neurons of the spinal cord, brainstem, and subcortical regions of the brain (Figure 15.1). The relaxation produced by centrally acting relaxants is not as profound as that produced by peripherally acting muscle relaxants. Other anesthetic agents that provide muscle relaxation include α₂-adrenoceptor agonists, anticonvulsants such as gabapentin and pregabalin and inhalant anesthetics. These compounds are reviewed elsewhere in the text.

Guaifenesin

Guaifenesin (glyceryl guaiacolate, [GG]) was originally derived from the Guaiacum genus of trees and has been used as a therapeutic agent for more than 80 years (Pang 2015). Historically, it was used in humans both as an anesthetic agent and in the management of tetanus but is currently only used as a cough expectorant (Pang 2015). It was introduced as an alternative to succinylcholine for anesthesia in the horse in 1949 and has been used in the US since 1965. At therapeutic doses, it was found to relax skeletal muscles without significant effects on the respiratory muscles or diaphragm compared to succinylcholine (Muir 2009; Posner 2018). Although the mechanism of action remains largely unknown, early evidence suggests that it acts centrally by depressing or blocking nerve impulse transmission at the internuncial neuron level of the subcortical areas of the brain, brainstem, and spinal cord (Funk 1970; Muir 2009; Pang 2015; Posner 2018; Plumb 2018a). GG produces effects similar to benzodiazepines, decreasing transmission at the level of the internuncial or inter-neurons of polysynaptic reflexes at the level of the spinal cord (Posner 2018). It relaxes laryngeal and pharyngeal muscles, allowing for easier oral tracheal intubation. A prominent feature is the ability to decrease impulse transmission in the internuncial neurons of the spinal cord without significantly impairing respiratory ventilation (Muir 2009). Guafenesin produces recumbency and some sedative-hypnotic effects by binding to specific inhibitory neurotransmitter receptor sites in the reticular formation, brainstem and subcortical areas of the brain activated by GABA (Plumb 2018a). However, it does not cause unconsciousness nor provide analgesia sufficient for painful stimuli. When used alone, animals may obtain recumbency, but surgical anesthesia is not attained. Guaifenesin is still used as an adjunct anesthetic, usually co-administered with ketamine with or without an α-2 agonist, for its sedative and muscle relaxation properties in equine, ruminant and camelid species. It can be used as an adjunct for both induction and total or partial intravenous (IV) anesthesia. It smooths induction and recovery as well as decreases the amount of other induction drugs required.

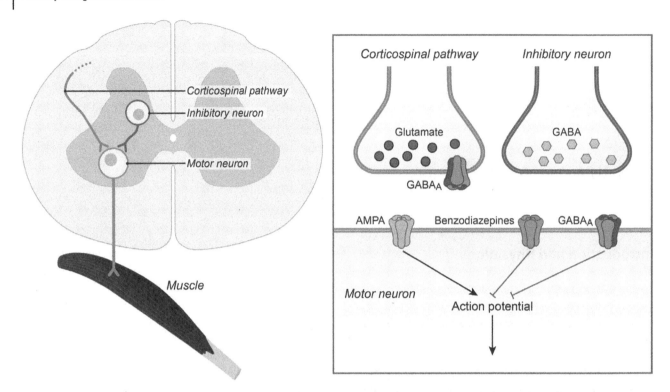

Figure 15.1 Higher brain centers control muscle activity through the ventral horn cells of the spinal cord. Central muscle relaxants, including guafenesin and benzodiazepines, increase the inhibitory effects of GABA thereby decreasing transmission at the level of the inter-nuncial or interneurons of the ventral horn of the spinal cord. (modified using Adobe Illustrator, attributed to Bill Connelly (http://en.wikipedia.org/wiki/Muscle_relaxant#/media/File:Spasticity2.svg), link to licence site at CreativeCommons Attribution-ShareAlike: http://creativecommons.org/licenses/by-sa/3.0/)

Guaifenesin is a white crystalline powder compatible with sterile water or D5W. Currently, there are no commercially available injectable products marketed in the US. Therefore, the only way to obtain an injectable agent is by compounding from USP grade powder by pharmacies with the appropriate facilities and procedures (Plumb 2018a). It is recommended that compounding pharmacies use the formula of the previously available commercial products (per ml): Guaifenesin (50 mg), dextrose (50 mg), propylene glycol (20 mg), dimethyl acetamide (50 mg), edetate disodium (0.75 mg), and water for injection or another validated formula (Plumb 2018a). Although a 10% solution is stable at room temperature for one week, it is recommended that the solution be prepared freshly prior to use (Plumb 2018a). Precipitation can occur at ≤22 °C (72 °F) which can be eliminated by warming and agitation. Guaifenesen is not a controlled substance and is approved as a skeletal muscle relaxant for use in horses. Its use in production animals is extra-label with a withdrawal time of 48 hours for milk and three days for meat (Posner 2018).

Guaifenesin has a concentration-related risk of hemolysis. Concentrations greater than 5% cause clinically significant hemolysis in cattle (Wall and Muir 1990). Glucose solutions are reported to protect the red blood cell against the hemolytic effects of GG. Equine RBCs are less susceptible to the hemolysis, occurring at concentrations exceeding 15%, however, a high incidence of jugular vein thrombosis is associated with concentrations greater than 5% (Herschl et al. 1992). Stabilized 15% guaifenesin solutions available in some countries may be less likely to cause hemolysis in horses but may still be associated with jugular vein thrombosis (Lerche 2013). Urticarial reactions can be observed in horses administered high GG concentration (10–15%) of either commercially available or compounded solutions (Muir 2009). The mechanism is unknown. Perivascular injection causes tissue damage resulting in inflammation, tissue swelling, thrombophlebitis and sloughing (Muir 2009; Pang 2015).

Guaifenesin has a reported therapeutic index of two to four times the dose required to produce recumbency in horses (Funk 1970). Clinical signs of overdose include opisthotonus, irregular/apneustic breathing, nystagmus, hypotension, and muscle rigidity and occur at an average dose of 180 mg/kg (Funk 1973; Plumb 2018a). The toxic signs may be attributed, in part, to the catechol compound formed during biotransformation of GG as it is known to produce convulsions followed by paralysis and death caused by respiratory and circulatory failure (Davis and Wolf 1970). Treatment of toxicity should be based on supportive care until plasma levels decrease. The veterinary label indicates that physostigmine is contraindicated in horses receiving guafenesin but no explanation of the actual interaction is noted (Plumb 2018a). Other anticholinesterase agents may also be contraindicated.

When GG is administered as a single agent, recumbency occurs in two minutes and lasts approximately six minutes. Sedation has a duration of 15–30 minutes and muscle relaxation persists for 10–20 minutes (Plumb 2018a). IV GG undergoes rapid equilibration in 5–10 minutes, followed by a longer elimination phase. GG is metabolized by the liver where it is conjugated with glucuronide and excreted in the urine (Muir 2009). Catechol is an intermediary compound. Plasma half-life in ponies and horses is ~60–80 minutes (Davis and Wolf 1970; Hubbell et al. 1980). There is a significant gender difference in the half-lives of ponies; where males have a $T_{1/2}$ of ~85 minutes and female $T_{1/2}$ is ~60 minutes (Davis and Wolf 1970). The half-life in donkeys is also longer because of lower clearance (Matthews et al. 1997).

When administered as a single agent, GG has minimal cardiovascular effects. At clinical doses, guaifenesin does not significantly affect ventilation, heart rate (HR), pulmonary arterial pressure and cardiac output (CO) (Hubbell et al. 1980; Muir 2009). Arterial blood pressure decreases but only minimally so. Cardiac contractility is not decreased and may slightly increase after recumbency. Heart rate, cardiac contractile force, right atrial pressure, pulmonary arterial pressure, and CO remain unchanged, however, a transient decrease in blood pressure is observed (Hubbell et al. 1980). Xylazine decreases the dose of GG required for recumbency, however, it also causes a decrease in HR, CO, respiratory rate (RR) and further decreases in blood pressure and the partial pressure of arterial oxygen (PaO_2) (Hubbell et al. 1980). Horses maintained in the upright position have minimal blood gas alterations; the arterial partial pressure of carbon dioxide ($PaCO_2$) remains unchanged. However, after induction to lateral recumbency, RR increases but minute volume and PaO_2 decrease and with continued infusion; $PaCO_2$ significantly increases leading to acidosis (Schatzmann et al. 1978). A high incidence of apnea occurs when GG is infused before a bolus of barbiturate for induction and may be avoided by co-administration of barbiturate or ketamine with GG (Hubbell et al. 1980). Serum chemistry and hematologic values remain unchanged as long as solutions below those that induce hemolysis are used. Laryngeal and pharyngeal muscles become relaxed, facilitating intubation of the trachea. The additional CNS depression and muscle relaxation provided by guaifenesin may allow for smaller doses of

more cardiovascular depressing drugs, therefore preserving cardiovascular function. GG crosses the placental barrier producing concentrations ~30% of that found in the maternal circulation, but foals reportedly do not show signs of significant depression (Hubbell et al. 1980). Guaifenesin does not predispose to premature delivery or abortion in the mare (Muir 2009). Detrimental effects on pregnant animals have not been reported but fetal movements are suppressed in cattle.

Although the approved dose in horses is 2.2 ml/kg (110 mg/kg), significantly less is used when GG is administered with other CNS depressants (Posner 2018). Guaifenesin is most commonly used as a co-induction agent for anesthesia induction and/or as part of a total IV anesthesia or partial IV anesthesia regimen for maintenance of anesthesia after induction. GG helps in producing a smooth induction and recovery from anesthesia as well as decreases the doses of other drugs. The primary disadvantage in using GG is the large volume required to produce relaxation. The recommended adjunct induction dose of 30–50 mg/kg (~300–500 ml of a 5% solution) requires use of large-bore IV catheters and a method for rapid administration such as a pressure bag. Typical use for equine induction includes premedication with an α-2 agonist or phenothiazine, with or without an opioid. After the horse is sedated, guaifenesin is rapidly infused using pressurization until marked sedation and muscle relaxation is achieved which is clinically evident by buckling of the limbs. GG is then discontinued or slowed and the induction agent is administered. Ketamine at 2.2 mg/kg (or thiopental where available) can be administered as a bolus and recumbency usually occurs within 60 seconds. For compromised patients, the dose of α-2 agonist should be reduced and guaifenesin is administered initially at a slower rate to create the desired level of sedation and to allow adequate time for the centralization of cardiac output. Since guaifenesin has a slow onset of action, this initial slow rate of administration avoids making the patient overly ataxic while waiting for centralization (Plumb 2018a). Guaifenesin is then rapidly infused using pressurization until marked sedation and muscle relaxation is achieved evidenced by buckling of front limbs and lowered head carriage. The ketamine bolus dose may be reduced in compromised patients or the calculated induction dose may be added to the infusion bag of GG to allow better titration of induction doses.

More recently, GG has been used as an adjunct prior to induction with the newer injectable anesthetic agents propofol and alfaxalone. In unpremedicated healthy adult horses, GG (70–90 mg/kg IV) was able to decrease the adverse anesthetic induction events (excitation, myotonus, paddling, rigidity) associated with propofol induction in horses (Brosnan et al. 2011). Preliminary trials with alfaxalone induction after premedication with an α-2 agonist alone resulted in excitation and uncontrolled inductions (Goodwin et al. 2011, 2019). The addition of GG (35 mg/kg IV) in horses premedicated with acepromazine 0.03 mg/kg and xylazine 1.0 mg/kg IV prior to induction with alfaxalone (1.0 mg/kg) significantly improved induction quality to good–excellent (Goodwin et al. 2011, 2019). Induction quality was evaluated as good to excellent (4–5 out of 5) and recoveries were also assessed as good (Goodwin et al. 2011, 2019).

Guafenesin is also frequently used as part of total or partial IV anesthetic regimens. It is usually combined in "Triple Drips" that also contain ketamine and an α-2 agonist (xylazine, detomidine, romifidine, medetomidine, or dexmedetomidine) and are reviewed elsewhere (Lerche 2013; Valverde 2013) (Table 15.1). The standard

"GKX" recipe contains GG (50 mg/ml, 5%), ketamine 1–2 mg/ml (use 2 mg/ml for longer or more painful procedures) and xylazine 0.5 mg/ml. The triple drip CRI is administered at a rate of 1.5–2.2 ml/kg/hour (75–110 mg/kg/hr) but can be higher when administered "to effect" depending on the procedure, patient response, and ketamine concentration (Plumb 2018a). The average dose at which clinical signs of overdosage can occur is 180 mg/kg (1.8 l of 5% GG for 500 kg horse) (Funk 1973). Therefore, time and dose should be limited to ~1 hour and 1–1.5 l of 5% GG to avoid GG toxicity. Horses should be intubated and provided oxygen supplementation via demand valve or nasal insufflation of oxygen at a rate of 10–15 l/min when available to counter the respiratory depression and decrease in PaO$_2$ associated with GG and recumbency. Recovery after guaifenesen administration is generally uneventful with horses rolling into a sternal position and standing in one or two attempts.

In cattle, guaifenesin produces muscle relaxation and ataxia at dose of ~50 mg/kg (Lin 2014a). Significant decreases in arterial pressure and respiratory acidosis were observed in buffalo calves administered guaifenesin. However, the dose was quite high at 165 mg/kg (Singh et al. 1981). Guaifenesin can be used alone at doses of 15–25 mg/kg IV for standing sedation in large ruminants and camelids (Lin 2014a). The dose should be carefully titrated to avoid excessive muscle relaxation and recumbency; analgesics should be administered for painful procedures or conditions. Triple drip contains GG, ketamine, and xylazine and can be used for induction and short-term (<30–60 minutes) maintenance of anesthesia in large and small ruminants, calves, and camelids (Table 15.1). Camelids are less sensitive to xylazine and therefore, the dose of xylazine should be higher. GKX (GG 5%, ketamine 1.0 mg/ml, xylazine 0.1 mg/ml) was compared to isoflurane for induction and maintenance of anesthesia in 2–26-day-old calves ventilated on 100% oxygen (Kerr et al. 2007). A smooth induction was accomplished with ~0.5 ml/kg of GKX and calves were maintained with ~2.5 ml/kg/hr for laparoscopic bladder surgery (Kerr et al. 2007). Heart rate was significantly lower but blood pressure was significantly higher in the GKX group compared to the isoflurane group, however, there were no significant differences in cardiac index nor blood gas values (Kerr et al. 2007). GKX (GG 5%, ketamine 1.0 mg/ml, xylazine 0.1 mg/ml) has also been used to induce (~1.2 ml/kg) and maintain (~2.6 ml/kg) Suffolk sheep (Lin et al. 1993). There were no significant differences in heart rate or noninvasive blood pressure from baseline. Intubation and supplementation with 100% oxygen is recommended to counter respiratory depression resulting in high partial pressure of carbon dioxide (PaCO$_2$) and low partial

Table 15.1 "Triple Drip" can be used for total intravenous or partial intravenous anesthesia after induction in horses and for induction and/or maintenance in cattle, small ruminants, camelids, and swine. Due to species and breed variation in sensitivity to xylazine, it is important to adjust the concentration and rate of administration accordingly.

TIVA/PIVA preparation	Final concentration	Infusion rate
Equine triple drip		
GKX	G: 50 mg/ml	1–2 ml/kg/hr
Add 50 gm GG to 1.0 l 5% dextrose, 1–2 gm ketamine, 500 mg xylazine	K: 1–2 mg/ml X: 0.5 mg/ml	
GKD	D: 20 mg/mL	1 – 2 mL/kg/hr
Same as above, substitute 20 mg detomidine for xylazine		
Bovine triple drip		
GKX	G: 50 mg/ml	Induction:
Add 50 gm GG to 1.0 l 5% dextrose, 1–2 gm ketamine, 50–100 mg xylazine	K: 1–2 mg/ml X: 0.05– 0.1 mg/ml	0.5–1.0 ml/kg Maintenance: 1–2 ml/kg/hr
Sheep		
Same as Bovine, except only 1.0 gm ketamine		
Camelid	X: 0.1 –	
Same as Bovine, except 100–250 mg xylazine	0.25 mg/ml	
Swine triple drip[a]		
Add 50 gm GG to 1.0 l 5% dextrose, 1–2 gm ketamine, xylazine 1.0 gm (1000 mg = 10 ml)	G: 50 mg/ml K: 1–2 mg/ml X: 1.0 mg/ml	Induction: 0.5–1.0 ml/kg Maintenance: 1.0–2.0 ml/kg/hr

[a] Note: swine xylazine dose 2× horse and 10× bovine dose.

pressure of oxygen (PaO$_2$) (Lin et al. 1993). Triple drip can be used in properly restrained adult cattle without premedication and induction of anesthesia is smooth with good muscle relaxation. Tracheal intubation is recommended to prevent aspiration of ruminal contents. Supplementation with O$_2$ (10–15 l/min) during prolonged procedures may help prevent hypoxemia caused by hypoventilation and recumbency. Recovery to standing usually occurs within 40–45 minutes after discontinuation of the infusion (Lin 2014a).

Guaifenesin is not used routinely in dogs due to the large volume requirement. It has been combined with xylazine and ketamine in situations where inhalant anesthesia is unavailable. The GKX mixture is made with 2.0 ml of 5% ketamine and 1.25 ml of 2% xylazine added to 100 ml of 5% guaifenesin and infused at 2.2 ml/kg IV (Benson et al. 1985; Mezerová et al. 1992).

Benzodiazepines

Benzodiazepines, as a group, provide five pharmacologic effects in slightly varying degrees: sedation and hypnosis, anxiolysis, anterograde amnesia, anti-convulsant activity, and spinal-cord-mediated skeletal muscle relaxation (Rathmell and Rosow 2015; Vuyk et al. 2020). Benzodiazepines were first discovered in the 1950s and chlordiazepoxide (Librium) was the first benzodiazepine patented (Posner 2018; Vuyk et al. 2020). Diazepam was synthesized in 1963 and used for induction of anesthesia in human medicine and oxazepam (Seresta), which is a metabolite of diazepam, also became available (Vuyk et al. 2020). Lorazepam (Ativan) became available in the 1970s in an attempt to produce a more potent benzodiazepine. Midazolam (Versed, Dormicum) was synthesized in 1976 and became the first benzodiazepine primarily used for anesthesia (Vuyk et al. 2020). Remimazolam is a new ultra-short-acting benzodiazepine that is rapidly degraded in the plasma by nonspecific esterases and is presently undergoing phase III trials (Vuyk et al. 2020). Benzodiazepines are widely prescribed in human medicine for anxiety and sleep disturbances and have added to addiction concerns worldwide. Ongoing research is focused on the neural mechanisms of the reward-related effects of benzodiazepines, which appear related to the α-2 and α-3 subunits of GABA$_A$ receptors (Vuyk et al. 2020). The common benzodiazepines used in human anesthesia include midazolam (the most common), diazepam, lorazepam, and temazepam (Vuyk et al. 2020). Midazolam is classified as short-acting, lorazepam and temazepam as intermediate and diazepam as long-acting, according to their metabolism and plasma clearance (Vuyk et al. 2020). In veterinary medicine, benzodiazepines are used for their anti-convulsant properties (diazepam,

midazolam, clonazepam, and clorazepate), management of behavioral issues (diazepam, clorazepate, alprazolam, lorazepam, oxazepam, and orazepam) and as adjuncts in veterinary anesthesia (diazepam, midazolam, lorazepam, and zolazepam). This discussion will focus on the use of benzodiazepines in veterinary anesthesia, however, reference to other uses will be included where appropriate. The benzodiazepine effects of sedation/hypnosis, anxiolysis, and spinal-cord-mediated skeletal muscle relaxation contribute to their beneficial use as anesthetic adjuncts. In humans, benzodiazepines also have an antegrade amnesic effect which is even more potent than the sedative effects. Stored information (retrograde amnesia) is not altered (Rathmell and Rosow 2015). Although difficult to assess in animals, the antegrade amnesic properties may be especially useful in veterinary patients, where the recognition of fear and anxiety associated with veterinary visits and procedures has recently gained significant concern and attention.

Benzodiazepines produce their pharmacologic effects by facilitating the actions of GABA at the GABA$_A$ receptor (Figure 15.2). GABA is the primary inhibitory neurotransmitter in the CNS. GABA$_A$ is a large macromolecule that has α, β, and γ subunits and separate binding sites (Rathmell and Rosow 2015). The benzodiazepines do not directly

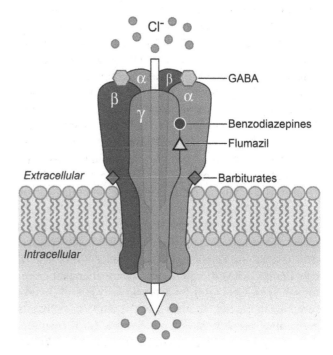

Figure 15.2 GABAA receptor is a ligand-gated chloride channel with separate binding sites for GABA, benzodiazepines, barbiturates, propofol and neurosteroid anesthetics. Benzodiazepines interact with the site between the α and γ subunits and enhances the binding of GABA which increases chloride conductance and hyperpolarizes the post-synaptic cell membranes.

activate GABA$_A$ receptors but bind at their specific site and then allosterically enhance the affinity to GABA which increases chloride conductance and hyperpolarizes the post-synaptic cell membrane. This renders it resistant to excitation which is the mechanism by which benzodiazepines exert their effects (Rathmell and Rosow 2015; Vuyk et al. 2020). The α-subunit (α1, α2, α3, α5) and β-subunit must be co-expressed with the γ subunit for the GABA$_A$ receptors to be sensitive to benzodiazepines (Mohler 2014). The GABA binding site is located between the α- and β-subunits. Benzodiazepines do not bind to the same receptor site on the GABA$_A$ receptor complex as GABA. They bind to distinct benzodiazepine binding sites situated at the interface between the α- and γ-subunits of α- and γ-subunit containing GABA$_A$ receptors. Also, they do not activate the receptor directly, but allosterically enhance the affinity of the receptors for GABA. This causes a greater frequency of channel openings, increased chloride conductance and hyperpolarization of the post-synaptic cell membrane leading to less excitation of the post-synaptic neurons. Hyperpolarization and resistance to excitation is presumed to be the mechanism by which benzodiazepines produce anxiolysis, sedation, amnesia, anti-convulsant and skeletal muscle relaxant effects (Rathmell and Rosow 2015). The GABA$_A$ receptor has a pentameric structure that is built from 18 or more subunits (Vuyk et al. 2020). Different combinations of the pentameric structure occur in different parts of the brain. The α subunit occurs in six isoforms (α1–α6) (Vuyk et al. 2020). The four subtypes of benzodiazepine-sensitive GABA$_A$ receptors are distinguished by their α subunits: α1, α2, α3, and α5 which show distinct expression patterns in the CNS (Mohler 2014). The GABA$_A$ subtypes mediate the different pharmacologic effects of benzodiazepines. α-1 subunits containing GABA$_A$ receptors are important for the sedative, anti-convulsant, anti-grade amnesia, and dependence actions (Mohler 2014). Muscle relaxation is mediated via α2 subunits (Vuyk et al. 2020). Anxiolysis is mediated by α2 and α3 at high receptor occupancy (Mohler 2014). α2 subunit containing receptors are also thought to be involved in pain suppression through α2 spinal receptors (Mohler 2014). The α$_1$ containing GABA$_A$ receptors are the most abundant receptor subtypes, accounting for approximately 60% of GABA$_A$ receptors in the human brain (Mohler 2014). α-2 subunits containing receptors have a more restricted distribution, principally in the hippocampus and amygdala. The α$_5$-containing GABA$_A$ receptors are primarily extra-synaptic and are responsible for modulation of the resting membrane potential (Rathmell and Rosow 2015). The benzodiazepine receptors are found in highest numbers in the cerebral cortex, cerebellum, hippocampus, substantia nigra, inferior colliculus and olfactory bulb, whereas lower numbers of receptors are found in the striatum, lower brainstem, and spinal cord (Reves et al. 2009; Vuyk et al. 2020). In addition to GABA and benzodiazepine binding sites, the GABA$_A$ receptor contains separate binding for barbiturates, etomidate, propofol, neurosteroids, and alcohol. Since these compounds all act on a single receptor, albeit at different binding sites, they can produce synergistic effects to increase GABA$_A$ receptor-mediated inhibition in the CNS. This synergy is also the basis for pharmacologic cross-tolerance with these drugs (Rathmell and Rosow 2015).

Based on their effects at the benzodiazepine binding site on the GABA$_A$ receptor, compounds may be classified as agonists, partial agonists, antagonists, partial inverse agonists and inverse agonists. Agonists increase binding affinity of GABA opening the chloride channel leading to agonist effects such as sedation, anxiolysis or anti-convulsant actions. Inverse agonists decrease the amount of chloride current generated by GABA$_A$ receptor activation and decrease inhibitory GABAnergic synaptic transmission leading to CNS excitation. Agonists, such as midazolam, shift the GABA concentration-response curve to the left whereas inverse agonists shift the curve to the right. Both these effects are blocked by antagonists such as flumazenil at the benzodiazepine binding site. In the absence of an agonist or inverse agonist for the benzodiazepine binding site, antagonists do not affect GABA$_A$ receptor function (Reves et al. 2009).

Pharmacokinetics – Human

Differences in onset and duration of action of benzodiazepines are due to differences in potency (which is related to receptor-binding affinity), lipid solubility (the ability to cross the blood–brain barrier and redistribute to peripheral tissues) and pharmacokinetics (uptake, distribution, metabolism, and elimination). All benzodiazepines are highly lipid soluble and highly protein bound; hypoalbuminemia may result in enhanced clinical effects (Rathmell and Rosow 2015). The plasma disappearance curves of all benzodiazepines can be described by a two- or three-compartment model (Vuyk et al. 2020). Protein binding and volumes of distribution are very similar for the different benzodiazepines; however, the clearance is significantly different for specific drugs and between species. Factors that may influence the pharmacokinetics include age, gender, race, enzyme induction and hepatic or renal disease (Vuyk et al. 2020). Pharmacokinetics of benzodiazepines are also influenced by obesity as the volume of distribution increases as the drug diffuses from plasma to fat. Although clearance is not affected, elimination half-lives are prolonged due to the increased volume of distribution and the delay in drug returning to the plasma in obese patients (Vuyk et al. 2020). Additional factors may contribute to increased "sensitivity" of elderly patients to benzodiazepines since pharmacokinetics are minimally altered (Vuyk et al. 2020).

Midazolam has a unique solubility profile due to its fused imidazole ring. It has pH-dependent solubility: it is water soluble as formulated in its buffered acidic medium (pH ~3.5) but is highly lipid soluble at normal physiologic pH. Midazolam has a higher lipid solubility resulting in faster onset and shorter duration of action compared to diazepam. It also has a higher affinity for benzodiazepine receptors, making it three to six times as potent as diazepam (Reves et al. 2009; Rathmell and Rosow 2015).

Metabolism – Humans

In general, benzodiazepines are metabolized by two types of reactions. Phase I oxidase reactions form metabolites that are still pharmacologically active, although this varies with specific metabolites. Phase II reactions are conjugation reactions, primarily with glucuronide. Glucuronidation is a very important mechanism in the elimination of benzodiazepines because it inactivates the metabolites, makes them more water soluble and accelerates their renal excretion (Driessen et al. 1987).

Midazolam is rapidly distributed after IV administration, with a distribution half-life of 6–15 minutes; it is highly protein bound (94–98%) (Vuyk et al. 2020). The hepatic extraction ratio is intermediate (0.3–0.44), thus, metabolic clearance may be susceptible to changes in both hepatic enzyme activity and blood flow (Vuyk et al. 2020). The elimination half-life is 1.7–3.5 hours and plasma clearance ranges from 5.8–9.0 ml/kg/min, higher than other benzodiazepines (Vuyk et al. 2020). Midazolam is metabolized by CYP3A4 and CYP3A5 hepatic microsomal isoenzymes to form 1-hydroxymethylmidazolam (the primary metabolite) and 4-hydroxymidazolam (Rathmell and Rosow 2015; Vuyk et al. 2020). The 1-hydroxymethylmidazolam metabolite has about half the activity of the parent compound. It is rapidly conjugated with glucuronide and then subsequently eliminated by the kidney (Rathmell and Rosow 2015). The glucuronide metabolite has significant pharmacologic activity, especially if present in high concentrations as in patients with renal insufficiency or critically ill patients. Metabolism of midazolam may be decreased with co-administration of other drugs that inhibit CYP450 enzymes such as cimetidine, erythromycin, calcium channel blockers, and antifungal drugs leading to increased CNS depression (Rathmell and Rosow 2015). Fentanyl is also

metabolized by CYP3A and therefore co-administration of these drugs may influence hepatic clearance (Rathmell and Rosow 2015).

Diazepam has a large volume of distribution (0.7–4.7 l/kg) and a plasma clearance of 0.2–0.5 ml/kg/min and is highly protein bound (Vuyk et al. 2020). The elimination half-life is prolonged, averaging ~40 hours in healthy individuals (Rathmell and Rosow 2015). The pharmacokinetics of diazepam are affected by liver dysfunction, age, and obesity (Vuyk et al. 2020). Hypoalbuminemia increases the unbound fraction of diazepam and can increase drug-related side effects (Rathmell and Rosow 2015). Metabolism is mediated primarily by CYP2C19 and CYP3A4 hepatic microsome enzymes to N-desmethyldiazepam which has pharmacodynamic properties similar to diazepam but has a much slower elimination half-life of 48–96 hours. Thus, plasma concentrations of the parent drug diazepam decrease more rapidly than the pharmacologically active metabolite which can accumulate with chronic use (Rathmell and Rosow 2015). N-desmethyldiazepam is further metabolized to oxazepam which is also pharmacologically active and a lesser amount is metabolized to temazepam (Rathmell and Rosow 2015; Vuyk et al. 2020). These active metabolites can prolong the drug effects. These metabolites are then conjugated with glucuronic acid and excreted in the urine (Rathmell and Rosow 2015).

Lorazepam is a more potent sedative and amnesic than midazolam and diazepam, whereas its effects on ventilation, cardiovascular variables and skeletal muscle relaxation are similar to the other benzodiazepines (Rathmell and Rosow 2015). Lorazepam has a slower onset of action and a longer duration of action due, in part, to the lower lipid solubility and slower passage in and out of the CNS (Rathmell and Rosow 2015). After IV administration, effects occur within 1–2 minutes but peak effect does not occur until 20–30 minutes and may last 6–30 hours (Rathmell and Rosow 2015). This slow onset of action limits its usefulness for induction of anesthesia or as an anticonvulsant. The extended duration of action may delay emergence from sedation/anesthesia and weaning from mechanical ventilation. Lorazepam has a large volume of distribution (0.8–1.3 l/kg) and a clearance of 0.8–1.8 ml/kg/min and is highly protein bound. Lorazepam is conjugated with glucuronic acid in the liver to form inactive metabolites that are excreted by the kidneys. This differs from midazolam and diazepam which both have pharmacologically active metabolites. The elimination half time is ~14 hours; ~80% of lorazepam is excreted as lorazepam glucuronide. Hepatic glucuronidation is slower than the oxidative reactions of the CYP enzymes, however, it is less likely to be influenced by age or drugs that affect the CPY450 enzymes (Rathmell and Rosow 2015).

Dog Metabolism

Midazolam is rapidly and widely distributed from the central compartment after IV administration, has a mean volume of distribution of 3.0 l/kg and a clearance of 27 ml/kg/min (Court and Greenblat 1992). It is highly protein bound (94–97%) and plasma elimination is ~77 minutes which is significantly faster compared to humans (1.9–2.5 hours). Midazolam is very rapidly and completely absorbed following IM administration in dogs. Peak levels of midazolam are reached within 10–15 minutes and systemic availability values are greater than 90% at doses of 0.5 mg/kg but IM availability decreases to ~50–70% at 0.2 mg/kg (Court and Greenblat 1992; Schwartz et al. 2012). Oral administration results in peak plasma concentrations within 10 minutes and a bioavailability of 69%. Rectal administration in dogs yields very low systemic availability (Court and Greenblat 1992; Schwartz et al. 2012). Due to its high lipid solubility at normal body pH, it rapidly crosses the blood–brain barrier resulting in a fast onset of action (Court and Greenblat 1992; Schwartz et al. 2012). Although hydroxylated and glucuronidated metabolites have been identified in dog plasma and the glucuronide conjugates have been identified in dog urine, only small quantities of hydroxylated midazolam are measurable (Court and Greenblat 1992). The elimination half-life of hydroxylated metabolites is very short (only ~11 minutes) which suggests they undergo rapid glucuronidation in dogs (Court and Greenblat 1992). In contrast to humans, excretion of hydroxylated and conjugated metabolites in urine of dogs appears to be low (<5% of dose after seven hours) suggesting an extra-renal route of metabolite elimination, perhaps through the bile (Court and Greenblat 1992). Midazolam is metabolized in the liver by CYP450 isoenzymes CYP2B11 and CYP3A and its elimination may be affected by co-administration of other drugs that inhibit these enzymes such as ketoconazole and medetomidine (Baratta et al. 2009; KuKanich and Hubin 2010).

Diazepam

In dogs, diazepam (2.0 mg/kg) has a terminal half-life of ~80 minutes and is primarily converted to N-desmethyldiazepam (nordiazepam) in both *in-vivo* and *in-vitro* studies and to a smaller extent to temazepam in *in-vitro* studies (Schwartz 1965; Vree et al. 1979; Chenery et al. 1987; Seddon 1989). Nordiazepam is slowly eliminated ($t_{1/2} = 10$ hours) by hydroxylation to oxazepam which is conjugated with glucuronide and has a $t_{1/2}$ of ~8 hours (Vree et al. 1979). Nordiazepam and temazepam are catalyzed primarily by CYP2B11 and CYP3A12, respectively

and temazepam is also further biotransformed to oxazepam by CYP2B11 (Shou et al. 2003; Lu et al. 2005).

Cats

Midazolam hydroxylated metabolites (1- and 4-hydroxymidazolam) have been found to be metabolized by CYP3A isoenzymes and female cats have lower CYP3A activity than male cats (Shah et al. 2007). Midazolam hydroxylation is significantly decreased by ketoconazole, a known CYP3A inhibitor (Shah et al. 2009). A recent study evaluated the pharmacokinetics of midazolam (0.3 mg/kg IV) and its presumed major metabolite 1-hydroxymidazolam in cats anesthetized with sevoflurane (Dholakia et al. 2020). The elimination half-life was ~79 minutes and the clearance rate was 11.4 ml/kg/min which is consistent with those reported for other species (Dholakia et al. 2020). Peak plasma concentrations of 1-hydroxymidazolam occurred within 15 minutes. Elimination of this metabolite, which is known to be an active metabolite in humans, occurred at a much slower rate with plasma concentrations still present at six hours (Dholakia et al. 2020). This is in contrast to metabolism in dogs, where 1-hydroxymidazolam is rapidly conjugated with glucuronide (Court and Greenblat 1992). One cat in the study did not produce any measurable 1-hydroxymidazolam, indicating that there may be individual pharmacogenetic variability even within species (Dholakia et al. 2020). Although 1-hydroxymidazolam undergoes glucuronidation in dogs and humans, the metabolic pathway for 1-hydroxymidazolam in cats has not been described. Currently, there is no specific evidence regarding the glucuronidation of commonly used benzodiazepines such as midazolam, diazepam or alprazolam (Schillings et al. 1975; Court 2013). However, despite the well-known feline deficiency in UDP-glucuronosyltransferase (UGT) enzymes, cats are able to conjugate lorazepam as efficiently as other species (Court 2013).

Diazepam

In *in-vivo* studies in cats, approximately 50% of diazepam is biotransformed to N-desmethyldiazepam (nordiazepam) and a smaller amount is converted to temazepam (Colter et al. 1984; Driessen et al. 1987). Diazepam has a total body clearance of 4.7 ml/kg/min and is eliminated relatively quickly with a $t_{1/2}$ of 210 minutes, indicating that formation of nordiazepam is a rapid process in the cat (Driessen et al. 1987). Elimination of the parent compound is approximately six times that of nordiazepam (0.85 ml/kg/min). The elimination half-life of nordiazepam is approximately

21 hours, which is over four times slower than diazepam. Nordiazepam can be further hydroxylated to form oxazepam but this is a very slow process in the cat (Driessen et al. 1987). Glucuronide conjugates were found in very small amounts, even after eight hours, indicating that cats have poor ability to glucuronidate hydroxylated benzodiazepine metabolites.

A more recent *in-vitro* study using feline and canine hepatic microsomes showed some quantitative differences in metabolite formation in cats. Although incubations with a concentration range of diazepam resulted in formation of both nordiazepam and temazepam, cat-liver microsomes mainly produced temazepam, whereas dog microsomes produced relatively more nordiazepam (van Beusekom et al. 2015). The decreased formation of nordiazepam and oxazepam in feline-liver microsomes compared to dogs may suggest that differences exist in the feline CYP2B ortholog gene expression and/or substrate interactions. The formation of nordiazepam and oxazepam was much lower in this *in-vitro* study using liver microsomes compared to plasma levels found in previous *in-vivo* studies, suggesting extra-hepatic biotransformation (Colter et al. 1984; Driesson et al. 1987; van Beusekom et al. 2015). A high formation of the R-temazepam was observed in feline-liver microsome incubations, however, the S-temazepam and both isoforms of oxazepam were formed with much lower affinity and capacity compared to canine-liver microsomes (van Beusekom et al. 2015). Since oxazepam is conjugated by UGT2B15 and UGT2B7 in humans, this may give further evidence to low activity of these UGT homolog activities in the cat. The authors also suggest that the conjugation of temazepam in cats may be dependent on UGT1A3 in cats (Court and Greenblat 2000; van Beusekom et al. 2015). Differences in the pattern of phase I metabolites and low glucuronidation capacity increases the risk of accumulation of diazepam and its metabolites in the liver cells which may result in inhibition of the bile acid efflux system and accumulation of bile within hepatocytes and may contribute to the clinical observation of drug-induced liver injury in cats (van Beusekom et al. 2015). Decreasing the dose and especially increasing the dosing interval may reduce the incidence of this side effect.

Horses – Midazolam

Midazolam, administered at 0.05 and 0.1 mg/kg IV to adult horses has a rapid onset of action (within five minutes), likely due to its high lipid solubility and brain uptake (Hubbell et al. 2013). It has a large volume of distribution (>2 l/kg) and a high plasma clearance of ~10 ml/kg/min. The doses of 0.05 and 0.1 mg/kg have median terminal half-lives of 216 and 408 minutes, respectively. Cardiorespiratory

parameters do not change significantly. Also, sedation scores did not change and horses exhibited signs of agitation, ataxia, and weakness (Hubbell et al. 2013). The metabolic pathways have not been elucidated in horses.

Alpacas – Midazolam

After administration of midazolam (0.5 mg/kg) IV or IM, the median maximal plasma concentrations were 1394 and 411 ng/ml, respectively (Aarnes et al. 2013). The distribution half-life was ~19 minutes after IV administration and 41 minutes after IM administration and the elimination half-lives were 98 minutes for IV and 234 minutes for IM administration (Aarnes et al. 2013). Total clearance after IV administration was 11.3 ml/kg/min and steady state volume of distribution was 525 ml/kg/min (Aarnes et al. 2013). Peak onset of sedation occurs in less than one minute after IV administration. Midazolam is well absorbed after IM administration with a bioavailability of 92% (Aarnes et al. 2013). Mean heart rate and respiratory rates both increased after IV administration. Midazolam provides moderate levels of sedation when used as a sole agent in alpacas without signs of agitation or excitation. Alpacas assume sternal or lateral recumbency after IV administration, whereas they become quieter and more approachable within 15 minutes of IM administration, making IM administration particularly useful in animals that are difficult to handle or restrain (Aarnes et al. 2013).

Pharmacodynamics

Benzodiazepines decrease cerebral metabolic oxygen requirement ($CMRO_2$) and cerebral blood flow in a dose-related manner and maintain the ratio of CBF to $CMRO_2$ (Vuyk et al. 2020). Cerebral vasomotor responsiveness to carbon dioxide is preserved with midazolam and patients with decreased intracranial compliance display little to no change in intracranial pressure (ICP) (Rathmell and Rosow 2015).

Midazolam, diazepam, and lorazepam increase the seizure threshold of local anesthetics and increase survival in mice exposed to lethal doses of local anesthetics. Benzodiazepines increase the seizure threshold to local anesthetics (Vuyk et al. 2020).

Benzodiazepines produce dose-related centrally mediated respiratory depression. They flatten the respiratory response curve to carbon dioxide and also depress hypoxic ventilatory drive (Rathmell and Rosow 2015; Vuyk et al. 2020). The peak onset of respiratory depression occurs in about three minutes, is directly related to rate of administration and lasts 60–120 minutes. The incidence of apnea at induction is similar to thiopental but the duration of respiratory depression is longer with benzodiazepines. Other respiratory depressant drugs increase the incidence of apnea and respiratory depression, especially opioids which have an additive or supra-additive (synergistic) effect on respiratory depression (Reves et al. 2009; Rathmell and Rosow 2015). Benzodiazepines affect the muscular tone and may increase the risk of upper airway obstruction (Rathmell and Rosow 2015; Vuyk et al. 2020).

Benzodiazepines have mild but dose-related hemodynamic effects, which are primarily lowered arterial blood pressure due to decreased systemic vascular resistance (Rathmell and Rosow 2015; Vuyk et al. 2020). Heart rate, ventricular filling pressures and cardiac output are maintained (Vuyk et al. 2020). Benzodiazepines maintain relatively stable hemodynamics through preservation of homeostatic reflex mechanisms. Recent studies using heart rate variability indicate a biphasic effect of benzodiazepines on autonomic neurocardiac regulation (Vuyk et al. 2020). Vagal tone is first decreased and then the cardiac pacemaker decreases after IV doses (Vuyk et al. 2020). Benzodiazepines do not inhibit the sympathetic response and subsequent increases in heart rate, blood pressure or ICP invoked by laryngoscopy and intubation (Rathmell and Rosow 2015; Vuyk et al. 2020).

Reproductive/Nursing Safety

Diazepam, but not midazolam, has been implicated in causing congenital abnormalities in humans when administered during the first trimester of pregnancy (Plumb 2018b, 2018d). Infants born to mothers receiving large doses of benzodiazepines prior to delivery can have respiratory depression, impaired thermoregulation and difficulty feeding. Infants may exhibit withdrawal symptoms if the mother was chronically administered benzodiazepines (Plumb 2018b). The significance in veterinary patients is unclear. However, caution should be used in the use of these drugs in the first trimester of pregnancy and should occur only when the benefit outweighs the possible risks (Plumb 2018b). In humans, the FDA categorizes diazepam as a category D for use during pregnancy indicating there is evidence of human fetal risk but the potential benefit in pregnant women may be acceptable despite the potential risk (Plumb 2018b). Studies of lorazepam in animals generally suggest that the drug is safe for use during pregnancy at usual doses (Plumb 2018c). A study in mice administered 400 times the dose produced offspring with an increased incidence of cleft palate (Plumb 2018c).

Benzodiazepines and their metabolites are excreted into milk and may cause CNS effects in nursing neonates. The significance of these effects in veterinary patients is unclear but caution should be used during the first trimester of pregnancy and in lactating/nursing animals (Plumb 2018b, 2018d).

Drug Interactions

Ketoconazole, which is an inhibitor of CYP3A12 microsomal enzymes decreases the elimination of midazolam in dogs (KuKanich and Hubin 2010). Using cloned canine p450 cytochromes, medetomidine has been demonstrated to be an extremely potent inhibitor of CYP2B1 and may affect the clearances of both midazolam and ketamine which are CYP2B11 substrates with high intrinsic clearances (Baratta et al. 2009). Healthy dogs treated with fluconazole and subsequently anesthetized with ketamine (7.0 mg/kg) and midazolam (0.25 mg/kg) had a significantly longer time to standing and the clearance of both ketamine and midazolam were significantly slower (~50%) and the area under the curves were approximately twofold higher (Berke et al. 2019). Horses treated with fluconazole for fungal keratitis had significantly longer anesthesia recovery times (109 vs. 50 minutes) when midazolam was used as part of the anesthetic-induction protocol compared to an anesthetic-induction protocol without midazolam (Krein et al. 2014).

Veterinary Medicine – Uses and Specific Agents

The primary benzodiazepine drugs used in veterinary anesthesia are midazolam and diazepam (Table 15.2). Currently, midazolam has largely replaced diazepam in veterinary anesthesia due to better availability and lower cost. Benzodiazepines are used as premedication sedatives and co-induction agents. The degree to which they provide sedation is dependent on the specific species, patient age and physiologic status. In general, benzodiazepines produce greater sedative effects in pediatric (neonatal foals, dogs, and cats <3 months of age) and geriatric patients, whereas they can cause paradoxical excitement in healthy adults. Comparatively, benzodiazepines provide more reliable sedation, even when used as a sole agent in small ruminants and camelids of any age. Benzodiazepines are useful premedications and co-induction agents in debilitated and critically ill patients due to their minimal effect on cardiovascular depression. An additional advantage is the ability to antagonize their effects with flumazenil (0.02–0.1 mg/kg IV).

Table 15.2 Differences between diazepam and midazolam (Plumb 2018b, 2018d; Ko 2019).

Characteristic	Diazepam	Midazolam
Formulation	Formulated with propylene glycol	Water soluble but lipid soluble at body pH
Absorption	Rapidly with IV, slow with IM	Rapid IV or IM
Pain on injection	Yes with IM injection	Less pain with IM injection
Compatibility (Plumb 2018b, 2018d)	• Not recommended to mix with other drugs due to precipitation and microcrystal formation • Adsorbs to plastic; do not store in plastic syringes, IV bags/tubing	• compatible with: D5W, LRS, normal saline, atricurium, atropine, buprenorphine, butorphanol, cefuroxime, ciprofloxacin, fentanyl, gentamicin, glycopyrrolate, hydromorphone, ketamine, meperidine, metoclopramide, morphine, nalbuphine, ondansetron, promethazine, sufentanil, scopolamine • incompatible with: dexamethasone SP, heparin, pantoprazole, pentobarbital, ranitidine
Cost	Currently more expensive due to decreased manufacturing	Less expensive due to increased manufacturing and availability of generic formulations

Midazolam

Midazolam is used in veterinary patients for its sedative, anxiolytic, and muscle relaxant properties as an anesthetic premedication or co-induction agent in a variety of veterinary species. It does not provide predictable sedation on its own in dogs, cats or horses but may provide adequate sedation in goats, alpacas, rabbits, ferrets, some avian species, and swine. Patients may become sedate or dysphoric and excited. Cats may be more prone to the "disinhibition" or excitement effects than dogs. Midazolam provides more predictable sedation when combined with other drugs such as opioids, dexmedetomidine, ketamine, or acepromazine. Sedation is also more reliable in neonatal/pediatric, geriatric and critically ill ("very young, old or sick") veterinary patients. Benzodiazepines typically cause sedation and recumbency in small ruminants, depending on dose and patient status. Unlike in humans, it cannot be used alone for anesthetic induction.

Dosages and Usage

Dogs

When administered alone, healthy dogs exhibit muscle weakness, ataxia but minimal sedation and may display paradoxical excitement or agitation and hyperresponsiveness (Court and Greenblat 1992). Therefore, midazolam is usually combined with an opioid for anesthetic premedication and usually reserved for use in pediatric, geriatric or debilitated patients. It can also be used as a co-induction agent to provide muscle relaxation and reduction of induction agent.

Sedation Protocols:

1) Midazolam (0.3 mg/kg) + either butorphanol (0.3 mg/kg) or morphine (0.3 mg/kg) IM did not cause clinically relevant changes in echocardiographic (ECG) variables in healthy dogs. Therefore, these combinations may be used for sedation of uncooperative dogs during ECG evaluation (Possidonia et al. 2021).

2) Midazolam (0.3 mg/kg) combined with medetomidine (10 or 20 mcg/kg) did not provide adequate sedation for routine radiologic diagnostics compared to butorphanol (0.3 mg/kg) combined with medetomidine at the same doses (Le Chevallier et al. 2018).

Premedication: 0.1–0.3 mg/kg IM or IV is used most commonly in combination with opioids.

1) Midazolam (0.2 mg/kg) combined with alfaxalone (2.0 mg/kg) and butorphanol (0.4 mg/kg) IM produced reliable sedation in healthy young adult dogs with no significant effects on heart rate, cardiac output, or oxygen delivery. However, recovery quality was poor (Murdock et al. 2020).

2) Midazolam (0.5 mg/kg) combined with alfaxalone (1.0 mg/kg) and methadone (0.5 mg/kg) in healthy dogs resulted in significantly less sedation and was approximately five times more likely to show excitement than dogs premedicated without midazolam. Therefore, it is not recommended to add midazolam to an IM combination of methadone and alfaxalone in healthy dogs (Micieli et al. 2019).

3) Midazolam (0.2–0.3 mg/kg) added to medetomidine (5–10 mcg/kg) IV in healthy dogs resulted in a high incidence of undesirable behavioral effects including agitation, excitement, restlessness, aggression and vocalization, which was different from pre-sedation and did not have a sparing effect on the propofol induction dose (Le Chevallier et al. 2019).

4) Midazolam (0.3 mg/kg) IM does not enhance the sedation provided by dexmedetomidine (5 mcg/kg) and does not decrease the induction dose of propofol in healthy dogs (Canfran et al. 2016).

5) Midazolam (0.25 mg/kg) IM to healthy dogs caused behavioral changes including pacing, restlessness, chewing/licking, excitement, panting, and vocalization that were not ameliorated by acepromazine (0.03 mg/kg) or methadone (0.75 mg/kg) (Simon et al. 2014).

6) Midazolam (0.5 mg/kg) added to acepromazine (0.05 mg/kg) and morphine (0.5 mg/kg) IM resulted in more intense sedation and provides the greatest propofol sparing effects in healthy dogs compared to premedication with acepromazine + morphine or midazolam + morphine (Monteiro et al. 2014).

Co-induction Agent:

1) Midazolam (0.2 mg/kg) combined with ketamine 4.0 mg/kg can be used for induction of anesthesia.

2) Midazolam (0.2–0.4 mg/kg) can be administered as a co-induction agent to reduce the dose of propofol by ~20–47%. It is best to administer the midazolam after administration of 1.0 mg/kg of propofol to avoid excitement and to maximize the propofol sparing effect. Diazepam at the same doses does not have the same propofol sparing effect (Robinson and Borer-Weir 2013; Sanchez et al. 2013; Hopkins et al. 2014).

3) Midazolam (0.2 mg/kg) significantly decreased (46%) the induction and maintenance dose (32%) of alfaxalone in healthy dogs (Bustamante et al. 2020).

4) Midazolam (0.4 mg/kg IV) administered after 0.5 mg/kg of alfaxalone in healthy client-owned dogs that were premedicated with acepromazone (0.02 mg/kg) and methadone (0.3 mg/kg) had a significant dose-sparing effect on the dose of alfaxalone required for intubation. Although there were no significant differences in HR or BP, post-induction apnea was significantly more prevalent in dogs receiving midazolam (Miller et al. 2019).

5) Midazolam (0.3 or 0.5 mg/kg) administered after 0.5 mg/kg of alfaxalone IV to healthy dogs premedicated with acepromazine (0.01 mg/kg) and methadone (0.2 mg/kg) significantly decreased the total induction dose of alfaxalone and improved the ease of endotracheal intubation (ET) (Italiano and Robinson 2018).

6) Midazolam (0.25 mg/kg) IV administered after an initial dose of 0.5 mg/kg of alfaxalone in healthy dogs premedicated with acepromazine (0.02 mg/kg) and morphine (0.4 mg/kg) significantly decreased the total induction dose of alfaxalone. Administering midazolam prior to the administering an initial dose of alfaxalone resulted in a significant increase in the incidence of excitement and did not have a sparing effect on the induction dose of alfaxalone. However, there was no significant difference in cardiorespiratory values between groups (Zapata et al. 2018).

7) Midazolam (0.3 mg/kg IV) after premedication with acepromazine (0.02 mg/kg), hydromorphone (0.1 mg/kg), and alfaxalone (0.25 mg/kg) IM significantly decreased the total induction dose of alfaxalone in healthy client-owned dogs, however, differences in cardiopulmonary variables were minor (Munoz et al. 2017).

8) Midazolam (0.2 mg/kg) IV significantly decreased the propofol target controlled infusion dose required for ET in healthy client-owned dogs premedicated with acepromazine (0.03 mg/kg) and morphine (0.2 mg/kg) IM compared to saline control or lidocaine (2.0 mg/kg). However, there were no significant differences in cardiopulmonary variables (Minghella et al. 2016).

Critical Patient Premedication/Induction: Due to the minimal cardiovascular effects of opioids and benzodiazepines, they provide a good option for induction protocol for critical and severely debilitated patients. Fentanyl 5.0–10.0 mcg/kg slowly over two to five minutes followed by midazolam 0.2 mg/kg. If desired, lidocaine 2.0 mg/kg IV slowly over two minutes can be administered prior to fentanyl administration. Due to the likelihood of bradycardia and hypoventilation during this prolonged induction process, ECG, blood pressure, and SpO2 should be monitored and oxygen supplementation provided. Patients can be arousable and stimulated by noise and movement but the majority of patients can be intubated with careful handling.

1) Midazolam (0.3 mg/kg IV) significantly decreases the total propofol induction dose (1.1 vs. 1.9 mg/kg) in critically ill dogs (ASA >3). However, no significant differences were found in cardiorespiratory variables (Aguilera et al. 2020).

Constant Rate Infusion (CRI): Midazolam CRI can be used as part of a sedation/analgesia protocol for dogs maintained on assisted ventilation in the intensive care unit (ICU).

1) A comparison of two protocols for ventilation in the ICU: midazolam (0.5 mg/kg/hour) + morphine (0.6 mg/kg/hour) or fentanyl (18 mcg/kg/hr) + medetomidine (1.0 mcg/kg/hour) or propofol (2.5 mg/kg/hr). Both

protocols were effective in facilitating mechanical ventilation in healthy dogs. Both protocols caused a reduction in cardiac index due to bradycardia, however, there was no negative effect on oxygen delivery and global tissue perfusion (Ethier et al. 2008).

Cats

When administered alone, healthy cats exhibit minimal sedation and may display paradoxical excitement or aggression therefore, it is usually combined with ketamine. If used as a premedication in geriatric or debilitated patients, midazolam is usually combined with an opioid analgesic.

Premedication: Midazolam (0.1–0.3 mg/kg) IV, IM can be used in combination with opioids. Doses of 0.1–0.5 mg/kg IV, IM can be used in combination with ketamine 3.0–10 mg/kg. Ketamine causes sympathetic stimulation resulting in tachycardia and increased blood pressure, profuse salivation, and airway secretions necessitating co-administration of an anti-cholinergic with this combination, emergence delirium with uncoordinated movements of the head and neck, vocalization and agitation can occur during recovery, risking patient injury, or requiring sedation.

1) Midazolam (0.2 mg/kg) added to hydromorphone (0.1 mg/kg) and alfaxalone (1.5 mg/kg) IM produces more profound sedation and greater ease of IV catheter placement in healthy client-owned cats compared to IM hydromorphone and alfaxalone alone (Wheeler et al. 2021).
2) Intra-nasal administration – midazolam 0.5 mg/kg + ketamine 14 mg/kg administered intranasally (IN) showed no difference in time to onset or duration of sedation compared to the same doses administered IM. The time to sternal recumbency was significantly shorter for IN administration (~22 vs. 32 minutes). Behavioral reaction to IN administration was sneezing/snorting compared to excessive vocalization in response to IM administration. Intra-nasal administration may provide a less painful and less stressful invasive route of administration of this drug combination (Marjani et al. 2015).

Co-induction Agent: Midazolam (0.2 mg/kg) combined with ketamine 4.0 mg/kg for anesthesia induction.

1) Midazolam (0.08 mg/kg) IV allowed smooth ET in 50% of healthy cats after premedication with dexmedetomidine (3 mcg/kg), methadone (0.3 mg/kg) IM followed by alfaxalone (0.25 mg/kg) IV (Lagos-Carvajal et al. 2019).
2) Midazolam (0.2–0.5 mg/kg) and diazepam (0.3–0.5 mg/kg) both significantly reduce the propofol dose required for ET in cats when administered after 2 mg/kg of propofol IV (Robinson and Borer-Weir 2015).

Constant Rate Infusion: Midazolam CRI can be used as part of a sedation/analgesia protocol for cats maintained on assisted ventilation in the intensive care unit.

Fentanyl (10 mcg/kg/hr) and midazolam (0.5 mg/kg/hr) plus one of the following:

Ketamine (5.0 mg/kg/hr) or propofol (0.1 mg/kg/min) or ketamine (2.5 mg/kg/hr) + propofol (0.05 mg/kg/min)

Cardiovascular stability and recovery times were most favorable with the protocol using a combination of propofol and ketamine. Recoveries are prolonged 0.5–2.0 hours for extubation and 10–36 hours until standing/walking in healthy cats (Boudreau et al. 2012).

Rabbits, Rodents, Small Mammals: Difficulty obtaining IV access in small mammals and rodents often necessitates using combinations of drugs via SC, IM, or TN routes rather than IV titration to achieve the necessary objective. Inability or difficult intubation requires balancing sedation needs with respiratory depression. Midazolam provides good sedation in rabbits and small mammals and, when used alone, has minimal effect of the cardiovascular and respiratory systems. Therefore, it may decrease the adverse effect profile of co-administered drugs when used as an adjunct for sedation, premedication or total injectable anesthesia since it allows lower doses of other drugs and is reversible.

Sedation or Pre-anesthetic: Midazolam 0.5–5 mg/kg can be administered IV, IM, SC, or transnasally. It is usually combined with other drugs such as α-2 agonists, opioids, and/or ketamine.

1) For sedation or anesthetic premedication, midazolam (2.0 mg/kg) can be combined with butorphanol (0.3 mg/kg) or buprenorphine (0.03 mg/kg) to facilitate IV catheter access for anesthetic induction (Schroeder and Smith 2011).
2) Lower doses of midazolam (0.2 mg/kg) can be combined with dexmedetomidine (25 mcg/kg) or ketamine (30 mg/kg) to facilitate diagnostic procedures such as abdominal ultrasound (Bellini et al. 2014).
3) A combination of dexmedetomidine (0.1 mg/kg), midazolam (2.0 mg/kg), and butorphanol (0.2 mg/kg) administered via transnasal catheter provides deep sedation and analgesia within approximately one minute of administration and lasting for 45–60 minutes. This protocol is appropriate for diagnostics or minor surgery in healthy rabbits (Santangelo et al. 2016). Oxygen supplementation and monitoring of blood pressure and SpO2 is highly recommended.
4) Gastric and small intestinal transit times were significantly longer in rabbits administered ketamine (15 mg/kg) and

medetomidine (0.25 mg/kg) IM (despite reversal with atipamazole) compared to IM administration of ketamine (15 mg/kg) and midazolam (3.0 mg/kg) (Botman et al. 2020).

5) Midazolam (1.0 mg/kg) combined with alfaxalone (6.0 mg/kg) IM has an onset of sedation of two to five minutes and provides approximately 60 minutes of sedation in healthy rabbits (Bradley et al. 2019).

Rodents: Inhalant anesthetics are commonly used for induction and maintenance of general anesthesia in both laboratory and pet rodents. Disadvantages include a lack of analgesia and, when used alone, the necessity for high doses thus potentiating adverse effects. A recent study used midazolam 2.5 mg/kg and butorphanol 2.0 mg/kg for premedication prior to isoflurane inhalant anesthesia. Premedication decreased the minimum alveolar concentration (MAC) of isoflurane by 32% and provided a more stable respiratory rate and SpO2 with few adverse effects compared to isoflurane alone (Tsukamoto et al. 2016).

Horses

Benzodiazepines are rarely used as a sole agent in horses and are usually combined with tranquilizers, opioids and/or combined with dissociative anesthetics for induction of anesthesia.

Clinical doses (0.05–0.1 mg/kg) of diazepam or midazolam have minimal cardiorespiratory effects (Hubbell et al. 2013). Respiratory rate, tidal volume, blood gas variables, heart rate, cardiac output, and mean arterial pressures do not change but ataxia, muscle fasiculations, and recumbency may be observed. Ataxia and recumbency can be seen with doses greater than 0.1 mg/kg (Hubbell et al. 2013). Diazepam has a relatively long plasma half-life (7–21 hours) compared to midazolam (median terminal half-life 216–408 minutes) (Hubbell et al. 2013). Muscle relaxation and concomitant ataxia are not desirable effects during equine anesthetic recovery, therefore, the shorter duration of action of midazolam may be advantageous in equine patients. Midazolam is currently being used as a substitute for diazepam at equal dose rates in equine anesthesia based on current drug availability and decreased cost of generic midazolam formulations.

Sedation in Neonatal Foals

Foals less than one month of age can be sedated with 0.1–0.2 mg/kg IV to produce recumbency for non-painful procedures.

Co-induction Agent in Horses: The recommended dose of midazolam or diazepam for co-induction with ketamine is 0.05–0.1 mg/kg.

1) Induction with propofol (0.5 mg/kg) and ketamine (3.0 mg/kg) provides better recovery and may be preferable for short procedures (<60 minutes) compared to induction with midazolam (0.1 mg/kg) and ketamine (3.0 mg/kg) (Jarrett et al. 2018).

2) Co-induction with midazolam (0.06 mg/kg) IV in ponies sedated with detomidine (2.0 mcg/kg) and induced with ketamine (2.2 mg/kg) improved induction scores, intubation and surgical relaxation and required fewer additional rescue anesthetic administration compared to detomidine and ketamine alone. Time to sternal and standing was longer in ponies receiving midazolam, but there was no difference in the quality of recovery (Allison et al. 2018).

3) Horses treated with fluconazole for fungal keratitis have significantly longer anesthesia recovery times (109 vs. 50 minutes) when midazolam is included as part of the anesthetic induction protocol compared to a protocol without midazolam (Krein et al. 2014).

Total Intravenous Anesthesia (TIVA):

1) A combination of ketamine (3.0 mg/kg/hr), medetomidine (5mcg/kg/hr), and midazolam (0.1 mg/kg/hr) can be used as part of a balanced anesthesia regimen to maintain anesthesia in horses for routine castration. This protocol provided good surgical conditions; recoveries were good with the horses standing in ~30 minutes (Cunneen et al. 2021).

2) Recovery scores were significantly better for weanling horses for computed tomography (CT) administered the TIVA regimen of ketamine (3 mg/kg/hr) + medetomidine (5 mcg/kg/hr) + midazolam (0.1 mg/kg/hr) compared to the same protocol using guafenesin (100 mg/kg/hr) instead of midazolam. However, there were no significant differences in cardiopulmonary variables or recovery times (Pratt et al. 2019).

3) A TIVA regimen of midazolam (25 mg), ketamine (650 mg), and xylazine (325 mg) added to a 500 ml bag of 0.9% saline can be used for short-term TIVA in horses for a variety of procedures including: castration, bone marrow aspirate, wound debridement/flushing, cast application, etc. Recovery scores were good with horses standing at ~30 minutes after discontinuation (Aarnes et al. 2018).

4) The addition of midazolam (0.06 mg/kg/hr) to horses receiving romifidine bolus (0.03 mg/kg) followed by romifidine CRI (0.05 mg/kg/hr) had improved conditions for standing dental surgery with decreased

chewing and tongue activity, however, horses were significantly more ataxic than with romifidine alone or romifidine with butorphanol (Muller et al. 2017).

Camelids

Midazolam (0.5 mg/kg) IV or IM provides moderate levels of sedation when used as a sole agent in alpacas without signs of agitation or excitation. Alpacas assume sternal or lateral recumbency after IV administration, whereas they become quieter and more approachable within 15 minutes of IM administration, making IM administration particularly useful in animals that are difficult to handle or restrain (Aarnes et al. 2013).

Small Ruminants

Midazolam (0.3 mg/kg IV or 0.4–0.6 mg/kg IM) produces 10–20 minutes of recumbency; increasing the dose to 1.2 mg/kg increased the duration of recumbency to 30 minutes (Lin 2014b).

1) Midazolam (0.3 mg/kg) IM alone or in combination with butorphanol (0.3 mg/kg) IM produces a degree of sedation that significantly reduces the dose of alfaxalone required for induction of general anesthesia in goats, without causing any major adverse cardiorespiratory effects (Dzikiti et al. 2014).

Diazepam

Diazepam has been the most widely used benzodiazepine in veterinary medicine. However, as in human medicine, use of midazolam may be supplanting diazepam due to the availability of cost-effective generic formulations, a solubility profile that allows administration via multiple routes and shorter elimination half-time. Diazepam is insoluble in water and parenteral formulations contain 40% propylene glycol (Posner and Burns 2009). Therefore, it should not be mixed with other drugs (ketamine is the exception) or given IM since it is poorly absorbed and irritating to tissues. In dogs, the elimination half-life of diazepam is ~3 hours, active metabolites nordiazepam and oxazepam peak within

two hours and have elimination half-lives of three to six hours (Plumb 2018b). In cats, the elimination half-time of diazepam is 5.5 hours but that of nordiazepam may be as long as 21 hours (Plumb 2018b). In horses, the elimination half-life ranges from 7 to 22 hours; hydroxylated metabolites are rapidly conjugated with glucuronide and are not detectable in plasma (Plumb 2018b). Diazepam is not a reliable sedative in most species but it can be administered to decrease the dose of induction agents or to decrease the MAC of inhalant by 20–30% in dogs and horses.

Co-Induction:

1) Midazolam 0.3 and 0.5 mg/kg and diazepam 0.4 mg/kg co-administered at anesthetic induction allow alfaxalone dose reduction in healthy dogs. Use of benzodiazepines improved the ease of ET (Italiano and Robinson 2018).
2) Midazolam or diazepam (0.06 mg/kg) can be used interchangeably as a co-induction agent with ketamine (2.2 mg/kg) in ponies sedated with detomidine (20 mcg/kg) and undergoing field castration. Surgical conditions were good with either drug, and time to standing was not significantly different with minimal ataxia (De Vries et al. 2015).

Small Ruminants

Diazepam (0.25–0.5 mg/kg) IV produces standing sedation without analgesia (Lin 2014b).

Flumazenil

Flumazenil is the only benzodiazepine receptor antagonist available for clinical use and is used to reverse the sedative and muscle relaxant effects of benzodiazepines. It is highly selective and has a strong affinity but minimal intrinsic activity and will reverse the sedative and muscle relaxant effects of benzodiazepines. Doses of 0.008–0.04 mg/kg can be administered via IV, IM, submucosal, ET, or rectal routes in dogs. In horses, the recommended dose for foals and adults is 0.01–0.02 mg/kg IV (Posner and Burns 2009). However, titration of much smaller doses are effective in reversing residual effects of clinical doses. The elimination half-life in dogs is 0.4–1.3 hours, significantly shorter than benzodiazepines and their active metabolites. Caution should be used in patients receiving tricyclic antidepressants as fatal arrhythmias may develop (Posner and Burns 2009).

References

Aarnes, T.K., Fry, P.R., Hubbell, J.A.E. et al. (2013). Pharmacokinetics and pharmacodynamics of midazolam after intravenous and intramuscular administration in alpacas. *Am. J. Vet. Res.* 74: 294–299.

Aarnes, T.K., Lerche, P., Bednarski, R.M. et al. (2018). Total intravenous anesthesia using a midazolam-ketamine-xylazine infusion in horses: 46 cases (2011–2014). *Can. Vet. J.* 59 (5): 500–504.

Aguilera, R., Sinclair, M., Valverde, A. et al. (2020). Dose and cardiopulmonary effects of propfol alone or with midazolam for induction of anesthesia in critically ill dogs. *Vet. Anaesth. Analg.* 47 (4): 472–480.

Allison, A., Robinson, R., Jolliffe, C. et al. (2018). Evaluation of the use of midazolam as a co-induction agent with ketamine for anaesthesia in sedated ponies undergoing field castration. *Equine Vet. J.* 50 (3): 321–326.

Baratta, M.T., Zaya, M.J., White, J.A., and Locuson, C.W. (2009). Canine CYP2B11 metabolizes and is inhibited by anesthetic agents often co-administered in dogs. *J. Vet. Pharmacol. Therap.* 33: 50–55.

Bellini, L., Banzato, T., Contiero, B., and Zotti, A. (2014). Evaluation of sedation and clinical effects of midazolam with ketamine or dexmedetomidine in pet rabbits. *Vet. Rec.* 175 (15): 372.

Benson, G.J., Thurmon, J.C., Tranquilli, W.J., and Smith, C.W. (1985). Cardiopulmonary effects of an intravenous infusion of guaifenesin, ketamine, and xylazine in dogs. *Am. J. Vet. Res.* 46 (9): 1896–1898.

Berke, K., KuKanich, B., Orchard, R. et al. (2019). Clinical and pharmacokinetic interactions between oral fluconazole and intravenous ketamine and midazolam in dogs. *Vet. Anaesth. Analg.* 46 (6): 745–752.

van Beusekom, C.D., van den Heuvel, J.J.M.W., Koenderink, J.B. et al. (2015). Feline hepatic biotransformation of diazepam: differences between cats and dogs. *Res. Vet. Sci.* 103: 119–125.

Botman, J., Hontoir, F., Gustin, P. et al. (2020). Postanaesthetic effects of ketamine-midazolam and ketamine-medetomidine on gastrointestinal transit time in rabbits anaesthetised with isoflurane. *Vet. Rec.* 186 (8): 249.

Boudreau, A.E., Bersenas, A.M.E., Kerr, C.L. et al. (2012, 2012). A comparison of 3 anesthetic protocols for 24 hours of mechanical ventilation in cats. *J. Vet. Emerg. Crit. Care* 22 (2): 239–252.

Bradley, M.P., Doerning, C.M., Nowland, M.H. et al. (2019). Intramuscular Administration of alfaxalone alone and in combination for sedation and anesthesia of rabbits (*Oryctolagus cuniculus*). *J. Am. Assoc. Lab. Anim. Sci.* 58 (2): 216–222.

Brosnan, R.J., Steffey, E.P., Escobar, A. et al. (2011). Anesthetic induction with guaifenesin and propofol in adult horses. *Am. J. Vet. Res.* 72: 1569–1575.

Bustamante, R., Gomez de Segura, I., Canfran, S. et al. (2020). Effects of ketamine or midazolam continuous rate infusions on alfaxalone total intravenous anaesthesia requirements and recovery quality in healthy dogs: a randomized clinical trail. *Vet. Anaesth. Analg.* 47 (4): 437–446.

Canfran, S., Bustamante, R., Gonzalez, P. et al. (2016). Comparison of sedation scores and propofol induction

doses in dogs after intramuscular administration of dexmedetomidine alone or in combination with methadone, midazolam, or methadone plus midazolam. *Vet. J.* 210: 56–60.

Chenery, R.J., Ayrton, A., Oldham, H.G. et al. (1987). Diazepam metabolism in cultured hepatocytes from rat, rabbit, dog, guinea pig and man. *Drug Metab. Dispos.* 15 (3): 312–317.

Colter, S., Gustafson, J., and Colburn, W. (1984). Pharmacokinetics of diazepam and nordiazepam in the cat. *J Pharm Sci.* 73: 348–351.

Court, M.H. (2013). Feline drug metabolism and disposition: pharmacokinetic evidence for species differences and molecular mechanisms. *Vet. Clin. North Am. Small Anim. Pract.* 43 (5): 1039–1054.

Court, M.H. and Greenblatt, D.J. (1992). Pharmacokinetics and preliminary observations of behavioral changes following administration of midazolam to dogs. *J. Vet. Pharmacol. Therap.* 15: 343–350.

Court, M.H. and Greenblatt, D.J. (2000). Molecular genetic basis for deficient acetaminophen glucuronidation by cats: UGT1A6 is a pseudogene, and evidence for reduced diversity of expressed hepatic UGT1A isoforms. *Pharmacogenetics* 10: 355–369.

Cunneen, A., Pratt, S., Perkins, N. et al. (2021). Total intravenous anaesthesia with ketamine, medetomidine and midazolam as part of a balanced anaesthesia technique in horses undergoing castration. *Vet. Sci.* 8 (8): 142.

Davis, L.E. and Wolf, W.A. (1970). Pharmacokinetics and metabolism of glyceryl guaiacolate in ponies. *Am. J. Vet. Res.* 3 (31): 469–473.

De Vries, A., Thomson, S., and Taylor, P.M. (2015). Comparison of midazolam and diazepam as co-induction agents with ketamine for anaesthesia in sedated ponies undergoing field castration. *Vet. Anaesth. Analg.* 42 (5): 512–517.

Dholakia, U., Seddighi, R., Cox, S.K. et al. (2020). Pharmacokinetics of midazolam in sevoflure anesthetized cats. *Vet. Anaesth. Analg.* 47: 200–209.

Driessen, J.J., Vree, T.B., Van de Pol, F. et al. (1987). Pharmacokinetics of diazepam and four 3-hydroxybenzodiazepines in the cat. *Eur J Drug Metab Pharmacokinet.* 12 (3): 219–224.

Dzikiti, T.B., Zeiler, G.E., Dzikiti, L.N. et al. (2014). The effects of midazolam and butorphanol, administered alone or combined, on the dose and quality of anaesthetic induction with alfaxalone in goats. *J. S. Afr Vet. Assoc.* 85: 1–1047.

Ethier, M.R., Mathews, K.A., Valverde, A., and Kerr, C. (2008). Evaluation of the efficacy and safety for use of two sedation and analgesia protocols to facilitate assisted ventilation of healthy dogs. *Am. J. Vet. Res.* 69: 1351–1359.

Funk, K.A. (1970). Glyceryl guaiacolate: a centrally acting muscle relaxant. *Equine Vet. J.* 2: 173–177.

Funk, K.A. (1973). Glyceryl guaiacolate: some effects and indications in horses. *Equine Vet. J.* 5: 15–19.

Goodwin, W.A., Keates, H.L., Pasloske, K. et al. (2011). The pharmacokinetics and pharmacodynamics of the injectable anaesthetic alfaxalone in the horse. *Vet. Anaesth. Analg.* 38: 431–438.

Goodwin, W.A., Pasloske, K., and Keates, H.L. (2019). Alfaxalone for total intravenous anaesthesia in horses. *Vet. Anaesth. Analg.* 46: 188–199.

Herschl, M.A., Trim, C.M., and Mahaffey, E.A. (1992). Effects of 5% and 10% guaifenesin infusion on equine vascular endothelium. *Vet. Surg.* 21 (6): 494–497.

Hopkins, M., Giuffrida, M., and Larenza, M.P. (2014). Midazolam, as a co-induction agent, has propofol sparing effects but also decreases systolic blood pressure in healthy dogs. *Vet. Anesth. Analg.* 41: 64–72.

Hubbell, J.A., Muir, W.W., and Sams, R.A. (1980). Guafenesin: cardiopulmonary effects and plasma concentrations. *Am. J. Vet. Res.* 41 (11): 1751–1755.

Hubbell, J.A., Kelly, E.M., Aarnes, T.K. et al. (2013). Pharmacokinetics of midazolam after intravenous administration to horses. *Equine Vet. J.* 45: 721–725.

Italiano, M. and Robinson, R. (2018). Effect of benzodiazepines on the dose of alfaxalone needed for endotracheal intubation in healthy dogs. *Vet. Anaesth. Analg.* 45 (6): 720–728.

Jarrett, M.A., Bailey, K.M., Messenger, K.M. et al. (2018). Recovery of horses from general anesthesia after induction with propofol and ketamine versus midazolam and ketamine. *J. Am. Vet. Med. Assoc.* 253 (1): 101–107.

Kerr, C.L., Windeyer, C., Boure, L.P. et al. (2007). Cardiopulmonary effects of administration of a combination solution of xylazine, guaifenesin and ketamine or inhaled isoflurane in mechanically ventilated calves. *Am. J. Vet. Res.* 68: 1287–1293.

Ko, J. (2019). Preanesthetic medication: drugs and dosages. In: *Small Animal Anesthesia and Pain Management* (ed. J.C. Ko), 56–57. Boca Raton, FL: CRC Press, Taylor & Frances Group.

Krein, S.R., Lindsey, J.C., Blaze, C.A., and Wetmore, L.A. (2014). Evaluation of risk factors, including fluconazole administration, for prolonged anesthetic recovery times in horses undergoing general anesthesia for ocular surgery: 81 cases (2006–2013). *J. Am. Vet. Med. Assoc.* 244 (5): 577–581.

KuKanich, B. and Hubin, M. (2010). The pharmacokinetics of ketoconazole and its effects on the pharmacokinetics of midazolam and fentanyl in dogs. *J. Vet. Pharmacol. Ther.* 33 (1): 42–49.

Lagos-Carvajal, A., Queiroz-Williams, P., da Cunha, A. et al. (2019). Determination of midazolam dose for co-induction with alfaxalone in sedated cats. *Vet. Anaesth. Analg.* 46 (3): 299–307.

Le Chevallier, D., Slingsby, L., and Murrell, J.C. (2018). Randomised clinical trial comparing clinically relevant sedation outcome measures in dogs after intramuscular administration of medetomidine in combination with midazolam or butorphanol for routine diagnostic imaging procedures. *Vet. J.* 239: 30–34.

Le Chevallier, D., Slingsby, L., and Murrell, J. (2019). Use of midazolam in combination with medetomidine for premedication in healthy dogs. *Vet. Anaesth. Analg.* 46 (1): 74–78.

Lerche, P. (2013). Total intravenous anesthesia in horses. *Vet. Clin. Equine* 29: 123–129.

Lin, H. (2014a). Injectable anesthetics and field anesthesia. In: *Farm Animal Anesthesia* (ed. H. Lin and P. Walz), 60–94. Ames, IA: Wiley.

Lin, H. (2014b). Standing sedation and chemical restraint. In: *Farm Animal Anesthesia* (ed. H. Lin and P. Walz), 39–59. Ames, IA: Wiley.

Lin, H.C., Tyler, J.W., Welles, E.G. et al. (1993). Effects of anesthesia induced and maintained by continuous intravenous administration of guaifenesin, ketamine, and xylazine in spontaneously breathing sheep. *Am. J. Vet. Res.* 54 (11): 1913–1916.

Lu, P., Singh, S.B., and Carr, B.A. (2005). Selective inhibition of dog hepatic CYP2B11 and CYP3A12. *J. Pharmacol. Exp. Therap.* 313: 518–528.

Marjani, M., Akbarinejad, V., and Bagheri, M. (2015). Comparison of intranasal and intramuscular ketamine midazolam combination in cats. *Vet. Anaesth. Analg.* 42: 178–118.

Matthews, N.S., Peck, K.E., Mealy, K.L. et al. (1997). Pharmacokinetics and cardiopulmonary effects of guafenesin in donkeys. *J. Vet. Pharmacol. Therap.* 20: 442–446.

Mezerová, J., Němecek, L., and Snásil, M. (1992). Continuous intravenous anesthesia in dogs using a combination of xylazine, ketamine and guaifenesin. *[Article in Czech] Vet. Med. (Praha)* 37 (5, 6): 341–347.

Micieli, F., Chiavaccini, L., Pare, M.D. et al. (2019). Comparison of the sedative effects of alfaxalone and methadone with or without midazolam in dogs. *Can. Vet. J.* 60 (10): 1060–1064.

Miller, C., Hughes, E., and Gurney, M. (2019). Co-induction of anaesthesia with alfaxalone and midazolam in dogs: a randomized, blinded clinical trial. *Vet. Anaesth. Analg.* 46 (5): 613–619.

Minghella, E., Auckburally, A., Pawson, P. et al. (2016). Clinical effects of midazolam or lidocaine co-induction with a propofol target-controlled infusion (TCI) in dogs. *Vet. Anaesth. Analg.* 43 (5): 472–481.

Mohler, H. (2014). The legacy of the benzodiazepine receptor: from flumazenil to enhancing cognition in down syndrome and social interaction in autism. *Adv. Pharmacol.* 72: 7–8.

Monteiro, E.R., Nunes-Junior, J.S., and Bressan, T.F. (2014). Randomized clinical trial of the effects of a combination of acepromazine with morphine and midazolam on sedation, cardiovascular variables and the propofol dose requirements for induction of anesthesia in dogs. *Vet. J.* 200 (1): 157–161.

Muir, W.W. (2009). Intravenous anesthetic drugs. In: *Equine Anesthesia: Monitoring and Emergency Therapy* (ed. W.W. Muir and H. JAE), 243–259. St. Louis, MO: Saunders Elsevier.

Muller, T.M., Hopster, K., Bienert-Zeit, A. et al. (2017). Effect of butorphanol, midazolam or ketamine on romifidine based sedation in horses during standing cheek tooth removal. *BMC Vet. Res.* 13 (1): 381.

Munoz, K., Robertson, S.A., and Wilson, D.V. (2017). Alfaxalone alone or combined with midazolam or ketamine in dogs: intubation dose and select physiologic effects. *Vet. Anaesth. Analg.* 44 (4): 766–774.

Murdock, M., Ricco, C.H., Aarnes, T.K. et al. (2020). Sedative and cardiorespiratory effects of intramuscular administration of alfaxalone and butorphanol combined with acepromazine, midazolam, or dexmedetomidine in dogs. *Am. J. Vet. Res.* 81 (1): 65–76.

Pang, D. (2015). Anesthetic and analgesic adjunctive drugs. In: *Veterinary Anesthesia and Analgesia, The 5th edition of Lumb and Jones* (ed. K.A. Grimm, L.A. Lamont, W.J. Tranquilli, et al.), 247. Ames, IA: Wiley.

Plumb, D.C. (2018a). Guafenesin. In: *Plumb's Veterinary Drug Handbook*, 9e (ed. D.C. Plumb), 560–563. Hoboken, NJ: Wiley.

Plumb, D.C. (2018b). Diazepam. In: *Plumb's Veterinary Drug Handbook*, 9e (ed. D.C. Plumb), 357–360. Hoboken, NJ: Wiley.

Plumb, D.C. (2018c). Lorazepam. In: *Plumb's Veterinary Drug Handbook*, 9e (ed. D.C. Plumb), 709–711. Hoboken, NJ: Wiley.

Plumb, D.C. (2018d). Midazolam. In: *Plumb's Veterinary Drug Handbook*, 9e (ed. D.C. Plumb), 722–725. Hoboken, NJ: Wiley.

Posner, L.P. (2018). Sedatives and tranquilizers. In: *Veterinary Pharmacology & Therapeutics*, 10e (ed. J.E. Riviere and M.G. Papich), 324–368. Hoboken, NJ: Wiley.

Posner, L.P. and Burns, P. (2009). Injectable anesthetic agents. In: *Veterinary Pharmacology & Therapeutics*, 9e (ed. J.E. Riviere and M.G. Papich), 287–289. Ames, IA: Wiley.

Possidonia, G., Santos, C.A., Ferreira, M.A. et al. (2021). Echocardiographic assessment of healthy midazolam/Butorphanol or midazolam/morphine sedated dogs. *Top Companion Anim. Med.* 45: 100553. https://doi.org/10.1016/j.tcam.2021.100553. Online ahead of print.

Pratt, S., Cunneen, A., Perkins, N. et al. (2019). Total intravenous anaesthesia with ketamine, medetomidine and guaifenesin compared with ketamine, medetomidine and midazolam in young horses anaesthetised for computerised tomography. *Equine Vet. J.* 51 (4): 510–516.

Rathmell, J.P. and Rosow, C.E. (2015). Intravenous sedatives and hypnotics. In: *Stoelting's Pharmacology and Physiology* (ed. P. Flood, J.P. Rathmell and S. Shafer), 171–182. Philadelphia, PA: Wolters Kluwer.

Reves, J.G., Glass, P.S.A., Lubarsky, D.A. et al. (2009). Intravenous anesthetics. In: *Miller's Anesthesia*, 7e (ed. R.D. Miller), 1191–1200. Philadelphia, PA: Churchill Livingston, Elsevier.

Robinson, R. and Borer-Weir (2015). The effects of diazepam or midazolam on the dose of propofol required to induce anaesthesia in cats. *Vet. Anaesth. Analg.* https://doi.org/10.1111/vaa.12244. [Epub ahead of print].

Robinson, R. and Borer-Weir. (2013). A dose titration study into the effects of diazepam or midazolam on the propofol dose requirements for induction of general anaesthesia in client owned dogs, premedicated with methadone and acepromazine. *Vet. Anaesth. Analg.* 40: 455–463.

Sanchez, A.S., Belda, E., Escobar, M. et al. (2013). Effects of altering the sequence of midazolam and propofol during co-induction of anaesthesia. *Vet. Anaesth. Analg.* 40: 359–366.

Santangelo, B., Micieli, F., Mozzillo, T. et al. (2016). Transnasal administration of a combination of dexmedetomidine, midazolam and butorphanol produces deep sedation in New Zealand White rabbits. *Vet. Anaesth. Analg.* 43 (2): 209–214.

Schatzmann, U., Tschudi, P., Held, J.P., and Muhlebach, B. (1978). An investigation of the action and haemolytic effect of glyceral guaiacolate in the horse. *Equine Vet. J.* 10 (4): 224–228.

Schillings, R.T., Sisenwine, S.F., Schwartz, M.H. et al. (1975). Lorazepam: glucuronide formation in the cat. *Drug Metab. Dispos.* 3 (2): 85–88.

Schroeder, C.A. and Smith, L.J. (2011). Respiratory rates and arterial blood-gas tensions in healthy rabbits given buprenorphine, butorphanol, midazolam, or their combinations. *J. Am. Assoc. Lab. An. Sci.* 50 (2): 205–211.

Schwartz, M.A. (1965). Metabolism of diazepam in rat, dog and man. *J. Pharmacol. Exp. Therap.* 149 (3): 423–435.

Schwartz, M., Munana, K.R., Nettifee-Osborne, J.A. et al. (2012). The pharmacokinetics of midazolam after intravenous, intramuscular, and rectal administration in healthy dogs. *J. Vet. Pharmacol. Therap.* 36: 471–477.

Seddon, T., Michelle, I., Chenery, M. (1989). Comparative Drug Metabolism of Diazepam in hepatocytes isolated from man, rat, monkey and dog. *Biochem. Pharmacol.* 38(10): 1657–1665.

Shah, S.S., Sanda, S., Regmi, N.L. et al. (2007). Characterization of cytochrome P450-mediated drug metabolism in cats. *J. Vet. Pharmacol. Therap.* 30: 422–428.

Shah, S.S., Sasaki, K., Hayashi, Y. et al. (2009). Inhibitory effects of ketoconazole, cimetidine and erythromycin on hepatic CYP3A activities in cats. *J. Vet. Med. Sci.* 71 (9): 1151–1159.

Shou, M., Norcross, R., Sandig, G. et al. (2003). Substrate specificity and kinetic properties of seven heterologously expressed dog cytochromes p450. *Drug Metab. Dispos.* 31: 1161–1169.

Simon, B., Scallan, E.M., Siracusa, C. et al. (2014). Effects of acepromazine or methadone on midazolam-induced behavioral reactions in dogs. *Can. Vet. J.* 55 (9): 875–885.

Singh, J., Sobti, V., Kohli, R. et al. (1981). Evaluation of glycerol guaicolate as a muscle relaxant in buffalo calves. *Zentralbl Veterinarmed A.* 28: 60–69.

Tsukamoto, A., Uchida, K., Maesato, S. et al. (2016). Combining isoflurane anesthesia with midazolam and butorphanol in rats. *Exp. Anim.*, Feb 12. [Epub ahead of print] 65 (3): 223–230.

Valverde, A. (2013). Balanced anesthesia and constant-rate infusions in horses. *Vet. Clin. Equine* 29: 89–122.

Vree, T.B., Baars, A.M., Hekster, Y.A. et al. (1979). Simultaneous determination of diazepam and its metabolites N-desmethyldiazepam, oxydiazepam and oxazepam in plasma and urine of man and dog by means of high-performance liquid chromatography. *J. Chromatogr.* 162: 605–614.

Vuyk, J., Sitsen, E., and Reekers, M. (2020). Intravenous anesthetics. In: *Miller's Anesthesia*, 9e (ed. M.A. Gropper), 638–653. Philadelphia, PA: Elsevier.

Wall, R. and Muir, W.W. (1990). Hemolytic potential of guafenesin in cattle. *Cornell Vet.* 80: 209–216.

Wheeler, E.P., Abelson, A.L., Lindsey, J.C. et al. (2021). Sedative effects of alfaxalone and hydromorphone with or without midazolam in cats: a pilot study. *J. Feline Med. Surg.* 2021 Mar 3;1098612X21996155, Online ahead of print. https://doi.org/10.1177/1098612X21996155.

Zapata, A., Laredo, F.G., Eschobar, M. et al. (2018). Effects of midazolam before or after alfaxalone for co-induction of anaesthesia in healthy dogs. *Vet. Anaesth. Analg.* 45 (5): 609–617.

16

Neuromuscular Blocking Agents

Manuel Martin-Flores and Daniel M. Sakai

Introduction

Skeletal muscle contraction is dependent on the interaction between A-alpha nerve fibers and muscle fibers. When depolarization reaches the nerve terminal, an influx of Ca^{2+} mobilizes acetylcholine (ACh), which is stored in synaptic vesicles after being synthesized by the neuron. ACh is then released into the synaptic space (or synaptic cleft) of the neuromuscular junction (NMJ) (Figure 16.1) (Rahamimoff et al. 1980). Nicotinic acetylcholine receptors (nAChR) are ionic channels situated primarily in the folds of the synaptic space. These receptors are activated when two molecules of ACh interact with specific binding sites. The activated nAChR undergoes a conformational change that allows an influx of Na^+, which depolarizes the end-plate terminal (Auerbach 2015). Adjacent voltage-gated Na^+ channels are then activated and the action potential propagates along the muscle fiber. This is the signaling of muscle contraction. The action of ACh in the NMJ terminates almost immediately and free ACh is hydrolyzed by the acetylcholinesterase (AChE) enzyme (Booij et al. 1981). Neuromuscular blocking agents (NMBAs) relax the skeletal musculature by interrupting the normal process of neuromuscular transmission described above. NMBAs may act as agonists (depolarizing) or competitive antagonists (non-depolarizing) agents at the nAChR.

NMBAs are unique among drugs used during general anesthesia in that they do not produce sedation, hypnosis or analgesia (Smith and Brown 1947); NMBAs are administered solely to produce transient muscle relaxation (paralysis) as an adjunct of general anesthesia. This specific effect is useful to improve surgical conditions, prevent sudden movement, or aid tracheal intubation and mechanical ventilation. The lack of effects in the central nervous system (CNS) implies that other agents must be used to produce hypnosis, analgesia and/or amnesia, and that the equipment and skills required to intubate and ventilate must be available.

Despite the limited effects of NMBAs, these agents can play a vital role in balanced anesthetic protocols. Inclusion of NMBAs typically results in a decrease in the dose of general anesthetics administered, as the hypnotic dose of general anesthetics is substantially lower than the dose required to prevent movement (i.e. $MAC_{awake} < MAC$) (Stoelting et al. 1970). Consequently, the cardiovascular depressant effects of volatile anesthetics can be reduced (Kumazawa and Merin 1975; Kazama and Ikeda 1988; Conzen et al. 1989). However, the use of NMBAs is accompanied by its own potential risks, such as the risk of residual paralysis; this potential problem will be addressed in Chapter 17. NMBAs can be classified according to their mechanism of action (depolarizing and non-depolarizing agents); chemical structure (benzylisoquinolines and aminosteroids); and duration of action (short, intermediate and long).

General Concepts and Nomenclature Regarding NMBAs

Potency is measured by the dose that reduces the evoked muscular contraction by 50% (ED50) or 95% (ED95). Dosing can be referred to in terms of multiples of the ED95 (e.g. $2 \times ED95$). The *onset time* is the time interval between administration of the agent and > 95% depression of the evoked muscle contraction. *Clinical (or surgical) blockade* is commonly defined as the period of complete blockade, until force of contraction returns to 10% (some authors will allow 25%) of baseline. Recovery from neuromuscular blockade is a gradual process, not an all-or-none phenomenon. The *recovery index* represents the slope (or speed) of recovery, and it is the time interval between 25% and 75% recovery of the evoked muscular response. More details on monitoring are provided below.

Pharmacology in Veterinary Anesthesia and Analgesia, First Edition. Edited by Turi Aarnes and Phillip Lerche.

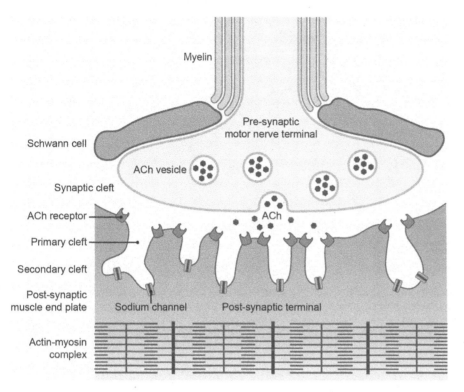

Figure 16.1 The neuromuscular junction. The motor neuron, muscle cell, and Schwan cell are shown. Acetylcholine (ACh) is produced and stored by the nerve cell and released into the synaptic cleft. Nicotinic acetylcholine receptors (nAChRs) are found primarily in the muscle cell, although presynaptic receptors are also found in the nerve cell. Under normal circumstances, the interaction between ACh and nAChR results in muscular activation. Neuromuscular blocking agents prevent this process.

Monitoring of Neuromuscular Function

Monitoring is integral to the clinical use of NMBAs, and is required for assessing depth of blockade, redosing, or deciding whether pharmacologic reversal is needed before emergence from general anesthesia. Moreover, monitoring is necessary to avoid residual neuromuscular blockade. Several monitoring modalities exist, but they all share the same principle: stimulation of a motor nerve with a peripheral nerve stimulator, and evaluation of the evoked response. Commonly, the ulnar or peroneal (fibular) nerves are used in animals (Figure 16.2). It is important that the stimulus be supramaximal, so that decreases in response can be attributed to the effects of the agent, and not a decrease in the magnitude of the stimulus. Supramaximal current also ensures that all muscle fibers are recruited during stimulation. The evoked response can be evaluated in several ways: muscular twitches can simply be observed or palpated. This subjective evaluation can easily be performed, however it cannot detect intermediate and shallow levels of residual neuromuscular blockade

(Martin-Flores et al. 2008). The gold standard for measuring evoked responses is mechanomyography (MMG) (Figure 16.3), where the isometric force of contraction is measured. Alternatively, acceleromyography (AMG) or electromyography (EMG) can be used as surrogates. Both AMG and EMG are better suited for clinical use.

Although several patterns of stimulation exist, train-of-four (TOF) is the one most commonly used in a clinical setting. The main advantage of TOF stimulation is that no baseline value is required: every TOF acts as its own control. A fade (progressive decrease in response magnitude) during TOF can be measured in the presence of nondepolarizing neuromuscular blockade (Figure 16.4). In the absence of neuromuscular blockade, all four responses to TOF stimulation are equal; the TOF ratio (T4/T1) = 1.0. A TOF ratio < 1.0 indicates that neuromuscular transmission is decreased. As blockade becomes deeper, all responses to TOF will disappear. Clinical (surgical) blockade usually requires that ≤1 response to TOF is present. A TOF ratio ≥ 0.9 is typically used in people to indicate that

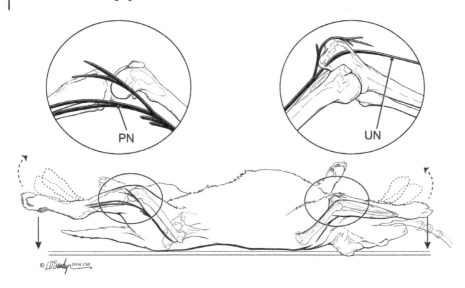

Figure 16.2 Illustration of motor nerves commonly used for peripheral nerve stimulation. The ulnar nerve (UN) and peroneal nerve (PN) are indicated. Stimulating subcutaneous needles or cutaneous patches can be placed over these nerves for stimulation. Isometric force of contraction of the innervated muscles (mechanomyography; MMG), electrical activation of those muscles (electromyography; EMG), or peak acceleration of the evoked movements (acceleromyography; AMG), can be used to quantify the response (Source: Lauren D. Sawchyn, DVM, CMI).

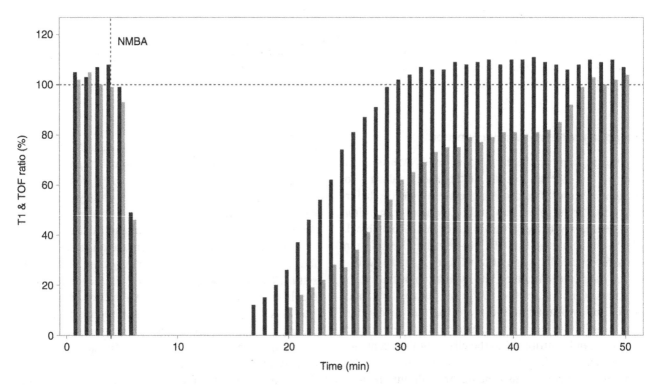

Figure 16.3 Time-course representation of the onset and offset of nondepolarizing neuromuscular blockade measured with train-of-four (TOF) stimulation every minute. The blue bars (first in a pair) represent the magnitude of the first twitch (T1) of the TOF and the pink bars (second in a pair) represent the TOF ratio (T4/T1). Administration of the NMBA occurs at minute 4. Note that values are expressed as percentages rather than absolute measurements. T1 is measured as the percentage change from baseline, while the TOF ratio is calculated within each train. A dashed horizontal line indicates 100% and shows that recovery occurs earlier (30 minutes) for T1 than for TOF ratio (47 min in this case), making the latter a more sensitive indicator of residual blockade. Similar traces can be obtained with acceleromyography (AMG), mechanomyography (MMG), or electromyography (EMG)..

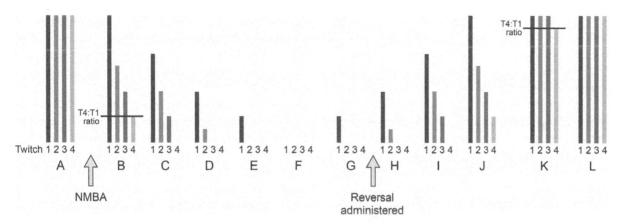

Figure 16.4 Response to train-of-four (TOF) stimulation during non-depolarizing neuromuscular block. Prior to injection of the NMBA, no fade during TOF is observed (left). A progressive fade (TOF ratio <1.0) and disappearance of responses occurs during onset of neuromuscular block. A progressive reappearance of the responses occurs as neuromuscular transmission is restored. A TOF ratio of 1.0 should be measured when complete recovery of neuromuscular function occurs (right).

recovery of neuromuscular function is sufficient for extubation (Lien and Kopman 2014).

Depolarizing Neuromuscular Blocking Agents

Succinylcholine (SCh) is the only depolarizing NMBA in clinical use. It is composed of two ACh molecules linked at the acetyl group (Castillo and De 1950).

Mechanism of action – When SCh binds with the nAChR, it causes an initial depolarization; SCh is an *agonist* to the nAChR. Since SCh is not hydrolyzed by the AChE enzyme, the interaction between SCh and the nAChR is much longer (minutes) than that of the natural neurotransmitter, ACh (<1 ms). The initial depolarization produced by SCh manifests as muscular fasciculations (Meadows 1971) which are caused by a desynchronized depolarization of muscle membranes. These fasciculations are short lived (typically <1 minute) and are followed by a longer period of flaccid relaxation. This relaxation is the result of the prolonged interaction between SCh and the nAChR, which renders the receptor inactive to ACh. The effects of SCh are terminated once the drug diffuses out of the NMJ into the systemic circulation and is metabolized by plasma cholinesterase (Appiah-Ankam and Hunter 2004). Despite the many drawbacks of SCh (see below), this agent remains in clinical use due to its fast onset and short duration of action. These characteristics make SCh a unique agent, and a useful one as an aid for intubation, especially during rapid sequence induction.

Metabolism - Succinylcholine is rapidly hydrolyzed in plasma to succinylmonocholine, succinic acid and

choline, by the pseudocholinesterase (or butyrylcholinesterase) enzyme, a protein synthesized by the liver. The neuromuscular blocking effects of succinylmonocholine are substantially less than those of SCh (estimated 1/20 to 1/80), and hence this metabolite does not substantially contribute to neuromuscular blockade (Foldes et al. 1954). The efficiency of this enzyme is such that most of the SCh (90%) administered is hydrolyzed before it reaches the neuromuscular junction (Gissen et al. 1966). The AChE enzyme present in the NMJ does not hydrolyze SCh. The fast hydrolysis in the plasma decreases the plasma concentration of SCh and creates a concentration gradient, so that SCh diffuses back to the systemic circulation. The decrease in SCh at the NMJ leaves more nAChR available, terminating neuromuscular blockade (Appiah-Ankam and Hunter 2004).

Genetic mutations resulting in atypical forms of the pseudocholinesterase enzyme can gravely increase the duration of action of SCh, as the activity of the atypical enzyme is much lower. The duration of action can increase up to 4 h or more, instead of the expected 5–15 minutes in healthy patients (Soliday et al. 2010). Severe hepatic disease can also increase the duration of action of SCh, as the pseudocholinesterase enzyme is produced by that organ (Birch et al. 1956). Prolonged duration of SCh, due to a reduced concentration of regular pseudocholinesterase enzyme, is treated with plasma transfusion. Pseudocholinesterase levels, and the activity of the pseudocholinesterase enzyme can be assessed perianesthetically, in patients at risk, by measuring the dibucaine number (DN). In short, the DN is the percentage of the enzyme's activity inhibited by dibucaine (Kalow and Staron 1957).

Clinical use – In veterinary anesthesiology, orotracheal intubation is commonly achieved without the use of relaxants, therefore SCh is seldom used. The same characteristics that have kept this agent in clinical use when humans are anesthetized (fast onset and short duration) might not provide any advantages when animals require neuromuscular blockade. Intermediate-acting non-depolarizing NMBAs are more frequently used when animals are anesthetized. Notwithstanding some species-specific differences, SCh generally produces a short duration of neuromuscular blockade. In dogs, SCh 0.3 mg/kg will consistently produce neuromuscular blockade of approximately 20–30 minutes (Cullen et al. 1980) (Martin-Flores et al. 2015b). In cats and horses, SCh-induced blockade is of shorter duration, and better resembles what is observed in people. Doses as low as 0.15 mg/kg will commonly produce neuromuscular blockade in horses lasting approximately 5–10 minutes. Similar results have been observed in cats (Martin-Flores M and Sakai DM, unpublished observations) and rats (Ginsburg et al. 1971). A dose of 1 mg/kg administered to cats produced apnea that lasted no more than 15 minutes (Rex 1971). Larger doses are used in pigs; 3 mg/kg produced complete paralysis with a recovery time < 15 minutes (Loughren et al. 2014).

Effects on Organ Systems

Cardiovascular system – SCh can interact as an agonist with cardiac muscarinic receptors and precipitate bradyarrhythmias (sinus bradycardia, junctional rhythm and sinus arrest). However, interaction of SCh with sympathetic autonomic ganglia can produce the opposite effect by increasing the concentration of circulating catecholamines. Therefore, tachycardia and arterial hypertension might also occur. In pentobarbital-anesthetized dogs, hemodynamic parameters were not significantly altered when doses of 5 and 15 mg/kg of SCh were administered (Länsimies et al. 1971). However, Leighton (1971) described a consistent decrease in arterial blood pressure, but stable cardiac output, after administration of 4 mg/kg of succinylcholine to dogs. It should be noted that those doses are supraclinical, and complete neuromuscular blockade can be achieved with 0.3 mg/kg IV. No arrhythmias were observed when 0.3 mg/kg was used in healthy or myopathic dogs, however, a small and short-lived decrease in arterial blood pressure was reported in two myopathic dogs (Martin-Flores et al. 2015b). In

halothane-anesthetized horses, SCh 0.3 mg/kg resulted in mild increases in heart rate and arterial blood pressure (Benson et al. 1979). However, 0.1 mg/kg produced severe tachycardia when administered to ponies (Hildebrand and Howitt 1983).

Central nervous system and eye – Although SCh has no direct effect on CNS function or vision, intracranial (Minton et al. 1986) and intraocular hypertension (Chiu et al. 1999) have been reported in humans with its use. SCh increased intracranial pressure (ICP) in cats and dogs (Cottrell et al. 1983; Lanier et al. 1986), and caused a steep increase in extraocular muscle tension and intraocular pressure (IOP) in cats and rabbits (Collins and Bach-y-Rita 1972).

Other – SCh administration can result in increases in the circulating levels of histamine (Ertama 1978), which can in turn result in flushing, urticaria, arterial hypotension and bronchospasm (Moss 1995). SCh-induced hyperkalemia has also been reported and it can be severe when the drug is used in patients with muscle trauma (Cairoli et al. 1982) or motor neuron defects (Stone et al. 1970). In those patients, the use of SCh might be contraindicated. A recent study in a small group of dogs with centronuclear myopathy did not detect exaggerated increases in K^+ after SCh was administered (Martin-Flores et al. 2015b).

Interactions with other drugs – Neostigmine, an AChE inhibitor agent commonly used to reverse non-depolarizing neuromuscular blockade also produces substantial inhibition of plasma cholinesterase. As a result, the duration of action of SCh is increased when neostigmine is administered during recovery from SCh. A similar effect is observed in animals intoxicated with organophosphates (Himes et al. 1967).

Contraindications – SCh is contraindicated in hyperkalemic animals and those with myopathy, muscle trauma or burns due to the risk of life-threatening hyperkalemia. It is also prudent to avoid SCh in animals with arrhythmias or those at risk of having elevated intracranial or intraocular pressures. SCh is a known trigger of malignant hyperthermia and should be avoided in animals in which mutations responsible for that syndrome are confirmed or suspected.

Regrettably, SCh has been used in the past to immobilize unsedated horses or used as a sole agent for euthanasia. This practice is inhumane, as paralysis is not accompanied by depression of the CNS, and it is discouraged and condemned by the AVMA (www.avma.org) and these authors.

Non-depolarizing Neuromuscular Blocking Agents

Non-depolarizing NMBAs are used with much more frequency in veterinary anesthesiology than depolarizing agents.

Mechanism of action – All non-depolarizing agents share the same mechanism of action; non-depolarizing blockers are *competitive antagonists* of ACh at the nAChR.

When a molecule of a non-depolarizing NMBA binds to one of the two α-subunits of the nAChR, it renders this receptor unavailable to ACh. When enough nAChRs are bound with non-depolarizing NMBA, the influx of cations into the membrane is insufficient, and therefore, depolarization does not occur. As a result, skeletal muscular contraction is effectively prevented. It is estimated that at least 70% of the receptors need to be blocked before a decrease in neuromuscular transmission is measured (Waud and Waud 1972). This is to say, the number of available nAChR in the NMJ greatly exceeds the number required for effective neuromuscular transmission and evidences the wide safety margin of neuromuscular transmission. Once >70% of nAChR are occupied by the NMBA, further administration of the agent will produce measurable decreases in force of contraction. There are two clinical implications that follow this principle: (i) the *priming* technique consists of administering a small dose of a non-depolarizing NMBA. This first dose is designed to occupy a proportion of receptors so that only minimal (or no) measurable neuromuscular blockade occurs. A second dose is administered later with the intent of blocking the remaining "active" receptors, that is, those in which neuromuscular transmission now relies upon. The objective with the priming technique is to hasten the onset time of an otherwise slow-acting drug. Priming was used more commonly with slow acting drugs, such as pancuronium (Doherty et al. 1985). (ii) The second implication is that re-dosing an NMBA will produce an increasingly greater effect if the same amount of drug is given. Even when the effects of a first dose of an NMBA dissipate, it is expected that a number of receptors will still be occupied. A second dose of the NMBA will then act on the remaining "active" receptors and produce a greater interruption of neuromuscular transmission.

Metabolism and excretion of the non-depolarizing NMBA will result in a decrease in the plasma concentration of the agent, followed by a decrease in its concentration at the NMJ. When a sufficient amount of NMBA is removed from the NMJ, neuromuscular transmission is restored. However, because non-depolarizing NMBAs are competitive antagonists, reversal can be enhanced pharmacologically. This is commonly achieved with the use of AChE inhibitor agents (neostigmine and edrophonium) and it is the subject of Chapter 17.

Metabolism – While all non-depolarizing NMBAs share the same mechanism of action, metabolism of the two major chemical families of non-depolarizing NMBAs differ substantially.

Benzylisoquinolinium compounds in clinical use include atracurium and cisatracurium. Other agents such as mivacurium might be available in some countries.

Atracurium undergoes both enzymatic and non-enzymatic degradation. Enzymatic hydrolysis depends on nonspecific plasma esterases while non-enzymatic degradation occurs spontaneously at normal pH and temperature, a process named Hoffman elimination. Both pathways are independent from hepatic or renal function, which allows for atracurium to be infused with little accumulation (Ward and Weatherley 1986). Decreases in temperature will delay non-enzymatic degradation, however, it is unlikely that changes in pH encountered in clinical practice would produce a noticeable effect on duration of atracurium. Moreover, pH changes also affect ester hydrolysis but in the opposite direction, so that a delay in Hoffman elimination might be counterbalanced by an increase in enzymatic activity. It is estimated that enzymatic hydrolysis accounts for two thirds of the overall degradation process (Fisher et al. 1986).

Laudanosine is a byproduct of atracurium degradation, whether it occurs by enzymatic or non-enzymatic pathways (Agoston et al. 1992). Laudanosine has no neuromuscular blocking effects but it is a CNS stimulant at high concentrations. In rabbits, high laudanosine plasma concentrations increased MAC by 23–30% (Shi et al. 1985). Unlike atracurium, excretion of laudanosine depends primarily on hepatic function; 70% of laudanosine is excreted through the bile, and 30% through urine (Ward and Weatherley 1986). Therefore, while severe hepatic disease will not affect the duration of action of atracurium, biliary obstruction may result in increased levels of circulating laudanosine. Laudanosine, but not atracurium, was increased in plasma during an anhepatic phase of surgery in pigs (Pittet et al. 1990).

Cisatracurium is degraded by Hoffman elimination similar to atracurium, but it does not undergo enzymatic degradation (Welch et al. 1995). Like atracurium, elimination of cisatracurium does not depend on hepatic or renal function (Kisor et al. 1996). The higher potency of cisatracurium means that lower doses are used. As a result, less laudanosine is formed during degradation.

Mivacurium, also a non-depolarizing benzylisoquinolinium agent, is hydrolyzed by the pseudocholinesterase enzyme, similarly to SCh (Savarese et al. 1988). Accordingly, low enzymatic activity, or atypical pseudocholinesterase enzyme will result in prolongation of neuromuscular blockade (Cerf et al. 2002).

Aminosteroid NMBAs in clinical use are vecuronium, rocuronium, and pancuronium, although the latter is used with much less frequency. Clearance of aminosteroid NMBAs relies on organ function and hence, hepatic and/or renal disease can noticeably delay clearance and prolong their duration of action.

Vecuronium is only minimally metabolized by the liver, and it is excreted through the bile (46%) and kidneys (7.5%) (Upton et al. 1982). An active metabolite (3-OH) which retains about 80% of the neuromuscular blocking potency is formed during biotransformation. Prolonged administration and/or decreases in hepatic and renal function can contribute to the accumulation of vecuronium and its active metabolite (Wright et al. 1994). Hepatic metabolism of **pancuronium** is also limited, however, excretion of this agent occurs primarily through the kidneys (40–60%) and secondarily through the bile (11%). An active (3-OH) metabolite can also contribute to prolongation of neuromuscular blockade during prolonged infusions or repeated doses (Miller and Roderick 1978). **Rocuronium** does not undergo metabolism and is excreted primarily by the liver and secondarily by the kidneys (Proost et al. 1997). Liver disease affects elimination (van Miert et al. 1997), but kidney disease only marginally decreases it (Della Rocca et al. 2003). The absence of active metabolites (Muir et al. 1989) suggests that rocuronium is more suitable for infusions than its predecessors.

Clinical use and pharmacokinetics – Non-depolarizing NMBAs are used in veterinary anesthesia to permit mechanical ventilation, improve surgical conditions during thoracotomy, laparotomy, fracture repairs or ophthalmic surgeries (Auer and Moens 2011; Briganti et al. 2015) and to prevent sudden movements that could result in lesions. By producing immobility, these agents also participate in balanced anesthetic protocols, allowing a reduction in the dose of general anesthetics, and commonly resulting in less cardiovascular depression (Kumazawa and Merin 1975; Kazama and Ikeda 1988; Conzen et al. 1989). Less frequently, non-depolarizing blockers are used during induction of anesthesia to facilitate tracheal intubation (Moreno-Sala et al. 2013).

Recommended doses and approximated duration of action of several NMBAS in selected species are described in Table 16.1.

Unlike SCh, most non-depolarizing agents are intermediate-acting drugs, with effects lasting somewhere between 20 and 45 minutes. The onset time of these drugs is also slower than that of SCh; 1–5 minutes must elapse before complete blockade is attained, depending on the agent and the dose administered. In general, larger doses will result in faster onset and longer duration of action. Longer-acting drugs (also characterized by a slow onset) such as pancuronium, are rapidly losing popularity in anesthesiology. This chapter will emphasize the characteristics of modern, intermediate-acting agents commonly used in veterinary anesthesia.

Non-depolarizing NMBAs are quaternary ammonium compounds. The positive charge on the chemical structure renders the molecule insoluble in lipid, therefore there is minimal transfer of NMBAs across the blood–brain barrier and placenta. In people, the non-depolarizing NMBAs have low volumes of distribution (31–278 ml/kg), and elimination half-times that vary between 2 and 78 minutes (Flood et al. 2015). The characteristics of hepatic, enzymatic or Hoffmann biotransformation and the biliary or renal excretion of NMBAs and its metabolites are specific for each agent and are described below.

Table 16.1 Recommended doses and approximate duration of action of NMBAs in selected species.

	Succinylcholine		Atracurium		Cisatracurium		Mivacurium		Vecuronium		Rocuronium	
	Dose	Duration	Dose	Duration	Dose	Duration	Dose	Duration	Dose	Duration	Dose	Duration
Dog	0.3	20–30	0.2	20–40	0.05–0.15	20–40	0.1	30	0.05	17–75	0.6	22
Cat	0.15	5–10	0.2	20–40	0.06	20–30	0.08	12	0.05	27	0.2–0.6	15–20
Horse	0.15	5–10	0.07–0.15	20–60	0.05–0.01	30–40	NA		Not recommended		0.2–0.6	20–65
Sheep	0.04	15	0.5	30	NA		0.2	15	0.25	40	NA	
Pig	3	15	1.6–2.0	45	NA		0.27	11	0.6–1	20	0.67	6
Rabbit	0.1–0.2	NA	0.05	14	0.04	40	0.16	20	NA		0.07[a]	5

[a] ~ED50. NA: data not available. Doses are in mg/kg and duration in minutes.
Data compiled from scientific literature and clinical experience of the authors.

Benzylisoquinolines

As a group, benzylisoquinolines are characterized by their capacity to release histamine (at large doses) and for being susceptible to extra-hepatic metabolism.

Atracurium besylate is composed of a mixture of ten steroisomers, is likely the most commonly used NMBA in domestic animals, and there is extensive collective experience with this agent in dogs, cats, and horses. Atracurium is an intermediate-acting agent; clinical neuromuscular blockade lasts approximately 20 minutes, and complete recovery from atracurium occurs approximately 30–45 minutes after injection, depending on the dose administered and the presence of factors that might affect speed of recovery (i.e. body temperature).

In humans, the ED95 of atracurium approximates 0.2 mg/kg (Basta et al. 1982). The onset time ranges between three and five minutes. In dogs, the ED95 is approximately 0.12 mg/kg (Hughes and Chapple 1981) but doses up to 0.6 mg/kg can be found in the literature (Jones et al. 1983). Increasing the dose of atracurium carries a higher risk of histamine release. In cats, 0.12 mg/kg approximated the ED50, while 0.25 mg/kg produced 99% twitch depression (Hughes and Chapple 1981; Sutherland et al. 1983). However, in a different study on the same species, the ED95 was estimated at ~0.1 mg/kg, with an onset of four minutes and a duration of 12 minutes (Wastila et al. 1996). Discrepancies between potency studies may be due to differences in methodology and, more specifically, in how neuromuscular transmission was measured, or what anesthetic agents were used. In these authors' experience, atracurium 0.2 mg/kg consistently produces neuromuscular blockade in dogs and cats under inhalational anesthesia. In horses, doses as low as 0.07 mg/kg have shown to produce complete blockade (Hildebrand and Arpin 1988). However, a more recent experiment showed that at least one response during TOF stimulation could be observed even after 0.15 mg/kg was administered (Martin-Flores et al. 2008). Because reversal of neuromuscular blockade can be problematic in horses (see Chapter 17), it is probably a safe course of action to evaluate the response to a low dose of atracurium, and then increase the dose incrementally if complete blockade is not achieved. Neuromuscular transmission after 0.15 mg/kg in horses required approximately one hour to be restored spontaneously, however, in one horse it took 110 minutes (Martin-Flores et al. 2008).

While the dose of atracurium does not vary substantially among many domestic species, larger doses are used in pigs; the ED95 was estimated between 1.1 and 2.0 mg/kg (Pittet et al. 1990; Shorten and Gibbs 1993).

Cisatracurium is a stereoisomer of atracurium. Cisatracurium is a more potent agent and it does not cause histamine release; this is possibly its most important clinical advantage over atracurium and other benzylisoquinolines.

Cisatracurium was recently examined in dogs under isoflurane anesthesia (Sakai et al. 2015). While the ED95 was not calculated as part of that study, cisatracurium 0.05 mg/kg produced ~95% twitch depression, suggesting that the ED95 might approximate that dose. The onset time for that dose ranged between three and five minutes in most dogs. Clinical blockade lasted 10–20 minutes, and complete spontaneous recovery occurred 25–30 minutes after injection (Sakai et al. 2015). Cisatracurium was also evaluated in dogs with portosystemic shunts and compared with healthy animals (Adams et al. 2006). Onset time after a dose of 0.1 mg/kg was ~3 minutes, and neuromuscular blockade lasted ~30 minutes, regardless of whether dogs had shunts or not. In other words, the presence of a portosystemic shunt did not affect the time-course of cisatracurium.

In cats, the ED95 of cisatracurium was estimated at 0.06 mg/kg (Wastila et al. 1996). Cisatracurium at a dose of 0.075 and 0.1 mg/kg reliably produced neuromuscular blockade in isoflurane-anesthetized horses (Tutunaru et al. 2019), while doses of 0.05 produced blockade in 5/8 horses. Pilot data (Martin-Flores M; data not published) suggests that complete neuromuscular blockade can be attained in isoflurane-anesthetized horses with 0.05 mg/kg.

While atracurium and cisatracurium are considered intermediate-acting NMBAs, **mivacurium** is a shorter acting agent in people. An evaluation of mivacurium in dogs however, revealed that the agent is actually intermediate to long acting in this species (Smith et al. 1999). In that study, doses of 10, 20, and 50 µg/kg produced complete blockade lasting ~30 minutes for the lowest dose, and over 2 hours for the highest dose. The observation that mivacurium produces longer blockade in dogs than in humans is in accordance with results obtained with SCh in dogs, where duration of action is also longer than in people. In closer agreement with observations in people, duration of mivacurium blockade in sheep is short. Clutton and Glasby 1998 showed that recovery from 0.2 mg/kg mivacurium in sheep required only 15 minutes. That dose is also within the range of doses used in clinical practice in humans (Vanlinthout et al. 2014). In cats, spontaneous restoration of neuromuscular function after the administration of 1.5 × ED95 (0.08 mg/kg) mivacurium required ~12 minutes (Savarese et al. 2004).

Currently, mivacurium is unavailable in the United States.

Aminosteroids

As a group, aminosteroid agents are characterized by their cardiovascular stability. These agents do not typically release histamine. Pancuronium, vecuronium and rocuronium are examples of aminosteroid agents.

Vecuronium is an intermediate-acting monoquaternary aminosteroid. It is structurally similar to pancuronium. Vecuronium is devoid of cardiovascular effects and does not release histamine at clinically relevant doses (Morris et al. 1983). Vecuronium has been extensively used in small animals. In dogs, the ED90 of vecuronium has been reported at 0.09 mg/kg (Bom et al. 2009), however, a dose of 0.05 mg/kg has been shown to produce complete blockade under clinical settings (Kariman and Clutton 2008). Moreover, a small bolus of 0.025 mg/kg produced ~80% twitch depression in isoflurane anesthetized dogs (Martin-Flores et al. 2014).

The onset time after 0.05 mg/kg in dogs was close to two minutes, with a clinical duration (absence of response to neurostimulation) of ~17 minutes (Kariman and Clutton 2008). In a different experiment in beagles, vecuronium 0.05 mg/kg produced a longer duration of action; the period of clinical neuromuscular blockade (to return of 25% of twitch height) was just over 30 minutes, and the time to complete recovery of neuromuscular transmission was ~75 minutes (Martin-Flores et al. 2015c). Lorenzutti et al. (2014) showed that when a dose of 0.1 mg/kg was administered to isoflurane-anesthetized dogs, time to return of the second twitch during TOF stimulation was ~25 minutes. Complete recovery (without reversal) was reached ~43 minutes after injection of vecuronium. Taken together, data suggest that periods of 20–30 minutes of complete blockade, and 45–75 minutes until complete return of neuromuscular function are to be expected after 0.05–0.1 mg/kg are used.

There is far less literature on the use of vecuronium in cats. In pentobarbital-anesthetized cats, the ED90 was estimated at 22.5 μg/kg (Michalek-Sauberer et al. 2000). The onset time after that dose was slow (mean 5 minutes) and was almost halved when 2 x ED90 was administered (mean 2.8 minutes) (Michalek-Sauberer et al. 2000). Recovery after 2 × ED90 required approximately 27 minutes.

Little information also exists in horses. A study in a small number of isoflurane-anesthetized horses investigated the effects of 25, 50, and 100 μg/kg vecuronium (Martin-Flores et al. 2012a). In those animals, no effect was measured from the smallest dose. A median twitch depression of 25% was produced with a dose of 50 μg/kg, however, complete spontaneous return of neuromuscular function required ~45 minutes. A dose of 100 μg/kg produced ~95% twitch depression with a slow onset time (3.5 minutes). After that dose, recovery of neuromuscular transmission required more than two hours, even when edrophonium was administered. It appears that, in horses, vecuronium has the ability to produce long-lasting neuromuscular blockade.

The effects of vecuronium in sheep are also noteworthy. While doses of at least 50 μg/kg are commonly administered in humans and dogs, as little as 25 μg/kg produces complete block in sheep (Clutton and Glasby 1998). Duration of blockade after that dose was ~40 minutes. A dose–response study in sheep suggested that the ED95 might be as low as 13 μg/kg in this species (Martin-Flores et al. 2012b).

As occurs with benzylisoquinolinium agents, pigs are also resistant to aminosteroid NMBAs. The ED90 of vecuronium in pigs ranges between 75 and 100 μg/kg (Muir and Marshall 1987; Proost et al. 2008). Doses of 0.4–0.6 mg/kg have been used in pigs for research purposes (Grong et al. 2015). In a recent study involving isoflurane-anesthetized pigs, boluses of vecuronium 1 mg/kg were administered to maintain surgical relaxation. No cardiovascular effects were noted from that dose, and redosing with the same dose (guided by peripheral nerve stimulation) occurred at <20-minute intervals due to reappearance of responses to fibular nerve stimulation (Cisternas et al. 2015).

Rocuronium is a weaker non-depolarizing aminosteroid agent with a faster onset than vecuronium. The ED90 of rocuronium in dogs was estimated at 0.18 mg/kg (Cason et al. 1990; Bom et al. 2009). This lower potency compared with vecuronium might be, at least in part, responsible for rocuronium's faster onset time. For equipotent doses (e.g. 1 × ED95) a larger number of molecules of rocuronium is administered, which might facilitate diffusion into the NMJ. A similar observation can be made when atracurium and cisatracurium are compared (Mellinghoff et al. 1996). Due to its cardiovascular stability and relatively short onset time, large doses of rocuronium are commonly used in humans during rapid sequence inductions. In dogs, the onset time after 0.3 mg/kg was two minutes (Auer 2007). That time was halved when the dose was doubled in one study (Auer 2007) and it was measured at a mean of 37 seconds in a different study using 0.6 mg/kg (Mosing et al. 2012). The duration of complete blockade after 0.3 and 0.6 mg/kg was ~14 and 22 minutes, and complete recovery occurred at ~24 and 32 minutes after injection, respectively (Auer 2007). Alderson et al. (2007) investigated the effects of an infusion of rocuronium (0.5 mg/kg followed by 0.2 mg/kg/h). They found that recovery times increased and the duration of the infusion was longer, suggesting that, at this rate, some accumulation may occur.

In cats, rocuronium 0.6 mg/kg had an onset time of ~45 seconds (Auer and Mosing 2006), and the time of surgical blockade approximated 13 minutes. Complete recovery was achieved 20 minutes after injection. In a recent study (Martin-Flores et al. 2016), complete blockade in propofol anesthetized cats was achieved with as little as 0.2 mg/kg of rocuronium. Clinical duration of neuromuscular blockade was ~10 minutes after 0.2 mg/kg and 18 minutes after 0.6 mg/kg. Rocuronium was readily reversed with neostigmine in all cats, once the evoked response had returned to >25%.

In horses, rocuronium was evaluated at doses of 0.2, 0.4 and 0.6 mg/kg (Auer et al. 2007). Onset times (2.7, 2.3, and 1.5 minutes, respectively) were shorter than those obtained with vecuronium 100 μg/kg (3.5 minutes) (Martin-Flores et al. 2012a). Complete blockade was produced with 0.4 and 0.6 mg/kg; 0.2 mg/kg produced ~90% depression. Complete recovery occurred at ~17 minutes with the lowest dose and 65 minutes with the highest one.

The ED90 of rocuronium in pigs is ~0.6 mg/kg; significantly higher than in other species (Proost et al. 2008). Doses of ~3 mg/kg have been used to achieve complete blockade in pigs (Madsen et al. 2015).

Effects on organ systems – Unlike SCh, non-depolarizing NMBA used at clinical doses are not associated with arrhythmias (other than tachycardia with pancuronium or secondary to histamine release with benzylisoquinolines) or changes in ICP or IOP. Non-depolarizing NMBAs do not trigger malignant hyperthermia, nor do they produce hyperkalemia.

Interactions with other drugs – Certain antibiotics, most noticeable the aminoglycosides (i.e. gentamicin), can potentiate neuromuscular blockade by inhibiting the pre-synaptic release of ACh and by decreasing nAChR sensitivity to ACh (Singh et al. 1978). The same is true with inhalational anesthetics; Nagahama et al. (2006) showed that the infusion rate required to maintain a TOF count of one in dogs was lower with inhalational agents (both isoflurane and sevoflurane) than with propofol, that is, inhalational anesthesia potentiated neuromuscular blockade. Similarly, increases in Mg^{2+} can prolong the duration of neuromuscular blockade (Martin-Flores et al. 2011).

Novel Non-depolarizing NMBAs

Research in non-depolarizing NMBAs has recently focused on two objectives: the development of an agent with fast onset and short duration that could replace SCh, and a novel method to promptly and completely reverse neuromuscular blockade. The development of novel cysteine-inactivated agents (olefinic isoquinolinium diesters) might fulfill both needs. **Gantacurium** is a fast-acting, ultrashort agent. The rapid inactivation is the result of two processes; inactivation by cysteine adduction and pH-sensitive hydrolysis. In cats, duration to complete recovery from 5 × ED95 of gantacurium was ~7 minutes. The duration of apnea after that dose was <3 minutes (Martin-Flores et al. 2015a). **CW002** is a related intermediate-lasting compound. In dogs, 3 × ED95 of CW002 had an onset of 2.6 minutes and a duration of ~45 minutes (Heerdt et al. 2015). However, upon injection of L-cysteine, neuromuscular function is promptly restored (Heerdt et al. 2015). Injection of L-cysteine is devoid of the undesirable effects associated with the use of AChE inhibitors.

References

Adams, W.A., Mark Senior, J., Jones, R.S. et al. (2006). Cis-atracurium in dogs with and without porto-systemic shunts. *Vet. Anaesth. Analg.* 33: 17–23.

Agoston, S., Vandenbrom, R.H., and Wierda, J.M. (1992). Clinical pharmacokinetics of neuromuscular blocking drugs. *Clin. Pharmacokinet.* 22: 94–115.

Alderson, B., Senior, J.M., Jones, R.S. et al. (2007). Use of rocuronium administered by continuous infusion in dogs. *Vet. Anaesth. Analg.* 34: 251–256.

Appiah-Ankam, J. and Hunter, J. (2004). Pharmacology of neuromuscular blocking drugs. *Cont. Educ. Anaesth. Critic. Care Pain* 4: 2–7.

Auer, U. (2007). Clinical observations on the use of the muscle relaxant rocuronium bromide in the dog. *Vet. J.* (London, England: 1997) 173: 422–427.

Auer, U. and Moens, Y. (2011). Neuromuscular blockade with rocuronium bromide for ophthalmic surgery in horses. *Vet. Ophthalmol.* 14: 244–247.

Auer, U. and Mosing, M. (2006). A clinical study of the effects of rocuronium in isoflurane-anaesthetized cats. *Vet. Anaesth. Analg.* 33: 224–228.

Auer, U., Uray, C., and Mosing, M. (2007). Observations on the muscle relaxant rocuronium bromide in the horse—a dose-response study. *Vet. Anaesth. Analg.* 34: 75–81.

Auerbach, A. (2015). Activation of endplate nicotinic acetylcholine receptors by agonists. *Biochem. Pharmacol.* 97: 601–608.

Basta, S.J., Ali, H.H., Savarese, J.J. et al. (1982). Clinical pharmacology of atracurium besylate (BW 33A): a new non-depolarizing muscle relaxant. *Anesth. Analg.* 61: 723–729.

Benson, G.J., Hartsfield, S.M., Smetzer, D.L. et al. (1979). Physiologic effects of succinylcholine chloride in mechanically ventilated horses anesthetized with halothane in oxygen. *Am. J. Vet. Res.* 40: 1411–1416.

Birch, J.H., Foldes, F.F., and Rendell-Baker, L. (1956). Causes and prevention of prolonged apnea with succinylcholine. *Curr. Res. Anesth. Analg.* 35: 609–633.

Bom, A., Hope, F., Rutherford, S. et al. (2009). Preclinical pharmacology of sugammadex. *J. Critic. Care* 24: 29–35.

Booij, L.H., Vree, T.B., Hurkmans, F. et al. (1981). Pharmacokinetics and pharmacodynamics of the muscle relaxant drug org NC-45 and each of its hydroxy metabolites in dogs. *Der. Anaesthesist.* 30: 329–333.

Briganti, A., Barsotti, G., Portela, D.A. et al. (2015). Effects of rocuronium bromide on globe position and respiratory function in isoflurane-anesthetized dogs: a comparison between three different dosages. *Vet. Ophthalmol.* 18: 89–94.

Cairoli, V.J., Ivankovich, A.D., Vucicevic, D. et al. (1982). Succinylcholine-induced hyperkalemia in the rat following radiation injury to muscle. *Anesth. Analg.* 61: 83–86.

Cason, B., Baker, D.G., Hickey, R.F. et al. (1990). Cardiovascular and neuromuscular effects of three steroidal neuromuscular blocking drugs in dogs (ORG 9616, ORG 9426, ORG 9991). *Anesth. Analg.* 70: 382–388.

Castillo, J.C. and De, B.E. (1950). The neuromuscular blocking action of succinylcholine (diacetylcholine). *J. Pharmacol. Exp. Ther.* 99: 458–464.

Cerf, C., Mesguish, M., Gabriel, I. et al. (2002). Screening patients with prolonged neuromuscular blockade after succinylcholine and mivacurium. *Anesth. Analg.* 94: 461–466.

Chiu, C.L., Jaais, F., and Wang, C.Y. (1999). Effect of rocuronium compared with succinylcholine on intraocular pressure during rapid sequence induction of anaesthesia. *Br. J. Anaesth.* 82: 757–760.

Cisternas, A.F., Martin-Flores, M., and Gleed, R.D. (2015). Continuous minimally invasive cardiac output monitoring with the COstatus in a neonatal swine model: recalibration is necessary during vasoconstriction and vasodilation. *Paediatr. Anaesth.* 25: 852–859.

Clutton, R.E. and Glasby, M.A. (1998). A comparison of the neuromuscular and cardiovascular effects of vecuronium, atracurium and mivacurium in sheep. *Res. Vet. Sci.* 64: 233–237.

Collins, C.C. and Bach-y-Rita, P. (1972). Succinylcholine, ocular pressure, and extraocular muscle tension in cats and rabbits. *J. Appl. Phys.* 33: 788–791.

Conzen, P.F., Hobbhahn, J., Goetz, A.E. et al. (1989). Myocardial contractility, blood flow, and oxygen consumption in healthy dogs during anesthesia with isoflurane or enflurane. *J. Cardiothorac. Anesth.* 3: 70–77.

Cottrell, J.E., Hartung, J., Giffin, J.P. et al. (1983). Intracranial and hemodynamic changes after succinylcholine administration in cats. *Anesth. Analg.* 62: 1006–1009.

Cullen, L.K., Jones, R.S., and Snowdon, S.L. (1980). Neuro-muscular activity in the intact dog: techniques for recording evoked mechanical responses. *Br. Vet. J.* 136: 154–159.

Della Rocca, G., Pompei, L., Coccia, C. et al. (2003). Atracurium, cisatracurium, vecuronium and rocuronium in patients with renal failure. *Minerva. Anestesiol.* 69: 605–611, 612, 605.

Doherty, W.G., Breen, P.J., Donati, F. et al. (1985). Accelerated onset of pancuronium with divided doses. *Can. Anaesth. Soc. J.* 32: 1–4.

Ertama, P.M. (1978). Histamine release in rats after administration of five neuromuscular blocking agents. *Arch. Int. Pharmacodyn. Ther.* 233: 82–91.

Fisher, D.M., Canfell, P.C., Fahey, M.R. et al. (1986). Elimination of atracurium in humans: contribution of Hofmann elimination and ester hydrolysis versus organ-based elimination. *Anesthesiology* 65: 6–12.

Flood, P., Rathmell, J., and Shafer, S. (2015). Neuromuscular blocking drugs and reversal agents. In: *Stoelting's Pharmacology & Physiology in Anesthetic Practice*, 5e, 323–344. Philadelphia, PA: Wolter Kluwer Health.

Foldes, F.F., McNall, P.G., and Birch, J.H. (1954). The neuromuscular activity of succinylmonocholine iodide in anaesthetized man. *Br. Med. J.* 1: 967–968.

Ginsburg, S., Kitz, R.J., and Savarese, J.J. (1971). Neuromuscular blocking activity of a new series of quaternary N-substituted choline esters. *Br. J. Pharmacol.* 43: 107–126.

Gissen, A.J., Katz, R.L., Karis, J.H. et al. (1966). Neuromuscular block in man during prolonged arterial infusion with succinylcholine. *Anesthesiology* 27: 242–249.

Grong, K., Salminen, P.R., Stangeland, L. et al. (2015). Haemodynamic differences between pancuronium and vecuronium in an experimental pig model. *Vet. Anaesth. Analg.* 42: 242–249.

Heerdt, P.M., Sunaga, H., and Savarese, J.J. (2015). Novel neuromuscular blocking drugs and antagonists. *Curr. Opin. Anaesthesiol.* 28: 403–410.

Hildebrand, S.V. and Arpin, D. (1988). Neuromuscular and cardiovascular effects of atracurium administered to healthy horses anesthetized with halothane. *Am. J. Vet. Res.* 49: 1066–1071.

Hildebrand, S.V. and Howitt, G.A. (1983). Succinylcholine infusion associated with hyperthermia in ponies anesthetized with halothane. *Am. J. Vet. Res.* 44: 2280–2284.

Himes, J.A., Edds, G.T., Kirkham, W.W. et al. (1967). Potentiation of succinylcholine by organophosphate compounds in horses. *J. Am. Vet. Med. Assoc.* 151: 54–59.

Hughes, R. and Chapple, D.J. (1981). The pharmacology of atracurium: a new competitive neuromuscular blocking agent. *Br. J. Anaesth.* 53: 31–44.

Jones, R.S., Hunter, J.M., and Utting, J.E. (1983). Neuromuscular blocking action of atracurium in the dog and its reversal by neostigmine. *Res. Vet. Sci.* 34: 173–176.

Kalow, W. and Staron, N. (1957). On distribution and inheritance of atypical forms of human serum cholinesterase, as indicated by dibucaine numbers. *Can. J. Biochem. Physiol.* 35: 1305–1320.

Kariman, A. and Clutton, R.E. (2008). The effects of medetomidine on the action of vecuronium in dogs anaesthetized with halothane and nitrous oxide. *Vet. Anaesth. Analg.* 35: 400–408.

Kazama, T. and Ikeda, K. (1988). The comparative cardiovascular effects of sevoflurane with halothane and isoflurane. *J. Anesth.* 2: 63–68.

Kisor, D.F., Schmith, V.D., Wargin, W.A. et al. (1996). Importance of the organ-independent elimination of cisatracurium. *Anesth. Analg.* 83: 1065–1071.

Kumazawa, T. and Merin, R.G. (1975). Effects of inhalation anesthetics on cardiac function and metabolism in the intact dog. *Rec. Adv. Stud. Cardiac. Struct. Metab.* 10: 71–79.

Lanier, W.L., Milde, J.H., and Michenfelder, J.D. (1986). Cerebral stimulation following succinylcholine in dogs. *Anesthesiology* 64: 551–559.

Länsimies, E.A., Klossner, J.A., and Hirvonen, L. (1971). Cardiovascular response to muscle relaxation in the dog. *Lab. Anim.* 5: 173–177.

Leighton, K.M. (1971). Studies on the effects of succinylcholine upon the circulation of the anaesthetized dog. *Can. Anaesth. Soc. J.* 18: 100–109.

Lien, C.A. and Kopman, A.F. (2014). Current recommendations for monitoring depth of neuromuscular blockade. *Curr. Opin. Anaesthesiol.* 27: 616–622.

Lorenzutti, A.M., Martin-Flores, M., Baldivieso, J.M. et al. (2014). Evaluation of neostigmine antagonism at different levels of vecuronium-induced neuromuscular blockade in isoflurane anesthetized dogs. *Can. Vet. J.* 55: 156–160.

Loughren, M.J., Kilbourn, J., Worth, K. et al. (2014). Comparison of muscle paralysis after intravenous and intraosseous administration of succinylcholine in swine. *J. Spec. Oper. Med.* 14: 35–37.

Madsen, M.V., Donatsky, A.M., Jensen, B.R. et al. (2015). Influence of intense neuromuscular blockade on surgical conditions during laparotomy: a pig model. *J. Anesth.* 29: 15–20.

Martin-Flores, M., Campoy, L., Ludders, J.W. et al. (2008). Comparison between acceleromyography and visual assessment of train-of-four for monitoring neuromuscular blockade in horses undergoing surgery. *Vet. Anaesth. Analg.* 35: 220–227.

Martin-Flores, M., Boesch, J., Campoy, L. et al. (2011). Failure to reverse prolonged vecuronium-induced neuromuscular blockade with edrophonium in an anesthetized dog. *J. Am. Anim. Hosp. Assoc.* 47: 294–298.

Martin-Flores, M., Pare, M.D., Adams, W. et al. (2012a). Observations of the potency and duration of vecuronium in isoflurane-anesthetized horses. *Vet. Anaesth. Analg.* 39 (4): 385–389.

Martin-Flores, M., Pare, M.D., Campoy, L. et al. (2012b). The sensitivity of sheep to vecuronium: an example of the limitations of extrapolation. *Can. J. Anaesth.* 59: 722–723.

Martin-Flores, M., Sakai, D.M., Campoy, L. et al. (2014). Recovery from neuromuscular block in dogs: restoration of spontaneous ventilation does not exclude residual blockade. *Vet. Anaesth. Analg.* 41: 269–277.

Martin-Flores, M., Cheetham, J., Campoy, L. et al. (2015a). Effect of gantacurium on evoked laryngospasm and duration of apnea in anesthetized healthy cats. *Am. J. Vet. Res.* 76: 216–223.

Martin-Flores, M., Pare, M.D., Campoy, L. et al. (2015b). The kalaemic and neuromuscular effects of succinylcholine in centronuclear myopathy: a pilot investigation in a canine model. *Eur. J. Anaesthesiol.* 32: 666–671.

Martin-Flores, M., Pare, M.D., Tomak, E.A. et al. (2015c). Neuromuscular blocking effects of vecuronium in dogs with autosomal-recessive centronuclear myopathy. *Am. J. Vet. Res.* 76: 302–307.

Martin-Flores, M., Sakai, D.M., Portela, D.A. et al. (2016). Prevention of laryngospasm with rocuronium in cats: a dose-finding study. *Vet. Anaesth. Anlag.* 43 (5): 511–518.

Meadows, J.C. (1971). Fasciculation caused by suxamethonium and other cholinergic agents. *Acta. Neurol. Scand.* 47: 381–391.

Mellinghoff, H., Radbruch, L., Diefenbach, C. et al. (1996). A comparison of cisatracurium and atracurium: onset of neuromuscular block after bolus injection and recovery after subsequent infusion. *Anesth. Analg.* 83: 1072–1075.

Michalek-Sauberer, A., Gilly, H., Steinbereithner, K. et al. (2000). Effects of vecuronium and rocuronium in antagonistic laryngeal muscles and the anterior tibial muscle in the cat. *Acta Anaesthesiol. Scandinavica.* 44: 503–510.

van Miert, M.M., Eastwood, N.B., Boyd, A.H. et al. (1997). The pharmacokinetics and pharmacodynamics of rocuronium in patients with hepatic cirrhosis. *Br. J. Clin. Pharmacol.* 44: 139–144.

Miller, R.D. and Roderick, L.L. (1978). Acid-base balance and neostigmine antagonism of pancuronium neuromuscular blockade. *Br. J. Anaesth.* 50: 317–324.

Minton, M.D., Grosslight, K., Stirt, J.A. et al. (1986). Increases in intracranial pressure from succinylcholine: prevention by prior nondepolarizing blockade. *Anesthesiology* 65: 165–169.

Moreno-Sala, A., Ortiz-Martinez, R., Valdivia, A.G. et al. (2013). Use of neuromuscular blockade with rocuronium bromide for intubation in cats. *Vet. Anaesth. Analg.* 40: 351–358.

Morris, R.B., Cahalan, M.K., Miller, R.D. et al. (1983). The cardiovascular effects of vecuronium (ORG NC45) and pancuronium in patients undergoing coronary artery bypass grafting. *Anesthesiology* 58: 438–440.

Mosing, M., Auer, U., West, E. et al. (2012). Reversal of profound rocuronium or vecuronium-induced neuromuscular block with sugammadex in isoflurane-anaesthetised dogs. *Vet. J.* 192: 467–471.

Moss, J. (1995). Muscle relaxants and histamine release. *Acta. Anaesthesiol. Scand. Suppl.* 106: 7–12.

Muir, A.W. and Marshall, R.J. (1987). Comparative neuromuscular blocking effects of vecuronium, pancuronium, org 6368 and suxamethonium in the anaesthetized domestic pig. *Br. J. Anaesth.* 59: 622–629.

Muir, A.W., Houston, J., Green, K.L. et al. (1989). Effects of a new neuromuscular blocking agent (org 9426) in anaesthetized cats and pigs and in isolated nerve-muscle preparations. *Br. J. Anaesth.* 63: 400–410.

Nagahama, S., Nishimura, R., Mochizuki, M. et al. (2006). The effects of propofol, isoflurane and sevoflurane on vecuronium infusion rates for surgical muscle relaxation in dogs. *Vet. Anaesth. Analg.* 33: 169–174.

Pittet, J.F., Tassonyi, E., Schopfer, C. et al. (1990). Plasma concentrations of laudanosine, but not of atracurium, are increased during the anhepatic phase of orthotopic liver transplantation in pigs. *Anesthesiology* 72: 145–152.

Proost, J.H., Roggeveld, J., Wierda, J.M. et al. (1997). Relationship between chemical structure and physicochemical properties of series of bulky organic cations and their hepatic uptake and biliary excretion rates. *J. Pharmacol. Exp. Ther.* 282: 715–726.

Proost, J.H., Houwertjes, M.C., and Wierda, J.M. (2008). Is time to peak effect of neuromuscular blocking agents dependent on dose? Testing the concept of buffered diffusion. *Eur. J. Anaesthesiol.* 25: 572–580.

Rahamimoff, R., Lev-Tov, A., Meiri, H. et al. (1980). Regulation of acetylcholine liberation from presynaptic nerve terminals. *Monogr. Neu. Sci.* 7: 3–18.

Rex, M.A. (1971). The effects of other drugs on the stimulation of laryngospasm in the cat: atropine; thiopentone, suxamethonium; local analgesics. *Br. J. Anaesth.* 43: 117–121.

Sakai, D.M., Martin-Flores, M., Tomak, E.A. et al. (2015). Differences between acceleromyography and electromyography during neuromuscular function monitoring in anesthetized beagle dogs. *Vet. Anaesth. Analg.* 42: 233–241.

Savarese, J.J., Ali, H.H., Basta, S.J. et al. (1988). The clinical neuromuscular pharmacology of mivacurium chloride (BW B1090U). A short-acting nondepolarizing ester neuromuscular blocking drug. *Anesthesiology* 68: 723–732.

Savarese, J.J., Belmont, M.R., Hashim, M.A. et al. (2004). Preclinical pharmacology of GW280430A (AV430A) in the rhesus monkey and in the cat: a comparison with mivacurium. *Anesthesiology* 100: 835–845.

Shi, W.Z., Fahey, M.R., Fisher, D.M. et al. (1985). Laudanosine (a metabolite of atracurium) increases the minimum alveolar concentration of halothane in rabbits. *Anesthesiology* 63: 584–588.

Shorten, G.D. and Gibbs, N.M. (1993). Dose-response relationship of atracurium besylate in the halothane-anaesthetised pig. *Res. Vet. Sci.* 55: 392–393.

Singh, Y.N., Marshall, I.G., and Harvey, A.L. (1978). Some effects of the aminoglycoside antibiotic amikacin on neuromuscular and autonomic transmission. *Br. J. Anaesth.* 50: 109–117.

Smith, S.M. and Brown, H.O. (1947). The lack of cerebral effects of d-tubocurarine. *Anesthesiology* 8: 1–14.

Smith, L.J., Moon, P.F., Lukasik, V.M. et al. (1999). Duration of action and hemodynamic properties of mivacurium chloride in dogs anesthetized with halothane. *Am. J. Vet. Res.* 60: 1047–1050.

Soliday, F.K., Conley, Y.P., and Henker, R. (2010). Pseudocholinesterase deficiency: a comprehensive review of genetic, acquired, and drug influences. *Aana J.* 78: 313–320.

Stoelting, R.K., Longnecker, D.E., and Eger, E.I. (1970). Minimum alveolar concentrations in man on awakening from methoxyflurane, halothane, ether and fluroxene anesthesia: MAC awake. *Anesthesiology* 33: 5–9.

Stone, W.A., Beach, T.P., and Hamelberg, W. (1970). Succinylcholine-induced hyperkalemia in dogs with transected sciatic nerves or spinal cords. *Anesthesiology* 32: 515–520.

Sutherland, G.A., Squire, I.B., Gibb, A.J. et al. (1983). Neuromuscular blocking and autonomic effects of vecuronium and atracurium in the anaesthetized cat. *Br.J. Anaesth.* 55: 1119–1126.

Tutunaru, A., Dupont, J., Gougnard, A. et al. (2019). Retrospective evaluation of clinical use of cis-atracurium in horses. *PLoS One* 14 (8): e0221196.

Upton, R.A., Nguyen, T.L., Miller, R.D. et al. (1982). Renal and biliary elimination of vecuronium (ORG NC 45) and pancuronium in rats. *Anesth. Analg.* 61: 313–316.

Vanlinthout, L.E., Mesfin, S.H., Hens, N. et al. (2014). A systematic review and meta-regression analysis of mivacurium for tracheal intubation. *Anaesthesia* 69: 1377–1387.

Ward, S. and Weatherley, B.C. (1986). Pharmacokinetics of atracurium and its metabolites. *Br.J. Anaesth.* 58 (Suppl 1): 6S–10S.

Wastila, W.B., Maehr, R.B., Turner, G.L. et al. (1996). Comparative pharmacology of cisatracurium (51W89), atracurium, and five isomers in cats. *Anesthesiology* 85: 169–177.

Waud, B.E. and Waud, D.R. (1972). The relation between the response to "train-of-four" stimulation and receptor occlusion during competitive neuromuscular block. *Anesthesiology* 37: 413–416.

Welch, R.M., Brown, A., Ravitch, J. et al. (1995). The in vitro degradation of cisatracurium, the R, cis-R'-isomer of atracurium, in human and rat plasma. *Clin. Pharmacol. Ther.* 58: 132–142.

Wright, P.M., Hart, P., Lau, M. et al. (1994). Cumulative characteristics of atracurium and vecuronium. A simultaneous clinical and pharmacokinetic study. *Anesthesiology* 81: 59–68; discussion 27A.

17

Anticholinesterase Drugs and Reversal of Neuromuscular Blockade

Manuel Martin-Flores and Daniel M. Sakai

Introduction

Non-depolarizing neuromuscular blocking agents (NMBAs) interrupt neuromuscular transmission by acting as *competitive antagonists* of acetylcholine (ACh) at the nicotinic ACh receptors (nAChR) of the neuromuscular junction (NMJ) (see Chapter 16). Consequently, reversal of non-depolarizing neuromuscular block can be enhanced by increasing the local concentration of ACh. As mentioned in Chapter 16, depolarizing block cannot be reversed.

Acetylcholinesterase (AChE) inhibitors, such as neostigmine or edrophonium, are commonly used to aid faster recovery from neuromuscular blockade, and to avoid residual neuromuscular blockade after extubation. Mounting evidence in people and domestic animals shows that even low levels of neuromuscular block can produce serious consequences; accordingly, pharmacologic reversal of non-depolarizing blockade with AChE inhibitors is practiced with increasing frequency.

Mechanism of action – Neostigmine and edrophonium are the most commonly used acetylcholinesterase inhibitor agents (Jones et al. 2015). AChE inhibitors reduce the activity of the AChE enzyme at the NMJ. Under normal conditions, AChE hydrolyzes ACh into choline and acetate. Choline is recycled back into the nerve cell and used to synthetize new ACh. AChE enzyme is found in high concentrations at the NMJ (see Figure 16.1), and it is a very effective enzyme; it is estimated that 50% of the ACh released to the synaptic cleft is hydrolyzed before it reaches the nAChR (Rosenberry 1975; Naguib et al. 2002). By reducing the activity of AChE, neostigmine and edrophonium allow for the concentration of ACh to increase. Accumulation of ACh at the NMJ competes with the NMBA and reverses any residual neuromuscular block. In other words, AChE inhibitors enhance reversal of blockade

through an indirect mechanism. The indirect nature of this mechanism is important in understanding the limitations of reversal of neuromuscular blockade.

The maximal concentration of ACh that can be reached at the NMJ depends on the rate of synthesis and release of ACh. Once all of the AChE enzyme is completely inhibited, a ceiling effect is reached. However, the maximal (potential) concentration of a NMBA is limitless; it depends on how much is administered. This extreme hypothetical situation is useful to understand why deep neuromuscular blockade cannot readily be antagonized with AChE inhibitors. Simply put, the concentration of ACh that can be reached at the NMJ will be insufficient to compete for the nAChR against a very high concentration of a NMBA. Reversal of neuromuscular block with AChE inhibitors is therefore limited to speeding up the already ongoing process of spontaneous recovery.

The intimate mechanism of AChE inhibition differs between neostigmine and edrophonium. The AChE enzyme has two active subsites: an anionic site and an esteratic site (Naguib et al. 2002; Wilson and Bergmann 1950). Neostigmine (and also pyridostigmine, which has been used with less frequency to reverse neuromuscular block) inhibits the activity of the AChE enzyme by producing a reversible carbamyl-ester complex at the esteratic site; it competes with ACh as substrate for that site. The newly formed carbamylated AChE is unable to hydrolyze ACh until the carbamate-enzyme bond is broken. The carbamate-enzyme bond has a half-life that ranges between 7 and 30 minutes (Wilson 1955).

Edrophonium does not have a carbamyl group; instead, it inhibits the AChE enzyme by an electrostatic bond to the anionic site. This bond prevents ACh from interacting with AChE and allows its accumulation at the NMJ. The edrophonium-AChE bond is not a true chemical bond, therefore the nature of this interaction is weaker and can be reversed by ACh, making edrophonium a weaker inhibitor agent. The half-life of the interaction is less than 0.5 minute (Wilson 1955). This might explain the lower efficiency in reversing neuromuscular blockade when compared with neostigmine (Rupp et al. 1986).

Pharmacokinetics and metabolism – In humans, the pharmacokinetics of neostigmine and edrophonium do not differ substantially. Like NMBAs, these drugs have relatively limited volumes of distribution (0.7–1.0 l/kg) and an elimination half-time of 1–2 hours (Ansermino et al. 1996; Cronnelly and Morris 1982). Between 50% and 75% of neostigmine and edrophonium are excreted through the kidneys, therefore renal failure substantially delays elimination (Cronnelly and Morris 1982). Kidney disease may also delay elimination of the NMBA, however, the effect on NMBA elimination appears to be smaller than on neostigmine. As a result, recurarization (where the patient shows signs of NMB returning despite prior reversal) from delayed elimination of NMBAs, as a consequence of kidney disease, is unlikely. In addition to renal excretion, AChE inhibitors undergo hepatic metabolism. Active and inactive metabolites are formed through this process, but studies in dogs show that these metabolites do not contribute to antagonism of neuromuscular blockade (Hennis et al. 1984).

Hypothermia (body temperature less than 34.5 °C) delays the onset time of neostigmine in people. Muscle blood flow is decreased with hypothermia and this is probably responsible for delaying the onset of neostigmine (Heier et al. 2002). The clearance, maximum effect and duration of action are not affected by hypothermia. A longer time of reversal should be expected in hypothermic animals.

Clinical Use – Restoration of neuromuscular function occurs spontaneously as the plasma concentration of the NMBA decreases through redistribution, biotransformation and excretion. However, recovery times can vary substantially between individuals and can be affected by several factors, such as body temperature, electrolyte concentration and drug interactions. Hence, simply relying on expected recovery times to assume return of adequate neuromuscular function can result in animals being extubated with substantial levels of residual paralysis. Neostigmine and edrophonium are used routinely to enhance or accelerate reversal from non-depolarizing neuromuscular blockade.

Pharmacologic reversal of neuromuscular blockade is practiced to avoid residual paralysis. While the evidence of the negative impact of residual paralysis in animals is still scarce, an abundant body of evidence has been collected in humans. Residual neuromuscular blockade, even if mild, increases the incidence of negative respiratory events in the early post-anesthesia period, such as hypoxia and upper airway obstruction (Murphy et al. 2011). Moreover,

experiments in volunteers show that mild levels of residual blockade predispose to tracheal aspiration of solids (Eriksson et al. 1997; Sundman et al. 2000) and blunt the ventilatory response to hypoxia (Eriksson et al. 1992; Eriksson et al. 1993). These low levels of residual block cannot be diagnosed without the aid of an objective monitor (Martin-Flores et al. 2008). In addition, return of spontaneous ventilation does not indicate that neuromuscular function has been restored to adequate levels, and using that as an indicator to judge whether reversal from neuromuscular block is necessary can lead to erroneous decisions (Martin-Flores et al. 2014). A train-of-four (TOF) ratio ≥ 0.9 is commonly accepted as an indicator of adequate recovery of neuromuscular transmission (see Figure 16.4). However, it was recently shown in dogs that neuromuscular blockade of some laryngeal muscles lasts longer than blockade of the limbs, where it is commonly monitored (Sakai et al. 2014). Even when the TOF ratio (measured at the pelvic limb) has returned to 0.9, residual block persists at the larynx. As a consequence, AChE inhibitors are administered routinely to prevent residual block.

Several factors can affect the efficacy of AChE inhibitors; of greatest importance are the AChE inhibitor agent used, its dose, and the depth of neuromuscular block at the time of reversal, all of which affect the outcome. In addition, the NMBA used might also impact efficacy of reversal. Neostigmine has been used in dogs in various doses (from 0.0125 to 0.2 mg/kg), and under various conditions (Jones 1990). Two recent studies in dogs evaluated the effects of depth of neuromuscular block at time of reversal, and the effects of neostigmine dose, on time of reversal. Neostigmine 0.04 mg/kg was administered when either two or four responses had spontaneously returned from vecuronium-induced block. Recovery was faster when administration occurred when four responses were visible (Lorenzutti et al. 2014). A dose finding study showed that recovery was not only faster, but also less variable as the dose of neostigmine increased from 0.02 to 0.04 and 0.07 mg/kg (Martin-Flores et al. 2017). In some of those dogs, recovery required 10–12 minutes when either a low dose of neostigmine was used, or when neostigmine was administered early during recovery from vecuronium. Larger doses and administration at shallower blockade resulted in recovery times of approximately five minutes. In a different study, neostigmine 0.04 mg/kg was administered when two responses of the TOF had returned from cisatracurium blockade. Recovery time after neostigmine required 10–15 minutes (Martin-Flores et al. 2015). These combined data underline the slow time-to-peak of neostigmine and point out that this interval can be reduced by administering larger doses, or by attempting reversal at more superficial depths of block.

In contrast to neostigmine, edrophonium has a short onset. The time-to-peak of edrophonium in humans receiving tubocurarine was 0.8–2.0 minutes when administered at 90% twitch depression (surgical blockade). The time-to-peak for neostigmine was 7–11 minutes (Cronnelly et al. 1982). Edrophonium was also faster than neostigmine for antagonizing vecuronium-induced blockade in humans (Ferguson et al. 1980). Despite its faster onset, edrophonium has been shown to be less effective under some circumstances. For example, it was found that edrophonium was unpredictable for reversing neuromuscular blockade when <3 responses to TOF could be elicited in humans recovering from pancuronium-blockade (Kopman 1979). When neostigmine and edrophonium were compared for antagonism of profound blockade (T1 < 5%), recovery was faster and less variable with neostigmine (Rupp et al. 1986). Reversal with edrophonium was equal to neostigmine when either the dose was increased to 1.0 mg/kg, or when blockade was more shallow (Rupp et al. 1986). In dogs and cats, doses of edrophonium of 0.5–1.0 mg/kg are frequently used, with the lowest dose likely being the most commonly used one. The combined data in humans suggest that despite its slow onset, neostigmine might be more reliable as a reversal agent when profound neuromuscular block is present or when long-lasting NMBAs are used.

There are fewer reports of AChE inhibitors in cats. A small dose of edrophonium (0.25 mg/kg) was useful to completely and quickly reverse vecuronium-induced blockade when administered at 90–100% twitch depression. However, that same dose was insufficient to reverse pancuronium, underscoring the limitations of edrophonium to reverse profound blockade from a longer lasting relaxant (Baird et al. 1982). Increasing the dose of edrophonium to 0.5–0.75 mg/kg produced faster reversal, and it was concluded that edrophonium 0.6 mg/kg was equipotent to neostigmine 0.05 mg/kg for reversing vecuronium (Baird et al. 1982). That study suggested that doses of edrophonium between 0.5–1.0 mg/kg and neostigmine at approximately 0.05 mg/kg are likely to be useful in clinical scenarios. These authors routinely use edrophonium 0.5 mg/kg or neostigmine 0.02–0.04 mg/kg to reverse neuromuscular block in the clinical setting.

Both neostigmine and edrophonium have been studied in horses. A dose-response study in horses, under moderate pancuronium or gallamine block, suggested that doses of neostigmine between 0.03–0.04 might be sufficient to restore neuromuscular function. Atropine (0.01 mg/kg) was administered prior to the AChE inhibitor (Klein et al. 1983). Neostigmine (0.04 mg/kg) and edrophonium (1 mg/kg) were successfully used to antagonize pancuronium-induced block in anesthetized horses (Hildebrand and Howitt 1984). In this case, both AChE

Table 17.1 Doses of neostigmine and edrophonium (and anticholinergic agents) commonly used in several domestic species.

	Neostigmine (mg/kg)	Edrophonium (mg/kg)
Dogs and cats	0.02–0.07 with atropine 0.02–0.04 or glycopyrrolate 0.01	0.5–1 mg/kg with atropine 0.02 mg/kg
Horses	0.007–0.04 with or without atropine 0.01	0.2–1.0 with or without atropine 0.01 mg/kg
Rabbits	0.05 with atropine 0.01	NA
Sheep	0.05 with atropine 0.08	0.5–1.0 with atropine 0.04–0.08

Anticholinergic drugs are usually administered prior to the AChE inhibitor agent.

inhibitors were administered without atropine or glycopyrrolate (see cardiovascular effects below). Bradycardia was observed after edrophonium but not after neostigmine. The onset of edrophonium was faster. Lower doses have been used to reverse shallow block; neostigmine 0.007 mg/kg was administered to horses recovering from rocuronium (Auer et al. 2007). A recent study showed some limitations of edrophonium to restore neuromuscular function in horses receiving vecuronium (Martin-Flores et al. 2012) Table 17.1.

Effects on organ systems – Acetylcholinesterase inhibitors increase the circulating levels of ACh; the effects on other organs are primarily the result of this effect. Most noticeably, the use of AChE inhibiting agents is associated with bradyarrhythmias and gastrointestinal (GI) activation. As a general rule, to avoid these effects, the administration of AChE inhibitors is preceded by (or administered simultaneously with) atropine or glycopyrrolate. Due to its slower onset time, glycopyrrolate appears to better match the time-course of neostigmine. Atropine can be used safely with either AChE inhibitor agent. In dogs and cats, doses of atropine between 0.02–0.04 are commonly administered prior to reversal with neostigmine (Lorenzutti et al. 2014; Adams et al. 2006). Glycopyrrolate 0.01 mg/kg has also been used in dogs to prevent bradycardia from neostigmine 04 mg/kg (Martin-Flores et al. 2015).

In horses, AChE inhibitors have been administered with and without the use of atropine. When atropine was omitted, increased defecation, flatulence, salivation, and increased airway secretions were noticed (Hildebrand and Howitt 1984).

Physostigmine is a tertiary amine AChE inhibitor that permeates through the blood–brain-barrier. It has been used to treat central anticholinergic syndrome in people (Moos 2007), and to improve recovery quality in horses by decreasing emergence delirium (Wiese et al. 2014). The potential use of physostigmine for reversing neuromuscular block in veterinary medicine is currently unknown.

Novel agents – Important advances have been made to improve the way neuromuscular block can be reversed. As described above, reversal with AChE inhibitors has several limitations: the mechanism by which reversal occurs is indirect, which results in a ceiling effect determined by the rate of release of quanta. As a result, profound neuromuscular block cannot be reversed. Moreover, due to the undesirable side effects of AChE inhibitors, anticholinergic agents are commonly administered. The resultant changes in cardiovascular function might be deleterious to many patients. Unwanted GI effects may also occur both from the AChE inhibitor or the anticholinergic agent; this is of particular importance in horses.

Sugammadex presents a new concept to restore neuromuscular function. This agent is currently approved in more than 50 countries. Sugammadex is a modified γ-cyclodextrin that selectively binds to rocuronium (and also vecuronium) (Adam et al. 2002). Sugammadex encapsulates rocuronium in its lipophilic cavity; the new complex (sugammadex-rocuronium) has no neuromuscular blocking properties. By "capturing" rocuronium, the plasma concentration of free rocuronium is drastically and quickly decreased, so that neuromuscular function is restored (Bom et al. 2002). The sugammadex-rocuronium complex is then excreted by the kidneys. Sugammadex is devoid of direct effects on cholinergic transmission. Since sugammadex was specifically designed to encapsulate rocuronium, it is currently classified as a *selective relaxant binding agent* (SRBA). Due to its ability to quickly render rocuronium (and vecuronium) devoid of effects, sugammadex can re-establish neuromuscular transmission with little delay, even in the presence of profound neuromuscular block. Mosing et al. (2010) showed that sugammadex could reverse profound rocuronium-induced block in ponies in <4 minutes. In dogs, sugammadex restored function from profound rocuronium or vecuronium-induced block in <2 minutes (Mosing et al. 2012). These results are a substantial improvement from the results that could be obtained with neostigmine or edrophonium. Moreover, there is no need to administer anticholinergic drugs, an advantage that might prove especially important in patients with cardiac disease, or in horses.

Calabadion has recently been proposed as a new alternative for reversing NMBAs (Hoffmann et al. 2013). Calabadion is a member of the cucurbit[n]uril family. This molecular container has a high affinity for both aminosteroid and benzylisoquinoline NMBAs (Ma et al. 2012), and pre-clinical studies have shown that it can quickly and completely reverse rocuronium and cisatracurium block in rats (Hoffmann et al. 2013). Calabadion might therefore offer the unique opportunity to bind several NMBAs and promptly re-establish neuromuscular function.

The newly developed neuromuscular blocking agents, **gantacurium** and **CW002**, are susceptible to cysteine adduction (Heerdt et al. 2015). Interaction with cysteine renders these NMBAs inactive and terminates neuromuscular block. Studies in different animal models show that CW002 has an intermediate duration of action, but that the effects can be terminated upon injection of L-cysteine. In dogs, administration of 9 × ED95 of CW002 produced neuromuscular block for approximately 75 minutes. That duration was reduced to <5 minutes when cysteine was administered (Sunaga et al. 2010). These novel cysteine-inactivated NMBAs might offer two advantages for the practice of clinical anesthesia: An ultrashort-acting drug (gantacurium) that does not require reversal, or an intermediate acting agent (CW002), in which reversal could be performed at any time regardless of depth of blockade, by injecting L-cysteine.

References

Adam, J.M., Bennett, D.J., Bom, A. et al. (2002). Cyclodextrin-derived host molecules as reversal agents for the neuromuscular blocker rocuronium bromide: synthesis and structure-activity relationships. *J. Med. Chem.* 45: 1806–1816.

Adams, W.A., Mark Senior, J., Jones, R.S. et al. (2006). Cis-atracurium in dogs with and without porto-systemic shunts. *Vet. Anaesth. Analg.* 33: 17–23.

Ansermino, J.M., Sanderson, P.M., Bevan, J.C., and Bevan, D.R. (1996). Acceleromyography improves detection of residual neuromuscular blockade in children. *Can. J. Anaesth.* 43: 589–594.

Auer, U., Uray, C., and Mosing, M. (2007). Observations on the muscle relaxant rocuronium bromide in the horse—a dose-response study. *Vet. Anaesth. Analg.* 34: 75–81.

Baird, W.L., Bowman, W.C., and Kerr, W.J. (1982). Some actions of Org NC 45 and of edrophonium in the anaesthetized cat and in man. *Br. J. Anaesth.* 54: 375–385.

Bom, A., Clark, J.K., and Palin, R. (2002). New approaches to reversal of neuromuscular block. *Curr. Opin. Drug Discovery Dev.* 5: 793–800.

Cronnelly, R. and Morris, R.B. (1982). Antagonism of neuromuscular blockade. *Br. J. Anaesth.* 54: 183–194.

Cronnelly, R., Morris, R.B., and Miller, R.D. (1982). Edrophonium: duration of action and atropine requirement in humans during halothane anesthesia. *Anesthesiology* 57: 261–266.

Eriksson, L.I., Lennmarken, C., Wyon, N., and Johnson, A. (1992). Attenuated ventilatory response to hypoxaemia at vecuronium-induced partial neuromuscular block. *Acta. Anaesthesiol. Scandinavica.* 36: 710–715.

Eriksson, L.I., Sato, M., and Severinghaus, J.W. (1993). Effect of a vecuronium-induced partial neuromuscular block on hypoxic ventilatory response. *Anesthesiology* 78: 693–699.

Eriksson, L.I., Sundman, E., Olsson, R. et al. (1997). Functional assessment of the pharynx at rest and during swallowing in partially paralyzed humans: simultaneous videomanometry and mechanomyography of awake human volunteers. *Anesthesiology* 87: 1035–1043.

Ferguson, A., Egerszegi, P., and Bevan, D.R. (1980). Neostigmine, pyridostigmine, and edrophonium as antagonists of pancuronium. *Anesthesiology* 53: 390–394.

Heerdt, P.M., Sunaga, H., and Savarese, J.J. (2015). Novel neuromuscular blocking drugs and antagonists. *Curr. Opin. Anaesthesiol.* 28: 403–410.

Heier, T., Clough, D., Wright, P.M. et al. (2002). The influence of mild hypothermia on the pharmacokinetics and time course of action of neostigmine in anesthetized volunteers. *Anesthesiology* 97: 90–95.

Hennis, P.J., Cronnelly, R., Sharma, M. et al. (1984). Metabolites of neostigmine and pyridostigmine do not contribute to antagonism of neuromuscular blockade in the dog. *Anesthesiology* 61: 534–539.

Hildebrand, S.V. and Howitt, G.A. (1984). Antagonism of pancuronium neuromuscular blockade in halothane-anesthetized ponies using neostigmine and edrophonium. *Am. J. Vet. Res.* 45: 2276–2280.

Hoffmann, U., Grosse-Sundrup, M., Eikermann-Haerter, K. et al. (2013). Calabadion: a new agent to reverse the effects of benzylisoquinoline and steroidal neuromuscular-blocking agents. *Anesthesiology* 119: 317–325.

Jones, R.S. (1990). Reversal of atracurium neuromuscular block with neostigmine in the dog. *Res. Vet. Sci.* 48: 96–98.

Jones, R.S., Auer, U., and Mosing, M. (2015). Reversal of neuromuscular block in companion animals. *Vet. Anaesth. Analg.* 42: 455–471.

Klein, L., Hopkins, J., Beck, E., and Burton, B. (1983). Cumulative dose responses to gallamine, pancuronium, and neostigmine in halothane-anesthetized horses: neuromuscular and cardiovascular effects. *Am. J. Vet. Res.* 44: 786–792.

Kopman, A.F. (1979). Edrophonium antagonism of pancuronium-induced neuromuscular blockade in man: a reappraisal. *Anesthesiology* 51: 139–142.

Lorenzutti, A.M., Martin-Flores, M., Baldivieso, J.M. et al. (2014). Evaluation of neostigmine antagonism at different levels of vecuronium-induced neuromuscular blockade in isoflurane anesthetized dogs. *Can. Vet. J.* 55: 156–160.

Ma, D., Zhang, B., Hoffmann, U. et al. (2012). Acyclic cucurbit[n]uril-type molecular containers bind neuromuscular blocking agents in vitro and reverse neuromuscular block in vivo. *Angew. Chem. Int. Ed. Engl.* 51: 11358–11362.

Martin-Flores, M., Campoy, L., Ludders, J.W. et al. (2008). Comparison between acceleromyography and visual assessment of train-of-four for monitoring neuromuscular blockade in horses undergoing surgery. *Vet. Anaesth. Analg.* 35: 220–227.

Martin-Flores, M., Pare, M.D., Adams, W. et al. (2012). Observations of the potency and duration of vecuronium in isoflurane-anesthetized horses. *Vet. Anaesth. Analg.* 39: 385–389.

Martin-Flores, M., Sakai, D.M., Campoy, L., and Gleed, R.D. (2014). Recovery from neuromuscular block in dogs: restoration of spontaneous ventilation does not exclude residual blockade. *Vet. Anaesth. Analg.* 41: 269–277.

Martin-Flores, M., Pare, M.D., Campoy, L., and Gleed, R.D. (2015). Neuromuscular blocking effects of cisatracurium and its antagonism with neostigmine in a canine model of autosomal-recessive centronuclear myopathy. *Br. J. Anaesth.* 115: 927–931.

Martin-Flores, M., Lorenzutti, A.M., Litterio, N.J. et al. (2017). Speed of reversal of vecuronium neuromuscular block with different doses of neostigmine in anesthetized dogs. *Vet. Anaesth. Analg.* 44: 28–34.

Moos, D.D. (2007). Central anticholinergic syndrome: a case report. *J. Perianesth. Nurs.* 22: 309–321.

Mosing, M., Auer, U., Bardell, D. et al. (2010). Reversal of profound rocuronium block monitored in three muscle groups with sugammadex in ponies. *Bri. J. Anaesth.* 105: 480–486.

Mosing, M., Auer, U., West, E. et al. (2012). Reversal of profound rocuronium or vecuronium-induced neuromuscular block with sugammadex in isoflurane-anaesthetised dogs. *Vet. J.* 192: 467–471.

Murphy, G.S., Szokol, J.W., Avram, M.J. et al. (2011). Intra-operative acceleromyography monitoring reduces symptoms of muscle weakness and improves quality of recovery in the early postoperative period. *Anesthesiology* 115: 946–954.

Naguib, M., Flood, P., McArdle, J.J., and Brenner, H.R. (2002). Advances in neurobiology of the neuromuscular junction: implications for the anesthesiologist. *Anesthesiology* 96: 202–231.

Rosenberry, T.L. (1975). Acetylcholinesterase. *Adv. Enzymol. Relat. Areas Mol. Biol.* 43: 103–218.

Rupp, S.M., McChristian, J.W., Miller, R.D. et al. (1986). Neostigmine and edrophonium antagonism of varying intensity neuromuscular blockade induced by atracurium, pancuronium, or vecuronium. *Anesthesiology* 64: 711–717.

Sakai, D.M., Martin-Flores, M., Romano, M., Tseng, C.T. et al. (2017) Recovery from rocuronium-induced neuromuscular block was longer in the larynx than in the pelvic limb of anesthetized dogs. *Vet. Anaesth. Analg.* 44 (2): 246–253. doi:10.1016/j.vaa.2016.04.001.

Sunaga, H., Malhotra, J.K., Yoon, E. et al. (2010). Cysteine reversal of the novel neuromuscular blocking drug CW002 in dogs: pharmacodynamics, acute cardiovascular effects, and preliminary toxicology. *Anesthesiology* 112: 900–909.

Sundman, E., Witt, H., Olsson, R. et al. (2000). The incidence and mechanisms of pharyngeal and upper esophageal dysfunction in partially paralyzed humans: pharyngeal videoradiography and simultaneous manometry after atracurium. *Anesthesiology* 92: 977–984.

Wiese, A.J., Brosnan, R.J., and Barter, L.S. (2014). Effects of acetylcholinesterase inhibition on quality of recovery from isoflurane-induced anesthesia in horses. *Am. J. Vet. Res.* 75: 223–230.

Wilson, I.B. (1955). The interaction of tensilon and neostigmine with acetylcholinesterase. *Arch. Int. Pharmacodyn. Ther.* 104: 204–213.

Wilson, I.B. and Bergmann, F. (1950). Studies on cholinesterase. VII. The active surface of acetylcholine esterase derived from effects of pH on inhibitors. *J. Biolumin. Chemilumin.* 185: 479–489.

18

Sympathomimetics and Vasopressin

Phillip Lerche

Introduction

The autonomic nervous system regulates homeostasis and the body's response to stress, and as such is responsible for regulating systemic blood pressure. It is comprised of the sympathetic nervous system (SNS) and the parasympathetic nervous system (PNS), which work in tandem to regulate organ function. Many drugs used in the peri-anesthetic period can decrease SNS output. These include benzodiazepines, particularly when combined with mu opioid receptor agonists, alpha$_2$ adrenoceptor agonists, injectable anesthetic induction agents (propofol, barbiturates) and inhalant anesthetics (halothane, isoflurane, sevoflurane) (Neukirchen and Kienbaum 2008).

In addition to direct effects of anesthetic drugs on the cardiovascular system, a reduction in sympathetic tone during anesthesia can contribute to unfavorable hemodynamics (decreased myocardial contractility, bradycardia, hypotension). Inadvertent sympathetic blockade by local anesthetics can also decrease sympathetic output, resulting in hypotension (Peters et al. 1990). Additionally, hypotension is known to contribute to the development of anesthesia-related myopathy in horses (Grandy et al. 1987).

Bradycardia is most frequently treated with drugs having parasympatholytic effects, i.e. anticholinergics (see Chapter 13). Drugs with agonist activity at sympathetic adrenergic receptors (adrenoceptors) are commonly used intraoperatively to treat hypotension (mean arterial blood pressure <60–70 mmHg) that is anesthetic drug-induced or due to disease states (e.g. congestive heart failure, cardiomyopathy, autonomic dysfunction, sepsis), as well as during cardiopulmonary resuscitation (CPR). These drugs are called sympathomimetics, and include endogenous catecholamines, synthetic catecholamines and synthetic non-catecholamines.

Mechanism of Action and Main Effects

Like the PNS, the neurotransmitter in preganglionic sympathetic fibers is acetyl choline. Postganglionic fibers in the SNS store norepinephrine (noradrenaline) in synaptic vesicles and are referred to as adrenergic (noradrenergic) fibers. Adrenoceptors are stimulated by the endogenous catecholamines dopamine, epinephrine (adrenaline) and norepinephrine (noradrenaline). These three catecholamines share a common biosynthetic pathway (Flatmark 2000). Phenylalanine is transformed to L-tyrosine, which in turn, is transformed to L-dopa, from which dopamine is synthesized. Dopamine is a precursor for norepinephrine and epinephrine synthesis (see Figure 18.1). When stimulated, adrenergic fibers release norepinephrine, which interacts with adrenoceptors in the synaptic cleft. Cessation of action is mostly due to reuptake of norepinephrine, with some being metabolized. Additionally, epinephrine and norepinephrine are released via sympathetic activation of the adrenal medulla, in which case, they are considered to act as hormones rather than neurotransmitters.

Adrenergic receptors are G protein-coupled receptors and are divided into alpha and beta adrenoceptors with subtypes alpha$_1$, alpha$_2$, beta$_1$, beta$_2$, and beta$_3$. Alpha$_1$ and alpha$_2$ adrenoceptors are further divided into alpha$_{1A}$, alpha$_{1B}$, alpha$_{1D}$, alpha$_{2A}$, alpha$_{2B}$, and alpha$_{2C}$ subtypes (Skelding and Valverde 2020; Motiejunaite et al. 2021).

Alpha$_1$ adrenoceptors are coupled to excitatory G$_q$ proteins and are located in the smooth muscle of the vasculature, including the coronary artery. Via activation of phospholipase C and inositol triphosphate, intracellular calcium increases resulting in vasoconstriction. Alpha$_1$ adrenoceptors located in the heart increase inotropy.

Alpha$_2$ adrenoceptors are coupled to G$_i$ proteins and cause inhibition by deactivating adenylyl cyclase thus

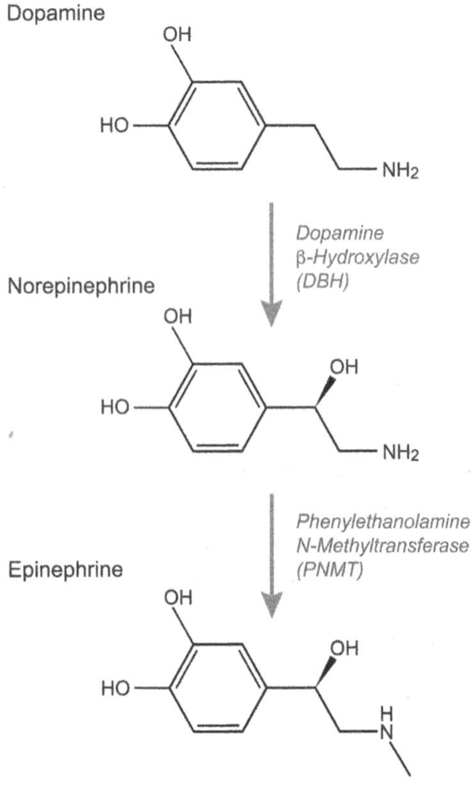

Dopamine

Norepinephrine

Epinephrine

Figure 18.1 The latter portion of the pathway of endogenous catecholamine synthesis.

preventing activation of phosphokinase A. They are present in the central nervous system (CNS) where they cause sedation, analgesia, and decrease sympathetic tone. In the vasculature, including coronary blood vessels, alpha$_2$ adrenoceptors cause vasoconstriction. They are also present on platelets (mediation of platelet aggregation) and in the Islets of Langerhans in the pancreas (inhibition of insulin release). See Chapter 4 for a discussion of alpha$_2$ adrenoceptor subtypes.

Beta$_1$ adrenoceptors located in the heart couple with excitatory G$_s$ proteins, exerting their action by increasing adenylyl cyclase, cyclic AMP, and protein kinase A. This results in increases in inotropy (contractile force of myocytes), chronotropy (heart rate), dromotropy (conduction through the atrioventricular node), and lusitropy (rate of myocyte relaxation).

Beta$_2$ adrenoceptors also couple with G$_s$ proteins. The effect on bronchial and vascular smooth muscle is relaxation. Beta$_2$ receptors in the heart contribute to increases in inotropy and chronotropy, as well as coronary artery vasodilation.

Beta$_3$ adrenoceptors are located in adipose tissue and are associated with lipolysis and associated thermogenesis. The general effect of sympathetic activation is an increased

metabolic rate. In the heart, beta$_3$ adrenoceptors are activated when sympathetic tone is high (e.g. due to congestive heart failure). Agonism of beta$_3$ adrenoceptors has been shown to be cardioprotective through decreasing inotropy, possibly acting as an endogenous beta receptor blockers (Niu et al. 2012).

Dopamine receptors have five subtypes, D$_1$ through D$_5$ (Beaulieu and Gainetdinov 2011). D$_1$ and D$_2$ receptors are relevant to mediation of vascular tone. D$_1$ receptors are found post-synaptically in several vascular beds (renal, mesenteric) as well as in coronary and cerebral blood vessels. They couple with G$_s$ proteins. D$_2$ receptors are found pre-synaptically, couple with G$_i$ proteins, and inhibit adenylyl cyclase and norepinephrine release.

Vasopressin (antidiuretic hormone) acts at vasopressin receptors (V$_{1A}$, V$_{1B}$, and V$_2$, which correlate to an alternate classification of V$_1$, V$_2$, and V$_3$) which are coupled to G$_q$ proteins. Vasopressin receptors are not sympathetic receptors. They are included here because V$_{1A}$ receptors on blood vessels cause vasoconstriction. V$_{1B}$ receptors located in the pituitary regulate mood and behavior, while V$_2$ receptors in the kidney promote water reabsorption (Zeynalov et al. 2020).

Location and effects of sympathetic and vasopressin receptors are given in Table 18.1. Drugs that have predominantly beta$_1$ adrenoceptor activity are frequently referred to as inotropes, while drugs that primarily increase blood pressure by causing vasoconstriction, i.e. acting predominantly on vascular alpha adrenoceptors or vasopressin receptors, are called vasopressors (or pressors). Alpha$_2$ adrenoceptors are included in Table 18.1, and this class of drugs is discussed in detail in Chapter 4.

Adrenoceptors can become desensitized or downregulated in the face of increased release of endogenous catecholamines (adrenergic overdrive) as occurs with congestive heart failure and septic shock (Wallukat 2002; Landry and Oliver 2001).

Catecholamines – Structure and Pharmacokinetics

Endogenous and exogenous sympathomimetics share the common structure of a catechol ring, which is comprised of a benzene ring with hydroxyl groups attached at C3 and C4. Amine side chains are attached at C1, therefore sympathomimetics sharing these two characteristics are referred to as catecholamines (Cannon 1983; Murrell 2015; Motiejunaite et al. 2021).

The onset of, and duration of action of most catecholamines is very short, typically in the range of a few minutes when given intravenously (IV). They are therefore frequently

Table 18.1 Location and effects of adrenergic, dopamine and vasopressin receptors.

Receptor	G-protein	Location	Effect
Alpha$_1$ adrenergic	G$_q$	Vasculature	Vasoconstriction
		Heart	↑ Inotropy
			Coronary artery vasoconstriction
Alpha$_2$ adrenergic	G$_i$	CNS	Sedation, analgesia, ↓ sympathetic tone
		Heart	Coronary artery vasoconstriction
		Vasculature	Vasoconstriction
		Platelets	↑ Aggregation
		Pancreas	↓ Insulin release
Beta$_1$ adrenergic	G$_s$	Heart	↑ Inotropy
			↑ Chronotropy
			↑ Dromotropy
			↑ Lusitropy
Beta$_2$ adrenergic	G$_s$	Bronchi	Bronchodilation
		Heart	↑ Inotropy
			↑ Chronotropy
			Coronary artery vasodilation
		Vasculature	Vasodilation
		Platelets	↓ Aggregation
		Hepatocytes	Glycogenolysis
D$_1$ dopamine	G$_s$	CNS	Modulates the extrapyramidal system
		Vasculature	Vasodilation
D$_2$ dopamine	G$_i$	CNS	↓ Norepinephrine release
			↓ Pituitary hormone release
		Vasculature	Vasodilation
V$_{1A}$ vasopressin	Gq	Vasculature	Vasoconstriction

CNS, central nervous system.

administered IV by constant rate infusion (CRI) for their hemodynamic effects during anesthesia. Boluses of epinephrine are used to treat severe anaphylaxis and during CPR (Odunayo et al. 2021; Fletcher et al. 2012). Ephedrine and phenylephrine have longer durations of action (10–20 minutes) and can also be given as bolus doses.

The action of catecholamines is terminated mostly due to reuptake by active transport mechanisms that ultimately return them to neuronal storage vesicles, which frequently involve intracytoplasmic metabolism (Eisenhofer et al. 2004). A small fraction of catecholamines undergo biotransformation to metabolites that are then excreted via the urine. In people, biotransformation is relatively complex with several possible pathways (Eisenhofer et al. 2001). The majority of catecholamine biotransformation is via initial deamination in the sympathetic neurons via monoamine oxidase (MAO). The resulting aldehyde intermediates are then transformed to alcohol or acid metabolites by aldehyde reductase (AR) or aldehyde dehydrogenase (AD). These intermediary alcohol and acid metabolites can be further metabolized by MAO, catechol-O-methyltransferase (COMT), AR, and AD. The final metabolites, produced in the liver, are homovanillic acid (dopamine) and vanillylmandelic acid (epinephrine and norepinephrine), which, along with other intermediary metabolites, are excreted in urine.

Exogenous catecholamines can undergo pulmonary clearance. In newborn lambs, approximately 25% of circulating norepinephrine and 10% of epinephrine was removed by the lungs (Smolich et al. 1997). In dogs, pulmonary clearance was similar (25% and 14% for norepinephrine and epinephrine, respectively), and occurred due to neuronal uptake of catecholamines within the lung, as well as via non-neuronal mechanisms (Eisenhofer et al. 1992). Non-neuronal pulmonary clearance can be attributed to uptake into endothelial cells with metabolism by MAO and COMT (Gillis and Pitt 1982).

Endogenous Catecholamines

Epinephrine (Adrenaline)

Epinephrine has a relatively indiscriminate adrenergic receptor profile and is an agonist at alpha and beta adrenoceptors (see Table 18.2). As such, it is not usually used for cardiovascular support during anesthesia, as drugs with more specific receptor profiles are preferred. Epinephrine is used to prolong the action of local anesthetics (see Chapter 12), to treat severe anaphylaxis, and during CPR (Odunayo et al. 2021; Fletcher et al. 2012). See Table 18.3 for recommended dosing of catecholamines.

Cardiovascular Effects

At lower doses (0.01 mg/kg IV) beta adrenergic effects result in increased cardiac output (beta$_1$), coronary dilation, and decreased systemic vascular resistance (beta$_2$). At higher doses (0.1 mg/kg IV) epinephrine also has alpha adrenergic effects resulting in increases in systemic vascular resistance. CRIs of epinephrine increased heart rate, systemic blood pressure, cardiac index and oxygen delivery in a dose-dependent fashion in cats (Pascoe et al. 2006). As with all catecholamines, epinephrine is pro-arrhythmogenic. In dogs, epinephrine (0.3–0.9 μg/kg/min IV) increased mean arterial blood pressure and caused ventricular arrhythmias (Deterling et al. 1954).

Ketamine, and xylazine plus ketamine decreased the arrhythmogenic dose of epinephrine in dogs (Wright et al. 1987). Compared to other inhalants, halothane sensitizes the myocardium to epinephrine-induced arrhythmias in most domestic species (Sumikawa et al. 1983; Bednarski and Majors 1986; Lees and Tavernor 1970; Rezakhani et al. 1977; Zahed et al. 1977; Stowe et al. 1988).

During CPR

High doses of epinephrine used during CPR in people resulted in an increase in rates of return to spontaneous circulation (ROSC) (Vandycke and Martens 2000). Survival to discharge was not different compared to a lower dose. In small animals, low-dose epinephrine (0.01 mg/kg IV) is preferred. High-dose epinephrine (0.1 mg/kg IV) should only be used if ROSC has not been achieved after prolonged CPR (Fletcher et al. 2012). Cardiopulmonary arrest results in increased circulating epinephrine in dogs, and it is recommended that administration of epinephrine be limited to every second advanced life support cycle in order to avoid overdosing (Huyghens et al. 1991; Fletcher et al. 2012). The resuscitation dose of epinephrine in horses is lower than in small animals – 0.003–0.005 mg/kg (Muir 2009).

Other Effects

Epinephrine infusion increased packed cell volume in cats, likely due to splenic contraction (alpha$_1$ adrenergic effect) (Pascoe et al. 2006). In the same study, body temperature increased due to a thermogenic effect.

Norepinephrine (Noradrenaline)

Norepinephrine acts at alpha$_1$, alpha$_2$, and beta$_1$ adrenoceptors, with no beta$_2$ activity (Table 18.2) Norepinephrine

Table 18.2 Receptor profiles of sympathomimetic drugs and vasopressin at clinical dosages.

Drug	Receptor activity					
	Alpha$_1$	Alpha$_2$	Beta$_1$	Beta$_2$	D$_1$/D$_2$	V$_{1A}$
Epinephrine low dose	0	0	+++	++	0	0
Epinephrine high dose	++	++	+++	++	0	0
Norepinephrine	+++	+++	++	0	0	0
Dopamine[a]	+++	++	++	+	+++	0
Isoproterenol	0	0	+++	+++	0	0
Dobutamine	0/+	0	+++	+	0	0
Phenylephrine	+++	0	0	0	0	0
Ephedrine	++	++	+	+	0	0
Vasopressin	0	0	0	0	0	++

Alpha$_1$, alpha$_2$, beta$_1$, beta$_2$, adrenoceptors; D$_1$, D$_2$, dopamine receptors; V$_{1A}$, vasopressin receptor. 0, no activity; +, ++, +++, relative increases in activity.
[a] Receptor activity of dopamine is dose and individual dependent, with alpha adrenoceptor effects typically occurring at high infusion rates (10–20 μg/kg/min).
Source: Table adapted from the following sources: (Muir 2009; Schauvliege and Gasthuys 2013; Murrell 2015; Skelding and Valverde 2020; Motiejunaite et al. 2021; Congdon 2022; Lorenzo 2022).

Table 18.3 Recommended dosages for sympathomimetics and vasopressin in small animals and horses during CPR and for treatment of hypotension during anesthesia.

Indication and main actions		Drug	Dose (IV) Dogs and cats	Dose (IV) Horses
CPR	Vasoconstriction	Epinephrine	—	0.001–0.005 mg/kg
	↑ Inotropy	Epinephrine low dose	0.01 mg/kg	—
	↑ Chronotropy	Epinephrine high dose	0.1 mg/kg	—
	Vasoconstriction	Vasopressin	0.8 U/kg	—
Hypotension	↑ Inotropy	Dobutamine	1–10 μg/kg/min	0.5–5 μg/kg/min
	↑ Inotropy ↑ Chronotropy	Dopamine low dose	5–10 μg/kg/min	1–5 μg/kg/min
	Vasoconstriction	Dopamine high dose	10–20 μg/kg/min	—
	↑ Inotropy	Isoproterenol	0.001–2 μg/kg/min	—
	Vasoconstriction ↑ Inotropy ↑ Chronotropy	Ephedrine	0.06–0.2 mg/kg 10–20 μg/kg/min	0.03–0.06 mg/kg
	Vasoconstriction ↑ Inotropy[a] ↑ Chronotropy[a]	Norepinephrine	0.05–2 μg/kg/min	0.05–1 μg/kg/min
	Vasoconstriction	Phenylephrine	1–5 μg/kg 0.5–3 μg/kg/min	0.01–0.02 mg/kg 0.25–2 μg/kg/min
		Vasopressin	0.1–0.6 U/kg 1–5 mU/kg/min	0.3–1 mU/kg/min[b]
Bradycardia due to sinus node dysfunction	↑ Chronotropy ↑ Inotropy Vasodilation	Isoproterenol	0.001–2 μg/kg/min	—

CPR, cardiopulmonary resuscitation.
[a] At higher doses.
[b] In foals.
Source: Adapted from Muir (2009), Fletcher et al. (2012), Schauvliege and Gasthuys (2013), Murrell (2015), and Skelding and Valverde (2020).

is used to manage hypotension due to decreased systemic vascular resistance as a result of drug effects (e.g. inhalant anesthetics) or diseases that result in excessive vasodilation (e.g. septic shock).

Pharmacodynamics

Norepinephrine causes a greater degree of vasoconstriction compared to epinephrine, while increases in contractility are less. Increases in blood pressure can cause decreased heart rate due to baroreceptor reflex. Norepinephrine (0.05–0.3 μg/kg/min IV) effectively maintained normotension in isoflurane-anesthetized cats (Kobluk and Pypendop 2022). In dogs, norepinephrine (0.3–0.9 μg/kg/min IV) increased mean arterial blood pressure and caused ventricular arrhythmias (Deterling et al. 1954). In an isoflurane-induced hypotension model, norepinephrine increased blood pressure and cardiac output while reducing the heart rate, with the most effective dose being 0.44 μg/kg/min IV (Henao-Guerrero et al. 2023). In a canine endotoxic shock model, norepinephrine (0.5–1 μg/kg/min IV) increased blood pressure, cardiac index and oxygen delivery (Bakker and Vincent 1993). Norepinephrine increased cardiac index, oxygen delivery and systemic vascular resistance during isoflurane-induced hypotension in 1–4-day old foals (Valverde et al. 2006). In 8–14-day old foals, norepinephrine increased mean arterial blood pressure, heart rate, partial pressure of oxygen, and systemic vascular resistance index, while cardiac index was not significantly different from the baseline (Craig et al. 2007). In isoflurane-anesthetized horses, norepinephrine increased blood pressure, and did not change GI perfusion (Dancker et al. 2018).

Other Effects

In sheep, where anesthesia was being maintained with a propofol CRI, a norepinephrine infusion dose-dependently increased cardiac output, and decreased propofol plasma concentration (Myburgh et al. 2001). This is likely as a result of increased hepatic blood flow causing an increased clearance of propofol.

Dopamine

Dopamine has dose-dependent activity at adrenergic and dopamine receptors. It is commonly used in cats and dogs to manage hypotension during anesthesia (see Table 18.3).

Pharmacodynamics

At lower doses (1–3 μg/kg/min IV) dopamine receptor effects predominate resulting in vasodilation and diuresis. As the dose range increases to 3–10 μg/kg/min IV, beta adrenergic effects tend to dominate, resulting in increases in chronotropy and inotropy. Above 10 μg/kg/min IV alpha adrenergic effects result in vasoconstriction and increased systemic vascular resistance (Murrell 2015). This general pattern is not consistent and, in people, there is considerable individual variation in plasma concentrations achieved from a given dose (MacGregor et al. 2000). Dopamine should therefore be titrated to effect.

In a canine model of isoflurane-induced hypotension that initially targeted a mean arterial pressure of 50 mmHg, dopamine increased blood pressure and cardiac index in a dose-dependent manner (Rosati and Dyson 2007). In that study, dopamine at 7 μg/kg/min IV achieved a mean blood pressure of 70 mmHg, however, the heart rate was not increased at that dose. Dopamine was effective at increasing mean arterial pressure in dogs anesthetized for orthopedic surgery when given at 10 μg/kg/min IV, but not at 5 μg/kg/min IV (Chen et al. 2007). The effects of acepromazine, an alpha₁ adrenergic antagonist, administered at 0.03 mg/kg IV prior to isoflurane anesthesia on dopamine infusion has been investigated (Monteiro et al. 2007). Cardiac output increased when dopamine was administered at 5 μg/kg/min IV, however blood pressure did not increase due to decreased systemic vascular resistance. Dopamine at 15 μg/kg/min IV increased blood pressure largely due to increased cardiac output. In that same study, when dopamine was given without acepromazine, systemic vascular resistance was reduced when dopamine at 5 and 10 μg/kg/min IV was infused. This was likely due to dopamine receptor agonism, thus demonstrating that there can be overlap of beta₁ adrenoceptor and dopamine receptor agonism at these doses of dopamine. Unexpected acute bradycardia and hypotension associated with dopamine infusion in dogs have been attributed to activation of the Bezold-Jarisch reflex, a vagal response which can result from acute increases in cardiac contractility (Tsompanidou et al. 2007).

Treatment with atropine and cessation of the dopamine infusion combined with an IV fluid bolus resulted in improved hemodynamics.

In cats, heart rate, blood pressure and inotropy increased when dopamine was administered at 10 μg/kg/min IV (Pascoe et al. 2006). Systemic vascular resistance did not increase in that study, even when the dose was 15 μg/kg/min IV, with oxygen delivery and cardiac output increases noted starting at 5 μg/kg/min IV. When dopamine was administered to isoflurane-anesthetized cats with hypertrophic myopathy, dose-dependent increases in mean arterial pressure, heart rate, and cardiac index were observed starting at 5 μg/kg/min IV (Wiese et al. 2012). Additionally, oxygen delivery was increased when 10 μg/kg/min IV dopamine was administered, and ventricular premature complexes were seen in all cats in the study. Dopamine at 25 μg/kg/min IV was ineffective at increasing blood pressure to 70 mmHg in isoflurane-anesthetized cats that also received a vatinoxan infusion, and a vatinoxan infusion with a low infusion rate of dexmedetomidine (Kobluk and Pypendop 2022).

Similar to other species, dopamine at 10 μg/kg/min IV increased mean arterial pressure, heart rate and cardiac index in ponies anesthetized with halothane (Lee et al. 1998). In the same study, dopamine at 20 μg/kg/min IV caused arrhythmias and muscle tremors. Dopamine at 4 μg/kg/min IV resulted in increases in cardiac output, heart rate, and decreases in aortic mean blood pressure in halothane-anesthetized horses (Young et al. 1998). In another study, dopamine at 5 and 10 μg/kg/min increased cardiac output whereas a 3 μg/kg/min IV dose did not (Swanson et al. 1985). Further, peripheral resistance decreased only with the 5 μg/kg/min IV dose, and heart rate did not increase during any dose. In a model of endotoxemia in halothane-anesthetized horses, dopamine at 5 μg/kg/min IV increased cardiac output and prevented hypotension, and had no effect on the development of hypoxemia and metabolic acidosis (Trim et al. 1991). Dopamine 5–6 μg/kg/min IV was effective in restoring normal sinus rhythm in foals that developed second-degree atrioventricular block during halothane anesthesia that was not atropine responsive (Whitton and Trim 1985).

In anesthetized, instrumented pigs dopamine at 15 μg/kg/min IV resulted in a 20% increase in mean blood pressure and a 30% increase in heart rate, with no change in systemic vascular resistance (Priebe et al. 1995). Global and splanchnic oxygen delivery was increased compared to the baseline. In addition to expected increases in mean arterial pressure, dopamine increased cerebral blood flow and intracranial pressure in awake and isoflurane-anesthetized sheep (Myburgh et al. 2002).

Other Effects

Like norepinephrine, dopamine decreased propofol concentrations in sheep (Myburgh et al. 2001).

Synthetic Catecholamines

Isoproterenol (Isoprenaline)

Isoproterenol is a synthetic catecholamine that is structurally related to epinephrine. It is a potent beta adrenoceptor agonist that is devoid of alpha adrenoceptor effects.

Pharmacodynamics

Beta$_1$ adrenoceptor agonism results in increases in heart rate, and inotropy (Nagao et al. 1984). Beta$_2$ adrenoceptor agonism results in decreased arterial blood pressure due to vasodilation, and decreased airway resistance as a result of bronchodilation (Boncyk et al. 1984). It is rarely used in clinical veterinary anesthesia due to its hypotensive effects. Due to its chronotropic effects, isoproterenol is recommended as an option for treating bradycardia in patients with sinus node dysfunction where the risk of coronary ischemia is low (Kusumoto et al. 2019). Isoproterenol has been used to increase heart rate in a cat anesthetized with isoflurane that developed transient third-degree atrioventricular block (Sunahara et al. 2021).

Dobutamine

Dobutamine is a derivative of isoproterenol. It was developed to retain the inotropic effects while decreasing the chronotropic, arrhythmogenic and vasodilatory effects of isoproterenol (Tuttle and Mills 1975). The structure of dobutamine is presented in Figure 18.2. Dobutamine is a racemic mixture of stereoisomers. The (+)-isomer is a strong beta$_1$ and beta$_2$ adrenoceptor agonist, while acting as an alpha adrenoceptor antagonist. The (−)-isomer is a strong alpha$_1$ adrenergic agonist and a weak beta$_1$ adrenergic agonist. Cardiovascular effects of dobutamine are therefore a result of the combined effects of the isomers, with the main effect being increased inotropy due to beta$_1$ and alpha$_1$ adrenoceptor agonism on myocytes. Systemic vascular resistance is often unchanged as a result of the opposing effects of alpha and beta$_2$ effects on the vasculature. Additionally, since the isomers have the same affinity, the (+)-isomer will act as a partial alpha$_1$ adrenoceptor antagonist although, clinically, this action is likely to be weak due to the high efficacy of the (−)-isomer at the alpha$_1$ adrenoceptor. The cardiac alpha$_1$ adrenoceptor effects of the (−)-isomer combined with the beta$_1$ effects of both isomers can explain the selectivity for inotropy over

chronotropy of the racemic mixture (Ruffolo and Yaden 1983). Chronotropy is evident at higher doses.

Pharmacodynamics

Similarly to dopamine, in a canine model of isoflurane-induced hypotension that initially targeted a mean arterial pressure of 50 mmHg, dobutamine increased heart rate and cardiac index in a dose-dependent manner (Rosati and Dyson 2007). Mean arterial pressure also increased, however, the effect was not as marked as with dopamine, and even at the high dose (8 µg/kg/min IV) a target mean arterial pressure of 70 mmHg was not reached, largely due to a decrease in systemic vascular resistance. There was also no benefit when co-infusing dobutamine (2 µg/kg/min IV) and dopamine (7 µg/kg/min IV). In another study in dogs, using a model of isoflurane-induced hypotension, dobutamine (5–15 µg/kg/min IV) increased cardiac output and oxygen delivery and decreased systemic vascular resistance, but was not successful in achieving a mean arterial blood pressure of 65 mmHg (Henao-Guerrero et al. 2023). The arrhythmogenic dose of dobutamine in halothane-anesthetized dogs was 10 µg/kg/min IV, and dobutamine was less arrhythmogenic than epinephrine and dopamine during pentobarbital anesthesia (Bednarski and Muir 1985). In a canine model of mitral valve insufficiency, dobutamine was effective in combating depression of myocardial contractility associated with isoflurane anesthesia (Goya et al. 2018). Systolic aortic blood pressure increased at doses of dobutamine above 4 µg/kg/min IV, however, mean aortic blood pressure only increased in that model when dobutamine was administered at 8 µg/kg/min IV.

In cats, dobutamine dose-dependently increased heart rate and cardiac index with a decrease in systemic vascular resistance and no statistically significant change in mean arterial pressure, although mean arterial pressure remained above 70 mmHg when infusion rates were ≥5 µg/kg/min IV (Pascoe et al. 2006).

Dobutamine is a first-line treatment for anesthesia-induced hypotension in horses, improving blood pressure via its positive inotropic effect (Muir 2009; Schauvliege and Gasthuys 2013). Dobutamine increases inotropy, cardiac output, and arterial blood pressure in horses anesthetized with halothane, isoflurane, and sevoflurane (Swanson et al. 1985; Dancker et al. 2018; Ohta et al. 2013). Dobutamine has variable effects on systemic vascular resistance, including decreases, increases, or no change (Dancker et al. 2018; Schauvliege and Gasthuys 2013). Whether chronotropic effects are noted with dobutamine also varies among studies, and bradyarrhythmias, most commonly a baroreceptor reflex response to increasing arterial pressure, and tachycardia, a direct chronotropic effect,

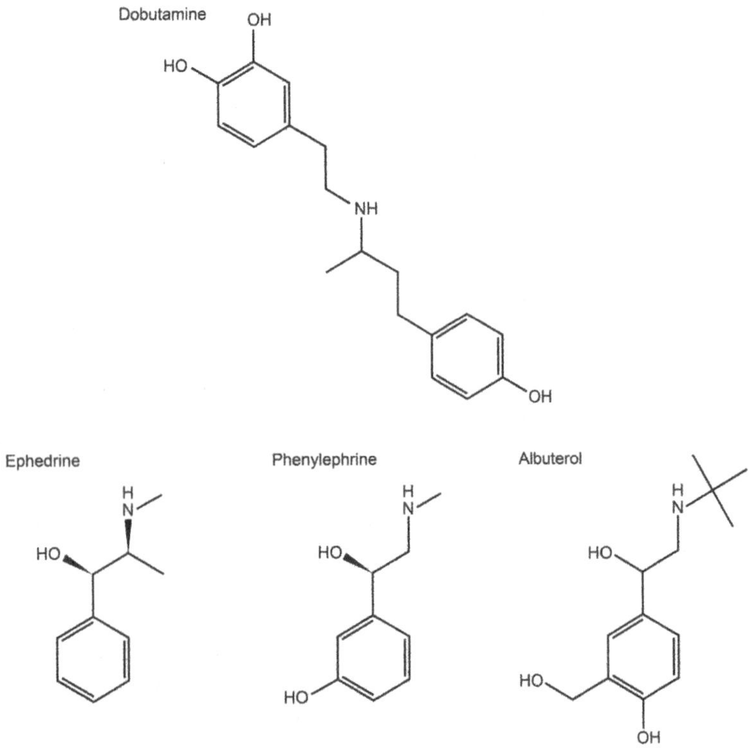

Figure 18.2 Chemical structures of selected sympathomimetic drugs.

are also seen, particularly at higher doses (3–5 μg/kg/min IV). Dobutamine improved systemic hemodynamics as well as GI tract microperfusion (Dancker et al. 2018). Compared to dopamine, and phenylephrine, dobutamine was most consistent in improving intramuscular blood flow, including blood flow to muscles of the dependent limb in laterally recumbent ponies (Lee et al. 1998). In a model of isoflurane-induced hypotension (mean arterial pressure of 30–34 mmHg) in 1–5-day old foals, dobutamine (4 and 8 μg/kg/min IV) increased cardiac index, stroke volume index, heart rate, systemic vascular resistance and oxygen delivery in a dose-dependent manner (Valverde et al. 2006). In 8–14-day old foals, dobutamine (2.5–10 μg/kg/min IV) increased cardiac index, stroke volume index and heart rate, arterial blood pressure increases were mild, and systemic vascular resistance decreased (Craig et al. 2007). Dobutamine increased packed cell volume in horses anesthetized with inhalant anesthetics (Hellyer et al. 1998).

Synthetic Non-catecholamines

Phenylephrine (m-Synephrine, Neosynephrine)

Phenylephrine has a chemical structure similar to epinephrine, however, due to the lack of a 4-hydroxyl group on the benzene ring it is classified as a non-catecholamine (Figure 18.2) It is metabolized via deamination, sulfation and glucuronidation, with its main metabolites being phenylephrine 3-O-sulfate, m-hydroxymandelic acid, and phenylephrine 3-O-β-D-glucuronide which are excreted in the urine (Ibrahim et al. 1983). In people, the half-life is longer than for the catecholamines at two to three hours (Hengstmann and Goronzy 1982).

At clinical doses, phenylephrine is a pure $alpha_1$ agonist, resulting in vasoconstriction. Arterial vasoconstriction increases systemic vascular resistance and systemic blood pressure. This increase in afterload may lead to a bradycardia due to a baroreceptor reflex. Increased afterload decreases cardiac output, although venous constriction promotes increases in venous return which contributes to improved cardiac output (Rebet et al. 2016). Norepinephrine is preferred over phenylephrine as the vasopressor of choice in cases of septic shock (Silverstein and Beer 2015). It may be advantageous in patients that are refractory to norepinephrine, when side effects (e.g. arrythmias) of norepinephrine are severe, or in patients with hypertrophic obstructive cardiomyopathy (Kislitsina et al. 2019). In horses with colic due to nephrosplenic entrapment of part of the large colon, phenylephrine can be administered as an IV bolus to shrink the size of the spleen (Hardy et al. 1994, 2000). Phenylephrine can be given to horses intranasally to decrease nasal congestion that frequently develops during general anesthesia (Lukasik et al. 1997).

Pharmacodynamics

Phenylephrine (3–6 µg/kg/min IV) increased blood pressure, decreased heart rate, and did not cause arrhythmias in dogs (Deterling et al. 1954). A high dose of phenylephrine (50 µg/kg/min IV) caused hypertension and ventricular arrhythmias in isoflurane- and halothane-anesthetized dogs (Tucker et al. 1974). Administration of propranolol abolished the ventricular arrhythmias, indicating that phenylephrine at extremely high doses has beta$_1$ adrenoceptor activity. The use of phenylephrine-containing eyedrops resulted in increased arterial blood pressure in dogs, likely due to systemic absorption (Martin-Flores et al. 2010).

In cats, a phenylephrine infusion increased mean arterial pressure, cardiac index, stroke volume index, systemic vascular resistance index, and packed cell volume, with no changes in heart rate (Pascoe et al. 2006). The positive inotropic effects of phenylephrine in cats is likely due to cardiac alpha$_1$ adrenoceptor agonism (Rodrigues-Pereira and Wagner 1975). In cats with hypertrophic myopathy, similar effects on blood pressure were noted, however, cardiac output was not changed (Wiese et al. 2012).

In sevoflurane-anesthetized horses, phenylephrine increased blood pressure but decreased cardiac output due to increased systemic vascular resistance (Ohta et al. 2013). Phenylephrine decreased blood flow to the GI tract and did not improve muscle blood flow in anesthetized horses (Dancker et al. 2018; Lee et al. 1998). An infusion of phenylephrine (2 µg/kg/min) increased blood pressure to targeted levels within 10 minutes, and blood pressure remained within clinically acceptable parameters for 90 minutes after the end of the infusion (Fantoni et al. 2013).

Phenylephrine has traditionally been used to decrease the size of the spleen in horses presenting with colic due to nephrosplenic entrapment prior to jogging, as well as prior to rolling in anesthetized horses (Baker et al. 2011; Gillen et al. 2019). These strategies are used to avoid the need for abdominal surgery. Phenylephrine can also be given during anesthesia for colic surgery to make surgical correction of entrapment easier (Hardy et al. 2000). A recent meta-analysis showed that medical resolution of nephrosplenic entrapment (rolling, jogging) was not more likely to occur if phenylephrine was administered, although none of the studies included in the analysis were prospective randomized trials (Gillen et al. 2019). Phenylephrine can be used at a low infusion rate alongside dobutamine for its alpha effects (Schauvliege and Gasthuys 2013).

As mentioned above, phenylephrine (4–6 ml) has been used intranasally to decrease upper airway obstruction due to congestion of mucosae that occurs when horses are recumbent during anesthesia (Lukasik et al. 1997). Equipment to establish a patent airway in horses recovering from anesthesia should always be available regardless of whether phenylephrine is used in recovery.

Cardiovascular effects of phenylephrine in pigs are similar to those seen in other species (Cannesson et al. 2012).

Ephedrine

Ephedrine (L-ephedrine) is an alkaloid found in many plants of the *Ephedra* genus. It can also be chemically synthesized, and its anti-hypotensive and bronchodilatory effects have been known for over a century (Chen 1927). Ephedrine acts mostly indirectly by competitively reducing norepinephrine reuptake from adrenergic nerve endings at all alpha and beta adrenoceptors. It exerts some of its effects through direct adrenoceptor agonism (Inchiosa 2011; Stohs et al. 2020). Due to its indirect action, onset may take several minutes, and the duration of action is sustained for up to 20 minutes. Tachyphylaxis may be seen with repeat doses of ephedrine as a result of depletion of vesicular norepinephrine (Liles et al. 2006). Norephedrine is the main metabolite of ephedrine, and both it and the parent compound are excreted in urine. Due to its lipophilicity, ephedrine readily crosses the blood-brain barriers and can cause CNS excitement (Kalix 1991). General cardiovascular effects due to ephedrine's alpha and beta adrenoceptor activity include increased blood pressure and increases in heart rate.

In isoflurane-anesthetized dogs ephedrine (0.1 mg/kg IV) increased mean arterial pressure, cardiac index, stroke volume and oxygen delivery (Wagner et al. 1993). Cardiovascular effects of ephedrine in another study in isoflurane-anesthetized dogs were similar, although the dose-dependent duration of action was shorter, likely due to premedication with acepromazine (Chen et al. 2007). A higher dose (0.25 mg/kg) also increased systemic vascular resistance with decreased heart rate, and the effects lasted longer. The dose required to cause ventricular arrythmias during inhalant anesthesia in dogs is relatively high (0.8–4 mg/kg IV) (Tucker et al. 1974). Ephedrine (0.1 mg/kg IV) was more effective at increasing blood pressure than crystalloid or colloid fluid administration in isoflurane-anesthetized dogs that were premedicated with acepromazine (0.05 mg/kg IV) (Sinclair and Dyson 2012). Inclusion of ephedrine with premedication in dogs and cats delayed the onset of anesthetic-related hypotension by 40 and 25 minutes respectively (Egger et al. 2009). Ephedrine increased the minimum alveolar concentration (MAC) of halothane in dogs by 50% (Steffey and Eger 1975).

Ephedrine (0.06 mg/kg IV) increased cardiac output, stroke volume and systolic arterial blood pressure in horses that were anesthetized with two different end-tidal concentrations of halothane (Grandy et al. 1989). In horses anesthetized with isoflurane, an ephedrine infusion (20 μg/kg/min IV) cardiac index, systemic vascular resistance and heart rate increased, and the targeted increase in blood pressure was reached in 10 minutes (Fantoni et al. 2013). In that study, after the infusion was discontinued, blood pressure remained elevated compared to the baseline for 90 minutes. In another study comparing ephedrine and dobutamine infusions, results were similar (Garcia Filho et al. 2023). Interestingly, the time to correct blood pressure to 70 mmHg in that study did not differ from dobutamine. Tachyphylaxis was not observed in either infusion study, however, the duration of observation of effect was short (10–15 minutes). In addition to improving arterial pressure and cardiac index, ephedrine also increased intramuscular blood flow in the dependent and non-dependent forelimb of halothane-anesthetized ponies (Lee et al. 2002).

Like other sympathomimetics with beta adrenoceptor activity, ephedrine has thermogenic and lipolytic effects (Astrup et al. 1995).

Vasopressin (Arginine Vasopressin, Anti-Diuretic Hormone)

Vasopressin is an endogenous nonapeptide neurohormone synthesized in the hypothalamus and stored in the posterior pituitary gland. It is released in response to increased osmolarity and marked decreases in blood pressure and blood volume (Mitra et al. 2011). It is included here since exogenous vasopressin (8-arginine vasopressin) is used to treat hypotension that is refractory to intervention with sympathomimetics (septic shock), and it may have benefits during CPR (Park and Yoo 2017; Fletcher et al. 2012). Vasopressin can also enhance the actions of other pressors (Holmes et al. 2001). Vasopressin acts at G protein-coupled vasopressin receptors, which have three subtypes (Holmes et al. 2001). V_{1A} (also classified as V_1) receptors are located on vascular smooth muscle and cause vasoconstriction. V_2 receptors in the kidney are responsible for vasopressin's antidiuretic effect. V_{1B} (or V_3) receptors are found in the pituitary gland and likely play a role in regulation of adrenocorticotropic hormone, body temperature regulation and memory. Vasopressin also binds to oxytocin receptors which are present in vascular smooth muscle and the uterus. The release of endogenous vasopressin is mediated by osmoreceptors, which are very sensitive to small changes in osmolarity of extracellular fluid (Baylis and

Robertson 1980). Vasopressin release is much less sensitive to decreases in mean arterial blood pressure and plasma volume, with release of vasopressin requiring respective decreases of 20–30% and 8–10% of blood pressure and blood volume (Park and Yoo 2017). Vasopressin has a half-life of 24 minutes, with clearance via the kidney and tissue peptidase (Baumann and Dingman 1976). At the time of writing, the cost of vasopressin has fluctuated considerably, having, at one time, cost approximately US$ 200/ml. This may make vasopressin financially nonviable as a treatment option in many veterinary patients.

In a hemorrhagic shock model in isoflurane-anesthetized dogs, vasopressin (0.4 U/kg IV) administered prior to crystalloid fluid resuscitation restored systolic arterial blood pressure, cardiac output, and oxygen delivery, and was more effective than when given after fluid resuscitation (Yoo et al. 2007). This is in contrast to an isoflurane anesthetic-induced hypotension model (mean arterial pressure <45 mmHg) in euvolemic dogs where vasopressin did not increase blood pressure to target levels (>65 mmHg) despite increases in systemic vascular resistance and decreased cardiac output and oxygen delivery (Henao-Guerrero et al. 2023).

Vasopressin was less effective than norepinephrine and dobutamine at improving cardiovascular parameters in an isoflurane-induced hypotension model in euvolemic neonatal foals (Valverde et al. 2006). See Table 18.3 for recommended dosing of vasopressin.

Use in CPR

In a randomized, blinded, study in dogs, return of spontaneous circulation was similar between vasopressin and epinephrine (Buckley et al. 2011). Vasopressin (0.8 U/kg IV) can be used either in place of epinephrine or given every second cycle of basic life support (Fletcher et al. 2012).

Use in Septic Shock

Sepsis can lead to vasodilatory shock and lactic acidosis. In addition to other vasodilatory mediators like nitric oxide, lactic acidosis activates ATP-sensitive potassium channels on vascular smooth muscle (Landry and Oliver 2001). This leads to hyperpolarization of the smooth muscle fibers, which prevents intracellular calcium from increasing, making catecholamines like norepinephrine much less effective at treating hypotension. Increased plasma concentrations of norepinephrine that are present as part of the autonomic stress response to sepsis can also downregulate adrenoceptors, further decreasing the effectiveness of norepinephrine. Additionally, significant hypotension causes endogenous vasopressin to be released in large amounts initially. In the face of continued severe hypotension, depletion of vasopressin stores occurs, as synthesis of vasopressin takes a few hours. Administering vasopressin to patients with septic shock can be effective in treating severe hypotension for two main reasons. Firstly, since endogenous stores are depleted, administering vasopressin will have vasoconstrictive action at V_{1A} receptors, and secondly, vasopressin inactivates ATP-sensitive potassium channels, thus enhancing the effects of norepinephrine in vascular smooth muscle.

Selective Beta₂ Adrenoceptor Agonists

Agents that have selective beta₂ adrenoceptor activity are used for their effect of relaxing bronchiolar smooth muscle.

Albuterol (Salbutamol)

Albuterol is a short-acting beta₂ adrenoceptor agonist effective in relieving bronchospasm. In people given IV albuterol, it is eliminated by renal clearance and metabolism to 4'-O-sulphate which is excreted in urine (Morgan et al. 1986). Inhaled albuterol is used to treat horses with recurrent airway obstruction, with minimal side effects (Derksen et al. 1999). Albuterol is supplied as a metered dose inhaler that delivers 90 μg per depression of the inhaler. When delivered at 90 μg per 45 kg (2 μg/kg, rounded up) into the breathing system of the anesthetic machine at the start of patient inhalation in halothane- and isoflurane-anesthetized horses, PaO_2 was significantly increased 20 minutes after drug administration that lasted up to 1 hour, accompanied by a decrease in $PaCO_2$ (Robertson and Bailey 2002). No undesirable cardiovascular effects were noted in that study, whereas Casoni, et al. reported tachycardia and profuse sweating in five horses after inhaled albuterol administration (Casoni et al. 2014). Ventricular tachycardia was observed in one horse, and variable changes in blood pressure, with all horses recovering uneventfully. Inhaled albuterol improved PaO_2 in isoflurane-anesthetized horses breathing a reduced fraction of inspired oxygen ($FiO_2 = 0.5$). The effect lasted for 40 minutes, with tachycardia and sweating noted in some horses (Clark-Price et al. 2022). The side effects of sweating and increased heart rate are likely due to systemic absorption of albuterol, which acts at beta₂ adrenoceptors in the heart and on sweat glands. Albuterol treatment in anesthetized horses resulted in a small but significant decrease in serum potassium (Loomes 2021). Albuterol administration can result in hypokalemia due to beta₂ adrenoceptor mediated sodium/potassium ATPase pump activity moving potassium from the extracellular to the intracellular space. No sequelae of hypokalemia were observed, and the clinical impact remains unclear.

Albuterol attenuated histamine-induced bronchoconstriction in halothane-anesthetized dogs (Tobias and Hirshman 1990). Albuterol administered with ipratropium (an anticholinergic bronchodilator), but not albuterol alone, decreased the bronchoconstriction response to broncho-alveolar lavage in cats (Kirschvink et al. 2005).

Terbutaline

Terbutaline is a short-acting synthetic selective beta₂ agonist used to treat bronchoconstriction. In people, it is excreted unchanged in the urine, and can also be metabolized to sulfate and glucuronidate conjugates (Domínguez-Romero and García-Reyes 2013). In cats, bronchospasmolytic effects have been demonstrated after both IV and inhaled administration of terbutaline (Andersson 1976). In one study in cats, terbutaline (0.01 mg/kg^2) given BID or TID 12–24 hours prior to bronchoscopy, with the final dose given 2–4 hours prior to induction of anesthesia had fewer overall complications (Johnson and Drazenovich 2007). In another study, terbutaline-treated cats had a lower incidence of desaturation during bronchoscopy (Tucker and MacFarlane 2019).

Terbutaline (2 μg/kg IV) given to horses anesthetized with guaifenesin-ketamine-xylazine did not improve oxygenation, and was associated with decreased blood pressure and increased heart rate (Arcaro et al. 2017).

Drug Interactions

Tricyclic antidepressants (TCAs), e.g. amitriptyline, act by inhibiting norepinephrine reuptake inhibition (see Chapter 22 for details). This results in an increase in norepinephrine activity in the synaptic cleft of adrenergic nerve fibers. Ephedrine, which acts indirectly by competitively reducing norepinephrine reuptake, can cause severe hypertension when given with TCAs, and should be avoided. Direct-acting sympathomimetics should be given cautiously if needed to provide hemodynamic support (Peck et al. 2010).

MAOs metabolize catecholamines, therefore MAO inhibitors, e.g. selegiline, can result in elevations in catecholamine neurotransmitters. The indirect-acting sympathomimetic ephedrine should not be used at the same time as MAOs (see Chapter 22). If needed, direct-acting sympathomimetics can be used at two thirds of the typical dose (Wells and Bjorksten 1989).

References

Andersson, P. (1976). Bronchospasmolytic and cardiovascular effects in anaesthetized cats of ibuterol and terbutaline given intravenously and after inhalation: drug and prodrug compared. *Acta. Pharmacol. Toxicol.* 39: 225–231.

Arcaro, I., Fischer, B.L. et al. (2017). Effects of intravenous terbutaline on heart rate, arterial pressure and blood gases in anesthetized horses breathing air. *Vet. Anaesth. Analg.* 44: 70–76.

Astrup, A., Breum, L., and Toubro, S. (1995). Pharmacological and clinical studies of ephedrine and other thermogenic agonists. *Obes. Res.* 4: 537S–540S.

Baker, W.T., Frederick, J. et al. (2011). Reevaluation of the effect of phenylephrine on resolution of nephrosplenic entrapment by the rolling procedure in 87 horses. *Vet. Surg.* 40: 825–829.

Bakker, J. and Vincent, J.L. (1993). Effects of norepinephrine and dobutamine on oxygen transport and consumption in a dog model of endotoxic shock. *Crit. Care Med.* 21: 425–432.

Baumann, G. and Dingman, J.F. (1976). Distribution, blood transport, and degradation of antidiuretic hormone in man. *J. Clin. Invest.* 57: 1109–1116.

Baylis, P.H. and Robertson, G.L. (1980). Plasma vasopressin response to hypertonic saline infusion to assess posterior pituitary function. *J. R. Soc. Med.* 73: 255–260.

Beaulieu, J.M. and Gainetdinov, R.R. (2011). The physiology, signaling, and pharmacology of dopamine receptors. *Pharmacol. Rev.* 63: 182–217.

Bednarski, R.M. and Majors, L.J. (1986). Ketamine and the arrhythmogenic dose of epinephrine in cats anesthetized with halothane and isoflurane. *Am. J. Vet. Res.* 47: 2122–2125.

Bednarski, R.M. and Muir, W.W. (1985). Catecholamine infusion in vagotomized dogs during thiamylal-halothane and pentobarbital anesthesia. *Cornell Vet.* 75: 512–523.

Boncyk, J., Redon, D., and Rusy, B. (1984). Hemodynamic effects of amrinone in dogs anesthetized with halothane: comparison with isoproterenol and dobutamine. *Res. Commun. Chem. Pathol. Pharmacol.* 44: 347–354.

Buckley, G.J., Rozanski, E.A., and Rush, J.E. (2011). Randomized, blinded comparison of epinephrine and vasopressin for treatment of naturally occurring cardiopulmonary arrest in dogs. *J. Vet. Intern. Med.* 25: 1334–1340.

Cannesson, M., Jian, Z. et al. (2012). Effects of phenylephrine on cardiac output and venous return depend on the position of the heart on the Frank-Starling relationship. *J. Appl. Physiol.* 113: 281–289.

Cannon, J.G. (1983). Structure-activity relationships of dopamine agonists. *Annu. Rev. Pharmacol. Toxicol.* 23: 103–129.

Casoni, D., Spadavecchia, C., and Adami, C. (2014). Cardiovascular changes after administration of aerosolized salbutamol in horses: five cases. *Acta Vet. Scand.* 56 (1): 49.

Chen, K. (1927). A study of ephedrine. *Br. Med. J.* 2: 593.

Chen, H.C., Sinclair, M.D., and Dyson, D.H. (2007). Use of ephedrine and dopamine in dogs for the management of hypotension in routine clinical cases under isoflurane anesthesia. *Vet. Anaesth. Analg.* 34: 301–311.

Clark-Price, S.C., Lascola, K.M. et al. (2022). The effect of inhaled albuterol on PaO2 in anesthetized horses receiving a FiO2 of 0.5 or >0.95. *J. Equine Vet. Sci.* 113: 103944.

Congdon, J.M. (2022). Cardiovascular disease. In: *Canine and Feline Anesthesia and Co-existing Disease*, 2e (ed. R.A. Johnson, L.B.C. Snyder, and C.A. Schroeder), 1–85. Hoboken, NJ: Wiley.

Craig, C.A., Haskins, S.C., and Hildebrand, S.V. (2007). The cardiopulmonary effects of dobutamine and norepinephrine in isoflurane-anesthetized foals. *Anaesth. Analg.* 34: 377–387.

Dancker, C., Hopster, K. et al. (2018). Effects of dobutamine, dopamine, phenylephrine and noradrenaline on systemic haemodynamics and intestinal perfusion in isoflurane anaesthetised horses. *Equine Vet. J.* 50: 104–110.

Derksen, F.J., Olszewski, M.A. et al. (1999). Aerosolized albuterol sulfate used as a bronchodilator in horses with recurrent airway obstruction. *Am. J. Vet. Res.* 60: 689–693.

Deterling, R.A., Ngai, S.H. et al. (1954). The cardiovascular effects of continuous intravenous infusion of norepinephrine, epinephrine and neosynephrine during cyclopropane and ether anesthesia in the dog. *Anesthesiology* 15: 11–18.

Domínguez-Romero, J.C. and García-Reyes, J.F. (2013). Detection of main urinary metabolites of β2-agonists clenbuterol, salbutamol and terbutaline by liquid chromatography high resolution mass spectrometry. *Chromatogr. B. Analyt. Technol. Biomed. Life Sci.* 923–924: 128–135.

Egger, C., McCrackin, M.A. et al. (2009). Efficacy of preanesthetic intramuscular administration of ephedrine for prevention of anesthesia-induced hypotension in cats and dogs. *Can. Vet. J.* 50: 179–184.

Eisenhofer, G., Smolich, J.J., and Esler, M.D. (1992). Different desipramine-sensitive pulmonary removals of plasma epinephrine and norepinephrine in dogs. *Am. J. Phys.* 262: L360–L365.

Eisenhofer, G., Huynh, T.T. et al. (2001). Understanding catecholamine metabolism as a guide to the biochemical diagnosis of pheochromocytoma. *Rev. Endocr. Metab. Disord.* 2: 297–311.

Eisenhofer, G., Kopin, I.J., and Goldstein, D.S. (2004). Catecholamine metabolism: a contemporary view with implications for physiology and medicine. *Pharmacol. Rev.* 56: 331–349.

Fantoni, D.T., Marchioni, G.G. et al. (2013). Effect of ephedrine and phenylephrine on cardiopulmonary parameters in horses undergoing elective surgery. *Vet. Anaesth. Analg.* 40: 367–374.

Flatmark, T. (2000). Catecholamine biosynthesis and physiological regulation in neuroendocrine cells. *Acta Physiol. Scand.* 68: 1–17.

Fletcher, D.J., Boller, M. et al. (2012). RECOVER evidence and knowledge gap analysis on veterinary CPR. Part 7: clinical guidelines. *J. Vet. Emerg. Crit. Care* 22 (Suppl. 1): S102–S131.

Garcia Filho, S.G., de Andrade, F.S.R.M. et al. (2023). Comparison of hemodynamic effects of dobutamine and ephedrine infusions in isoflurane-anesthetized horses. *Vet. Sci.* 10: 278.

Gillen, A.M., Munsterman, A.S., and Reid Hanson, R. (2019). Evaluation of phenylephrine and exercise with or without trocarization for treatment of suspected nephrosplenic entrapment in horses. *Am. Vet. Med. Assoc.* 254: 1448–1453.

Gillis, C.N. and Pitt, B.R. (1982). The fate of circulating amines within the pulmonary circulation. *Annu. Rev. Physiol.* 44: 269–281.

Goya, S., Wada, T. et al. (2018). Dose-dependent effects of isoflurane and dobutamine on cardiovascular function in dogs with experimental mitral regurgitation. *Vet. Anaesth. Analg.* 45: 432–442.

Grandy, J.L., Steffey, E.P. et al. (1987). Arterial hypotension and the development of postanesthetic myopathy in halothane-anesthetized horses. *Am. J. Vet. Res.* 48: 192–197.

Grandy, J.L., Hodgson, D.S. et al. (1989). Cardiopulmonary effects of ephedrine in halothane-anesthetized horses. *J. Vet. Pharmacol. Ther.* 12: 389–396.

Hardy, J., Bednarski, R.M., and Biller, D.S. (1994). Effect of phenylephrine on hemodynamics and splenic dimensions in horses. *Am. J. Vet. Res.* 55: 1570–1578.

Hardy, J., Minton, M. et al. (2000). Nephrosplenic entrapment in the horse: a retrospective study of 174 cases. *Equine Vet. J.* 32: 95–97.

Hellyer, P.W., Wagner, A.E. et al. (1998). The effects of dobutamine and ephedrine on packed cell volume, total protein, heart rate, and blood pressure in anaesthetized horses. *J. Vet. Pharmacol. Ther.* 21: 497–499.

Henao-Guerrero, N., Ricco-Pereira, C.H. et al. (2023). A comparison of dobutamine, norepinephrine, vasopressin, and hetastarch for the treatment of isoflurane-induced hypotension in healthy, normovolemic dogs. *Animals (Basel)* 13: 2674.

Hengstmann, J.H. and Goronzy, J. (1982). Pharmacokinetics of 3H-phenylephrine in man. *Eur. J. Clin. Pharmacol.* 21: 335–341.

Holmes, C.L., Patel, B.M. et al. (2001). Physiology of vasopressin relevant to management of septic shock. *Chest* 120: 989–1002.

Huyghens, L.P., Calle, P.A. et al. (1991). Plasma concentrations of epinephrine during CPR in the dog. *Ann. Emerg. Med.* 20: 239–242.

Ibrahim, K.E., Midgley, J.M. et al. (1983). The mammalian metabolism of R-(−)-m-synephrine. *J. Pharm. Pharmacol.* 35: 144–147.

Inchiosa, M.A. (2011). Experience (mostly negative) with the use of sympathomimetic agents for weight loss. *J. Obes.* 764584. https://doi.org/10.1155/2011/764584.

Johnson, L.R. and Drazenovich, T.L. (2007). Flexible bronchoscopy and bronchoalveolar lavage in 68 cats (2001-2006). *J. Vet. Intern. Med.* 21: 219–225.

Kalix, P. (1991). The pharmacology of psychoactive alkaloids from ephedra and catha. *J. Ethnopharmacol.* 32: 201–208.

Kirschvink, N., Leemans, J. et al. (2005). Bronchodilators in bronchoscopy-induced airflow limitation in allergen-sensitized cats. *J. Vet. Intern. Med.* 19: 161–167.

Kislitsina, O.N., Rich, J.D. et al. (2019). Shock – classification and pathophysiological principles of therapeutics. *Curr. Cardiol. Rev.* 15: 102–113.

Kobluk, K. and Pypendop, B.H. (2022). Effects of dopamine, norepinephrine or phenylephrine on the prevention of hypotension in isoflurane-anesthetized cats administered vatinoxan or vatinoxan and dexmedetomidine. *Vet. Anaesth. Analg.* 49: 54–64.

Kusumoto, F.M., Schoenfeld, M.H. et al. (2019). 2018 ACC/AHA/HRS guideline on the evaluation and management of patients with bradycardia and cardiac conduction delay: a report of the American College of Cardiology/American Heart Association task force on clinical practice guidelines and the Heart Rhythm Society. *Circulation* 140: e382–e482.

Landry, D.W. and Oliver, J.A. (2001). The pathogenesis of vasodilatory shock. *N. Engl. J. Med.* 345: 588–595.

Lee, Y.H., Clarke, K.W. et al. (1998). Effects of dopamine, dobutamine, dopexamine, phenylephrine, and saline solution on intramuscular blood flow and other cardiopulmonary variables in halothane-anesthetized ponies. *Am. J. Vet. Res.* 59: 1463–1472.

Lee, Y.L., Clarke, K.W. et al. (2002). The effects of ephedrine on intramuscular blood flow and other cardiopulmonary parameters in halothane-anesthetized ponies. *Vet. Anaesth. Analg.* 29: 171–181.

Lees, P. and Tavernor, W.D. (1970). Influence of halothane and catecholamines on heart rate and rhythm in the horse. *Br. J. Pharmacol.* 39: 149–159.

Liles, J.T., Dabisch, P.A. et al. (2006). Pressor responses to ephedrine are mediated by a direct mechanism in the rat. *J. Pharmacol. Exp. Ther.* 316: 95–105.

Loomes, K. (2021). Effect of aerosolised salbutamol administration on arterial potassium concentration in anaesthetised horses. *J. Equine Vet. Sci.* 103: 103667.

Lorenzo, J. (2022). Sympathomimetic drugs. In: *Stoelting's Pharmacology and Physiology in Anesthetic Practice 6e* (ed. P. Flood, J.P. Rathmell, and R.D. Urman), 450–470. Philadelphia, PA: Wolters Kluwer.

Lukasik, V.M., Gleed, R.D. et al. (1997). Intranasal phenylephrine reduces post anesthetic upper airway obstruction in horses. *Equine Vet. J.* 29: 236–238.

MacGregor, D.A., Smith, T.E. et al. (2000). Pharmacokinetics of dopamine in healthy male subjects. *Anesthesiology* 92: 338–346.

Martin-Flores, M., Mercure-McKenzie, T.M. et al. (2010). Controlled retrospective study of the effects of eyedrops containing phenylephrine hydrochloride and scopolamine hydrobromide on mean arterial blood pressure in anesthetized dogs. *Am. J. Vet. Res.* 71: 1407–1412.

Mitra, J.K., Roy, J., and Sengupta, S. (2011). Vasopressin: its current role in anesthetic practice. *Indian J. Crit. Care Med.* 15: 71–77.

Monteiro, E.R., Teixeira Neto, F.J. et al. (2007). Effects of acepromazine on the cardiovascular actions of dopamine in anesthetized dogs. *Vet. Anaesth. Analg.* 34: 312–321.

Morgan, D.J., Paull, J.D. et al. (1986). Pharmacokinetics of intravenous and oral salbutamol and its sulphate conjugate. *Br. J. Clin. Pharmacol.* 22: 587–593.

Motiejunaite, J., Amar, L., and Vidal-Petiot, E. (2021). Adrenergic receptors and cardiovascular effects of catecholamines. *Ann. Endocrinol. (Paris)* 82: 193–197.

Muir, W.W. (2009). Cardiopulmonary resuscitation. In: *Equine Anesthesia Monitoring and Emergency Therapy*, 2e (ed. W.W. Muir and J.A.E. Hubbell), 418–429. St. Louis, MO: Saunders Elsevier.

Muir, W.W. and Hubbell, J.A.E. (2009). Anesthetic-associated complications. In: *Equine Anesthesia Monitoring and Emergency Therapy*, 2e (ed. W.W. Muir and J.A.E. Hubbell), 397–417. St. Louis, MO: Saunders Elsevier.

Murrell, J. (2015). Adrenergic agents. In: *Veterinary Anesthesia and Analgesia*, 5e (ed. K.A. Grimm, L.A. Lamont, W.J. Tranquilli, et al.), 183–195. Ames, IA: Wiley Blackwell.

Myburgh, J.A., Upton, R.N. et al. (2001). Epinephrine, norepinephrine and dopamine infusions decrease propofol concentrations during continuous propofol infusion in an ovine model. *Intensive Care Med.* 27: 276–282.

Myburgh, J.A., Upton, R.N. et al. (2002). The cerebrovascular effects of adrenaline, noradrenaline and dopamine infusions under propofol and isoflurane anaesthesia in sheep. *Anaesth. Intensive Care* 30: 725–733.

Nagao, T., Ikeo, T. et al. (1984). Cardiovascular effects of a new positive inotropic agent, (−)-(R)-1-(p-hydroxyphenyl)-2-[(3,4-dimethoxyphenethyl)amino]-ethanol (TA-064) in the anesthetized dog and isolated guinea pig heart. *Jpn. J. Pharmacol.* 35: 415–423.

Neukirchen, M. and Kienbaum, P. (2008). Sympathetic nervous system: evaluation and importance for clinical general anesthesia. *Anesthesiology* 109: 1113–1131.

Niu, X., Watts, V.L. et al. (2012). Cardioprotective effect of beta-3 adrenergic receptor agonism: role of neuronal nitric oxide synthase. *J. Am. Coll. Cardiol.* 59: 1979–1987.

Odunayo, A., Nash, K.J. et al. (2021). Association of Veterinary Hematology and Transfusion Medicine (AVHTM) transfusion reaction small animal consensus statement (TRACS). Part 3: diagnosis and treatment. *J. Vet. Emerg. Crit. Care* 31: 189–203.

Ohta, M., Kurimoto, S. et al. (2013). Cardiovascular effects of dobutamine and phenylephrine infusion in sevoflurane-anesthetized thoroughbred horses. *J. Vet. Med. Sci.* 75: 1443–1448.

Park, K.S. and Yoo, K.Y. (2017). Role of vasopressin in current anesthetic practice. *Korean J. Anesthesiol.* 70: 245–257.

Pascoe, P.J., Ilkiw, J.E., and Pypendop, B.H. (2006). Effects of increasing infusion rates of dopamine, dobutamine, epinephrine, and phenylephrine in healthy anesthetized cats. *Am. J. Vet. Res.* 67: 1491–1499.

Peck, T., Wong, A., and Norman, E. (2010). Anaesthetic implications of psychoactive drugs. *BJA Education* 10: 177–181.

Peters, J., Schlaghecke, R. et al. (1990). Endogenous vasopressin supports blood pressure and prevents severe hypotension during epidural anesthesia in conscious dogs. *Anesthesiology* 73: 694–702.

Priebe, H.J., Nöldge, G.F. et al. (1995). Differential effects of dobutamine, dopamine, and noradrenaline on splanchnic haemodynamics and oxygenation in the pig. *Acta Anaesthesiol. Scand.* 39: 1088–1096.

Rebet, O., Andremont, O. et al. (2016). Preload dependency determines the effects of phenylephrine on cardiac output in anaesthetised patients: a prospective observational study. *Eur. J. Anaesthesiol.* 33: 638–644.

Rezakhani, A., Edjtehadi, M. et al. (1977). Prevention of thiopental and thiopental/halothane cardiac sensitization to epinephrine in the sheep. *Can. J. Comp. Med.* 41: 389–395.

Robertson, S.A. and Bailey, J.E. (2002). Aerosolized salbutamol (albuterol) improves PaO2 in hypoxaemic anaesthetized horses – a prospective clinical trial in 81 horses. *Vet. Anaesth. Analg.* 29: 212–218.

Rodrigues-Pereira, E. and Wagner, J. (1975). Stimulation by phenylephrine of myocardial alpha-adrenoceptors in the left ventricle of the cat. *Res. Exp. Med. (Berl.)* 166: 165–171.

Rosati, M. and Dyson, D.H. (2007). Response of hypotensive dogs to dopamine hydrochloride and dobutamine hydrochloride during deep isoflurane anesthesia. *Am. J. Vet. Res.* 68: 483–494.

Ruffolo, R.R. Jr. and Yaden, E.L. (1983). Vascular effects of the stereoisomers of dobutamine. *J. Pharmacol. Exp. Ther.* 224: 46–50.

Schauvliege, S. and Gasthuys, F. (2013). Drugs for cardiovascular support in anesthetized horses. *Vet. Clin. North Am. Equine Pract.* 29: 19–49.

Silverstein, D.C. and Beer, K.A. (2015). Controversies regarding choice of vasopressor therapy for management of septic shock in animals. *J. Vet. Emerg. Crit. Care* 25: 48–54.

Sinclair, M.D. and Dyson, D.H. (2012). The impact of acepromazine on the efficacy of crystalloid, dextran or ephedrine treatment in hypotensive dogs under isoflurane anesthesia. *Vet. Anaesth. Analg.* 39: 563–573.

Skelding, A.M. and Valverde, A. (2020). Sympathomimetics in veterinary species under anesthesia. *Vet. J.* 258: 105455. https://doi.org/10.1016/j.tvjl.2020.105455.

Smolich, J.J., Cox, H.S. et al. (1997). Pulmonary clearance and release of norepinephrine and epinephrine in newborn lambs. *Am. J. Phys.* 273: L264–L274.

Steffey, E.P. and Eger, E.I. (1975). The effect of seven vasopressors on halothane MAC in dogs. *Br. J. Anaesth.* 47: 435–438.

Stohs, S.J., Shara, M., and Ray, S.D. (2020). p-Synephrine, ephedrine, p-octopamine and m-synephrine: comparative mechanistic, physiological and pharmacological properties. *Phytother. Res.* 34: 1838–1846.

Stowe, D.F., Bosnjak, Z.J. et al. (1988). Effects of halothane with and without histamine and/or epinephrine on automaticity, intracardiac conduction times, and development of dysrhythmias in the isolated guinea pig heart. *Anesthesiology* 68: 695–706.

Sumikawa, K., Ishizaka, N., and Suzaki, M. (1983). Arrhythmogenic plasma levels of epinephrine during halothane, enflurane, and pentobarbital anesthesia in the dog. *Anesthesiology* 58: 322–325.

Sunahara, H.T., Tani, K. et al. (2021). Transient third-degree atrioventricular block during anesthesia in a cat. *Open Vet. J.* 11: 662–666.

Swanson, C.R., Muir, W.W. et al. (1985). Hemodynamic responses in halothane-anesthetized horses given infusions of dopamine or dobutamine. *Am. J. Vet. Res.* 46: 365–370.

Tobias, J.D. and Hirshman, C.A. (1990). Attenuation of histamine-induced airway constriction by albuterol during halothane anesthesia. *Anesthesiology* 72: 105–110.

Trim, C.M., Moore, J.N. et al. (1991). Effects of an infusion of dopamine on the cardiopulmonary effects of *Escherichia coli* endotoxin in anaesthetised horses. *Res. Vet. Sci.* 50: 54–63.

Tsompanidou, P.P., Kazakos, G.M., and Anagnostou, T.L. (2007). Dopamine-induced bradycardia in two dogs under isoflurane anaesthesia. *J. Small Anim. Pract.* 54: 672–674.

Tucker, P.K. and MacFarlane, P. (2019). Incidence of perianaesthetic complications experienced during feline bronchoscopy: a retrospective study. *J. Feline Med. Surg.* 21: 959–966.

Tucker, W.K., Rackstein, A.D., and Munson, E.S. (1974). Comparison of arrhythmic doses of adrenaline, metaraminol, ephedrine and phenylephrine during isoflurane and halothane anaesthesia in dogs. *Br. J. Anaesth.* 46: 392–396.

Tuttle, R.R. and Mills, J. (1975). Dobutamine: development of a new catecholamine to selectively increase cardiac contractility. *Circ. Res.* 36: 185–196.

Valverde, A., Giguère, S. et al. (2006). Effects of dobutamine, norepinephrine, and vasopressin on cardiovascular function in anesthetized neonatal foals with induced hypotension. *Am. J. Vet. Res.* 67: 1730–1737.

Vandycke, C. and Martens, P. (2000). High dose versus standard dose epinephrine in cardiac arrest – a meta-analysis. *Resuscitation* 45: 161–166.

Wagner, A.E., Dunlop, C.I., and Chapman, P.L. (1993). Effects of ephedrine on cardiovascular function and oxygen delivery in isoflurane-anesthetized dogs. *Am. J. Vet. Res.* 54: 1917–1922.

Wallukat, G. (2002). The beta-adrenergic receptors. *Herz* 27: 683–690.

Wells, D.G. and Bjorksten, A.R. (1989). Monoamine oxidase inhibitors revisited. *Can. J. Anaesth.* 36: 64–74.

Whitton, D.L. and Trim, C.M. (1985). Use of dopamine hydrochloride during general anesthesia in the treatment of advanced atrioventricular heart block in four foals. *J. Am. Vet. Med. Assoc.* 187: 1357–1361.

Wiese, A.J., Barter, L.S. et al. (2012). Cardiovascular and respiratory effects of incremental doses of dopamine and phenylephrine in the management of isoflurane-induced hypotension in cats with hypertrophic cardiomyopathy. *Am. J. Vet. Res.* 73: 908–916.

Wright, M., Heath, R.B., and Wingfield, W.E. (1987). Effects of xylazine and ketamine on epinephrine-induced arrhythmia in the dog. *Vet. Surg.* 16: 398–403.

Yoo, J.H., Kim, M.S. et al. (2007). Vasopressor therapy using vasopressin prior to crystalloid resuscitation in irreversible hemorrhagic shock under isoflurane anesthesia in dogs. *J. Vet. Med. Sci.* 69: 459–464.

Young, L.E., Blissitt, K.J. et al. (1998). Haemodynamic effects of a sixty minute infusion of dopamine hydrochloride in horses anaesthetised with halothane. *Equine Vet. J.* 30: 310–316.

Zahed, B., Miletich, D.J. et al. (1977). Arrhythmic doses of epinephrine and dopamine during halothane, enflurane, methoxyflurane, and fluroxene anesthesia in goats. *Anesth. Analg.* 56: 207–210.

Zeynalov, E., Jones, S.M., and Elliott, J.P. (2020). Vasopressin and vasopressin receptors in brain edema. *Vitam. Horm.* 113: 291–312.

19

Antihypertensives
Gianluca Bini

Introduction

Systemic hypertension can be classified as situational, secondary or idiopathic. While situational hypertension can be due to environmental or temporary stressors (i.e. being hospitalized) and normally the animal is otherwise normotensive, secondary hypertension defines a persistent increase in blood pressure pathologically caused by a disease, toxic substance or iatrogenically. Lastly, idiopathic hypertension occurs in the absence of a disease process, and it is often referred as primary hypertension (Acierno et al. 2018).

Antihypertensive drugs have multiple sites of action but, in general, they decrease blood pressure by regulating the autonomic nervous system, the renin–angiotensin–aldosterone system (RAAS) or by causing peripheral vasodilation. The classes of drugs commonly used to treat systemic hypertension include sympatholytics, angiotensin converting enzyme (ACE) inhibitors, angiotensin receptor blockers, calcium channel blockers and vasodilators (Acierno et al. 2018; Oparil et al. 2018), other drugs are discussed later in this chapter for completeness.

Sympatholytic Drugs

These are drugs inducing vasodilation by acting on adrenergic receptors, preventing the actions of sympathomimetic amines on adrenergic receptors. This class of drug can be subdivided depending on whether a drug is selective at α- or β-adrenergic receptors, while others have combined α- or β- adrenergic receptor antagonism. It is important to recognize that although most sympatholytic drugs are antagonists at the adrenergic receptors, α_2-agonists are an exception to this.

Selective α_1-Adrenergic Receptor Antagonists

These drugs prevent the activation of the α1-adrenergic receptor prevent the activation of the G_q protein phospholipase C and subsequent synthesis of diacylglycerol (DAG) and 1,4,5-inositol triphosphate (IP3) which, in turn, inhibits intracellular Ca^{2+} increase in the vascular smooth muscle, ultimately leading to a decrease in arterial and venous vascular resistance and reduction in blood pressure (Kellar et al. 1984; Singal et al. 2004; Han et al. 2018).

Prazosin

Prazosin is a highly selective postsynaptic α_1-receptor antagonist (Oates et al. 1977; Adams 1984). Prazosin can be administered either orally or intravenously (IV), but the oral formulation is the only one commercially available at the moment. A significant decrease in blood pressure has been reported after IV administration in cats and dogs (Ramage 1984; Fischer et al. 2003). The recommended dosages are 0.5–2 mg/kg q8–12h PO in dogs and 0.25–0.5 mg/cat q24h PO in cats (Acierno et al. 2018). Patients with chronic kidney disease have an increased drug sensitivity, therefore, dosages should be reduced (Lameire and Gordts 1986; Aronoff et al. 2007).

The lack of activity on the presynaptic α_2-receptor, preserves the negative feedback regulating norepinephrine release in the synaptic cleft, therefore no significant reflex increase in heart rate and cardiac output is evoked (Langer et al. 1977; Saeed et al. 1982). This makes the use of prazosin favorable in reducing cardiac workload in congestive heart failure, (Atwell 1979; Antani et al. 1991).

Prazosin and other selective α_1-adrenoceptor antagonists are used to treat hypertension (rarely as first-line [Heran et al. 2012]), benign prostatic hypertrophy as well as neurogenic and non-neurogenic urinary bladder outflow obstruction in humans (Lepor 1990; Foglar et al. 1995; Donohoe et al. 2005). Prazosin has also been investigated for a wide variety of conditions including treatment of post-traumatic stress disorder (PTSD) (Reist et al. 2021), alcoholism (Simpson et al. 2015), cytokine release syndrome (Staedtke et al. 2018) and it has been shown to significantly reduce the mortality rate after Indian red scorpion (*Mesobuthus tamulus*) sting (Bawaskar and Bawaskar 2011; Pandi et al. 2014).

Although prazosin can be used as an antihypertensive treatment in dogs and cats (Massingham and Hayden 1975; Fischer et al. 2003; Acierno et al. 2018), prazosin is mainly used for the treatment of vesico-urethral reflex dyssynergia (VURD), otherwise known as "detrusor-urethral dyssynergia" or "functional urethral obstruction", in these species (Díaz Espiñeira et al. 1998; Haagsman et al. 2013). VURD is a condition caused by inappropriate activation of α1-receptors in the smooth muscle of bladder neck and proximal urethra; their contraction during micturition leads to dysuria. Additionally, its use has also been recommended for treatment of urinary retention in dogs with supra-sacral spinal cord lesions in order to reduce sphincter tone (Granger et al. 2020), although some studies did not show a significant effect in that patient population (Barnes et al. 2019). There is contrasting evidence about prazosin rather than phenoxybenzamine decreasing the incidence of recurrent urethral obstruction in cats (Eisenberg et al. 2013; Hetrick and Davidow 2013). Prazosin has also been investigated to increase limb perfusion in horses affected by laminitis, with poor results (Galey et al. 1990).

Due to its long duration of action and lack of titratability, prazosin is not currently used for the management of blood pressure under anesthesia, nonetheless, the reader should be familiar with its effects when anesthetizing a patient receiving prazosin therapy. While, in the past, veterinary literature has anecdotally suggested to withhold prazosin 12–24 hours before induction of anesthesia to decrease the risk of hypotension during the anesthetic event (Murrell 2017), recommendations in human medicine suggest otherwise (Hollevoet et al. 2011), although, because of the low quality of evidence on which these recommendations are based (Halperin et al. 2016), the reader is invited to evaluate the risk/benefit of discontinuing prazosin before general anesthesia on a case-by-case basis.

Prazosin as well as terazosin and doxazosin have been used to perioperatively hemodynamically stabilize patients with pheochromocytoma in humans and in veterinary medicine (Knapp and Fitzgerald 1984; Hull 1986; Maher and McNiel 1997; Fang et al. 2020).

Phenoxybenzamine, a non-competitive, non-selective α1- and α2-receptor antagonist, further discussed below, is more commonly used in pheochromocytoma patients (Spencer 2020), hypertensive crisis and inadequate blood pressure control have been reported when patients were treated with prazosin alone (Nicholson et al. 1983; Knapp and Fitzgerald 1984).

Prazosin has a low (38%) bioavailability after oral administration in dogs (Rubin et al. 1979), lower than what is reported in humans (57%) (Vincent et al. 1985). Prazosin undergoes extensive first-pass hepatic metabolism, with only 6% being excreted unchanged in the urine (Taylor et al. 1977). The elimination half-time is about 2.5 hours in dogs, while this and its bioavailability are increased in patients with congestive heart failure (Jaillon et al. 1979; Rubin et al. 1979), that is not the case in patients with renal dysfunction (Lowenthal et al. 1980). P-glycoprotein 1, has been reported as the major prazosin efflux transporter, therefore an interference in patients with ABCB1 (previously referred as multidrug resistance mutation 1 [MDR1]) mutation could be speculated (Janani 2020) and care should be taken in adjusting dosages in these patients.

Several side effects have been reported in human medicine, including lethargy, headache, nausea, dizziness, postural hypotension, syncope and exaggerated hypotension during epidural anesthesia (Lepor 1990; Lydiatt et al. 1993; Kirsten et al. 1998). The veterinary literature is limited in this regard; lethargy occurred in a dog receiving prazosin (Haagsman et al. 2013), while another study with six Beagle dogs reported the same, but the incidence in the prazosin group was not different than that in the placebo group (Fischer et al. 2003). Lethargy, ptyalism, diarrhea and anorexia have been reported in cats (Reineke et al. 2017).

Terazosin and Doxazosin

Similarly to prazosin, these α1-receptor antagonist have been used for the treatment of hypertension, VURD in both human and veterinary medicine, as well as delayed micturition in dogs with thoracolumbar spinal cord injury (Ramage 1984; Luther et al. 1986; Chancellor et al. 1993; Bennett et al. 2000; Haagsman et al. 2013; Skytte and Schmökel 2018). Their effects and side effects appear to be similar to prazosin, there is not enough evidence to support a significantly different efficacy between them (Heran et al. 2012), but they have a significantly longer half-life (11 hours terazosin; 9–12 hours doxazosin) (Jønler et al. 1994; Akduman and Crawford 2001). Lethargy, ataxia, nausea, diarrhea, vomiting and dyspnea have been reported in dogs undergoing a six-week treatment with terazosin (Haagsman et al. 2013). As with prazosin, dosages should be decreased in patients with chronic kidney disease, due to an increased drug sensitivity.

Non-Selective α₁- and α₂-Adrenergic Receptor Antagonists

Drugs in this class have antihypertensive action due to their antagonism at the α₁-adrenergic receptor, while their antagonism at the presynaptic α₂-adrenergic receptors neutralize the norepinephrine negative feedback. The result is an increased norepinephrine release from the presynaptic nerve endings, which then stimulates β₁-adrenergic receptors in the heart potentially causing an increase in heart rate and cardiac output (Langer et al. 1977; Saeed et al. 1982).

The non-selective blockade including the presynaptic α₂-receptor, neutralizes the norepinephrine negative feedback, resulting in higher norepinephrine being released from the presynaptic nerve endings, potentially causing a reflex increase in heart rate and cardiac output (Langer et al. 1977; Saeed et al. 1982).

Phenoxybenzamine

Phenoxybenzamine is a haloalkylamine derivative, which irreversibly alkylates the α-adrenergic receptors (Vardanyan and Hruby 2006), providing long-acting, non-competitive, non-selective α₁- and α₂-receptor antagonism. Phenoxybenzamine has two stereoisomers R- and S-phenoxybenzamine (Portoghese et al. 1971), but it is commercially available only as a racemic mixture. Phenoxybenzamine can be administered either orally or IV, but the oral formulation has been demonstrated to be poorly available in humans (Hoffman and Lefkowitz 1980). The recommended dosages are 0.25 mg/kg q8-12h or 0.5 mg/kg q24h PO in dogs; 2.5 mg/cat q8-12h or 0.5 mg/cat q24h PO in cats (Acierno et al. 2018) and 1 mg/kg q24h IV or 0.7 mg/kg q6h PO in horses (Papich 2021).

Phenoxybenzamine is used for the perioperative hemodynamic stabilization of pheochromocytoma and paraganglioma in patients before surgery in both humans (Russell et al. 1998; Wachtel et al. 2015; Naranjo et al. 2017; Fang et al. 2020) and veterinary patients (Maher and McNiel 1997). A pheochromocytoma is a tumor arising from chromaffin cells, in the adrenal medulla, that commonly produces one or more catecholamines, but, in some rare instances, these tumors can be biochemically silent (Lenders et al. 2014). Paragangliomas, also called chemodectomas, on the other hand, are tumors derived from chromaffin cells outside the adrenal medulla (Lenders et al. 2014; Galac and Korpershoek 2017). Phenoxybenzamine's longer duration of action and its ability to provide a non-competitive blockade make it a more favorable choice for the perioperative management of these patients, compared to selective α1-adrenergic receptor antagonists like prazosin, avoiding the risk of hypertension in case of a spike in catecholamine plasma concentration (Knapp and Fitzgerald 1984; Hull 1986; Fang et al. 2020).

Dosages ranging from 0.1 mg to 2.5 mg/kg q12h PO in dogs undergoing presurgical treatment for pheochromocytoma have been reported, one study used a median dose of 0.6 mg/kg q12h PO for 20 days (Herrera et al. 2008), and another one suggested 2.5 mg/kg q12h PO for at least 14 days (Kyles et al. 2003). Another source suggested starting at 0.25 mg/kg q12h and increasing the dosage in a stepwise approach over the span of two to three weeks, until the final dosage of 1 mg/kg is reached, or side effects occur (Spencer 2020). Unfortunately, there is currently insufficient evidence to suggest an ideal dosage for presurgical treatment of pheochromocytoma in veterinary medicine.

Presurgical treatment with phenoxybenzamine for 20 days before adrenalectomy significantly decreased mortality in dogs (Herrera et al. 2008), and has been shown to improve cardiovascular stability and reduce mortality in humans (Russell et al. 1998; Wachtel et al. 2015). Recently, there has been some debate in the human literature on whether presurgical treatment with phenoxybenzamine is needed, mainly due to limited evidence, significant adverse effects of the α-adrenergic antagonists and availability of short-acting drugs that may be used to treat hypertension during anesthesia (Shao et al. 2011; Lafont et al. 2015; Wachtel et al. 2015; Groeben et al. 2017; Isaacs and Lee 2017; Neumann et al. 2019). Hypertension during surgery has been reported in several cases including patients with biochemically silent pheochromocytoma not receiving preoperative management (Song et al. 2011; Kota et al. 2012; El-Doueihi et al. 2019). The North American Neuroendocrine Tumor Society and the Endocrine Society recommend preparing patients with pheochromocytomas or paragangliomas, including the normotensive or biochemically silent ones, using phenoxybenzamine starting 10–14 days before surgery (Chen et al. 2010; Lenders et al. 2014). Ultimately, it has been suggested to be a collaborative decision with anesthetist and surgeon, taking into consideration the patient's cardiovascular status and intraoperative risks (Lenders et al. 2014; Isaacs and Lee 2017).

If blood pressure cannot be controlled by the sole means of a non-selective α-adrenergic receptor antagonist, a calcium channel blocker (e.g. doxazosin, amlodipine) is commonly added when treating patients with pheochromocytoma (Wimpole et al. 2010; Lenders et al. 2014). β-blockers are used in addition to phenoxybenzamine to control arrhythmias and tachycardia occurring during surgery for pheochromocytoma removal. I is important to recognize that phenoxybenzamine blocks only α- adrenergic receptors, therefore as other α₁-adrenergic antagonists, it may decrease the incidence of arrhythmias but it does not prevent them (Claborn and Szabuniewicz 1973; Wiersig et al. 1974; Benfey 1993; Myklejord 2004).

Phenoxybenzamine has been used to treat functional urethral obstruction in humans, dogs, and cats (Abrams et al. 1982; Moreau 1982; Oliver 1983; Barsanti et al. 1996; Díaz Espiñeira et al. 1998; Lane et al. 2000). Due to the availability of selective α_1-adrenergic receptor antagonists, the higher cost, and the potential carcinogenicity of phenoxybenzamine its use for functional urethral obstruction is nowadays considered obsolete (and off-label) in humans and veterinary patients (Lepor 1990; Breslin et al. 1993; Carruthers 1994; Jønler et al. 1994; Granger et al. 2020).

In horses, phenoxybenzamine has been suggested as a promising treatment for laminitis (Boosman and Németh 1988; Hood et al. 1993), as well as non-responsive diarrhea (Hood et al. 1982; Hunt and Gerring 1985), with mixed results.

The pharmacokinetic information for phenoxybenzamine is limited. In humans, it has a very low oral bioavailability ranging between 20% and 30% (Hoffman and Lefkowitz 1980) and, an half-life of about 24 hours when administered IV, while its half-life after oral administration is unknown (WellSpring Pharmaceutical Corporation [FDA Label] 2008). Phenoxybenzamine is metabolized by the liver and excreted in urine and bile (Mercury Pharmaceuticals Ltd [FDA Label] 2021). Phentolamine is highly lipophilic, therefore fat accumulation has been hypothesized (Adams 2009), but there is evidence of the contrary (Knapp and Fitzgerald 1984). The specific mechanism of action of phenoxybenzamine, creating a strong covalent bond with the α-adrenergic receptors, leads to a prolonged onset of action, it has been reported that as little as three days, and up to 25 days may be required to achieve an optimal preoperative management in humans (Russell et al. 1998; Zhu et al. 2010). Its duration of action is linked to the synthesis of new α-adrenergic receptors, and there is some evidence of different rate of recovery of α_1 and α_2-adrenergic receptors effects (Hamilton et al. 1984), where its effects can last up to four days (Hoffman and Lefkowitz 1980; WellSpring Pharmaceutical Corporation [FDA Label] 2008) but, in a study mean arterial pressure, was not significantly different from baseline after only 24 hours after phenoxybenzamine administration (Hamilton et al. 1984).

Persistent hypotension following pheochromocytoma removal has been reported. This is due to the mechanism of action of phenoxybenzamine (Nickerson 1962; Hamilton et al. 1984; Ramachandran and Rewari 2016), therefore, the anesthetist should plan accordingly for intra- and post-operative blood pressure support. Some veterinary literature suggests stopping administration of phenoxybenzamine 48 hours prior to surgery (Murrell 2017), while human guidelines suggest continuing treatment the day of surgery (Hollevoet et al. 2011).

As for all the non-selective α_1- and α_2-adrenergic receptor antagonists, phenoxybenzamine can cause a reflex increase in heart rate and cardiac output due to the non-selective blockade, including the presynaptic α_2-receptor, resulting in higher norepinephrine release from the presynaptic nerve endings (Langer et al. 1977; Saeed et al. 1982).

Postural hypotension with reflex tachycardia and arrhythmias, tiredness and dizziness have been reported with the use of phenoxybenzamine (Mulvihill-Wilson et al. n.d.; Caine et al. 1976; Jønler et al. 1994; Eri and Tveter 1995). While human literature suggests a higher incidence and severity of side effects including hypotension and dizziness, associated with non-selective α-antagonists compared to selective α_1-adrenergic receptor antagonists (Mulvihill-Wilson et al. n.d.; Caine et al. 1976; Jønler et al. 1994; Eri and Tveter 1995), a small study in six Beagle dogs found that phenoxybenzamine had less impact on blood pressure compared to prazosin (Fischer et al. 2003).

The availability of selective α_1-adrenergic receptor antagonists, the higher cost and the potential carcinogenicity of phenoxybenzamine made its use for functional urethral obstruction obsolete in humans (Lepor 1990; Breslin et al. 1993; Carruthers 1994; Jønler et al. 1994; Lane et al. 2000). The mutagenic activity of phenoxybenzamine has been demonstrated *in vitro* and in mice, moreover repeated use in laboratory animals has been associated with peritoneal, intestinal, and lung tumors and its mutagenicity (Hoffman and Lefkowitz 1980; Fischer et al. 2003; WellSpring Pharmaceutical Corporation [FDA Label] 2008).

Phentolamine

Phentolamine is a short-acting, competitive, non-selective α_1- and α_2-receptor antagonist.

Phentolamine can be administered IV, IM, submucosally and when used for treatment of extravasation of vasopressors, locally in the affected area of interest (Septodont Inc [FDA Label] 2016; West-Ward Pharmaceuticals Corp [FDA Label] 2018).

In human medicine, phentolamine is used in the management of hypertensive crisis due to β-blockade without adequate α-blockade or for patients with pheochromocytoma who have not been pretreated with phenoxybenzamine, as well as for prophylactic treatment before pheochromocytoma removal (McMillian et al. 2011; West-Ward Pharmaceuticals Corp [FDA Label] 2018; Yu et al. 2018; Fang et al. 2020).

Intraoperative hypertension during adrenalectomy for pheochromocytoma removal was successfully managed in dogs, administering a loading dose of 0.1 mg/kg IV followed by a constant rate infusion at a rate of 1–2 µg/kg/min IV (Kyles et al. 2003).

Phentolamine is the only treatment approved by the FDA for norepinephrine extravasation, although some alternatives have been evaluated (Plum and Moukhachen 2017). It is also recommended to treat and prevent tissue necrosis after extravasation of dopamine, epinephrine, phenylephrine and sympathomimetic vasopressors in general (Cooper 1989; Bey et al. 1998; Peberdy et al. 2010). No description of this use is currently available in the veterinary literature. The recommended doses for this treatment in adult humans are 5–10 mg of phentolamine diluted in 10 ml of saline injected into the area within 12 hours of vasopressors extravasation (Reynolds et al. 2014). On the other hand, in human pediatric patients, it is suggested to titrate subcutaneously 1–7.5 ml of phentolamine at a concentration of 0.5 mg/ml in the involved area (Aribit et al. 2000; Özalp Gerçeker et al. 2018; Hackenberg et al. 2021).

Phentolamine is also FDA approved for reversal of local anesthesia containing a vasoconstrictor for some dental procedures in humans, shortening the median time to return of sensation by up to 60% (Tavares et al. 2008).

Not surprisingly, phentolamine has also been evaluated for functional urethral obstruction in dogs, and it has with the greatest effect on the urethra of all the α-adrenergic receptor antagonist, while having the least impact on the cardiovascular system (Poirier et al. 1988).Unfortunately, its use is non practical due to its short duration of action (Rosin and Ross 1981).

Phentolamine has also been experimentally demonstrated to reduce frequency of ventricular premature complexes in dogs after coronary artery occlusion and reperfusion (Stewart et al. 1980).

The pharmacokinetic information for phentolamine is limited. In humans, it has a very fast onset of action (one to two minutes), a duration of action of 10–30 minutes (Chobanian et al. 2003) and a half-life of about 19 minutes when administered IV (West-Ward Pharmaceuticals Corp [FDA Label] 2018). Phentolamine is metabolized by the liver and only 13% of the drugs is excreted unchanged in the urine (West-Ward Pharmaceuticals Corp [FDA Label] 2018).

As for all the non-selective α$_1$- and α$_2$-adrenergic receptor antagonists, phentolamine can cause an increase in heart rate and cardiac output due to the blockade of the presynaptic α$_2$-adrenergic receptor (Langer et al. 1977; Saeed et al. 1982). The reported side effects in humans include tachycardia, vomiting and headache (Chobanian et al. 2003). In addition, phentolamine may elicit angina pectoris or myocardial infarction in patients with coronary artery disease (Grossman et al. 1998). β-blockers can be used to manage the compensatory tachycardia elicited by phentolamine.

Oral administration of very high doses of phentolamine to pregnant mice and rats during the period of organogenesis resulted in skeletal immaturity, decreased offspring growth and lower rate of implantation, but no malformations or embryofetal deaths were observed (Septodont Inc [FDA Label] 2016). It is important to recognize that these studies were performed with doses at least 20 times the recommended dose and, treating the pheochromocytoma is of paramount importance for the mother and fetus (Schenker and Chowers 1971; Schenker and Granat 1982). Therefore, the reader is invited to evaluate the risk/benefit of using phentolamine in pregnant patients on a case-by-case basis.

α$_2$-Adrenergic Receptor Agonists

Drugs in this class are widely used in veterinary medicine to provide sedation and analgesia, and can be reversed with administration of antagonists. These drugs act as agonists at the α$_2$-adrenergic receptor, activating the Gi protein thus inhibiting adenylate cyclase and the cAMP dependent pathway. This results in Ca^{2+}-channels closure in the presynaptic nerve ending which prevents the increase in intracellular Ca^{2+} necessary to release norepinephrine, thus decreasing sympathetic outflow, heart rate, contractility and systemic vascular resistance and consequently reducing blood pressure. Several α$_2$-adrenergic receptor subtypes have been identified, the clinically observed initial hypertensive phase is mediated by the agonist interaction with the α-$_{2B}$ subtype receptors found in the vascular smooth muscle, while the secondary hypotensive phase is mediated by activation of the α-$_{2A}$ which, together with α-$_{2C}$ receptor subtypes, are mainly located in the central nervous system (CNS) (Link et al. 1996; MacMillan et al. 1996; Buerkle and Yaksh 1998; Altman et al. 1999).

α$_2$-adrenergic receptor agonists are not considered first-line therapy for hypertension, due to their sedative side effects, which are mediated by the activation of the α-$_{2A}$ receptor subtype (Lakhlani et al. 1997). A more complete description of these drugs can be found elsewhere in the book.

Angiotensin Converting Enzyme (ACE) Inhibitors

Angiotensin II is a hormone which causes arteriolar vasoconstriction, sympathetic stimulation, water reabsorption and promotes the synthesis of aldosterone and vasopressin. When renal perfusion is decreased, the renin–angiotensin-aldosterone hormone system is triggered, this regulates blood pressure by altering systemic vascular resistance, as well as water retention. Angiotensin I is the result of the angiotensinogen conversion performed by renin, which is produced by the kidney in response to a decreased in perfusion. Angiotensin I is then converted to angiotensin II by ACEs in lungs capillaries as well as in endothelial and kidney epithelial cells (Kierszenbaum 2007). ACE inhibitors block the conversion of angiotensin I to angiotensin II (Soffer 1976) while also stopping the hydrolyzation of bradykinin (BK) a vasodilator, and N-acetyl-seryl-aspartyl-lysyl-proline (Ac-SDKP), a peptide with anti-inflammatory functions (Hrenak et al. 2015; Caballero 2020). The resulting bradykinin potentiation can lead to further vasodilation and natriuresis (Taddei and Bortolotto 2016). ACE inhibitors are mainly used to treat hypertension and congestive heart failure.

ACE inhibitors decrease glomerular efferent arteriolar resistance, normalizing the glomerular transcapillary hydrostatic pressure therefore decreasing proteinuria in patients with glomerulonephritis (Brown et al. 2001, 2003; King et al. 2006; Mizutani et al. 2006; Sent et al. 2015). The high incidence of chronic kidney disease and proteinuria in hypertensive dogs make ACE inhibitors a common and ideal initial therapy choice in this patient population (Acierno et al. 2018). While ACE inhibitors can be considered as a first-line therapy in dogs, this is not the case for cats (Acierno et al. 2018), due to their possible limited efficacy and worsening of renal function during treatment in this species (Brown et al. 2001; Sent et al. 2015; Lavallee et al. 2017). No effects on renal function have been demonstrated in dogs during long-term treatment with ACE inhibitors (Atkins et al. 2002). The ACE inhibitors most commonly used in veterinary medicine are benazepril and enalapril.

The oral bioavailability of benazepril and enalapril range between 20% and 40% in dogs, with a peak plasma concentration in about 40 minutes and have an elimination half-life of 40–60 minutes (Lefebvre et al. 2007). Benazepril it is partially metabolized by the liver which is advantageous in animals with renal dysfunction compared to enalapril which relies almost exclusively (95%) on renal excretion (Lefebvre et al. 2007). Hepatic clearance of benazepril is markedly higher in cats (85%) compared to dogs (55%) (Lefebvre et al. 2007).

Due to the risk of severe hypotension during general anesthesia in both human and veterinary patients receiving ACE inhibitors, it is recommended to withhold ACE inhibitors for 24 hours before general anesthesia (Coriat et al. 1994; Bertrand et al. 2001; Ishikawa et al. 2007; Uechi et al. 2007; Coleman et al. 2016a). A recent cohort study in a large number of humans withholding ACE inhibitors and angiotensin II receptor blockers before surgery was associated with a decreased risk of death and vascular events in the postoperative period (Roshanov et al. 2017).

Anorexia, diarrhea, vomiting, lethargy, hypotension, and hyperkalemia have been reported in dogs receiving ACE inhibitors (Sisson 1995). Additionally, ACE inhibitors can cause azotemia in some patients, especially if concurrently receiving diuretics, moreover acute worsening of azotemia has been reported with concurrent administration of ACE inhibitors and angiotensin receptor blockers. Therefore, it

is imperative that renal parameters should be closely monitored in these patients (Roudebush et al. 1994; Group CS 1995; Ettinger et al. 1998; Brown et al. 2001; King et al. 2006). The combination of ACE inhibitors and other antihypertensive drugs may exacerbate their hypotensive effect (Mignat and Unger 1995). Nonsteroidal anti-inflammatory drugs (NSAIDs) may reduce the efficacy of ACE inhibitors (Sahloul et al. 1990). Moreover, the combination of ACE inhibitors with NSAIDs may potentially lead to nephrotoxicity and renal insufficiency (Seelig et al. 1990; Shionoiri 1993). Although there is no report in veterinary medicine, lithium toxicity has been reported in humans receiving concomitant ACE inhibitors. The mechanism behind this interaction remains unknown, nonetheless, it is recommended to carefully monitor these patients (Shionoiri 1993). Lastly, ACE inhibitors can cross the placenta and have the potential of causing potentially fatal perinatal complications, therefore, they should be avoided in pregnant animals (Hanssens et al. 1991).

Benazepril

The recommended dosages are 0.5 mg/kg q12-24h PO and it can be increased up to a maximum of 2 mg/kg per day in dogs. It has been recommended to decrease the starting dose to 0.25 mg/kg in azotemic dogs (Brown et al. 2013; Acierno et al. 2018; Spencer 2020). The dosages for cats are 0.5 mg/kg q12h PO (Acierno et al. 2018).

Enalapril

The recommended dosages are 0.5 mg/kg q12-24h PO and it can be increased up to a maximum of 2 mg/kg per day in dogs. It has been recommended to decrease the starting dose to 0.25 mg/kg in azotemic dogs (Brown et al. 2013; Acierno et al. 2018; Spencer 2020). The dosages for cats are 0.5 mg/kg q24h PO (Acierno et al. 2018). Although enalapril has been experimentally used in horses, there are no clinically recommended doses for this species at the moment.

Angiotensin II Receptor Blockers

Angiotensin II receptors are G protein-coupled receptors. AT_1 is responsible for the vasoconstrictive effects, while AT_2 has multiple beneficial effects, including potentially limiting cardiac remodeling, although this has been debated in the literature and not all of its functions are entirely clear (D'Amore et al. 2005; Schnermann and Castrop 2013). Angiotensin II receptor blockers such as telmisartan and losartan, the most commonly used in veterinary species, have high affinity for the AT_1 receptor which allows for a reduction in blood pressure while maintaining normal bradykinin levels, as opposed to ACE inhibitors which, due to their different mechanism of action, can cause an increase in bradykinin levels over time (Tom et al. 2002; Taddei and Bortolotto 2016).

Telmisartan

Telmisartan is an angiotensin II receptor blocker, used to manage hypertension and proteinuria in cats with chronic kidney disease (Sent et al. 2015; Glaus et al. 2019), and it is more effective than benazepril or losartan in this species (Jenkins et al. 2015). Telmisartan has been reported to be as an effective antihypertensive agent as amlodipine in humans with chronic kidney disease (Nakamura et al. 2018), while there are veterinary reports of using telmisartan as a second-line treatment in dogs where amlodipine or a combination of amlodipine and benazepril failed (Caro-Vadillo et al. 2018; Kwon et al. 2018). A recent trial found telmisartan to be a potential first-line therapy to manage dogs with proteinuria (Lourenço et al. 2020), and it has been previously reported as a second-line treatment in dogs refractory to ACE inhibitors (Bugbee et al. 2014). The recommended dosage is 1 mg/kg q24h PO in both cats and dogs (Acierno et al. 2018).

The oral bioavailability of telmisartan is about 33% in cats, peak plasma level was reached in about 15–30 minutes, telmisartan is highly lipophilic and highly protein bound (98% in dogs). Telmisartan is mainly metabolized by the liver and largely excreted in bile, with an elimination half-life of about five hours in dogs and 8.5 hours in cats (Wienen et al. 2000; Boehringer Ingelheim Vetmedica Inc. [FDA FOI Summary] 2018)

Losartan

Losartan is an angiotensin II receptor blocker, the active drug metabolite (E-3174) is 10–40 times more potent than losartan. This is responsible for the antihypertensive effect. Dogs produce a limited amount of E-3174 (Christ et al. 1994). Losartan is also less efficacious than telmisartan in cats, and no better than placebo in cats and dogs (Brown et al. 2013; Coleman et al. 2014; Jenkins et al. 2015). The recommended dosages are 0.5–1 mg/kg q24h PO, while it has been recommended to reduce the dose to 0.125–0.25 mg/kg q24h PO in azotemic dogs (Brown et al. 2013).

The oral bioavailability of losartan ranges between 23% and 33% in dogs, peak plasma level was reached in about one hour and it is mainly metabolized by the liver and cleared by biliary excretion, with an elimination half-life of about 2.5 hours (Christ et al. 1994).

Similarly to ACE inhibitors, it is recommended to withhold angiotensin II receptor blockers for 24 hours or more, before induction of general anesthesia in human patients, due to the risk of severe or refractory hypotension in these patients (Wolf and McGoldrick 2011; Nabbi et al. 2013; Mets 2015; Hojo et al. 2020). The combination of angiotensin II receptor blockers and ACE inhibitors could increase the risk of side effects and worsening of kidney function (Misra and Stevermer 2009).

Hypotension, hypersalivation, weight loss, diarrhea, lethargy, anemia, and vomiting have been reported in cats receiving telmisartan (Boehringer Ingelheim Vetmedica Inc. [FDA FOI Summary] 2018). No side effects have been reported in dogs receiving telmisartan in the existing literature (Schierok et al. 2001; Bugbee et al. 2014; Coleman et al. 2016b; Caro-Vadillo et al. 2018; Konta et al. 2018; Kwon et al. 2018).

Calcium Channel Blocker

Amlodipine

Amlodipine is a dihydropyridine class, long-acting calcium blocker. It inhibits calcium entry from L-type voltage-gated calcium channels in the vascular smooth muscle, preventing contraction and causing vasodilation (Clusin and Anderson 1999). Amlodipine also has an inhibitory effect on N-type calcium channels, located presynaptically on neurons, decreasing norepinephrine release (Hirning et al. 1988; Westenbroek et al. 1992; Gohil et al. 1994; Elliott et al. 1995). This may be the reason for the comparatively lower increase in heart rate observed after amlodipine administration compared to other dihydropyridines (Furukawa et al. 1997). N-type calcium channels are also nociceptive signaling and, when blocked, may produce analgesic effects (Brose et al. 1997; Suh et al. 1997). The doses to obtain good analgesia are usually quite large and not devoid of significant side effect, making this a more a theoretical than clinical consideration (Brose et al. 1997).

The effect of amlodipine on the sympathetic nervous system has been debated in the human literature. Some studies reported a decrease, while others reported an increase in sympathetic nerve activity; the latter seems to be the case in hypertensive patients (Leenen et al. 2001; Toal et al. 2012). The antihypertensive effectiveness seems to overcome the risk of sympathetic activation (Toal et al. 2012).

Amlodipine, as well as ACE inhibitors and angiotensin II receptor blockers, is one of the most commonly used antihypertensive agents. Calcium channel blockers such as amlodipine are a first-line treatment for cats with systemic hypertension while, as discussed in a previous paragraph, RAAS inhibitors such as ACE inhibitors and angiotensin II receptor blockers are first-line treatments for systemic hypertension in dogs (Huhtinen et al. 2015; Acierno et al. 2018). Moreover, the combination of amlodipine and RAAS blocking agents is particularly useful in dogs with severe systemic hypertension, when systolic blood pressure is above 200 mmHg (Acierno et al. 2018).

Amlodipine is commercially available as an oral formulation while a less efficacious transdermal formulation has been investigated in cats (Helms 2007). The recommended dose for amlodipine is 0.1–0.25 mg/kg q24h PO and it can be increased up to a maximum of 0.5 mg/kg in both cats and dogs, alternatively, it could be dosed as 0.625–1.25 mg/cat q24h PO (Acierno et al. 2018).

There is no current evidence that administration of calcium channel blockers significantly increases anesthetic risk complications (Merin 1987; Schlanz et al. 1991). Therefore, perioperative medications guidelines in humans suggest continuing calcium channel blockers.

The oral bioavailability of amlodipine is 88% in dogs, it is extensively metabolized by the liver with only 5% of the drug excreted unchanged in the urine. The elimination half-life of amlodipine is about 30 hours in dogs (Stopher et al. 1988; Burges et al. 1989).

Hypotension, heart rate changes, lethargy, appetite, and weight loss are reported side effects of amlodipine. Dose-dependent gingival hyperplasia has also been reported in dogs, cats and humans, the mechanism of action is unknown, but several have been suggested (Thomason et al. 2009; Kaur et al. 2010; Desmet and van der Meer 2017). Moreover, the effects of neuromuscular blocking agents can be potentiated when calcium channel blockers are administered (Wolf and McGoldrick 2011).

β-Adrenergic Receptor Blockers

β-blockers (e.g. atenolol) may be useful to control heart rate in some tachycardic hypertensive cats (e.g. those with hyperthyroidism), but have negligible antihypertensive effect in such patients and therefore should not be used as a sole agent for the management of hypertension (Henik 1997; Maggio et al. 2000; Henik et al. 2008).

Vasodilators

Vasodilators such as hydralazine, nitroprusside and nitric oxide can be used as an antihypertensive and a description of this class of drugs can be found elsewhere in the book.

Others

Acepromazine

Acepromazine is a phenothiazine commonly used for sedation in many veterinary species. It decreases blood pressure by antagonizing $α_1$-adrenergic receptors. Oral administration could be used to manage hypertensive dogs, at the recommended dose of 0.5–2 mg/kg q8h PO in dogs and cats (Acierno et al. 2018). There are no reports of long-term use, and sedation. A more complete description of acepromazine can be found elsewhere in the book.

Magnesium Sulfate

Magnesium sulfate is commonly used for constipation, magnesium deficiency, torsade de pointe and ventricular tachycardia in small and large animals. Although not commonly used for this purpose, it is important to recognize that magnesium sulfate is also an effective arteriolar dilator with a sympatholytic effect. Multiple mechanisms of action seem to be involved including the blockade of on L-type calcium channels and calcium-dependent potassium channels on the vascular smooth muscle (Murata et al. 2016) and blockade of N-type and L-type calcium channels at adrenergic nerve terminals, hence inhibiting catecholamine release (Nakaigawa et al. 1997; Nakayama et al. 1999; Shimosawa et al. 2004; Elsharnouby and Elsharnouby 2006). The recommended dose for magnesium sulfate is 40 mg/kg followed by a continuous infusion of 15–30 mg/kg/h (Fang et al. 2020)

Diuretics

There is a high incidence of chronic kidney disease in the hypertensive dog population (Acierno et al. 2018), diuretics could cause dehydration, which could have detrimental consequences on this subset of population. Therefore, contrary to human patients, diuretics are not the first-choice drugs for antihypertensive treatment in veterinary patients, but they should be considered in hypertensive animals with a clinically significant volume overload (Acierno et al. 2018; Oparil et al. 2018). In this regard, furosemide, a loop diuretic at a dose of 2–4 mg/kg q12-24 h PO, hydrochlorothiazide, a thiazide diuretic at a dose of 1–4 mg/kg q8-24h PO and spironolactone, an aldosterone antagonist at a dose of 1.0–2.0 mg/kg q12h have been recommended in aiding hypertension treatment in dogs and cats (Acierno et al. 2018). A more complete description of these drugs can be found elsewhere in the book.

References

Abrams, P.H. et al. (1982). Bladder outflow obstruction treated with phenoxybenzamine. *Br. J. Urol.* 54 (5): 527–530. https://doi.org/10.1111/j.1464-410x.1982.tb13581.x.

Acierno, M.J. et al. (2018). ACVIM consensus statement: guidelines for the identification, evaluation, and management of systemic hypertension in dogs and cats. *J. Vet. Intern. Med.* 32 (6): 1803–1822. https://doi.org/10.1111/jvim.15331.

Adams, H.R. (1984). New perspectives in cardiopulmonary therapeutics: receptor-selective adrenergic drugs. *J. Am. Vet. Med. Assoc.* 185 (9): 966–974.

Adams, H.R. (2009). Adrenergic agonists and antagonists. In: *Veterinary Pharmacology and Therapeutics*, 9e (ed. J.E. Riviere and M.G. Papich), 125–155. Wiley: Hoboken, NJ, USA.

Akduman, B. and Crawford, E.D. (2001). Terazosin, doxazosin, and prazosin: current clinical experience. *Urology* 58 (6 Suppl. 1): 49–54. https://doi.org/10.1016/S0090-4295(01)01302-4.

Altman, J.D. et al. (1999). Abnormal regulation of the sympathetic nervous system in α2(a)-adrenergic receptor knockout mice. *Mol. Pharmacol.* 56 (1): 154–161. https://doi.org/10.1124/mol.56.1.154.

Antani, J.A., Antani, N.J., and Nanivadekar, A.S. (1991). Prazosin in chronic congestive heart failure due to ischemic heart disease. *Clin. Cardiol.* 14 (6): 495–500. https://doi.org/10.1002/clc.4960140608.

Aribit, F., Laville, J., and Baron, J. (2000). Extravasation injuries and subcutaneous aspiration in children. *Revue de chirurgie orthopedique et reparatrice de l'appareil moteur* 86 (1): 87–88.

Aronoff, G.R., Bennett, W.M., Berns, J.S., Brier, M.E., Kasbekar, N., Mueller, B.A. et al. (2007). *Drug Prescribing in Renal Failure: Dosing Guidelines for Adults and Children*, 5e (ed. G.R. Aronoff). Philadelphia, USA: American College of Physicians.

Atkins, C.E. et al. (2002). Effects of long-term administration of enalapril on clinical indicators of renal function in dogs with compensated mitral regurgitation. *J. Am. Vet. Med. Assoc.* 221 (5): 654–658. https://doi.org/10.2460/javma.2002.221.654.

Atwell, R.B. (1979). The use of alpha blockade in the treatment of congestive heart failure associated with dirofilariasis and mitral valvular incompetence. *Vet. Rec.* 104 (6): 114–116. https://doi.org/10.1136/vr.104.6.114.

Barnes, K.H., Aulakh, K.S., and Liu, C. (2019). Retrospective evaluation of prazosin and diazepam after thoracolumbar hemilaminectomy in dogs. *Vet. J.* 253: 105377. https://doi.org/10.1016/j.tvjl.2019.105377.

Barsanti, J.A. et al. (1996). Detrusor-sphincter dyssynergia. *Vet. Clin. N. Am. Small Anim. Pract.* 26 (2): 327–338. https://doi.org/10.1016/S0195-5616(96)50213-5.

Bawaskar, H.S. and Bawaskar, P.H. (2011). Efficacy and safety of scorpion antivenom plus prazosin compared with prazosin alone for venomous scorpion (Mesobuthus tamulus) sting: randomised open label clinical trial. *BMJ (Clin. Res. Ed.)* 342: c7136. https://doi.org/10.1136/bmj.c7136.

Benfey, B.G. (1993). Antifibrillatory effects of α1-adrenoceptor blocking drugs in experimental coronary artery occlusion and reperfusion. *Can. J. Physiol. Pharmacol.* 71 (2): 103–111. https://doi.org/10.1139/y93-015.

Bennett, J.K. et al. (2000). Terazosin for vesicosphincter dyssynergia in spinal cord-injured male patients. *Mol. Urol.* 4 (4): 415–420.

Bertrand, M. et al. (2001). Should the angiotensin II antagonists be discontinued before surgery? *Anesth. Analg.* 92 (1): 26–30. https://doi.org/10.1097/00000539-200101000-00006.

Bey, D. et al. (1998). The use of phentolamine in the prevention of dopamine-induced tissue extravasation. *J. Crit. Care* 13 (1): 13–20. https://doi.org/10.1016/S0883-9441(98)90024-7.

Boehringer Ingelheim Vetmedica Inc. (2018). Freedom of Information Summary. https://animaldrugsatfda.fda.gov/adafda/app/search/public/document/downloadFoi/3488 (accessed 30 June 2022).

Boosman, R. and Németh, F. (1988). Pathogenesis and drug therapy of acute laminitis in horses: a literature review. *Tijdschrift voor diergeneeskunde* 113 (22): 1237–1246.

Breslin, D. et al. (1993). Medical management of benign prostatic hyperplasia: a canine model comparing the in vivo efficacy of alpha-1 adrenergic antagonists in the prostate. *J. Urol.* 149 (2): 395–399. https://doi.org/10.1016/s0022-5347(17)36102-5.

Brose, W.G. et al. (1997). Use of intrathecal SNX-111, a novel, N-type, voltage-sensitive, calcium channel blocker, in the management of intractable brachial plexus avulsion pain. *Clin. J. Pain* 13 (3): 256–259. https://doi.org/10.1097/00002508-199709000-00012.

Brown, S.A. et al. (2001). Effects of the angiotensin converting enzyme inhibitor benazepril in cats with induced renal insufficiency. *Am. J. Vet. Res.* 62 (3): 375–383. https://doi.org/10.2460/ajvr.2001.62.375.

Brown, S.A. et al. (2003). Evaluation of the effects of inhibition of angiotensin converting enzyme with enalapril in dogs with induced chronic renal insufficiency. *Am. J. Vet. Res.* 64 (3): 321–327. https://doi.org/10.2460/ajvr.2003.64.321.

Brown, S. et al. (2013). Consensus recommendations for standard therapy of glomerular disease in dogs. *J. Vet. Intern. Med.* 27 (Suppl 1): S27–S43. https://doi.org/10.1111/jvim.12230.

Buerkle, H. and Yaksh, T.L. (1998). Pharmacological evidence for different alpha2-adrenergic receptor sites mediating analgesia and sedation in the rat. *Br. J. Anaesth.* 81 (2): 208–215. https://doi.org/10.1093/bja/81.2.208.

Bugbee, A.C. et al. (2014). Telmisartan treatment of refractory proteinuria in a dog. *J. Vet. Intern. Med.* 28 (6): 1871–1874. https://doi.org/10.1111/jvim.12471.

Burges, R.A., Dodd, M.G., and Gardiner, D.G. (1989). Pharmacologic profile of amlodipine. *Am. J. Cardiol.* 64 (17): https://doi.org/10.1016/0002-9149(89)90956-9.

Caballero, J. (2020). Considerations for docking of selective angiotensin-converting enzyme inhibitors. *Molecules (Basel, Switzerland)* 25 (2): 1–19. https://doi.org/10.3390/molecules25020295.

Caine, M., Pfau, A., and Perlberg, S. (1976). The use of alpha-adrenergic blockers in benign prostatic obstruction. *Br. J. Urol.* 48 (4): 255–263. https://doi.org/10.1111/j.1464-410x.1976.tb03013.x.

Caro-Vadillo, A. et al. (2018). Effect of a combination of telmisartan and amlodipine in hypertensive dogs. *Vet. Rec. Case Rep.* 6 (2): 1–6. https://doi.org/10.1136/vetreccr-2017-000471.

Carruthers, S.G. (1994). Adverse effects of α1-adrenergic blocking drugs. *Drug Saf.* 11 (1): 12–20. https://doi.org/10.2165/00002018-199411010-00003.

Chancellor, M.B., Erhard, M.J., and Rivas, D.A. (1993). Clinical effect of alpha-1 antagonism by terazosin on external and internal urinary sphincter function. *J. Am. Paraplegia Soc.* 16 (4): 207–214. https://doi.org/10.1080/01952307.1993.11735903.

Chen, H. et al. (2010). The North American neuroendocrine tumor society consensus guideline for the diagnosis and management of neuroendocrine tumors: pheochromocytoma, paraganglioma, and medullary thyroid cancer. *Pancreas* 39 (6): 775–783. https://doi.org/10.1097/MPA.0b013e3181ebb4f0.

Chobanian, A.V. et al. (2003). Seventh report of the joint National Committee on prevention, detection, evaluation, and treatment of high blood pressure. *Hypertension* 42 (6): 1206–1252. https://doi.org/10.1161/01.HYP.0000107251.49515.c2.

Christ, D.D. et al. (1994). The pharmacokinetics and pharmacodynamics of the angiotensin II receptor antagonist losartan potassium (DuP 753/MK 954) in the dog. *J. Pharmacol. Exp. Ther.* 268 (3): 1199–1205. https://jpet.aspetjournals.org/content/268/3/1199.

Claborn, L.D. and Szabuniewicz, M. (1973). Prevention of chloroform and thiobarbiturate cardiac sensitization to catecholamines in dogs. *Am. J. Vet. Res.* 34 (6): 801–804.

Clusin, W.T. and Anderson, M.E. (1999). Calcium Channel blockers: current controversies and basic mechanisms of action. *Adv. Pharmacol.* 46 (C): 253–296. https://doi.org/10.1016/S1054-3589(08)60473-1.

Coleman, A.S. et al. (2014). Attenuation of the pressor response to exogenous angiotensin by angiotensin receptor blockers in normal dogs. *J. Vet. Intern. Med.* 28: 976–1134.

Coleman, A.E. et al. (2016a). Effects of orally administered enalapril on blood pressure and hemodynamic response to vasopressors during isoflurane anesthesia in healthy dogs. *Vet. Anaesth. Analg.* 43 (5): 482–494. https://doi.org/10.1111/vaa.12338.

Cooper, B.E. (1989). High-dose phentolamine for extravasation of pressors. *Clin. Pharm.* 8 (10): 689.

Coriat, P. et al. (1994). Influence of chronic angiotensin-converting enzyme inhibition on anesthetic induction. *Anesthesiology* 81 (2): 299–307. https://doi.org/10.1097/00000542-199408000-00006.

D'Amore, A., Black, M.J., and Thomas, W.G. (2005). The angiotensin II type 2 receptor causes constitutive growth of cardiomyocytes and does not antagonize angiotensin II type 1 receptor-mediated hypertrophy. *Hypertension* 46 (6): 1347–1354. https://doi.org/10.1161/01.HYP.0000193504.51489.cf.

Desmet, L. and van der Meer, J. (2017). Antihypertensive treatment with telmisartan in a cat with amlodipine-induced gingival hyperplasia. *J. Feline Med. Surg. Open Rep.* 3 (2): 205511691774523. https://doi.org/10.1177/2055116917745236.

Díaz Espiñeira, M.M., Viehoff, F.W., and Nickel, R.F. (1998). Idiopathic detrusor-urethral dyssynergia in dogs: a retrospective analysis of 22 cases. *J. Small Anim. Pract.* 39 (6): 264–270. https://doi.org/10.1111/j.1748-5827.1998.tb03648.x.

Donohoe, J.M., Combs, A.J., and Glassberg, K.I. (2005). Primary bladder neck dysfunction in children and adolescents II: results of treatment with α-adrenergic antagonists. *J. Urol.* 173 (1): 212–216. https://doi.org/10.1097/01.ju.0000135735.49099.8c.

Eisenberg, B.W. et al. (2013). Evaluation of risk factors associated with recurrent obstruction in cats treated medically for urethral obstruction. *J. Am. Vet. Med. Assoc.* 243 (8): 1140–1146. https://doi.org/10.2460/javma.243.8.1140.

El-Doueihi, R.Z. et al. (2019). Bilateral biochemically silent pheochromocytoma, not silent after all. *Urol. Case Rep.* 24: 100876. https://doi.org/10.1016/j.eucr.2019.100876.

Elliott, E.M., Malouf, A.T., and Catterall, W.A. (1995). Role of calcium channel subtypes in calcium transients in hippocampal CA3 neurons. *J. Neurosci.* 15 (10): 6433–6444. https://doi.org/10.1523/jneurosci.15-10-06433.1995.

Elsharnouby, N.M. and Elsharnouby, M.M. (2006). Magnesium sulphate as a technique of hypotensive anaesthesia. *Br. J. Anaesth.* 96 (6): 727–731. https://doi.org/10.1093/bja/ael085.

Eri, L.M. and Tveter, K.J. (1995). Alpha-blockade in the treatment of symptomatic benign prostatic hyperplasia. *J. Urol.* 154 (3): 923–934.

Ettinger, S.J. et al. (1998). Effects of enalapril maleate on survival of dogs with naturally acquired heart failure. The long-term investigation of veterinary Enalapril (LIVE) study group. *J. Am. Vet. Med. Assoc.* 213 (11): 1573–1577.

Fang, F. et al. (2020). Preoperative Management of Pheochromocytoma and Paraganglioma. *Front. Endocrinol.* 11 (September): 1–10. https://doi.org/10.3389/fendo.2020.586795.

Fischer, J.R., Lane, I.F., and Cribb, A.E. (2003). Urethral pressure profile and hemodynamic effects of phenoxybenzamine and prazosin in non-sedated male beagle dogs. *Can. J. Vet. Res.* 67 (1): 30–38.

Foglar, R. et al. (1995). Use of recombinant alpha 1-adrenoceptors to characterize subtype selectivity of drugs for the treatment of prostatic hypertrophy. *Eur. J. Pharmacol.* 288 (2): 201–207. https://doi.org/10.1016/0922-4106(95)90195-7.

Furukawa, T. et al. (1997). Voltage and pH dependent block of cloned N-type Ca^{2+} channels by amlodipine. *Br. J. Pharmacol.* 121 (6): 1136–1140. https://doi.org/10.1038/sj.bjp.0701226.

Galac, S. and Korpershoek, E. (2017). Pheochromocytomas and paragangliomas in humans and dogs. *Vet. Comp. Oncol.* 15 (4): 1158–1170. https://doi.org/10.1111/vco.12291.

Galey, F.D. et al. (1990). Gamma scintigraphic analysis of the distribution of perfusion of blood in the equine foot during black walnut (*Juglans nigra*)-induced laminitis. *Am. J. Vet. Res.* 51 (4): 688–695.

Glaus, T.M. et al. (2019). Efficacy of long-term oral telmisartan treatment in cats with hypertension: results of a prospective European clinical trial. *J. Vet. Intern. Med.* 33 (2): 413–422. https://doi.org/10.1111/jvim.15394.

Gohil, K. et al. (1994). Neuroanatomical distribution of receptors for a novel voltage-sensitive calcium-channel antagonist, SNX-230 (ω-conopeptide MVIIC). *Brain Res.* 653 (1–2): 258–266. https://doi.org/10.1016/0006-8993(94)90398-0.

Granger, N., Olby, N.J., and Nout-Lomas, Y.S. (2020). Bladder and bowel Management in Dogs with Spinal Cord Injury. *Front. Vet. Sci.* 7 (November): 1–19. https://doi.org/10.3389/fvets.2020.583342.

Groeben, H. et al. (2017). Perioperative α-receptor blockade in phaeochromocytoma surgery: an observational case series. *Br. J. Anaesth.* 118 (2): 182–189. https://doi.org/10.1093/bja/aew392.

Grossman, E., Ironi, A.N., and Messerli, F.H. (1998). Comparative tolerability profile of hypertensive crisis treatments. *Drug Saf.* 19 (2): 99–122. https://doi.org/10.2165/00002018-199819020-00003.

Group CS (1995). Controlled clinical evaluation of Enalapril in dogs with heart failure: results of the cooperative veterinary Enalapril study group the COVE study group.

J. Vet. Intern. Med. 9 (4): 243–252. https://doi.org/10.1111/j.1939-1676.1995.tb01075.x.

Haagsman, A.N. et al. (2013). Comparison of terazosin and prazosin for treatment of vesico-urethral reflex dyssynergia in dogs. *Vet. Rec.* 173 (2): https://doi.org/10.1136/vr.101326.

Hackenberg, R. et al. (2021). Extravasation injuries of the limbs in neonates and children—development of a treatment algorithm. *Deutsches Arzteblatt Int.* 118 (33–34): 547–554. https://doi.org/10.3238/arztebl.m2021.0220.

Halperin, J.L. et al. (2016). Further evolution of the ACC/AHA clinical practice guideline recommendation classification system: a report of the American College of Cardiology/American Heart Association task force on clinical practice guidelines. *J. Am. Coll. Cardiol.* 67 (13): 1572–1574. https://doi.org/10.1016/j.jacc.2015.09.001.

Hamilton, C.A. et al. (1984). The recovery of α-adrenoceptor function and binding sites after phenoxybenzamine – an index of receptor turnover? *Naunyn-Schmiedeberg's Arch. Pharmacol.* 325 (1): 34–41. https://doi.org/10.1007/BF00507051.

Han, J.S. et al. (2018). The change of signaling pathway on the electrical stimulated contraction in streptozotocin-induced bladder dysfunction of rats. *Korean J. Physiol. Pharmacol.* 22 (5): 577–584. https://doi.org/10.4196/kjpp.2018.22.5.577.

Hanssens, M. et al. (1991). Fetal and neonatal effects of treatment with angiotensin-converting enzyme inhibitors in pregnancy. *Obstet. Gynecol.* 78 (1): 128–135.

Helms, S.R. (2007). Treatment of feline hypertension with transdermal amlodipine: a pilot study. *J. Am. Anim. Hosp. Assoc.* 43 (3): 149–156. https://doi.org/10.5326/0430149.

Henik, R. A. (1997) 'Diagnosis and treatment of feline systemic hypertension', *The Compendium on continuing education for the practicing veterinarian (USA)*.

Henik, R.A. et al. (2008). Efficacy of atenolol as a single antihypertensive agent in hyperthyroid cats. *J. Feline Med. Surg.* 10 (6): 577–582. https://doi.org/10.1016/j.jfms.2007.11.008.

Heran, B.S., Galm, B.P., and Wright, J.M. (2012). Blood pressure lowering efficacy of alpha blockers for primary hypertension. *Cochrane Database Syst. Rev.* 8: CD004643. https://doi.org/10.1002/14651858.CD004643.pub3.

Herrera, M.A. et al. (2008). Predictive factors and the effect of phenoxybenzamine on outcome in dogs undergoing adrenalectomy for pheochromocytoma. *J. Vet. Intern. Med.* 22 (6): 1333–1339. https://doi.org/10.1111/j.1939-1676.2008.0182.x.

Hetrick, P.F. and Davidow, E.B. (2013). Initial treatment factors associated with feline urethral obstruction recurrence rate: 192 cases (2004–2010). *J. Am. Vet. Med. Assoc.* 243 (4): 512–519. https://doi.org/10.2460/javma.243.4.512.

Hirning, L.D. et al. (1988). Dominant role of N-type Ca^{2+} channels in evoked release of norepinephrine from sympathetic neurons. *Science* 239 (4835): 57–61. https://doi.org/10.1126/science.2447647.

Hoffman, B. and Lefkowitz, R. (1980). Adrenergic agonists and antagonists. In: *Goodman & Gilman's: The Pharmacological Basis of Therapeutics*, 8e (ed. A.G. Gilman, T.W. Rall, A.S. Nies and P. Taylor), 221–243. New York, NY: Pergamon Press.

Hojo, T. et al. (2020). Refractory hypotension during general anesthesia despite withholding Telmisartan. *Anesth. Prog.* 67 (2): 86–89. https://doi.org/10.2344/anpr-67-02-02.

Hollevoet, I. et al. (2011). Medication in the perioperative period: stop or continue? A review. *Acta Anaesthesiol. Belg.* 62 (4): 193–201.

Hood, D.M., Stephens, K.A., and Bowen, M.J. (1982). Phenoxybenzamine for the treatment of severe nonresponsive diarrhea in the horse. *J. Am. Vet. Med. Assoc.* 180 (7): 758–762.

Hood, D.M. et al. (1993). The role of vascular mechanisms in the development of acute equine laminitis. *J. Vet. Intern. Med.* 7 (4): 228–234. https://doi.org/10.1111/j.1939-1676.1993.tb01012.x.

Hrenak, J., Paulis, L., and Simko, F. (2015). N-acetyl-seryl-aspartyl-lysyl-proline (Ac-SDKP): potential target molecule in research of heart, kidney and brain. *Curr. Pharm. Des.* 21 (35): 5135–5143. https://doi.org/10.2174/1381612821666150909093927.

Huhtinen, M. et al. (2015). Randomized placebo-controlled clinical trial of a chewable formulation of amlodipine for the treatment of hypertension in client-owned cats. *J. Vet. Intern. Med.* 29 (3): 786–793. https://doi.org/10.1111/jvim.12589.

Hull, C.J. (1986). Phaeochromocytoma: diagnosis, preoperative preparation and anaesthetic management. *Br. J. Anaesth.* 58 (12): 1453–1468. https://doi.org/10.1093/bja/58.12.1453.

Hunt, J.M. and Gerring, E.L. (1985). Effect of phenoxybenzamine in a pony with idiopathic diarrhoea. *Equine Vet. J.* 17 (5): 399–400. https://doi.org/10.1111/j.2042-3306.1985.tb02534.x.

Isaacs, M. and Lee, P. (2017). Preoperative alpha-blockade in phaeochromocytoma and paraganglioma: is it always necessary? *Clin. Endocrinol.* 86 (3): 309–314. https://doi.org/10.1111/cen.13284.

Ishikawa, Y. et al. (2007). Effect of isoflurane anesthesia on hemodynamics following the administration of an angiotensin-converting enzyme inhibitor in cats. *J. Vet. Med. Sci.* 69 (8): 869–871. https://doi.org/10.1292/jvms.69.869.

Jaillon, P. et al. (1979). Influence of congestive heart failure on prazosin kinetics. *Clin. Pharmacol. Ther.* 25 (6): 790–794. https://doi.org/10.1002/cpt1979256790.

Janani, M. (2020). Models for predicting efflux transport over the blood-brain barrier (Dissertation). Uppsala University.

Jenkins, T.L. et al. (2015). Attenuation of the pressor response to exogenous angiotensin by angiotensin receptor blockers and benazepril hydrochloride in clinically normal cats. *Am. J. Vet. Res.* 76 (9): 807–813. https://doi.org/10.2460/ajvr.76.9.807.

Jønler, M., Riehmann, M., and Bruskewitz, R.C. (1994). Benign prostatic hyperplasia: current pharmacological treatment. *Drugs* 47 (1): 66–81. https://doi.org/10.2165/00003495-199447010-00005.

Kaur, G. et al. (2010). Association between calcium channel blockers and gingival hyperplasia. *J. Clin. Periodontol.* 37 (7): 625–630. https://doi.org/10.1111/j.1600-051X.2010.01574.x.

Kellar, K.J. et al. (1984). Comparative effects of urapidil, prazosin, and clonidine on ligand binding to central nervous system receptors, arterial pressure, and heart rate in experimental animals. *Am. J. Med.* 77 (4A): 87–95. https://doi.org/10.1016/s0002-9343(84)80042-x.

Kierszenbaum, A.L. (2007). *Histology and Cell Biology: An Introduction to Pathology*, 2e. Maryland Heights, MO: Mosby.

King, J.N. et al. (2006). Tolerability and efficacy of benazepril in cats with chronic kidney disease. *J. Vet. Intern. Med.* 20 (5): 1054–1064. https://doi.org/10.1892/0891-6640(2006)20[1054:TAEOBI]2.0.CO;2.

Kirsten, R. et al. (1998). Clinical pharmacokinetics of vasodilators. Part II. *Clin. Pharmacokinet.* 35 (1): 9–36. https://doi.org/10.2165/00003088-199835010-00002.

Knapp, H.R. and Fitzgerald, G.A. (1984). Hypertensive crisis in prazosin-treated pheochromocytoma. *South. Med. J.* 77 (4): 535–536. https://doi.org/10.1097/00007611-198404000-00038.

Konta, M. et al. (2018). Evaluation of the inhibitory effects of telmisartan on drug-induced renin–angiotensin–aldosterone system activation in normal dogs. *J. Vet. Cardiol.* 20 (5): 376–383. https://doi.org/10.1016/j.jvc.2018.07.009.

Kota, S.K. et al. (2012). Pheochromocytoma: an uncommon presentation of an asymptomatic and biochemically silent adrenal incidentaloma. *Malays. J. Med. Sci.* 19 (2): 86–91.

Kwon, Y.-J. et al. (2018). Successful management of proteinuria and systemic hypertension in a dog with renal cell carcinoma with surgery, telmisartan, and amlodipine. *Can. Vet. J. = La revue veterinaire canadienne* 59 (7): 759–762. http://www.ncbi.nlm.nih.gov/pubmed/30026623.

Kyles, A.E. et al. (2003). Surgical management of adrenal gland tumors with and without associated tumor thrombi in dogs: 40 cases (1994–2001). *J. Am. Vet. Med. Assoc.* 223 (5): 654–662. https://doi.org/10.2460/javma.2003.223.654.

Lafont, M. et al. (2015). Per-operative hemodynamic instability in normotensive patients with incidentally discovered pheochromocytomas. *J. Clin. Endocrinol. Metab.* 100 (2): 417–421. https://doi.org/10.1210/jc.2014-2998.

Lakhlani, P.P. et al. (1997). Substitution of a mutant α2a-adrenergic receptor via "hit and run" gene targeting reveals the role of this subtype in sedative, analgesic, and anesthetic-sparing responses in vivo. *Proc. Natl. Acad. Sci. U.S.A.* 94 (18): 9950–9955. https://doi.org/10.1073/pnas.94.18.9950.

Lameire, N. and Gordts, J. (1986). A pharmacokinetic study of prazosin in patients with varying degrees of chronic renal failure. *Eur. J. Clin. Pharmacol.* 31 (3): 333–337. https://doi.org/10.1007/BF00981133.

Lane, I.F. et al. (2000). Functional urethral obstruction in 3 dogs: clinical and urethral pressure profile findings. *J. Vet. Intern. Med./Am. Coll. Vet. Intern. Med.* 14 (1): 43–49. https://doi.org/10.1111/j.1939-1676.2000.tb01498.x.

Langer, S.Z., Adler-Graschinsky, E., and Giorgi, O. (1977). Physiological significance of α-adrenoceptor-mediated negative feedback mechanism regulating noradrenaline release during nerve stimulation. *Nature* 265 (5595): 648–650. https://doi.org/10.1038/265648a0.

Lavallee, J.O. et al. (2017). Safety of benazepril in 400 azotemic and 110 non-azotemic client-owned cats (2001–2012). *J. Am. Anim. Hosp. Assoc.* 53 (2): 119–127. https://doi.org/10.5326/JAAHA-MS-6577.

Leenen, F.H.H., Ruzicka, M., and Huang, B.S. (2001). Central sympathoinhibitory effects of calcium channel blockers. *Curr. Hypertens. Rep.* 3 (4): 314–321. https://doi.org/10.1007/s11906-001-0094-7.

Lefebvre, H. et al. (2007). Angiotensin-converting enzyme inhibitors in veterinary medicine. *Curr. Pharm. Des.* 13 (13): 1347–1361. https://doi.org/10.2174/138161207780618830.

Lenders, J.W.M. et al. (2014). Pheochromocytoma and paraganglioma: an endocrine society clinical practice guideline. *J. Clin. Endocrinol. Metab.* 99 (6): 1915–1942. https://doi.org/10.1210/jc.2014-1498.

Lepor, H. (1990). Role of long-acting selective alpha-1 blockers in the treatment of benign prostatic hyperplasia. *Urol. Clin. N. Am.* 17 (3): 651–659.

Link, R.E. et al. (1996). Cardiovascular regulation in mice lacking α2-adrenergic receptor subtypes b and c. *Science* 273 (5276): 803–805. https://doi.org/10.1126/science.273.5276.803.

Lourenço, B.N. et al. (2020). Efficacy of telmisartan for the treatment of persistent renal proteinuria in dogs: a double-masked, randomized clinical trial. *J. Vet. Intern. Med.* 34 (6): 2478–2496. https://doi.org/10.1111/jvim.15958.

Lowenthal, D.T. et al. (1980). Prazosin kinetics and effectiveness in renal failure. *Clin. Pharmacol. Ther.* 27 (6): 779–783. https://doi.org/10.1038/clpt.1980.110.

Luther, R.R. et al. (1986). Terazosin: a new alpha 1-blocker for the treatment of hypertension: a review of randomized, controlled clinical trials of once-daily administration as monotherapy. *J. Hypertens. Suppl.* 4 (5): S494–S497.

Lydiatt, C.A., Fee, M.P., and Hill, G.E. (1993). Severe hypotension during epidural anesthesia in a prazosin-treated patient. *Anesth. Analg.* 76 (5): 1152–1153. https://doi.org/10.1213/00000539-199305000-00043.

MacMillan, L.B. et al. (1996). Central hypotensive effects of the alpha2a-adrenergic receptor subtype. *Science (New York, N.Y.)* 273 (5276): 801–803. https://doi.org/10.1126/science.273.5276.801.

Maggio, F. et al. (2000). Ocular lesions associated with systemic hypertension in cats: 69 cases (1985–1998). *J. Am. Vet. Med. Assoc.* 217 (5): 695–702. https://doi.org/10.2460/javma.2000.217.695.

Maher, J. and McNiel, E.A. (1997). Pheochromocytoma in dogs and cats. *Vet. Clin. N. Am. Small Anim. Pract.* 27 (2): 359–380. https://doi.org/10.1016/s0195-5616(97)50037-4.

Massingham, R. and Hayden, M.L. (1975). A comparison of the effects of prazosin and hydrallazine on blood pressure, heart rate and plasma renin activity in conscious renal hypertensive dogs. *Eur. J. Pharmacol.* 30 (1): 121–124. https://doi.org/10.1016/0014-2999(75)90213-7.

McMillian, W.D. et al. (2011). Phentolamine continuous infusion in a patient with pheochromocytoma. *Am. J. Health-Syst. Pharm.* 68 (2): 130–134. https://doi.org/10.2146/ajhp090619.

Mercury Pharmaceuticals Ltd [FDA Label] (2021). Dibenyline® (Phenoxybenzamine hydrochloride capsules) 10mg.

Merin, R.G. (1987). Calcium channel blocking drugs and anesthetics: is the drug interaction beneficial or detrimental? *Anesthesiology* 66 (2): 111–113.

Mets, B. (2015). To stop or not? *Anesth. Analg.* 120 (6): 1413–1419. https://doi.org/10.1213/ANE.0000000000000758.

Mignat, C. and Unger, T. (1995). ACE inhibitors: drug interactions of clinical significance. *Drug Saf.* 12 (5): 334–347. https://doi.org/10.2165/00002018-199512050-00005.

Misra, S. and Stevermer, J.J. (2009). ACE inhibitors and ARBs: one or the other – not both – for high-risk patients. *J. Fam. Pract.* 58 (1): 24–28.

Mizutani, H. et al. (2006). Evaluation of the clinical efficacy of benazepril in the treatment of chronic renal insufficiency in cats. *J. Vet. Intern. Med.* 20 (5): 1074–1079. https://doi.org/10.1892/0891-6640(2006)20[1074:EOTCEO]2.0.CO;2.

Moreau, P.M. (1982). Neurogenic disorders of micturition in the dog and cat. *Compend. Contin. Educ. Pract. Vet.* 4: 12–21.

Mulvihill-Wilson, J. et al. (n.d.). Comparative effects of prazosin and phenoxybenzamine on arterial blood pressure, heart rate, and plasma catecholamines in essential hypertension. *J. Cardiovasc. Pharmacol.* 1 (6 Suppl): S1–S7. http://www.ncbi.nlm.nih.gov/pubmed/94635.

Murata, T. et al. (2016). Mechanisms of magnesium-induced vasodilation in cerebral penetrating arterioles. *Neurosci. Res.* 107 (12): 57–62. https://doi.org/10.1016/j.neures.2015.12.005.

Murrell, J.C. (2017). Adrenergic agents. In: *Veterinary Anesthesia and Analgesia, The 5th of Lumb and Jones*, 5e (ed. K.A. Grimm, L.A. Lamont, W.J. Tranquilli, et al.), 183–195. Hoboken, NJ, USA: Wiley.

Myklejord, D.J. (2004). Undiagnosed pheochromocytoma: the anesthesiologist nightmare. *Clin. Med. Res.* 2 (1): 59–62. http://www.pubmedcentral.nih.gov/articlerender.fcgi?artid=1069072&tool=pmcentrez&rendertype=abstract.

Nabbi, R., Woehlck, H.J., and Riess, M.L. (2013). Case report: refractory hypotension during general anesthesia despite preoperative discontinuation of an angiotensin receptor blocker. *F1000Research* 2: 12. https://doi.org/10.12688/f1000research.2-12.v1.

Nakaigawa, Y. et al. (1997). Effects of magnesium sulphate on the cardiovascular system, coronary circulation and myocardial metabolism in anaesthetized dogs. *Br. J. Anaesth.* 79 (3): 363–368. https://doi.org/10.1093/bja/79.3.363.

Nakamura, R. et al. (2018). Changes in renal peritubular capillaries in canine and feline chronic kidney disease. *J. Comp. Pathol.* 160: 79–83. https://doi.org/10.1016/j.jcpa.2018.03.004.

Nakayama, T. et al. (1999). Hemodynamic and electrocardiographic effects of magnesium sulfate in healthy dogs. *J. Vet. Intern. Med./Am. Coll. Vet. Intern. Med.* 13 (5): 485–490. https://doi.org/10.1111/j.1939-1676.1999.tb01467.x.

Naranjo, J., Dodd, S., and Martin, Y.N. (2017). Perioperative management of pheochromocytoma. *J. Cardiothor. Vasc. Anesth.* 31 (4): 1427–1439. https://doi.org/10.1053/j.jvca.2017.02.023.

Neumann, H.P.H., Young, W.F., and Eng, C. (2019). Pheochromocytoma and paraganglioma. *N. Engl. J. Med.* 381 (6): 552–565. https://doi.org/10.1056/nejmra1806651.

Nicholson, J.P. et al. (1983). Pheochromocytoma and prazosin. *Ann. Intern. Med.* 99 (4): 477–479. https://doi.org/10.7326/0003-4819-99-4-477.

Nickerson, M. (1962). Mechanism of the prolonged adrenergic blockade produced by haloalkylamines. *Archives internationales de pharmacodynamie et de therapie* 140: 237–250.

Oates, H.F., Graham, R.M., and Stokes, G.S. (1977). Mechanism of the hypotensive action of prazosin. *Archives internationales de pharmacodynamie et de*

therapie 227 (1): 41–48. http://europepmc.org/abstract/MED/901072.

Oliver, J.E. (1983). Dysuria caused by reflex dyssynergia. In: *Current Veterinary Therapy XIII* (ed. R. Kirk), 1088. WB Saunders: Philadelphia, USA.

Oparil, S. et al. (2018). Hypertension. *Nat. Rev. Dis. Primers* 4 (4): 18014. https://doi.org/10.1038/nrdp.2018.14.

Özalp Gerçeker, G. et al. (2018). Infiltration and extravasation in pediatric patients: a prevalence study in a children's hospital. *J. Vasc. Access* 19 (3): 266–271. https://doi.org/10.1177/1129729817747532.

Pandi, K. et al. (2014). Efficacy of scorpion antivenom plus prazosin versus prazosin alone for Mesobuthus tamulus scorpion sting envenomation in children: a randomised controlled trial. *Arch. Dis. Childh.* 99 (6): 575–580. https://doi.org/10.1136/archdischild-2013-305483.

Papich, M.G. (2021). Phenoxybenzamine hydrochloride. In: *Papich Handbook of Veterinary Drugs (Fifth Edition)*, 5e (ed. M.G. Papich), 723–725. St. Louis (MO): W.B. Saunders https://doi.org/10.1016/B978-0-323-70957-6.00419-2.

Peberdy, M.A. et al. (2010). Part 9: Post-cardiac arrest care: 2010 American Heart Association guidelines for cardiopulmonary resuscitation and emergency cardiovascular care. *Circulation* 122 (Suppl. 3): 768–786. https://doi.org/10.1161/CIRCULATIONAHA.110.971002.

Plum, M. and Moukhachen, O. (2017). Alternative pharmacological management of vasopressor extravasation in the absence of phentolamine. *P T* 42 (9): 581–586.

Poirier, M. et al. (1988). Effects of five alpha-blockers on the hypogastric nerve stimulation of the canine lower urinary tract. *J. Urol.* 140 (1): 165–167. https://doi.org/10.1016/S0022-5347(17)41519-9.

Portoghese, P.S., Riley, T.N., and Miller, J.W. (1971). Stereochemical studies on medicinal agents. 10. The role of chirality in alpha-adrenergic receptor blockage by (plus)-and(minus)-phenoxybenzamine hydrochloride. *J. Med. Chem.* 14 (17): 561–564. https://doi.org/10.1021/jm00289a001.

Ramachandran, R. and Rewari, V. (2016). Preoperative optimization in pheochromocytoma: phenoxybenzamine may be redundant but not alpha blockade. *Can. J. Anesth.* 63 (5): 629. https://doi.org/10.1007/s12630-015-0557-y.

Ramage, A.G. (1984). The effect of prazosin, indoramin and phentolamine on sympathetic nerve activity. *Eur. J. Pharmacol.* 106 (3): 507–513. https://doi.org/10.1016/0014-2999(84)90054-2.

Reineke, E.L. et al. (2017). The effect of prazosin on outcome in feline urethral obstruction. *J. Vet. Emerg. Crit. Care* 27 (4): 387–396. https://doi.org/10.1111/vec.12611.

Reist, C. et al. (2021). Prazosin for treatment of post-traumatic stress disorder: a systematic review and meta-analysis. *CNS Spectr.* 26 (4): 338–344. https://doi.org/10.1017/S1092852920001121.

Reynolds, P.M. et al. (2014). Management of extravasation injuries: a focused evaluation of noncytotoxic medications. *Pharmacotherapy* 34 (6): 617–632. https://doi.org/10.1002/phar.1396.

Roshanov, P.S. et al. (2017). Withholding versus continuing angiotensin-converting enzyme inhibitors or angiotensin II receptor blockers before noncardiac surgery: an analysis of the vascular events in noncardiac surgery patIents cOhort evaluatioN prospective cohort. *Anesthesiology* 126 (1): 16–27. https://doi.org/10.1097/ALN.0000000000001404.

Rosin, A.H. and Ross, L. (1981). Diagnosis and pharmacological management of disorders of urinary continence in the dog. *Compend. Contin. Educ. Pract. Vet.* 3 (7): 601–610.

Roudebush, P. et al. (1994). The effect of combined therapy with captopril, furosemide, and a sodium-restricted diet on serum electrolyte concentrations and renal function in normal dogs and dogs with congestive heart failure. *J. Vet. Intern. Med.* 8 (5): 337–342. https://doi.org/10.1111/j.1939-1676.1994.tb03246.x.

Rubin, P. et al. (1979). Prazosin first-pass metabolism and hepatic extraction in the dog. *J. Cardiovasc. Pharmacol.* 1 (6): 641–647. https://doi.org/10.1097/00005344-197911000-00005.

Russell, W.J. et al. (1998). The preoperative management of phaeochromocytoma. *Anaesth. Intensive Care* 26 (2): 196–200. https://doi.org/10.1177/0310057x9802600212.

Saeed, M. et al. (1982). Alpha-adrenoceptor blockade by phentolamine causes beta-adrenergic vasodilation by increased catecholamine release due to presynaptic alpha-blockade. *J. Cardiovasc. Pharmacol.* 4 (1): 44–52. https://doi.org/10.1097/00005344-198201000-00008.

Sahloul, M.Z. et al. (1990). Nonsteroidal anti-inflammatory drugs and antihypertensives. Cooperative malfeasance. *Nephron* 56 (4): 345–352. https://doi.org/10.1159/000186173.

Schenker, J.G. and Chowers, I. (1971). Pheochromocytoma and pregnancy. Review of 89 cases. *Obst. Gynecol. Surv.* 26 (11): 739–747. https://doi.org/10.1097/00006254-197111000-00001.

Schenker, J.G. and Granat, M. (1982). Phaeochromocytoma and pregnancy — an updated appraisal. *Aust. N. Z. J. Obst. Gynaecol.* 22 (1): 1–10. https://doi.org/10.1111/j.1479-828X.1982.tb01388.x.

Schierok, H. et al. (2001). Effects of telmisartan on renal excretory function in conscious dogs. *J. Int. Med. Res.* 29 (2): 131–139. https://doi.org/10.1177/147323000102900210.

Schlanz, K.D., Myre, S.A., and Bottorff, M.B. (1991). Pharmacokinetic interactions with calcium channel antagonists (part II). *Clin. Pharmacokinet.* 21 (6): 448–460. https://doi.org/10.2165/00003088-199121060-00005.

Schnermann, J. and Castrop, H. (2013). Function of the juxtaglomerular apparatus: control of glomerular hemodynamics and renin secretion. In: *Seldin and Giebisch's the Kidney*, 5e (ed. R. Alpern, O. Moe and M. Caplan), 757–801. Academic Press.

Seelig, C.B., Maloley, P.A., and Campbell, J.R. (1990). Nephrotoxicity associated with concomitant ACE inhibitor and NSAID therapy. *South. Med. J.* 1144–1148. https://doi.org/10.1097/00007611-199010000-00007.

Sent, U. et al. (2015). Comparison of efficacy of long-term oral treatment with Telmisartan and benazepril in cats with chronic kidney disease. *J. Vet. Intern. Med.* 29 (6): 1479–1487. https://doi.org/10.1111/jvim.13639.

Septodont Inc [FDA Label] (2016). OraVerse™ (Phentolamine Mesylate) Injection.

Shao, Y. et al. (2011). Preoperative alpha blockade for normotensive pheochromocytoma: is it necessary? *J. Hypertens.* 29 (12): 2429–2432. https://doi.org/10.1097/HJH.0b013e32834d24d9.

Shimosawa, T. et al. (2004). Magnesium inhibits norepinephrine release by blocking N-type calcium channels at peripheral sympathetic nerve endings. *Hypertension* 44 (6): 897–902. https://doi.org/10.1161/01.HYP.0000146536.68208.84.

Shionoiri, H. (1993). Pharmacokinetic drug interactions with ACE inhibitors. *Clin. Pharmacokinet.* 25 (1): 20–58. https://doi.org/10.2165/00003088-199325010-00003.

Simpson, T.L. et al. (2015). A pilot trial of prazosin, an alpha-1 adrenergic antagonist, for comorbid alcohol dependence and posttraumatic stress disorder. *Alcohol.: Clin. Exp. Res.* 39 (5): 808–817. https://doi.org/10.1111/acer.12703.

Singal, T., Dhalla, N.S., and Tappia, P.S. (2004). Phospholipase C may be involved in norepinephrine-induced cardiac hypertrophy. *Biochem. Biophys. Res. Commun.* 320 (3): 1015–1019. https://doi.org/10.1016/j.bbrc.2004.06.052.

Sisson, D.D. (1995). Acute and short-term hemodynamic, echocardiography, and clinical effects of Enalapril maleate in dogs with naturally acquired heart failure: results of the invasive multicenter PROspective veterinary evaluation of Enalapril study: the IMPROVE study group. *J. Vet. Intern. Med.* 9 (4): 234–242. https://doi.org/10.1111/j.1939-1676.1995.tb01074.x.

Skytte, D. and Schmökel, H. (2018). Relationship of preoperative neurologic score with intervals to regaining micturition and ambulation following surgical treatment of thoracolumbar disk herniation in dogs. *J. Am. Vet. Med. Assoc.* 253 (2): 196–200. https://doi.org/10.2460/javma.253.2.196.

Soffer, R.L. (1976). Angiotensin converting enzyme and the regulation of vasoactive peptides. *Annu. Rev. Biochem.* 45 (4): 73–94. https://doi.org/10.1146/annurev.bi.45.070176.000445.

Song, G. et al. (2011). Risk of catecholamine crisis in patients undergoing resection of unsuspected pheochromocytoma. *Int. Braz. J. Urol.* 37 (1): 35–40. discussion 40–1. https://doi.org/10.1590/s1677-55382011000100005.

Spencer, S. (2020). Management of hypertension in dogs. In: *Hypertension in the Dog and Cat*, 1e (ed. J. Elliott, H.M. Syme and R.E. Jepson), 331–367. Cham: Springer International Publishing https://doi.org/10.1007/978-3-030-33020-0_13.

Staedtke, V. et al. (2018). Disruption of a self-amplifying catecholamine loop reduces cytokine release syndrome. *Nature* 564 (7735): 273–277. https://doi.org/10.1038/s41586-018-0774-y.

Stewart, J.R. et al. (1980). Electrophysiologic and antiarrhythmic effects of Phentolamine in experimental coronary artery occlusion and reperfusion in the dog. *J. Cardiovasc. Pharmacol.* 2 (1): 77–92. https://doi.org/10.1097/00005344-198001000-00009.

Stopher, D.A. et al. (1988). The metabolism and pharmacokinetics of amlodipine in humans and animals. *J. Cardiovasc. Pharmacol.* 12 Suppl. 7: S55–S59. https://doi.org/10.1097/00005344-198812007-00012.

Suh, H.W. et al. (1997). Effects of intrathecal injection of nimodipine, ω-conotoxin GVIA, calmidazolium, and KN-62 on the antinociception induced by cold water swimming stress in the mouse. *Brain Res.* 767 (1): 144–147. https://doi.org/10.1016/S0006-8993(97)00702-6.

Taddei, S. and Bortolotto, L. (2016). Unraveling the pivotal role of bradykinin in ACE inhibitor activity. *Am. J. Cardiovasc. Drugs* 16 (5): 309–321. https://doi.org/10.1007/s40256-016-0173-4.

Tavares, M. et al. (2008). Reversal of soft-tissue local anesthesia with phentolamine mesylate in pediatric patients. *J. Am. Dent.Assoc.* 139 (8): 1095–1104. https://doi.org/10.14219/jada.archive.2008.0312.

Taylor, J.A., Twomey, T.M., and Schach Von Wittenau, M. (1977). The metabolic fate of prazosin. *Xenobiotica* 7 (6): 357–364. https://doi.org/10.3109/00498257709035794.

Thomason, J.D. et al. (2009). Gingival hyperplasia associated with the administration of amlodipine to dogs with degenerative valvular disease (2004–2008). *J. Vet. Intern. Med.* 23 (1): 39–42. https://doi.org/10.1111/j.1939-1676.2008.0212.x.

Toal, C.B., Meredith, P.A., and Elliott, H.L. (2012). Long-acting dihydropyridine calcium-channel blockers and sympathetic nervous system activity in hypertension: a literature review comparing amlodipine and nifedipine GITS. *Blood Press.* 21 (Suppl. 1): 3–10. https://doi.org/10.3109/08037051.2012.690615.

Tom, B. et al. (2002). Bradykinin potentiation by ACE inhibitors: a matter of metabolism. *Br. J. Pharmacol.* 137 (2): 276–284. https://doi.org/10.1038/sj.bjp.0704862.

Uechi, M. et al. (2007). Effects of isoflurane anesthesia on hemodynamics following administration of an angiotensin-converting enzyme inhibitor in dogs. *J. Vet. Int. Med.* 634.

Vardanyan, R.S. and Hruby, V.J. (2006). Adrenoblocking drugs. *Synth. Essent. Drugs* 161–177. https://doi.org/10.1016/b978-044452166-8/50012-1.

Vincent, J. et al. (1985). Clinical pharmacokinetics of prazosin – 1985. *Clin. Pharmacokinet.* 10 (2): 144–154. https://doi.org/10.2165/00003088-198510020-00002.

Wachtel, H. et al. (2015). Preoperative Metyrosine improves cardiovascular outcomes for patients undergoing surgery for Pheochromocytoma and Paraganglioma. *Ann. Surg. Oncol.* 22: 646–654. https://doi.org/10.1245/s10434-015-4862-z.

WellSpring Pharmaceutical Corporation [FDA Label] (2008). *DIBENZYLINE® (Phenoxybenzamine Hydrochloride Capsules USP) 10mg*. FL: Bradenton https://www.accessdata.fda.gov/drugsatfda_docs/label/2008/008708s025lbl.pdf (

Westenbroek, R.E. et al. (1992). Biochemical properties and subcellular distribution of an N-type calcium channel alpha 1 subunit. *Neuron* 9 (6): 1099–1115. https://doi.org/10.1016/0896-6273(92)90069-p.

West-Ward Pharmaceuticals Corp [FDA Label] (2018). Phentolamine Mesylate Injection.

Wienen, W. et al. (2000). A review on telmisartan: a novel, long-acting angiotensin II-receptor antagonist. *Cardiovasc. Drug Rev.* 18 (2): 127–154. https://doi.org/10.1111/j.1527-3466.2000.tb00039.x.

Wiersig, D.O., Davis, R.H.J., and Szabuniewicz, M. (1974). Prevention of induced ventricular fibrillation in dogs anesthetized with ultrashort acting barbiturates and halothane. *J. Am. Vet. Med. Assoc.* 165 (4): 341–345.

Wimpole, J.A. et al. (2010). Plasma free metanephrines in healthy cats, cats with non-adrenal disease and a cat with suspected phaeochromocytoma. *J. Feline Med. Surg.* 12 (6): 435–440. https://doi.org/10.1016/j.jfms.2009.10.010.

Wolf, A. and McGoldrick, K.E. (2011). Cardiovascular pharmacotherapeutic considerations in patients undergoing anesthesia. *Cardiol. Rev.* 19 (1): 12–16. https://doi.org/10.1097/CRD.0b013e3182000e11.

Yu, M. et al. (2018). Clinical effects of prophylactic use of phentolamine in patients undergoing pheochromocytoma surgery. *J. Clin. Anesth.* 44: 119. https://doi.org/10.1016/j.jclinane.2017.11.030.

Zhu, Y. et al. (2010). Selective α1-adrenoceptor antagonist (controlled release tablets) in preoperative management of pheochromocytoma. *Endocrine* 38 (2): 254–259. https://doi.org/10.1007/s12020-010-9381-x.

20

Antiarrhythmic Therapies and Calcium Channel Blockers
Lance C. Visser

Introduction

Cardiac arrhythmias are common in the perianesthetic period. Therefore, when considering treatment, detailed knowledge of the pharmacologic properties of antiarrhythmic drugs is vital for successful management of anesthetized patients. A practical approach to choosing antiarrhythmic therapy incorporates knowledge of the drug's mechanism of action, known clinical efficacy, pharmacokinetics, adverse effects, drug interactions, and hemodynamic effects. However, deciding if/when to intervene is perhaps just as important as choosing which antiarrhythmic drug to intervene with. This decision should always be tailored to the individual patient. In the author's opinion, this decision should be primarily based on clinical signs and functional/hemodynamic consequences of the arrhythmia and not necessarily based on the quantity or morphology of the abnormal beats. In human medicine, there is a noticeable trend toward avoiding antiarrhythmic drug therapy, primarily due to proarrhythmic and sudden death risk, and thus implantable devices and ablation therapy are on the rise (Nattel et al. 2013). It is ultimately unknown whether veterinary medicine will follow suit, but drug therapy currently remains the most clinically feasible option and will likely remain so in the perianesthetic period. This chapter will specifically discuss antiaarrhythmic therapies in addition to the more vascular selective (dihydropyridine [DHP]) calcium channel blockers (CCBs).

General Properties of Antiarrhythmic Drugs

Classification of Antiarrhythmic Drugs

Drugs used for the management of tachyarrhythmias are traditionally classified according to the Vaughn-Williams classification scheme, which categorizes a drug into one of four major classes based on its blocking effects of cardiac sodium (class I), potassium (class III), and calcium channels (class IV), and β-adrenergic receptors (class II) (Table 20.1). Unfortunately, the Vaughn-Williams classification scheme significantly oversimplifies drug effects. Antiarrhythmic drug effects are often complex and depend on numerous factors such as tissue type, degree of acute or chronic tissue injury, heart rate, membrane potential, ionic composition of the extracellular space, and genetics (Miller and Zipes 2012). An alternate, more elaborate classification scheme (Sicilian gambit classification) was created and is based on arrhythmogenic mechanism and vulnerable parameters of arrhythmias for which drugs may be selected (European Society of Cardiology 1991). However, the arrhythmogenic mechanism (i.e. triggered activity, enhanced automaticity, or reentry) is rarely determined with certainty in veterinary species. Thus, current classification schemes may not provide ideal guidance in determining which drug to select to treat a specific cardiac arrhythmia. Some prefer an alternate division of drugs used chiefly in the therapy of supraventricular tachyarrhythmias (e.g. diltiazem) and those used predominantly for ventricular tachyarrhythmias (e.g. lidocaine) (Nattel et al. 2013). Yet, this classification is also flawed by oversimplification of drug effects. Due to its simplicity and usefulness for communication, the Vaughn-Williams classification scheme will be used throughout this chapter.

Use Dependence

Some antiarrhythmic drugs exhibit greater antiarrhythmic effect at higher heart rates and prolonged periods of stimulation, a drug characteristic called use dependence (Miller and Zipes 2012). This is a desirable trait in the setting of managing tachyarrhythmias, as the higher the heart rate, the more life-threatening a tachyarrhythmia tends to be.

Pharmacology in Veterinary Anesthesia and Analgesia, First Edition. Edited by Turi Aarnes and Phillip Lerche.
© 2024 John Wiley & Sons, Inc. Published 2024 by John Wiley & Sons, Inc.

Table 20.1 Drugs used for treatment of tachyarrhythmias.

Class	MOA[a]	Drug	Clinical use	Dose	Hemodynamic effects	Half-life (hours)	Elimination	Adverse effects
IA	++Na⁺-blocker; Prolongs RT	Quinidine	SVA (and VA)	H: 0.5–2 mg/kg quinidine gluconate IV; 0.1–0.2 mcg/kg/min CRI 22 mg/kg quinidine sulfate PO by NGT, don't exceed six doses PO q2	++Cardiodepressant; vasodilation	H: 6–8	Liver	Numerous, GI upset, proarrhythmia
		Procainamide	VA and SVA	D: 4–10 mg/kg IV slow; 25–50 mcg/kg/min CRI C: 1–2 mg/kg IV slow; 10–20 mcg/kg/min H: 1 mg/kg/min, up to 20 mg/kg total dose	+Cardiodepressant; vasodilation	D, H: 3	Kidney	See quinidine (less frequent)
IB	+Na⁺-blocker of diseased tissue; Shortens RT	Lidocaine	VA	D: 2 mg/kg IV; 50–100 mcg/kg/min CRI C: 0.2–1 mg/kg IV; 10–15 mcg/kg/min CRI H: 0.25–0.5 mg/kg IV slow, 0.02–0.05 mg/kg/min CRI	Minimal; prolonged clearance; cardiodepressant in cats	D, H: 1 C: 1.5	Liver	Nausea, GI upset, neurologic (C and H are sensitive)
		Mexiletine	VA	D: 4–6 mg/kg PO q8	Minimal	D: 4–7	Liver	See lidocaine
		Phenytoin	VA	H: 5–10 mg/kg IV	Minimal	H: 8	Liver	Excitement, recumbency (H)
IC	+++ Na⁺-blocker; Unchanged RT	Flecainide	SVA (and VA)	D: 1–2 mg/kg PO q8–12 H: 1–2 mg/kg IV at 0.2 mg/kg/min or 4 mg/kg PO q2 for 4–6 doses	++Cardiodepressant	H: 4–5	Kidney	Proarrhythmia, sudden death
		Propafenone	SVA (and VA)	H: 0.5–2 mg/kg in 5% dextrose IV slow	++Cardiodepressant	H: 1–2	Liver	Proarrhythmia

(Continued)

Table 20.1 (Continued)

Class	MOA[a]	Drug	Clinical use	Dose	Hemodynamic effects	Half-life (hours)	Elimination	Adverse effects
II	+++Beta-blockers	Propranolol	SVA (and VA)	D and C: 0.02–0.06 mg/kg IV slow H: 0.03–0.1 mg/kg IV slow	+++Cardiodepressant	D, H: 1–2	Liver	Hypoglycemia, bronchial constriction, cardiodepressant
		Esmolol	SVA (and VA)	D and C: 0.05–0.2 mg/kg IV; 50–200 mcg/kg/min CRI		D, C: 10 min	Plasma esterases	Cardiodepressant
		Atenolol	SVA	D and C: 0.2–1 mg/kg PO q12		D, C: 4–5	Kidney	
		Metoprolol	SVA				Liver	
III	+++K+-blocker	Amiodarone	SVA and VA	D: 3–5 mg/kg IV slow H: 5 mg/kg IV over 1 hr, then 0.83 mg/kg over 23 hrs	Minimal/+cardiodepressant	D, H: 60	Liver	Numerous (see text)
		Sotalol	VA (and SVA)	D and C: 1–3 mg/kg PO q12	Minimal/+cardiodepressant	D: 5	Kidney	Rare, proarrhythmia
IV	Nodal Ca²⁺-blocker	Diltiazem	SVA	D and C: 0.1–0.2 mg/kg IV slow; 1–4 mcg/kg/min; H: 0.125 mg/kg IV slow	++Cardiodepressant; vasodilation	D, C: 2–3 H: 1.5	Liver	Cardiodepressant
Other	Na⁺-K⁺ pump blocker; vagomimetic	Digoxin	SVA + HF	D: 0.003 mg/kg PO q12 H: 0.0022 mg/kg IV q12	Bradycardia	D: 15–50 H:17–20	Kidney	GI upset, proarrhythmia

MOA = mechanism of action; + = mild potency; ++ = moderate potency; +++ = marked potency; RT = repolarization time; SVA = supraventricular tachyarrhythmias; VA = ventricular tachyarrhythmias; HF = heart failure; D = dog; C = cat; H = horse (refer to the text for other species); GI = gastrointestinal; CRI = constant rate infusion; NGT = nasogastric tube.
[a]Drug mechanisms are oversimplified. Refer to the text for details and additional effects.

During times of slower heart rates, a greater proportion of receptors become drug free. Use dependence correlates with the rapidity of onset–offset kinetics of drug binding to its receptor, which accounts for some of the differences among sodium channel blocking drugs (class I).

Reverse use dependence is also possible and occurs when a drug exhibits a greater antiarrhythmic effect at slower heart rates. This may be an undesirable trait because the antiarrhythmic effect is lessened during tachycardia. Reverse use dependence often occurs in drugs that prolong repolarization (e.g. sotalol).

Proarrhythmia

Virtually all antiarrhythmic drugs have the potential to induce or exacerbate cardiac arrhythmias (proarrhythmia) (Anderson 1990). Although the frequency of proarrhythmia is unknown in veterinary species, 5–10% of humans receiving antiarrhythmic drugs experience proarrhythmic events (Miller and Zipes 2012). Circumstances that may increase the likelihood of proarrhythmia, include high doses of antiarrhythmic drugs, congestive heart failure, high-dose diuretics, depressed myocardial function, hypokalemia or hypomagnesemia (Moise 1999). Some of the sodium (class I) and potassium (class III) channel blocking drugs have the greatest likelihood of inducing tachyarrhythmias and proarrhythmic sudden death, whereas the beta-blockers (class II) and CCBs (class IV) may induce bradyarrhythmias.

Class I Antiarrhythmic Drugs

The class I antiarrhythmic drugs chiefly block fast sodium channels decreasing sodium influx during phase 0 of the action potential. This reduces the rate of rise of action potential upstroke (V_{max}), which thereby decreases conduction velocity. These drugs work best in cells dependent on fast sodium channels for their action potential, i.e. non-nodal tissue, including normal and ischemic Purkinje cells and myocardial tissue. Many of the drugs in this class are local anesthetics and most fail to function adequately in the setting of hypokalemia. Class I drugs are subclassified (IA, IB, IC) according to their effects on repolarization.

Class IA Drugs

In addition to reducing conduction velocity in normal and abnormal cardiac tissue (class I effect), these agents also lengthen action potential duration by prolonging repolarization (class III effect). This mild class III effect lengthens the effective (or absolute) refractory period during which no stimuli can evoke an action potential. Many drugs within this subclass also possess a vagolytic effect. The kinetics of onset-offset sodium channel blocking is considered intermediate (seconds) within this subclass (Miller and Zipes 2012).

Quinidine

Mechanism of action – Quinidine is considered the prototypical class IA antiarrhythmic drug and produces a profound decrease in sodium influx through fast sodium channels during phase 0 of the action potential. This results in a decrease in cardiac electrical impulse conduction velocity. Quinidine also prolongs action potential duration (class III effect), which results in a marked prolongation of the effective refractory period. It is important to note that quinidine's antiarrhythmic efficacy is highly dependent on serum potassium concentrations. Hyperkalemia decreases resting membrane potential, which reduces sodium transmembrane conductance and the conduction velocity of the action potential. Thus, quinidine's effect of reducing impulse conduction is enhanced in the setting of hyperkalemia. Conversely, hypokalemia counteracts the depressant effects of quinidine on conduction velocity. Quinidine antagonizes cholinergic receptors (vagolytic effect), which may increase sinus node automaticity and AV node conduction. This is particularly important when considering quinidine for treatment of atrial fibrillation (see clinical use), as ventricular rate may markedly increase. Pre-treatment with drugs to slow AV node conduction can be considered.

Pharmacokinetics and metabolism – Quinidine is available in oral and intravenous (IV) formulations, although the oral formulation is most frequently utilized. Species–specific pharmacokinetic data is available for the dog (Clohisy and Gibson 1982; Neff et al. 1972), rabbit (Ueda and Nickols 1980), horse (McGuirk et al. 1981b), and cow (McGuirk et al. 1981a). Quinidine is highly (>80%) protein-bound and has a large volume of distribution. Its oral formulation is rapidly absorbed and reaches peak effect within one to two hours of administration. In dogs, it has a half-life of five to six hours and reaches steady state in approximately 24 hours (Neff et al. 1972; Clohisy and Gibson 1982). Reported serum half-lives in other species include six to eight hours in horses, five to six hours in pigs, approximately one hour in goats, and two hours in cows, cats, and rabbits (Plumb 2008). It is partially excreted by the kidneys and metabolized by the liver.

Clinical use – Quinidine can be utilized to treat supraventricular or ventricular arrhythmias. In small animal species, its clinical use is rare due to the availability of safer and more effective alternatives. However, in large animal species, it is often a first-line therapy for supraventricular tachyarrhythmias (e.g. atrial fibrillation) and, in some cases, ventricular tachyarrhythmias (Boon 2011). Oral (via nasogastric tube) or IV formulations may be used in horses, whereas IV administration is solely used in cattle (Reef and McGuirk 2009).

Effect on patients under general anesthesia – Quinidine can have profound hemodynamic effects when administered at therapeutic doses, which may affect a patient's cardiovascular status, particularly under general anesthesia. These effects include decreased contractility, vasodilatation, and hypotension, and may be exacerbated in patients with underlying cardiac disease or heart failure. The vasodilatory effects of quinidine are mediated by α1- and α2-adrenergic receptors (Schmid et al. 1974).

Side (other) effects – Side effects are well documented in dogs and horses and can potentially be extrapolated to other species. Side effects include gastrointestinal (GI) upset (colic, diarrhea, inappetence), ataxia, weakness, or signs of hypersensitivity reaction such as swelling of the nasal mucosa and upper airways (horses) and urticaria. Thrombocytopenia is a potential concern in humans. Potential signs of toxicity include widening of QRS complexes and Q-T interval prolongation, circulatory collapse, seizures, and sudden death. Therapeutic drug monitoring can be performed if side effects or signs of toxicity are noted.

Contraindications – Quinidine should be avoided in patients with myasthenia gravis (due to its vagolytic effect), in the setting of pre-existing cardiac conduction disorders (AV block and bundle branch blocks), and in patients with uncorrected hypokalemia or acid-base derangements. As previously mentioned, caution is advised when quinidine is administered to animals with concurrent structural cardiac disease or heart failure. Caution is also advised in patients with concurrent renal or hepatic disease, which may induce drug accumulation and signs of toxicity.

Drug interactions – Quinidine has numerous drug interactions, which largely stem from its inhibition of the hepatic microsomal enzyme cytochrome p450. Thus, numerous drugs that also rely on cytochrome p450 for metabolism (e.g. antacids) may alter (increase or decrease) quinidine serum levels. Quinidine also has a well-known interaction with digoxin. It displaces digoxin from its binding sites and reduces renal clearance thereby potentiating toxicity. Concurrent use of other class I or class III antiarrhythmic drugs should be avoided.

Procainamide

Mechanism of action – Procainamide has nearly identical antiarrhythmic properties to those of quinidine (see above) and its electrophysiologic effects are also highly dependent on extracellular potassium concentration. Although documented in the dog (Pearle et al. 1983), procainamide's vagolytic effects appear to be minimal and the least of the class IA drugs (Miller and Zipes 2012).

Pharmacokinetics and metabolism –Only parenteral formulations will be discussed due to the declining availability of oral formulations. Parenteral administration (IM/IV) results in nearly immediate action that is widely distributed to the tissues. Protein binding is relatively low (15% in dogs). Plasma half-life in dogs(Dreyfuss et al. 1971; Papich et al. 1986a, 1986b) and horses (Ellis et al. 1994) is relatively short at approximately three hours. With the exception of dogs (Papich et al. 1986b), procainamide is metabolized by the liver to an active metabolite, N-acetylprocainamide, which partly prolongs action potential duration (class III effect) and is excreted by the kidneys directly proportional to creatinine.

Clinical use – Like quinidine, procainamide features a broad spectrum of antiarrhythmic efficacy but has fewer side effects. It demonstrates antiarrhythmic properties in atrial and ventricular tissue and therefore can be used for supraventricular and ventricular tachyarrhythmias. It is most commonly utilized for acute cardioversion of ventricular tachyarrhythmias refractory to lidocaine and can be considered for acute onset supraventricular tachyarrhythmias (e.g. atrial flutter or fibrillation).

Effect on patients under general anesthesia – Depressed cardiac contractility, vasodilation, and hypotension are potential concerns in anesthetized patients but to a lesser extent than quinidine. These effects are exacerbated by rapid IV infusions. Procainamide's vasodilatory mechanism is unclear. Anesthetics appear to alter procainamide pharmacokinetics (Orszulak-Michalak 1995) (see drug interactions).

Side (other) effects – Dose-related side effects are similar to but less frequent than quinidine (see above). Doses should be reduced in patients with renal disease.

Contraindications – Similar to quinidine (see above).

Drug interactions – Procainamide does not interact with digoxin but drug interactions are otherwise similar to quinidine (see above). In rabbits, midazolam appears to decrease procainamide plasma concentration and enhances elimination (Orszulak-Michalak et al. 2002a), whereas injectable anesthetics, including propofol and ketamine, appear to prolong drug clearance times (Orszulak-Michalak 1995).

Class IB Drugs

These drugs produce little-to-no effect on phase 0 of the action potential in normal cardiac tissue but target and significantly decrease conduction velocity in diseased or ischemic cardiac tissue that tend to be partially depolarized (Nattel et al. 2013). Class IB drugs also shorten action potential duration (accelerate repolarization) in normal tissue, which can be proarrhythmic. Class IB drugs are notoriously ineffective against atrial arrhythmias probably due to their very rapid onset-offset kinetics (milliseconds) of sodium channel binding coupled with the already shortened action potential of the atrial myocardial tissue (Nattel et al. 2013).

Lidocaine

Mechanism of action – In contrast to the class IA drugs, lidocaine shortens repolarization, lacks a vagolytic effect, and exhibits no effect on normal cardiac tissue but selectively decreases cardiac electrical conduction velocity in diseased/ischemic cardiac tissue (see above). Despite shortening repolarization, lidocaine paradoxically lengthens the effective refractory period whereby no stimulus can propagate an action potential. It also reduces phase 4 (diastolic) depolarization and thus is efficacious against arrhythmias due to increased automaticity. Lidocaine exhibits use dependence. Like the class IA antiarrhythmics, lidocaine's efficacy is dependent on extracellular potassium concentration, with decreased efficacy noted with hypokalemia.

Pharmacokinetics and metabolism – Species–specific pharmacokinetic data for lidocaine is available for rabbits (Orszulak-Michalak et al. 2002b), cats (Thomasy et al. 2005), horses (Feary et al. 2005), dogs (Maes et al. 2007; Wilcke et al. 1983), pigs (Satas et al. 1997), and birds (chickens) (Da Cunha et al. 2012). Lidocaine is only used parenterally and is rapidly and extensively distributed to the tissues. Its onset of action should be within two minutes and duration of action is only 10–20 minutes. It is moderately protein bound (primarily α_1-acid glycoprotein). Lidocaine is rapidly and extensively metabolized by the liver, which can be significantly affected by liver function and blood flow, and passive congestion. Thus, dose reduction should be considered in patients with hepatic disease and heart failure due to delayed clearance. Lidocaine's elimination half-life is around 30 minutes in anesthetized chickens, 60 minutes in dogs, horses and pigs, and 100 minutes in cats and rabbits.

Clinical use – Across species, lidocaine is often considered the first-choice therapy for acute treatment of ventricular tachyarrhythmias due to its safety, minimal hemodynamic effects, and efficacy. It is usually ineffective against supraventricular tachyarrhythmias (Johnson et al. 2006). One exception to note is vagally-mediated (often perianesthetic) atrial fibrillation (Moise et al. 2005; Pariaut et al. 2008).

Effect on patients under general anesthesia – At therapeutic antiarrhythmic doses, lidocaine has negligible hemodynamic effects in most species. However, in anesthetized cats, lidocaine was found to exhibit cardiodepressant effects (Pypendop and Ilkiw 2005). Lidocaine infusions have been shown to reduce minimum alveolar concentration of inhalant anesthetics in horses, rodents, rabbits, dogs, cats, and small ruminants (Schnellbacher et al. 2013). Conversely, anesthesia/anesthetics have been shown to affect the pharmacokinetics of lidocaine in rabbits (Orszulak-Michalak et al. 2002b), horses (Feary et al. 2005), dogs (Boyce et al. 1978), and cats (Thomasy et al. 2005). Anesthetics, likely via decreased hepatic blood flow, secondary to reduced cardiac output, slows metabolism and prolongs elimination half-life.

Effects on organ systems (CV, Resp, central nervous system [CNS]) – Lidocaine may also be utilized as a local anesthetic, adjunct analgesic agent, intestinal promotility agent, and as a scavenger of reactive oxygen species.

Side (other) effects – Side effects of lidocaine are often dose-related and include CNS signs of ataxia, depression, tremors, and seizures. Nausea, vomiting, and anorexia are not uncommon but usually transient. Cats and horses are particularly sensitive to the CNS side effects and therefore doses are reduced accordingly. Hypotension is possible if administered too rapidly.

Contraindications – Contraindications are minimal but include uncorrected hypokalemia, severe liver dysfunction, and concurrent bradyarrhythmias such as advanced AV block.

Drug interactions – Avoid use with other class I drugs. Use with propranolol should also be avoided as it decreases hepatic blood flow thereby increasing risk of toxicity. Midazolam has been shown to increase elimination and reduce the half-life of lidocaine in rabbits (Orszulak-Michalak et al. 2002b).

Mexiletine

Mechanism of action – Mexiletine can be considered the oral equivalent of lidocaine with the same mechanism of action.

Pharmacokinetics and metabolism – Mexiletine is only available orally and is rapidly absorbed from the gut. The majority of the drug is excreted by the kidney and metabolized by the liver, which is influenced by hepatic blood flow (Prescott et al. 1977). Plasma half-life is approximately four to seven hours, and renal excretion is prolonged by alkaline urine (Muir et al. 1999).

Clinical use – Mexiletine is used for chronic oral therapy of ventricular tachyarrhythmias and its use is primarily limited to dogs. Although expected, a positive response to lidocaine may not always translate to a positive response to mexiletine (Moise 1999). Combination therapy with beta-blockers may increase effectiveness.

Side (other) effects – Similar to lidocaine. Mexiletine should be administered with food to attempt to decrease side effects.

Drug interactions – Atropine, antacids, and opiates may reduce the rate of oral absorption. Mexiletine may reduce the metabolism of theophylline thereby increasing risk of toxicity.

Other pharmacologic properties are similar to lidocaine.

Phenytoin

Pharmacokinetics and metabolism – Pharmacokinetic data is limited but phenytoin is orally absorbed and metabolized by the liver and partially renally excreted. Half-life is eight hours in horses (Plumb 2008).

Clinical use – Clinical efficacy of oral phenytoin therapy has been demonstrated in horses with ventricular ectopy refractory to other antiarrhythmic drugs and may be considered accordingly (Wijnberg and Ververs 2004). Phenytoin is also used for management of seizures and neuromuscular disease in horses.

Side (other) effects –Toxicity can cause excitement and recumbency in horses (Wijnberg and Ververs 2004).

Other pharmacologic properties are similar to lidocaine.

Class IC Drugs

Class IC drugs are the most potent inhibitors of the fast sodium channels and thus markedly depress conduction velocity. They have no effect on repolarization. Class IC drugs have received a bad reputation in humans due to proarrhythmic tendencies, particularly in those with structural heart disease (The Cardiac Arrhythmia Suppression Trial (CAST) Investigators 1989; Siebels et al. 1993). Thus, similar concerns have surfaced in veterinary medicine and these drugs are often reserved for refractory cases (Dembek et al. 2014). Class IC drugs have the slowest onset and offset kinetics (10 seconds) of the class I drugs (Miller and Zipes 2012).

Flecainide

Mechanism of action – Flecainide has marked depressant and use-dependent effects on the fast sodium channel, which results in prolongation of the QRS. However, this prolongation is not uniform because flecainide shortens Purkinje fiber action potentials but prolongs action potentials in ventricular muscle (Miller and Zipes 2012). These disparate effects are thought to contribute to flecainide's potential proarrhythmic effects.

Pharmacokinetics and metabolism – There is limited pharmacokinetic data on flecainide, except in horses (Ohmura et al. 2000, 2001). It is available in an oral and IV formulation and the oral formulation reaches peak effect within one hour. The liver metabolizes flecainide into two active but less potent metabolites. It is renally excreted with a plasma half-life of approximately four to five hours in the horse.

Clinical use – In horses, flecainide can be considered for cardioversion of refractory atrial fibrillation, with the oral formulation demonstrating more favorable results (van Loon et al. 2004; Risberg and McGuirk 2006). It may also be considered for supraventricular and ventricular tachyarrhythmias resistant to other treatments in horses and dogs, although published canine data is lacking.

Effect on patients under general anesthesia – Flecainide depresses myocardial function and should be used with caution in patients with systolic dysfunction and in patients under general anesthesia.

Side (other) effects – Side effects of the drug include proarrhythmia, collapse, sudden death, and depressed myocardial function.

Contraindications – Flecainide should be used with caution in patients with systolic dysfunction and in patients already receiving negative inotropic drugs.

Drug interactions – Digoxin increases plasma levels of flecainide. Concurrent use with other negative inotropic drugs and other class I drugs should be avoided.

Propafenone

Mechanism of action – Propafenone's mechanism of action is similar to other class IC drugs, with the exception that it is a very weak beta-blocker (1/40 of the beta-blocking properties of propranolol) (Greenberg et al. 1989). Propafenone also decreases diastolic (Phase-4) depolarization in Purkinje fibers and decreases AV node conduction.

Pharmacokinetics and metabolism – Oral formulations appear to be slowly absorbed but elimination half-life is rapid (one to two hours) in horses (Puigdemont et al. 1990). The drug is metabolized by the liver and metabolites may contain varying degrees of the parent compound.

Drug interactions – Propafenone increases digoxin levels and quinidine may inhibit the metabolism of propafenone. Concurrent use with other negative inotropic drugs and other class I drugs should be avoided.

Other pharmacologic properties are similar to flecainide.

Class II Antiarrhythmic Drugs

The class II antiarrhythmic drugs are the β-adrenergic receptor blockers (β-blockers). β-adrenergic stimulation commonly exacerbates abnormal cellular physiology, which can initiate or worsen tachyarrhythmias. Consequently, their antiarrhythmic mechanisms are primarily indirect and "cardioprotective" by blocking catecholamine enhancement of arrhythmias and improving cellular electrophysiology, respectively. By reducing myocardial oxygen consumption, β-blockers may reduce myocardial ischemia and fibrosis, a potential proarrhythmic nidus. Antiarrhythmic effects of β-blockers are largely dependent upon prevailing sympathetic tone. β-blockers may be useful for supraventricular tachyarrhythmias for multiple reasons. For example, they increase conduction time through the atrioventricular (AV) node thereby increasing the time the AV node is refractory to depolarization. Thus, β-blockers may convert some supraventricular tachyarrhythmias (i.e. those reliant on the AV node to maintain the arrhythmia) to sinus rhythm or decrease the number of depolarizations reaching the ventricles in other supraventricular tachyarrhythmias (i.e. those that do not rely on the AV node to maintain the arrhythmias) such as atrial fibrillation. Clinical experience has revealed that beta-blockers may not be as effective for ventricular tachyarrhythmias when administered as monotherapy but they may act in a synergistic and beneficial manner when combined with class IA or IB drugs (Meurs et al. 2002). All beta-blockers may induce bradyarrhythmias and are potent negative inotropes, an important consideration in the perianesthetic period. Thus, caution is advised when these drugs are used in animals with bradyarrhythmias and impaired myocardial function. The mechanism of action, side effects, and clinical use of beta-blockers are relatively consistent and specific drug selection is primarily based upon desired pharmacokinetics, drug interactions, and availability.

Propranolol

Mechanism of action – Propranolol is the prototypical beta-blocker. It is a relatively short-acting nonselective (antagonizes β1 and β2 adrenergic receptors) beta-blocker. Propranolol and other beta-blockers decrease sinus rate, AV node conduction, and the rate of atrial and ventricular premature depolarizations.

Pharmacokinetics and metabolism – Propranolol is available in both oral and IV formulations. Oral absorption is rapid and it is highly protein bound, making the drug widely distributed to the tissues. There is an extensive first-pass effect, hence the difference in oral versus IV doses. The liver extensively metabolizes propranolol and hepatic clearance is proportional to hepatic blood flow. The reported half-life is relatively short (<2 hours) in dogs and horses (Plumb 2008).

Effect on patients under general anesthesia – As a nonselective beta-blocker and, in addition to decreasing inotropy and blood pressure (via reduced CO), propranolol increases systemic vascular resistance and contraction of bronchial smooth muscle (β2 effects on smooth muscle).

Side (other) effects – In addition to the typical side effects of beta-blockers, the β2 effects of propranolol should be considered. Propranolol has the potential to induce hypoglycemia and bronchial spasm.

Contraindications – Propranolol should be avoided in patients with overt liver disease, heart failure, bradyarrhythmias, lower airway disease/bronchospasm, and hypoglycemia.

Drug interactions – Antacids and fluoxetine may decrease the effectiveness of propranolol. Lidocaine may impair propranolol clearance. Propranolol may prolong the hypoglycemic effects of insulin.

Esmolol

Mechanism of action – Esmolol is an IV-only ultra-short acting selective (β1 effects only) beta-blocker.

Pharmacokinetics and metabolism – Esmolol is rapidly (terminal half-life of 10 minutes) metabolized by plasma esterases to an inactive metabolite in dogs and cats (Plumb 2008). Thus, esmolol is usually administered as an IV bolus (loading dose) followed by a constant rate infusion (CRI). Steady state blood levels occur within five-minutes if a bolus is administered (Plumb 2008).

Clinical use – Esmolol is often the preferred IV beta-blocker in small animals as can be titrated to effect.

Effect on patients under general anesthesia – Loading doses should be used cautiously in patients under general anesthesia due to potent hypotensive and cardiodepressant effects.

Drug interactions – Concurrent use with morphine may raise plasma esmolol concentration (Turlapaty et al. 1987).

Atenolol

Mechanism of action – Atenolol is a popular cardioselective β1-receptor-blocker used in small animals. Compared to propranolol, dosing interval and side effects are less frequent.

Pharmacokinetics and metabolism – Atenolol is a water-soluble, oral-only beta-blocker with equal potency compared to propranolol. Bioavailability is 80–90% in dogs and cats and it is rapidly absorbed with peak absorption occurring in two to three hours (McAinsh and Holmes 1983; Quinones et al. 1996; Macgregor et al. 2008). Low protein binding (10%) is noted and CNS distribution is absent. Half-life for dogs and cats is approximately four to five hours but beta-blocking effect persists for approximately 12 hours. Atenolol is eliminated unchanged in the urine.

Clinical use – Atenolol is most commonly used for chronic oral therapy of supraventricular arrhythmias in small animals. Increased efficacy against ventricular tachyarrhythmias is noted when combined with class IB drugs such as mexiletine. Atenolol is also commonly used for medical management of ventricular outflow tract obstructions. For example, atenolol is commonly administered to dogs with severe pulmonic stenosis, which may affect an anesthetic protocol prior to balloon pulmonary valvuloplasty.

Effect on patients under general anesthesia – Additive cardiodepressant and hypotensive effects may be noted when combined with anesthesia.

Contraindications – Atenolol should be used cautiously or dose-reduced in patients with renal insufficiency. Although less likely to cause problems given its β1-selectiveness, atenolol should still be used with caution in animals with lower airway / bronchospastic disease.

Drug interactions – Avoid with other cardiodepressant or hypotensive drugs.

Metoprolol

Mechanism of action – Metoprolol is a cardioselective (β1-specific) beta-blocker used for chronic oral therapy in small animals. With the exception of lipid solubility and hepatic elimination, metoprolol's clinical and pharmacologic characteristics are nearly identical to atenolol.

Class III Antiarrhythmic Drugs

Class III antiarrhythmic drugs prolong repolarization and action potential duration. This is accomplished by blocking the repolarizing potassium current, which prolongs phase 2 or 3 of the action potential and the effective (or absolute) refractory period during which no stimuli can evoke a response. A potential concern with these drugs is that they inevitably prolong the QT interval which, coupled with hypokalemia, hypomagnesemia, or bradycardia may predispose to torsades de pointes, a life-threatening polymorphic ventricular tachycardia (Nattel et al. 2013). Drugs in this class often possess additional antiarrhythmic

properties and thus are said to be "broad-spectrum" antiarrhythmics. Pure class III drugs (ibutilide, dofetilide) exist but experience is very limited in veterinary medicine.

Amiodarone

Mechanism of action – Amiodarone blocks repolarizing potassium channels and thus markedly prolongs action potential duration with an associated increase in refractory period in all cardiac tissues. Therapeutic doses decrease sinus rate and AV node conduction, potentially explained by amiodarone's weak calcium channel blocking (class IV) effect. Amiodarone also possesses a powerful use dependent class I (sodium channel blocking) antiarrhythmic effect in ventricular muscle. Lastly, amiodarone noncompetitively blocks α- and β-adrenergic receptors (class II effect), explaining its weak vasodilatory actions. Thus, amiodarone has properties of all antiarrhythmic drug classes (Miller and Zipes 2012). Amiodarone is structurally related to thyroxine, has high iodine content, and blocks the conversion of thyroxine (T4) to triiodothyroxine (T3).

Pharmacokinetics and metabolism – Amiodarone is available in parenteral and oral formulations. It possesses bizarre pharmacokinetic properties, which have been studied in dogs (Abdollah et al. 1990) and horses (De Clercq et al. 2006; Trachsel et al. 2004). Amiodarone is highly protein bound (96% in horses). Its oral bioavailability is low and without a loading oral dose onset of action may take weeks. IV onset of action is generally within one to two hours. The liver extensively metabolizes amiodarone into the active metabolite desethylamiodarone. Amiodarone is highly lipophilic, widely distributed, and may accumulate in selective tissues including fat, lung, liver, skin, and the heart. Elimination half-life is exceedingly long and is approximately 2.5 days in horses and dogs. Renal excretion of the drug is negligible.

Clinical use – Amiodarone is a potent, broad-spectrum antiarrhythmic whose clinical use is hindered by its numerous side effects (particularly with chronic oral therapy). Indications include refractory life-threatening ventricular tachyarrhythmias and management (and prevention) of supraventricular tachyarrhythmias such as atrial fibrillation. Amiodarone is preferred over lidocaine for malignant ventricular tachycardia or fibrillation that is refractory to electrical defibrillation during cardiopulmonary resuscitation (Fletcher and Boller 2013).

Effect on patients under general anesthesia – Amiodarone's hemodynamic effects appear to be mild in healthy anesthetized dogs (Bicer et al. 2000) but reduced myocardial function and vasodilation should be considered possible.

Side (other) effects – Side effects associated with acute IV administration of amiodarone are thought to be relatively few including skin reactions, GI upset and injection site pain. Of note, acute adverse skin reactions and hypotension secondary to IV amiodarone, specifically the formulation containing the solvent polysorbate 80, have been noted in dogs (Cober et al. 2009). In contrast, side effects related to chronic/oral administration are numerous and may include, GI upset, hepatopathy, thrombocytopenia, thyroid dysfunction, corneal deposits, and positive Coombs' tests with many more adverse effects reported in humans. Some adverse effects are reversible after discontinuation.

Drug interactions – Drug interactions are numerous and consultation with a formulary is advised. In general, co-administration with other antiarrhythmic drugs is ill-advised. Of note, anesthetics and fentanyl may perpetuate bradycardia and hypotension.

Sotalol

Mechanism of action – Sotalol is a racemic mixture of dextro and levo (l) isomers that prolongs repolarization (class III effect), with l-sotalol possessing nonselective beta-blocking properties (class II effect). Prolongation of repolarization is mediated through blocking of repolarizing potassium channels and is greater at slower rates (reverse use dependence). This occurs in atrial and ventricular tissue and thus increase in refractoriness is noted in both tissues. Prolongation of action potential duration with possibly increased calcium influx may explain why the negative inotropic (class II) effect is less than expected (Nattel et al. 2013). Sotalol's beta-blocker properties may cause a decrease in sinus rate and AV node conduction. Beta-blocking potency is thought to be approximately 30% of propranolol.

Pharmacokinetics and metabolism – The oral formulation is rapidly absorbed with peak effect usually by two hours post-ingestion and it is not metabolized (Schnelle and Garrett 1973). Protein binding is negligible. The drug is water-soluble and excreted unchanged by the kidneys. Dose reduction is required in patients with renal disease. In dogs, the elimination half-life is five hours.

Clinical use – Sotalol is a popular oral antiarrhythmic drug in small animals that is used primarily for chronic management of ventricular tachyarrhythmias. Sotalol may also be used by some clinicians to manage supraventricular tachyarrhythmias and, specifically, may be used to prevent recurrence of atrial fibrillation.

Effect on patients under general anesthesia – Although clinical significance of sotalol's negative inotropic effect is debated, it should be used with caution in patients with reduced cardiac function and in anesthetized patients (Seidler et al. 1999).

Side (other) effects – Side effects are rare but stem from sotalol's nonselective beta-blocker properties (reduced myocardial function, bronchoconstriction, bradyarrhythmias) and the prolongation of repolarization (QT prolongation) and its associated possible proarrhythmic effect (early afterdepolarizations).

Contraindications – Sotalol should be used with caution in patients with depressed cardiac function, QT prolongation, bradyarrhythmias, and asthma. Dose reduction is advised in patients with renal disease.

Drug interactions – Avoid with concurrent use of drugs that prolong QT interval (e.g. class IA or III drugs) and that have negative chronotropic and inotropic properties.

Class IV Antiarrhythmic Drugs

The class IV antiarrhythmics consist of the non-DHP calcium channel blocking drugs diltiazem and verapamil, which antagonize the L-type ("long-lasting" inward) calcium channels in cardiac cell membranes. These drugs selectively target cardiac cells (with some carry over to smooth muscle) whereas the DHP CCBs (amlodipine; discussed later) target vascular smooth muscle cells. Given that the L-type calcium channels are partly responsible for depolarization of sinoatrial and AV nodal tissue and for initiating myocardial cell contraction, these channels play a pivotal role in regulating cardiac electrical and mechanical activity. Class IV drugs act as antiarrhythmics by drastically slowing AV node conduction in a use-dependent manner by increasing the refractoriness of nodal tissue. Thus, they are predominantly used for management of supraventricular tachyarrhythmias. Like class II drugs, class IV drugs may induce bradyarrhythmias and depress myocardial function due to their direct effect on myocardial L-type calcium channels during phase 2 of the action potential (excitation-contraction coupling). Verapamil is rarely used in veterinary species and will not be discussed in detail.

Diltiazem

Mechanism of action – The primary mechanism of action is blockage of L-type (slow) calcium channels, with the most notable effects in nodal tissue. With higher doses, blockage of smooth muscle calcium channels and subsequent systemic vasodilation may be noted.

Pharmacokinetics and metabolism – Diltiazem comes in several formulations including IV and oral formulations, of which an extended-release form is available. Specific pharmacokinetic data are available in dogs (Yeung et al. 2001), cats (Johnson et al. 1996), and horses (Schwarzwald et al. 2006). The drug has an almost immediate onset of action when administered IV. The liver rapidly and nearly completely metabolizes diltiazem. Half-life in dogs and cats is two to three hours and is approximately 90 minutes in horses.

Clinical use – Non-DHP CCBs are primarily used for heart rate (by decreasing AV node conduction) or rhythm control (by interrupting reentry circuits that involve the AV node) in supraventricular tachyarrhythmias.

Effect on patients under general anesthesia – CCBs should be expected to have additive depressant effects on the cardiovascular system in patients under general anesthesia, including bradycardia, reduced contractility and vasodilation.

Side (other) effects – In general, side effects are associated with cardiodepression (bradyarrhythmias, decreased myocardial function and hypotension). IV administration must be slow and given over at least two minutes. Also, IV lines should be "flushed" slowly following administration.

Contraindications – Caution is advised in patients with bradyarrhythmias and reduced myocardial function.

Drug interactions – Diltiazem may increase benzodiazepine levels and concurrent use with beta-blockers should be avoided.

Additional Antiarrhythmic Therapies

Digoxin

Mechanism of action – Digoxin is a digitalis glycoside with weak positive inotropic properties (via sodium-potassium pump inhibition) and antiarrhythmic properties that involve baroreceptor sensitization and increased parasympathetic tone. The clinically desired consequence of which is usually prolongation of AV conduction and increased refractoriness of the AV node.

Pharmacokinetics and metabolism – Digoxin is one of the oldest and widely used cardiac medications across veterinary species. The parenteral formulation is rarely used and is becoming more difficult to acquire. Peak serum levels are usually noted 90 minutes post-ingestion, but following an initial dose, peak effect may not be for six to eight hours (Plumb 2008). Relatively low protein binding (20–30%) occurs. Digoxin undergoes minimal metabolism and is excreted by the kidneys. Thus, doses should be adjusted accordingly in patients with renal insufficiency. Elimination half-lives are long and variable and consist of 15–50 hours in dogs, 30–170 hours in cats, 17–20 hours in horses, and approximately 7 hours in cattle and sheep (Plumb 2008).

Clinical use – Digoxin is most often used for chronic therapy of supraventricular tachyarrhythmias (i.e. atrial fibrillation), particularly in patients with heart failure. In dogs, it is rarely used as a sole agent for this purpose. Its clinical use for chronic inotropic support in heart failure has markedly declined with the advent of other safer and effective drugs (pimobendan).

Effect on patients under general anesthesia – Digoxin's adverse hemodynamic effects are likely minimal but bradycardia may be noted.

Side (other) effects – Given digoxin's narrow therapeutic window, side effects may be common and primarily consist of GI upset and proarrhythmia (tachy- or bradyarrhythmia).

Contraindications – Digoxin should only be administered to normokalemic animals. Hyperkalemia displaces digoxin from its binding site and blunts its effects whereas hypokalemia exacerbates digoxin toxicity. Digoxin should be avoided in patients with ventricular tachyarrhythmias. Breeds susceptible to the multidrug resistance mutation 1(MDR1) mutation are at higher risk for digoxin toxicity, as p-glycoprotein pump transportation occurs.

Drug interactions – Drug interactions are numerous and consultation with a formulary is advised (Plumb 2008). Interactions relevant to the reader include that digoxin serum levels may be increased by amiodarone, anticholinergics, diazepam, high-dose furosemide, omeprazole, and quinidine.

Electrolytes – Magnesium and Potassium

Throughout this chapter maintenance of normokalemia has been emphasized, as potassium derangements can exacerbate proarrhythmic effects of certain antiarrhythmic drugs, particularly class I and class III drugs (El-Sherif and Turitto 2011). As a general consideration, most antiarrhythmic drugs are potentially toxic during hyperkalemia and either ineffective or progressively proarrhythmic in the setting of hypokalemia.

Hypomagnesemia may directly or indirectly induce ventricular tachyarrhythmias, although the exact mechanism is unclear (El-Sherif and Turitto 2011). Magnesium is vital for sodium–potassium pump function, cellular electrolyte homeostasis, and potassium channel function, which may affect action potential duration and resting membrane potential (El-Sherif and Turitto 2011). Magnesium is also a physiologic L-type CCB that may shorten action potential duration. Derangements in action potential duration and resting membrane potential may be conducive to tachyarrhythmias. Therefore, magnesium supplementation, particularly in the setting of hypomagnesemia, may be safe and potentially effective adjunct therapy for tachyarrhythmias.

Thus, serum electrolyte monitoring (particularly potassium, magnesium, and calcium) is strongly advised particularly at initiation of antiarrhythmic drug therapy.

Dihydropyridine Calcium Channel Blockers

Mechanism of action – The DHP L-type CCBs primarily differ from diltiazem and verapamil in their vascular smooth muscle selectivity. Their major action is arterial dilation and afterload reduction with less calcium channel antagonism in cardiac and nodal tissue. Nifedipine is considered the first-generation DHP CCB. Its half-life is relatively short and thus longer acting second-generation CCBs such as amlodipine were formulated. Amlodipine is the DHP CCB predominantly used in veterinary species and thus nifedipine with not be discussed further. Clevidipine is a relatively new ultra-short acting IV DHP CCB with a rapid onset of action (Ericsson et al. 1999; de Wolff et al. 2000). The author has very limited experience with this drug but has used the human starting dose of 1 mcg/kg/min titrated to effect to help manage refractory congestive heart failure in dogs.

Pharmacokinetics and metabolism – Amlodipine is only available in an oral formulation and its pharmacologic profile has only been evaluated in dogs (Burges et al. 1989). The drug is slowly but completely absorbed (with 88% bioavailability) with peak plasma concentrations (and peak arterial dilation) occurring between six and nine hours, post-administration. The drug exhibits a high degree of protein binding (+90%). Amlodipine gradually but extensively undergoes hepatic metabolism. Its plasma half-life is long at 30 hours in dogs and steady state is achieved after four to seven days of dosing (Burges et al. 1989).

Clinical use – Amlodipine is the treatment of choice for chronic therapy of moderate-to-severe systemic hypertension in dogs and cats. Amlodipine is also occasionally used in dogs for refractory heart failure secondary to degenerative mitral valve disease (afterload reduction).

Effect on patients under general anesthesia – Arterial vasodilation and hypotension, coupled with the possibility of a reflex-mediated tachycardia, should be anticipated in anesthetized patients. Mild negative inotropic effects are possible.

Side (other) effects – Aside from overzealous arterial vasodilation (hypotension, weakness, collapse, lethargy) and a reflex-mediated tachycardia, chronic side effects may include azotemia, peripheral edema, activation of the renin-angiotensin-aldosterone system (with higher doses), and gingival hyperplasia.

Contraindications/Drug interactions – Amlodipine is contraindicated in hypotensive animals and should be used with caution with other drugs that may reduce blood pressure (diuretics, beta-blockers, non-DHP CCBs, vasodilators, etc.)

References

Abdollah, H., Brien, J.F., and Brennan, F.J. (1990). Antiarrhythmic effect of chronic oral amiodarone treatment in dogs with myocardial infarction and reproducibly inducible sustained ventricular arrhythmias. *J. Cardiovasc. Pharmacol.* 15: 799–807.

Anderson, J.L. (1990). Reassessment of benefit-risk ratio and treatment algorithms for antiarrhythmic drug therapy after the cardiac arrhythmia suppression trial. *J. Clin. Pharmacol.* 30: 981–989.

Bicer, S., Schwartz, D.S., Nakayama, T., and Hamlin, R.L. (2000). Hemodynamic and electrocardiographic effects of graded doses of amiodarone in healthy dogs anesthetized with morphine/alpha chloralose. *J. Vet. Intern. Med.* 14: 90–95.

Boon, J.A. (ed.) (2011). *Hypertensive Heart Disease*. Ames, IA: Blackwell.

Boyce, J.R., Cervenko, F.W., and Wright, F.J. (1978). Effects of halothane on the pharmacokinetics of lidocaine in digitalis-toxic dogs. *Can. Anaesth. Soc. J.* 25: 323–328.

Burges, R.A., Dodd, M.G., and Gardiner, D.G. (1989). Pharmacologic profile of amlodipine. *Am. J. Cardiol.* 64: 10I–18I. discussion 18I-20I.

Clohisy, D.R. and Gibson, T.P. (1982). Comparison of pharmacokinetic parameters of intravenous quinidine and quinine in dogs. *J. Cardiovasc. Pharmacol.* 4: 107–110.

Cober, R.E., Schober, K.E., Hildebrandt, N. et al. (2009). Adverse effects of intravenous amiodarone in 5 dogs. *J. Vet. Intern. Med.* 23: 657–661.

Da Cunha, A.F., Messenger, K.M., Stout, R.W. et al. (2012). Pharmacokinetics of lidocaine and its active metabolite monoethylglycinexylidide after a single intravenous administration in chickens (*Gallus domesticus*) anesthetized with isoflurane. *J. Vet. Pharmacol. Ther.* 35: 604–607.

De Clercq, D., Baert, K., Croubels, S. et al. (2006). Evaluation of the pharmacokinetics and bioavailability of intravenously and orally administered amiodarone in horses. *Am. J. Vet. Res.* 67: 448–454.

De Wolff, M.H., Leather, H.A., and Wouters, P.F. (2000). Effect of clevidipine, an ultra-short acting 1,4-dihydropyridine calcium channel blocking drug, on the potency of isoflurane in rats and dogs. *Eur. J. Anaesthesiol.* 17: 506–511.

Dembek, K.A., Hurcombe, S.D., Schober, K.E., and Toribio, R.E. (2014). Sudden death of a horse with supraventricular tachycardia following oral administration of flecainide acetate. *J. Vet. Emerg. Crit. Care (San Antonio)* 24: 759–763.

Dreyfuss, J., Ross, J.J., and JR. & Schreiber, E. C. (1971). Absorption, excretion, and biotransformation of procainamide-C 14 in the dog and rhesus monkey. *Arzneimittelforschung* 21: 948–951.

Ellis, E.J., Ravis, W.R., Malloy, M. et al. (1994). The pharmacokinetics and pharmacodynamics of procainamide in horses after intravenous administration. *J. Vet. Pharmacol. Ther.* 17: 265–270.

El-Sherif, N. and Turitto, G. (2011). Electrolyte disorders and arrhythmogenesis. *Cardiol. J.* 18: 233–245.

Ericsson, H., Tholander, B., Bjorkman, J.A. et al. (1999). Pharmacokinetics of new calcium channel antagonist clevidipine in the rat, rabbit, and dog and pharmacokinetic/pharmacodynamic relationship in anesthetized dogs. *Drug Metab. Dispos.* 27: 558–564.

Feary, D.J., Mama, K.R., Wagner, A.E., and Thomasy, S. (2005). Influence of general anesthesia on pharmacokinetics of intravenous lidocaine infusion in horses. *Am. J. Vet. Res.* 66: 574–580.

Fletcher, D.J. and Boller, M. (2013). Updates in small animal cardiopulmonary resuscitation. *Vet. Clin. North Am. Small Anim. Pract.* 43: 971–987.

Greenberg, S., Cantor, E., and Paul, J. (1989). Beta-adrenoceptor blocking activity of diprafenone in anesthetized dogs: comparison with propafenone and propranolol. *J. Cardiovasc. Pharmacol.* 14: 444–453.

Johnson, L.M., Atkins, C.E., Keene, B.W., and Bai, S.A. (1996). Pharmacokinetic and pharmacodynamic properties of conventional and CD-formulated diltiazem in cats. *J. Vet. Intern. Med.* 10: 316–320.

Johnson, M.S., Martin, M., and Smith, P. (2006). Cardioversion of supraventricular tachycardia using lidocaine in five dogs. *J. Vet. Intern. Med.* 20: 272–276.

Macgregor, J.M., Rush, J.E., Rozanski, E.A. et al. (2008). Comparison of pharmacodynamic variables following oral versus transdermal administration of atenolol to healthy cats. *Am. J. Vet. Res.* 69: 39–44.

Maes, A., Weiland, L., Sandersen, C. et al. (2007). Determination of lidocaine and its two N-desethylated metabolites in dog and horse plasma by high-performance liquid chromatography combined with electrospray ionization tandem mass spectrometry. *J. Chromatogr. B Analyt. Technol. Biomed. Life Sci.* 852: 180–187.

Mcainsh, J. and Holmes, B.F. (1983). Pharmacokinetic studies with atenolol in the dog. *Biopharm. Drug Dispos.* 4: 249–261.

Mcguirk, S.M., Muir, W.W., and Sams, R.A. (1981a). Pharmacokinetic analysis of intravenously and orally administered quinidine in cows. *Am. J. Vet. Res.* 42: 1482–1487.

Mcguirk, S.M., Muir, W.W., and Sams, R.A. (1981b). Pharmacokinetic analysis of intravenously and orally administered quinidine in horses. *Am. J. Vet. Res.* 42: 938–942.

Meurs, K.M., Spier, A.W., Wright, N.A. et al. (2002). Comparison of the effects of four antiarrhythmic treatments for familial ventricular arrhythmias in Boxers. *J. Am. Vet. Med. Assoc.* 221: 522–527.

Miller, J.M. and Zipes, D.P. (ed.) (2012). *Therapy for Cardiac Arrhythmias*. Philadelphia: Elsevier Saunders.

Moise, N.S. (ed.) (1999). *Diagnosis and Management of Canine Arrhythmias*. Philadelphia: Saunders.

Moise, N.S., Pariaut, R., Gelzer, A.R. et al. (2005). Cardioversion with lidocaine of vagally associated atrial fibrillation in two dogs. *J. Vet. Cardiol.* 7: 143–148.

Muir, W.W., Sams, R.A., and Moise, N.S. (ed.) (1999). *Pharmacology and Pharmacokinetics of Antiarrhythmic Drugs*. Philadelphia: Saunders.

Nattel, S., Gersh, B.J., and Opie, L.H. (ed.) (2013). *Antiarrhythmic Drugs and Strategies*. Philadelphia: Elsevier Saunders.

Neff, C.A., Davis, L.E., and Baggot, J.D. (1972). A comparative study of the pharmacokinetics of quinidine. *Am. J. Vet. Res.* 33: 1521–1525.

Ohmura, H., Nukada, T., Mizuno, Y. et al. (2000). Safe and efficacious dosage of flecainide acetate for treating equine atrial fibrillation. *J. Vet. Med. Sci.* 62: 711–715.

Ohmura, H., Hiraga, A., Aida, H. et al. (2001). Determination of oral dosage and pharmacokinetic analysis of flecainide in horses. *J. Vet. Med. Sci.* 63: 511–514.

Orszulak-Michalak, D. (1995). The influence of selected general anesthetics on pharmacokinetic parameters of some antiarrhythmic drugs in rabbits. Part I. Procainamide and its active metabolite-N-acetylprocainamide. *Acta Pol. Pharm.* 52: 141–146.

Orszulak-Michalak, D., Owczarek, J., and Wiktorowska-Owczarek, A.K. (2002a). Influence of midazolam on pharmacokinetic parameters of procainamide in rabbits. *Pol. J. Pharmacol.* 54: 151–155.

Orszulak-Michalak, D., Owczarek, J., and Wiktorowska-Owczarek, A.K. (2002b). The influence of midazolam on plasma concentrations and pharmacokinetic parameters of lidocaine in rabbits. *Pharmacol. Res.* 45: 11–14.

Papich, M.G., Davis, L.E., and Davis, C.A. (1986a). Procainamide in the dog: antiarrhythmic plasma concentrations after intravenous administration. *J. Vet. Pharmacol. Ther.* 9: 359–369.

Papich, M.G., Davis, L.E., Davis, C.A. et al. (1986b). Pharmacokinetics of procainamide hydrochloride in dogs. *Am. J. Vet. Res.* 47: 2351–2358.

Pariaut, R., Moise, N.S., Koetje, B.D. et al. (2008). Lidocaine converts acute vagally associated atrial fibrillation to sinus rhythm in German Shepherd dogs with inherited arrhythmias. *J. Vet. Intern. Med.* 22: 1274–1282.

Pearle, D.L., Souza, J.D., and Gillis, R.A. (1983). Comparative vagolytic effects of procainamide and N-acetylprocainamide in the dog. *J. Cardiovasc. Pharmacol.* 5: 450–453.

Plumb, D.C. (2008). *Plumb's Veterinary Drug Handbook.* Ames, IA: Blackwell.

Prescott, L.F., Pottage, A., and Clements, J.A. (1977). Absorption, distribution and elimination of mexiletine. *Postgrad. Med. J.* 53 (Suppl 1): 50–55.

Puigdemont, A., Riu, J.L., Guitart, R., and Arboix, M. (1990). Propafenone kinetics in the horse. Comparative analysis of compartmental and noncompartmental models. *J. Pharmacol. Methods* 23: 79–85.

Pypendop, B.H. and Ilkiw, J.E. (2005). Assessment of the hemodynamic effects of lidocaine administered IV in isoflurane-anesthetized cats. *Am. J. Vet. Res.* 66: 661–668.

Quinones, M., Dyer, D.C., Ware, W.A., and Mehvar, R. (1996). Pharmacokinetics of atenolol in clinically normal cats. *Am. J. Vet. Res.* 57: 1050–1053.

Reef, V.B. and Mcguirk, S.M. (ed.) (2009). *Diseases of the Cardiovascular System.* St. Louis, MO: Elsevier.

Risberg, A.I. and Mcguirk, S.M. (2006). Successful conversion of equine atrial fibrillation using oral flecainide. *J. Vet. Intern. Med.* 20: 207–209.

Satas, S., Johannessen, S.I., Hoem, N.O. et al. (1997). Lidocaine pharmacokinetics and toxicity in newborn pigs. *Anesth. Analg.* 85: 306–312.

Schmid, P.G., Nelson, L.D., Mark, A.L. et al. (1974). Inhibition of adrenergic vasoconstriction by quinidine. *J. Pharmacol. Exp. Ther.* 188: 124–134.

Schnellbacher, R.W., Carpenter, J.W., Mason, D.E. et al. (2013). Effects of lidocaine administration via continuous rate infusion on the minimum alveolar concentration of isoflurane in New Zealand white rabbits (*Oryctolagus cuniculus*). *Am. J. Vet. Res.* 74: 1377–1384.

Schnelle, K. and Garrett, E.R. (1973). Pharmacokinetics of the - adrenergic blocker sotalol in dogs. *J. Pharm. Sci.* 62: 362–375.

Schwarzwald, C.C., Sams, R.A., and Bonagura, J.D. (2006). Pharmacokinetics of the calcium-channel blocker diltiazem after a single intravenous dose in horses. *J. Vet. Pharmacol. Ther.* 29: 165–171.

Seidler, R.W., Mueller, K., Nakayama, T., and Hamlin, R.L. (1999). Influence of sotalol on the time constant of isovolumic left ventricular relaxation in anesthetized dogs. *Am. J. Vet. Res.* 60: 717–721.

Siebels, J., Cappato, R., Ruppel, R. et al. (1993). Preliminary results of the Cardiac Arrest Study Hamburg (CASH). CASH Investigators. *Am. J. Cardiol.* 72: 109F–113F.

The Cardiac Arrhythmia Suppression Trial (CAST) Investigators (1989). Preliminary report: effect of encainide and flecainide on mortality in a randomized trial of arrhythmia suppression after myocardial infarction. *N. Engl. J. Med.* 321: 406–412.

Thomasy, S.M., Pypendop, B.H., Ilkiw, J.E., and Stanley, S.D. (2005). Pharmacokinetics of lidocaine and its active metabolite, monoethylglycinexylidide, after intravenous administration of lidocaine to awake and isoflurane-anesthetized cats. *Am. J. Vet. Res.* 66: 1162–1166.

Trachsel, D., Tschudi, P., Portier, C.J. et al. (2004). Pharmacokinetics and pharmacodynamic effects of amiodarone in plasma of ponies after single intravenous administration. *Toxicol. Appl. Pharmacol.* 195: 113–125.

Turlapaty, P., Laddu, A., Murthy, V.S. et al. (1987). Esmolol: a titratable short-acting intravenous beta blocker for acute critical care settings. *Am. Heart J.* 114: 866–885.

Ueda, C.T. and Nickols, J.G. (1980). Comparative pharmacokinetics of quinidine and its O-desmethyl metabolite in rabbits. *J. Pharm. Sci.* 69: 1400–1403.

Van Loon, G., Blissitt, K.J., Keen, J.A., and Young, L.E. (2004). Use of intravenous flecainide in horses with naturally-occurring atrial fibrillation. *Equine Vet. J.* 36: 609–614.

Wijnberg, I.D. and Ververs, F.F. (2004). Phenytoin sodium as a treatment for ventricular dysrhythmia in horses. *J. Vet. Intern. Med.* 18: 350–353.

Wilcke, J.R., Davis, L.E., and Neff-Davis, C.A. (1983). Determination of lidocaine concentrations producing therapeutic and toxic effects in dogs. *J. Vet. Pharmacol. Ther.* 6: 105–111.

Wilkins, L. and European Society of Cardiology (1991). The Sicilian gambit. A new approach to the classification of antiarrhythmic drugs based on their actions on arrhythmogenic mechanisms. Task force of the working group on arrhythmias of the European Society of Cardiology. *Circulation* 84: 1831–1851.

Yeung, P.K., Feng, J.D., and Buckley, S.J. (2001). Effect of administration route and length of exposure on pharmacokinetics and metabolism of diltiazem in dogs. *Drug Metabol. Drug Interact.* 18: 251–262.

21

Peripheral Vasodilators
Martin Kennedy

Introduction

Vascular tone is a key determinant of blood pressure and organ perfusion, making the control of vascular tone critical to organ function in both health and disease. Nitric oxide (NO) is thought to be the major effector molecule responsible for the modulation of arterial and venous tone (Ignarro et al. 1987; Palmer et al. 1987). Since the initial discovery of this pathway, much has been learned about the biological functions of NO and its role in various tissues (Moncada and Higgs 1993). NO is synthesized in the endothelium from the amino acid L-arginine in a series of reactions catalyzed by nitric oxide synthase (NOS), with the constitutive version of NOS (eNOS or NOS3) being the dominant isoform under normal conditions. NO then diffuses out of the endothelial cell and enters nearby smooth muscle cells and activates soluble guanylate cyclase, leading to decreased intracellular calcium and smooth muscle relaxation. Considering this understanding of NO function, drugs can manipulate this mechanism and produce vasodilation by providing an exogenous source of NO or by prolonging the effects of endogenous NO (Figure 21.1). Drugs and dosages are listed in Table 21.1.

Nitroglycerin

Nitroglycerin, also known as glyceryl trinitrate (GTN), is an organic nitrate ester with a three carbon chain. The chemical synthesis of nitroglycerin was first described by Italian chemist Ascanio Sobrero in 1847 (Sobrero 1847). Nitroglycerin is available in several formulations including ointments, patches, tablets, and injectable solutions.

Mechanism of Action

Nitroglycerin exerts its biological effects by serving as an exogenous source of NO. The metabolic activation and release of NO is thought to occur in association with the plasma membrane of vascular smooth muscle cells, however, the exact mechanism has yet to be fully elucidated (Chung and Fung 1990). Once NO is liberated, it activates soluble guanylate cyclase which, in turn, catalyzes the conversion of guanosine triphosphate (GTP) to cyclic guanosine monophosphate (cGMP). The increased levels of cGMP results in decreased intracellular calcium and decreased myosin light chain kinase activity ultimately leading to smooth muscle relaxation (Ignarro and Gruetter 1980).

Pharmacokinetics

The pharmacokinetics of nitroglycerin in conscious and pentobarbital anesthetized dogs is similar and has been described using a two-compartment open model (Miyazaki et al. 1982). After intravenous (IV) bolus administration to awaken dogs, there is a bi-exponential decrease in plasma concentrations characterized by a rapid initial decrease with a half-life of approximately 30 seconds, followed by a slower terminal phase with a half-life of approximately five minutes. The nitroglycerin plasma concentration similarly decreased after 30 minutes of a nitroglycerin constant rate infusion (CRI) in pentobarbital anesthetized dogs. Nitroglycerin clearance is high and exceeds cardiac output (CO). However, clearance has also been observed to be highly variable and appears to be both animal and dose dependent (Lee et al. 1990, 1993). In conscious dogs, the nitroglycerin clearance has been shown to decrease with increasing doses administered as an IV bolus. When a CRI

Pharmacology in Veterinary Anesthesia and Analgesia, First Edition. Edited by Turi Aarnes and Phillip Lerche.
© 2024 John Wiley & Sons, Inc. Published 2024 by John Wiley & Sons, Inc.

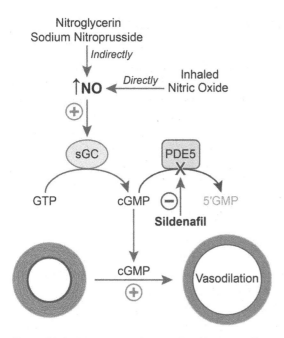

Figure 21.1 Mechanism of action for select vasodilating drugs.

was administered to conscious dogs it took approximately 60 minutes for nitroglycerin plasma levels to reach steady state, however, there was marked variability in the observed average steady-state plasma concentrations between dogs due to the high variability in clearance. In dogs, the oral bioavailability of nitroglycerin is reported to be low at only 1.5%, with oral administration resulting in detectable plasma concentrations for only a brief period of time.

In barbiturate anesthetized sheep, steady-state plasma concentrations of nitroglycerin were achieved approximately 20 minutes after beginning a CRI and dropped rapidly after the infusion was discontinued. The nitroglycerin plasma concentration declined in a bi-exponential manner with a terminal half-life of less than four minutes that appeared to be independent of CRI rate (Cossum et al. 1986). The nitroglycerin was highly cleared at all doses investigated, however, there was no consistent relationship between dose and clearance observed. In sheep blood, nitroglycerin was found to be moderately protein bound with approximately 60% being bound to plasma proteins. The oral bioavailability was also low in sheep and was estimated to be less than 3%.

The pharmacokinetics of nitroglycerin in hamsters, rats, guinea pigs, ferrets, and rabbits has been described using first-order kinetics for an open one-compartment model (Ioannides et al. 1982). For these laboratory animals, there was a correlation between the plasma half-life of nitroglycerin and body weight; following administration of 0.75 mg/kg IV, the shortest mean half-lives were observed in hamsters (3.7 ± 0.4 minute) while the longest were seen in rabbits (12.2 ± 2.5 minute). In rats, the half-life was also affected by route of administration and sex of the animal. In barbiturate anesthetized rats, the mean half-life was significantly longer in females vs. males (7.7 ± 1.2 vs. 4.4 ± 0.7 min, respectively). These effects of species and sex on pharmacokinetics were thought to be due to differences in the hepatic enzymes responsible for nitroglycerin metabolism.

Table 21.1 Reported doses and uses of select vasodilating drugs.

Drug	Dose	Route	Species	Context	References
Nitroglycerin	1–40 mcg/kg/min	IV	Canine	Left sided CHF	Kamijo et al. (1994), Achiel et al. (2020)
Nitroglycerin	2% ointment 2.5 cm/10 kg	Trans-dermal	Canine	Preload reduction	Parameswaran et al. (1999)
Nitroprusside	0.5–8.5 mcg/kg/min	IV	Canine	ICU setting	Tinker and Michenfelder (1976)
Sildenafil	1–4 mg/kg q12 hr or 1-3 mg/kg q8 hr	PO	Canine	PH	Akabane et al. (2020), Bach et al. (2006), Brown et al. (2010), Saetang and Surachetpong (2020)
Sildenafil	0.625–2.5 mg/kg	PO	Sheep	PH	Weimann et al. (2000)
Sildenafil	0.25–1 mg/kg over 15 min, followed by 0.3 mg/kg/hr for 30 min	IV	Canine	PH	Dias-Junior et al. (2005a, 2005b)
Nitric oxide	Pulse delivery: First 30–45% of inhalation, delivering ~39 ppm NO	Inhaled	Equine	Hypoxemia during anesthesia	Nyman et al. (2012), Grubb et al. (2013)

Abbreviations: Congestive heart failure (CHF). Pulmonary hypertension (PH). Intravenous (IV). Per Os (PO).

Sublingual administration to rats more than doubled the mean half-life (14.3 ± 3.4 minute) while oral administration increased it more than fourfold (30 ± 011 minute). The bioavailability of nitroglycerin in rats with sublingual administration was found to be high at 96%, however, it was less than 5% with oral administration.

Metabolism

Nitroglycerin is rapidly metabolized to 1,2-glycerol dinitrate (1,2-GDN), 1,3-glycerol dinitrate (1,3-GDN), and inorganic nitrite in varying amounts by the hepatic enzyme glutathione organic nitrate reductase (Needleman and Hunter 1965). Both 1,2-GDN and 1,3-GDN are active metabolites capable of producing cardiovascular effects, however, the magnitude of these effects are approximately one-tenth of GTN (Lee et al. 1990). In pentobarbital anesthetized rats, the metabolites' concentrations peaked within two to four minutes of GTN IV bolus administration (Johnson et al. 1972). In sheep and dogs, the 1,2-GDN has been reported to be the major metabolite produced during this first step (Miyazaki et al. 1982; Cossum et al. 1986; Lee et al. 1990, 1993). However, oral administration may result in increased levels of 1,3-GDN (Lee et al. 1990). Small amounts of these dinitrate metabolites are excreted by the kidney in varying degrees depending on species; rats excrete mainly 1,2-GDN with some 1,3-GDN, while rabbits excrete only 1,3-GDN (DiCarlo et al. 1968; Bogaert et al. 1969). Glutathione organic nitrate reductase then catalyzes the conversion of the GDN metabolites to glycerol mononitrate (GMN) and inorganic nitrite, however this second step at occurs at a much slower rate (Needleman and Hunter 1965). In dogs, the terminal half-lives of 1,2-GDN and 1,3-GDN are similar and have been reported to be approximately 40–50 minutes (Miyazaki et al. 1982; Lee et al. 1990, 1993). The GMN produced is the major metabolite excreted in urine (Needleman et al. 1971).

Clinical Use

William Murrel was the first to report on the medical use of nitroglycerin in 1879, when he described its sublingual and oral administration for the treatment of angina pectoris in humans (Murrel 1879). Both transdermal and IV GTN therapy have been recommended in dogs for acute preload reduction during emergency treatment of congestive heart failure (CHF) secondary to degenerative mitral valve disease (Parameswaran et al. 1999; Keene et al. 2019; Achiel et al. 2020). Transdermal nitroglycerin therapy has also been recommended for the acute treatment of grass-induced laminitis in horses and ponies (Hinckley et al. 1996a, 1996b).

Effect on Patients Under General Anesthesia

Given its cardiovascular effects, GTN administration may potentiate any vasodilation produced by anesthetic agents and other drugs administered in the perioperative period. In addition, the patient's anesthetic depth and/or cardiovascular status may not allow an appropriate autonomic response to prevent any hypotension. Continuous blood pressure monitoring should be used for careful titration of GTN to achieve the desired mean arterial pressure (MAP).

Effects on Organ Systems

Cardiovascular System

The overall cardiovascular effects of GTN are the result of smooth muscle relaxation in various circulatory beds and any autonomic reflexes that occur in response to these changes in vascular tone. Nitroglycerin administration decreases systemic vascular resistance (SVR) in a dose-dependent manner (Kadowitz et al. 1981), which may be manifested as decreased systemic arterial blood pressures and concomitant increases in heart rate (Vatner et al. 1972; Commarato et al. 1973; Chen et al. 1979; Lee et al. 1993; Morse and Rutlen 1994). Under these conditions of reduced afterload, CO may increase significantly above pretreatment values as a result of reflex increases in heart rate and inotropy (Vatner et al. 1972; Morse and Rutlen 1994). Smooth muscle relaxation in venous circulation increases capacitance and alters blood volume distribution, characterized by venous pooling in splanchnic circulation, which is thought to be the primary means of preload reduction (Chen et al. 1979; Morse and Rutlen 1994; Parameswaran et al. 1999). Under conditions of left sided CHF, these reductions in preload and afterload resulting from GTN treatment have been observed to significantly improve left ventricular performance (Kamijo et al. 1994). Left ventricular peak systolic and end-diastolic pressures are reported to decrease, while mean right atrial and left atrial pressures have been observed to decrease or remain unchanged with GTN treatment (Vatner et al. 1972; Kadowitz et al. 1981; Kamijo et al. 1994; Manohar 1995). Nitroglycerin is also a potent coronary vasodilator, producing a significant decrease in coronary vascular resistance and an increase in mean coronary blood flow (Vatner et al. 1972); coronary arterial–venous oxygen difference decreases as a result of increased blood flow and oxygen delivery. Pulmonary vascular resistance (PVR) and mean pulmonary arterial pressure (MPAP) also decrease with GTN administration in a dose-dependent fashion (Kadowitz et al. 1981; Manohar 1995).

Tachyphylaxis may develop from repeated GTN administration. The resulting shift in the dose response curve and magnitude of any producible cardiovascular effects appear to be affected by both the dose and duration of GTN treatment (Needleman 1970). Repeated administration of GTN may also render other vasodilating nitrates ineffective (Crandall 1933).

Respiratory System

Hypoxic pulmonary vasoconstriction (HPV) is inhibited by GTN administration (D'Oliveira et al. 1981; Kadowitz et al. 1981). When alveolar hypoxia is present, GTN may worsen gas exchange by increasing blood flow to nonventilated lung regions resulting in significantly decreased arterial oxygen tension (PaO_2) and hypoxemia.

Central Nervous System

Infusions of GTN may cause dose-dependent increases in intracranial pressure (ICP) due to cerebral vasodilation, and any increase in ICP becomes more pronounced when the ICP is already elevated prior to treatment with GTN (Morris et al. 1982). The combination of increased ICP with the potential for reductions in MAP could significantly decrease cerebral perfusion pressure, thus GTN is contraindicated in patients with elevated ICP.

Other Effects

Some investigators have reported increased hoof perfusion and improved lameness scores with GTN treatment in horses suffering from laminitis (Hinckley et al. 1996a, 1996b; Eades et al. 2006). However, others have reported conflicting results and did not observe a significant effect of GTN on hoof perfusion (Hoff et al. 2002; Gilhooly et al. 2005).

Contraindications

GTN is contraindicated in patients with elevated ICP, significant hemorrhage or hypovolemia, hypotension, pericardial tamponade, or restrictive cardiomyopathy. In addition, GTN is not currently recommended for the acute management of feline CHF (Luis Fuentes et al. 2020).

Drug Interactions

Chronic treatment with phenobarbital causes induction of the enzyme organic nitrate reductase, this may significantly increase the clearance of GTN and its metabolites (Needleman et al. 1971; Lee and Belpaire 1972). The vasodilating effects of GTN may be enhanced by the concurrent administration of other vasodilating drugs. The anti-coagulant effects of heparin may be impaired by IV GTN therapy (Becker et al. 1990). GTN absorption into IV infusion lines may cause substantial reductions in the dose actually delivered to the patient; non-absorption infusions sets will require significantly lower infusion rates of GTN to produce a given effect (Yuen et al. 1979).

Nitroprusside

Sodium nitroprusside (SNP) is an inorganic compound composed of an iron atom in its ferrous state at the center of five cyanide (CN) groups and a single NO group. It was initially discovered in 1849, however, SNP did not receive significant attention from the medical community until the 1950s and it eventually got FDA approval in 1974 for the control of severe hypertension (Ivankovich et al. 1978). It is formulated with 0.9% NaCl and supplied in single-use vials at a concentration of 0.5 mg/ml. Vials should be protected from light as SNP is susceptible to significant photodegradation and cyanide (CN) is a product of this process (Arnold et al. 1984).

Mechanism of Action

SNP spontaneously decomposes to release NO, thus it functions as a prodrug providing an exogenous source of NO causing smooth muscle relaxation and vasodilation via activation of soluble guanylate cyclase (Page et al. 1955; Ivankovich et al. 1978).

Pharmacokinetics

The dog has been deemed an adequate model for the studying the effects of SNP, thus most of the pharmacokinetic information available has been described in this species. No significant amount of SNP is likely absorbed following oral administration, making the IV route required for any therapeutic effects (Page et al. 1955). Due to the brief life of the prodrug molecule in circulation, most investigations instead focus on the fate of SNPs major metabolites, CN and thiocyanate (SCN), due to their potential for toxicity (Schulz 1984). In conscious dogs, when an SNP CRI was administered for one hour and titrated to maintain a 20% decrease in blood pressure, the whole blood CN concentration more than doubled (Behnia et al. 1978). The maximum CN concentrations observed were only a small percentage of that needed to cause signs of CN toxicity and levels returned to baseline within an hour of ending the infusion. When the same SNP doses were administered to the dogs under halothane anesthesia, the increase in whole blood levels of CN were significantly lower compared to awake conditions and there was no significant difference in SCN levels. Upon entering circulation, the decomposition of SNP is extremely rapid, the half-life in rats is approximately two minutes (Höbel and Raithelhuber 1976).

The released CN rapidly accumulates in red blood cells (RBCs) and accounts for more than 98% of the CN found in whole blood (Vesey et al. 1979). In barbiturate and nitrous oxide anesthetized dogs, the peak plasma CN concentration occurred 5–10 minutes after a SNP bolus (1 mg/kg IV), and the peak RBC CN concentration occurred within 20 minutes and both returned to baseline within three to four hours of injection (Vesey et al. 1979). The SCN concentration gradually increased in a linear fashion and peaked approximately 2.5 hours post SNP bolus. When the SNP was administered as a CRI (1.5 mg/kg/hr IV) both the plasma and RBC CN concentrations peaked at the end of the 60-minute infusion. Plasma and RBC CN concentrations then decreased rapidly during the first hour after stopping the infusion and both returned to baseline values within two to three hours. CN blood levels associated with toxicity were not achieved despite the high doses of SNP used in this investigation, likely due to the short duration of the CRI. The plasma SCN gradually increased during the CRI and peaked approximately two hours after ending the infusion. In humans, the half-life of SCN is approximately three days and is significantly prolonged with renal disease (Schulz et al. 1979).

Long duration and high-dose infusions of SNP have been investigated in dogs to model the effects of SNP in an intensive care setting (Tinker and Michenfelder 1976). Dogs were maintained with pancuronium and 70% nitrous oxide while being mechanically ventilated. Investigators found that dogs could safely be administered SNP at 0.5 mg/kg/hr (8.3 mcg/kg/min) for 48 hours without any adverse effects. Whole blood CN levels rapidly increased during the first hour and then plateaued at a steady state concentration of less than 2 mcg/ml for the duration of the infusion. The plasma SCN concentration increased linearly throughout the duration of infusion. In dogs that received higher doses of SNP, 0.75 or 1 mg/kg/hr, the whole blood CN concentration quickly increased in a linear fashion; all dogs developed CN toxicity and none survived beyond 38 hours of infusion. Signs of toxicity developed after approximately 20 hours of SNP CRI when whole blood CN concentrations reached 5–7 mcg/ml and death occurred at concentrations of 7–10 mcg/ml. The CN toxicity was characterized by progressive increases in mixed venous oxygen and the development of severe metabolic acidosis that eventually led to an isoelectric electroencephalogram (EEG) and/or hemodynamic collapse. Interestingly, dogs were able to maintain whole blood CN levels below 3 mcg/ml and avoid metabolic acidosis despite high-dose SNP infusions if they were simultaneously administered thiosulfate CRIs.

Metabolism

The specific pathways involved in the metabolism of SNP have been heavily researched and debated for almost 100 years (Page et al. 1955; Tinker and Michenfelder 1976; Ivankovich et al. 1978; Vesey et al. 1979; Friederich and Butterworth 1995). The current general understanding is that SNP interacts with oxyhemoglobin in a non-enzymatic

reaction to rapidly yield methemoglobin and an unstable SNP intermediate that then immediately decomposes to release NO and five CN ions. The fate of these liberated CN ions is crucial since any significant accumulation of CN can lead to toxicity, which may be fatal. The overwhelming majority of the CN released will be converted to SCN in the liver; this step requires thiosulfate as a sulfur donor and is catalyzed by the mitochondrial enzyme rhodanese. The availability of thiosulfate appears to be the rate limiting factor for this pathway of CN metabolism. The SCN is then excreted by the kidney, making this the major route of elimination. A portion of CN will react with the methemoglobin to yield cyanomethemoglobin, which then accumulates in erythrocytes. Some of the CN may bind to the ferric ion in the mitochondrial cytochrome oxidase system which inhibits oxidative phosphorylation and produces the cellular hypoxia that is the underlying mechanism for CN toxicity. Providing exogenous sources of thiosulfate or hydroxocobalamin have been reported to be effective treatments for CN toxicity (Reade et al. 2012).

Clinical Use

In humans, SNP was first used clinically for the management of hypertension (Page et al. 1955). SNP has also found routine use for the emergent treatment of left-sided CHF and for controlled hypotension during surgery in an effort to minimize hemorrhage.

Effect on Patients Under General Anesthesia

Inhalant anesthesia potentiates the vasodilating effects of SNP and reduces the dose required to achieve a given decrease in blood pressure (Bedford 1978, 1979).

Increasing concentrations of expired anesthetic may also decrease or abolish any sympathetic response to SNP induced hypotension (Bloor et al. 1989). As a result, the administration of SNP to patients under general anesthesia may cause profound hypotension, making continuous blood pressure monitoring and careful titration of SNP and/or any anesthetics critical for patient safety.

Effects on Organ Systems

Cardiovascular System

SNP administration produces arteriolar vasodilation resulting in dose-dependent decreases in SVR and MAP, with effects occurring rapidly and persisting for only a few minutes after IV bolus or discontinuation of CRI (Pagani et al. 1978; Pouleur et al. 1980; Kadowitz et al. 1981; Voss et al. 1985). The magnitude of reduction in SVR for a given dose is more profound during conditions of elevated arterial tone. Significant decreases in MAP may be accompanied by a marked reflex tachycardia that resolves shortly after stopping the infusion (Pagani et al. 1978). The vasodilation produced during SNP administration has also been observed to have differing effects on the blood flow to various organs; coronary blood flow had the largest relative increase, mesenteric and iliac blood flow showed moderate increases, and renal blood flow was minimally increased (Pagani et al. 1978). SNP also increases venous capacitance and alters blood volume distribution, as indicated by a significant downward shift of the venous return curve without changing the slope (Pouleur et al. 1980; Bower and Law 1993). PVR and MPAP both decrease with increasing doses of SNP, and the effects on PVR are more significant when there is some degree of pulmonary vasoconstriction (Kadowitz et al. 1981). The SNP induced vasodilation significantly decreases LV end-diastolic pressure in both normal hearts and those with LV dysfunction (Pagani et al. 1978; Saito et al. 1978; Pouleur et al. 1980; Hamaguchi et al. 1992). Left ventricular contractility has been reported to increase transiently after beginning an SNP CRI, while both LV end systolic and end-diastolic diameters remained significantly reduced for the duration of the SNP infusion.

The overall effects of SNP on CO are highly dependent on the pretreatment levels of arterial tone, venous tone, myocardial status, and the degree of baroreceptor response to any decreases in MAP, thus a wide range of effects on CO have been reported for SNP (Pagani et al. 1978; Saito et al. 1978; Pouleur et al. 1980; Kadowitz et al. 1981; Voss et al. 1985; Hamaguchi et al. 1992). In conscious dogs, with normal myocardial function, the combination of decreased SVR and a marked increase in heart rate produce a significant increase in CO during the initial five minutes of SNP infusion (Pagani et al. 1978). In anesthetized dogs, both increases and decreases in CO have been observed with SNP administration (Kadowitz et al. 1981; Voss et al. 1985; Hamaguchi et al. 1992). Under conditions of normal baseline arterial tone, CO may decrease with SNP administration in patients with normal hearts as venous return decreases, while CO increases in patients with decreased LV function as the decrease in venous return and afterload improve cardiac performance. When a normal myocardium is facing elevated afterload, then CO may increase with SNP administration.

In chloralose and urethane anesthetized dogs, SNP was observed to have significant anti-arrhythmic properties in the context of ischemia induced ventricular arrhythmias (Gönczi et al. 2009).

Respiratory System

Under conditions of normal oxygenation, SNP appears to have minimal effect on the respiratory system. Bolus or CRI administration of SNP did not significantly change PaO_2 in spontaneously breathing barbiturate anesthetized dogs (Kadowitz et al. 1981). High-dose SNP CRIs for 48 hours also did not significantly alter PaO_2 or arterial carbon dioxide tensions ($PaCO_2$) in dogs when mechanically ventilated with a mix of 30% oxygen and 70% nitrous oxide (Tinker and Michenfelder 1976). However, SNP administration may blunt or abolish HPV and could significantly worsen ventilation perfusion (V/Q) matching and decrease PaO_2 during conditions of alveolar hypoxia (Hill et al. 1979; D'Oliveira et al. 1981; Parsons et al. 1981). In barbiturate anesthetized dogs with left-sided atelectasis that were mechanically ventilated with 100% oxygen, SNP treatment increased the shunt fraction enough to produce a 40% reduction in PaO_2 (Colley and Cheney 1977).

Central Nervous System

SNP administration may impair cerebral autoregulation and increase ICP, thus it should not be used in patients with elevated ICP (Cottrell et al. 1978; Weiss et al. 1979; Thiagarajah et al. 1985).

Other Effects

The effects of SNP administration during cardiopulmonary resuscitation (CPR) have recently been explored in several animal models of cardiac arrest. The SNP-based protocols resulted in increased intracranial blood flow, increased return of spontaneous circulation, improved neurologic outcomes, and improved short-term survival compared to standard CPR protocols (Yannopoulos et al. 2011, 2017; Schultz et al. 2012). Additional investigations will likely determine the clinical utility of SNP-based CPR as more information is revealed.

SNP infusions may cause hypothyroidism due to the effects of CN and SCN on thyroid function (Philbrick et al. 1979).

Platelet function may be impaired during SNP administration, however, any dysfunction is rapidly reversed when the infusion is discontinued (Mehta and Mehta 1980; Rovin et al. 1993; Harris et al. 1995).

Contraindications

Profound hypotension and/or CN toxicity can result from SNP administration. SNP is contraindicated in patients with elevated ICP, hypotension, significant hemorrhage or hypovolemia, or any conditions where decreasing venous return would worsen cardiovascular status. In patients with reduced glomerular filtration rates, the maximum dose of SNP should be decreased accordingly due to risk of SCN accumulation and toxicity. Monitoring SCN levels should be considered in patients with renal impairment or those patients on high infusion rates of SNP for extended periods of time (Morris et al. 2017).

Drug Interactions

The vascular effects of SNP can be additive to those of other drugs producing vasodilation. Continuous blood pressure monitoring is critical for dose titration and avoiding excessive hypotension.

Sildenafil

Sildenafil is a nitrogen containing heterocyclic compound that was initially synthesized by Pfizer in 1989 as an intended therapy for angina, however, early clinical trials yielded disappointing results and the future of this drug became uncertain (Goldstein et al. 2019). Clinical development of sildenafil was almost discontinued until it was realized that sildenafil had potential for treating erectile dysfunction (ED) in men, after which the development of the drug took an entirely new direction. Sildenafil gained initial FDA approval in 1998 for the treatment of ED and is available in tablets, oral suspension, and an injectable formulation.

Mechanism of Action

Sildenafil is a selective phosphodiesterase-5 (PDE-5) inhibitor and exerts its biologic effects by prolonging the half-life of the second messenger molecule cGMP, resulting in selective smooth muscle relaxation in tissues with a high proportion of PDE-5 (Terrett et al. 1996).

Pharmacokinetics

Non-compartmental analysis has been used to describe select pharmacokinetic parameters for sildenafil in mice, rats, rabbits, and dogs (Walker et al. 1999). In mice after IV administration, sildenafil was highly cleared (91 ml kg/min), had a volume of distribution of 1 l/kg, and the elimination half-life was less than one hour. With oral administration, there was a significant first-pass effect, the bioavailability was 17% and time-to-peak concentration was 30 minutes. In mice, sildenafil was highly protein bound at 94%. In rats, the pharmacokinetics were gender dependent; male rats' clearance of sildenafil was almost four times faster than female rats (48 vs. 13 ml/kg/min). In female rats, the volume of distribution was nearly double (2.0 vs. 1.1 l/kg) and the elimination half-life was six times longer (1.9 vs. 0.3 hour) compared to male rats. Oral

administration resulted in greater bioavailability in female rats (44% vs. 23%), with much higher peak plasma concentrations achieved in less time compared to those reported in male rats. In rats, 95% of sildenafil was protein bound. In rabbits, only oral administration was investigated, with peak plasma concentrations observed two hours after administration. The terminal elimination half-life was 1.8 hours and the sildenafil was 91% protein bound.

In dogs, the clearance of sildenafil was similar to that of the female rat (12 ml/kg/min), however, dogs had a longer mean elimination half-life of 5.2 hours due to a larger mean volume of distribution (5.2 l/kg) attributed to only 86% of the drug being protein bound. In dogs, oral administration had a mean bioavailability of 54% and the peak plasma concentration was achieved in about one hour. Ideally, sildenafil should be administered in a fasted state, as administration to dogs with a meal has been shown to cause significant decreases in peak plasma concentration and bioavailability (Akabane et al. 2018). Rectal administration of sildenafil has also been investigated in healthy dogs (Yang et al. 2018). Compared to oral administration of the same dose, rectal administration produced 50% lower peak plasma concentrations and also halved the area under the curve (AUC). Rectal administration at five times the dose resulted in similar peak plasma concentrations, time-to-peak plasma concentration, and elimination half-life compared to oral administration. However, the AUC was more than double. The authors concluded that further investigations are needed to determine the optimal dose of sildenafil for rectal administration.

In thoroughbred horses, oral administration of sildenafil required relatively high doses (5 mg/kg) in order to produce mean plasma concentrations considered to be therapeutic in humans (Colahan et al. 2010). The time needed to reach peak plasma concentrations was approximately three hours.

Metabolism

Sildenafil's excretion is entirely dependent on hepatic metabolism involving the cytochrome P450 enzymes and requires NADPH (Walker et al. 1999). The performance of the cytochrome P450 system has been documented to be gender dependent in rats and this explains the marked difference in the observed pharmacokinetics between male and female rats (Kato and Yamazoe 1992). The metabolism of sildenafil is complex and involves five major pathways including aliphatic hydroxylation, pyrazole N-demethylation, piperazine N-demethylation, piperazine oxidation, or piperazine N,N-deethylation. Any administered sildenafil is ultimately excreted as small amounts of at least 16 different metabolites, with 87–98% of the administered dose being excreted within five days of administration in all species studied (Walker et al. 1999). Of the excreted metabolites, approximately 80–90% were found in the feces while only small amounts were present in urine.

Clinical Use

Sildenafil was initially FDA approved for treatment of ED in men, and since has also been approved for the treatment of pulmonary hypertension (PH) in humans. In veterinary medicine, sildenafil has mainly been used for the management of PH in dogs (Bach et al. 2006; Brown et al. 2010; Kellum and Stepien 2007; Toyoshima et al. 2007). Recently, there have been reports of sildenafil therapy for more nontraditional uses including the medical management of intracardiac heartworm infections, congenital megaesophagus, and myxomatous mitral valve degeneration (MMVD) (Kijtawornrat et al. 2017; Pirintr et al. 2017; Quintavalla et al. 2017; Tjostheim et al. 2019).

Effect on Patients Under General Anesthesia

Sildenafil administration may cause significant systemic vasodilation and associated hemodynamic changes in anesthetized patients. Supratherapeutic doses of sildenafil (3 mg/kg IV over 10 minutes) administered to halothane-anesthetized dogs produced transient decreases in SVR lasting 10–20 minutes that were accompanied by reflex increases in heart rate and inotropy that prevented any hypotension (Sugiyama et al. 2001). Similar changes in SVR, HR, and CO have been observed in dogs anesthetized with enflurane and nitrous oxide after receiving a 1 mg/kg IV sildenafil bolus (Yoo et al. 2002). In ketamine-xylazine anesthetized rabbits, an IV bolus of sildenafil (0.7 mg/kg) produced transient yet marked reductions in MAP resulting in hypotension, while oral administration (1.4 mg/kg) only produced mild yet sustained reductions in MAP that persisted for the entire 60 minute observation period (Ockaili et al. 2002). Significant increases in cardiac index (CI) with a minimal change in MAP were observed in propofol-anesthetized pigs following oral sildenafil administration, indicating that SVR had decreased compared to baseline values (Kleinsasser et al. 2001). In sufentanil- and α-chloralose-anesthetized dogs breathing a hypoxic mixture, sildenafil administration caused both systemic and pulmonic vasodilation that decreased MAP and MPAP both by approximately 12%; these effects on systemic circulation were not significantly different than those of a SNP CRI (Fesler et al. 2006).

Effects on Organ Systems

Cardiovascular System

Sildenafil's vasodilating effects are generally considered to be selective for the pulmonary vasculature due to its high concentration of PDE-5 (Corbin et al. 2005). Interestingly, when pressure vs. flow curves were used to assess the hemodynamic effects of sildenafil in dogs, there was no selectivity observed for pulmonary vs. systemic circulation (Fesler et al. 2006). The authors concluded that most of the apparent pulmonary selectivity reported in other studies was likely the result of differences in baroreceptor-mediated reflexes present in systemic vs. pulmonary circulation. Indeed, in most of the literature, sildenafil appears to have minimal impacts on systemic hemodynamics in awake animals. In conscious healthy dogs, oral sildenafil administration (3 mg/kg) did not produce any significant changes in MAP or heart rate (HR). However IV bolus administration of even low doses can result in transient decreases in MAP and reflex tachycardia (Kim et al. 2005; Zhao et al. 2006). No significant effects on HR or MAP were observed in dogs with naturally occurring MMVD receiving sildenafil treatment (1–3 mg/kg BID to TID) for short- or long-term therapy (Kijtawornrat et al. 2017; Saetang and Surachetpong 2020). Compared to the placebo group, sildenafil-treated horses (5 mg/kg PO) had significantly higher HR during submaximal exercise and during recovery, which was attributed to modest peripheral vasodilation caused by sildenafil treatment (Colahan et al. 2010). In a pig model of acute pulmonary embolism, sildenafil produced a 30% decrease in SVR that was accompanied by an increased CO and no change in MAP (Schultz et al. 2020).

Sildenafil does not appear to have significant effects on pulmonary circulation when baseline PVR and MPAP are normal (Kleinsasser et al. 2001; Yoo et al. 2002; Dias-Junior et al. 2005a). When pretreatment PVR and MPAP are elevated, sildenafil can produce marked decreases in PVR and MPAP with minimal effects on systemic circulation, as several animal models of PH have demonstrated. In a canine model of chronic embolic PH, sildenafil administration (1, 2, or 4 mg/kg PO BID) significantly reduced PVR and MPAP in a dose-dependent fashion without any significant effects on HR, SVR, or CO (Akabane et al. 2020). The 4 mg/kg dose decreased PVR by over 50% and decreased MPAP by 33% without any adverse effects. In a model of acute pulmonary embolism using xylazine ketamine anesthetized dogs, sildenafil infusions resulted in dose-dependent decreases in PVRI and MPAP without any significant changes in HR, MAP, SVRI, or CI (Dias-Junior et al. 2005a, 2005b). The high sildenafil infusion dose

(1 mg/kg IV over 15 minutes followed by 0.3 g/kg/hr for 30 minutes) decreased MPAP by 47% and PVRI by over 50% with the peak effects observed 45 minutes after finishing the infusion (Dias-Junior et al. 2005a). In dogs with naturally occurring PH, sildenafil therapy has been reported to significantly reduce severity of clinical signs and improve quality of life (Bach et al. 2006; Brown et al. 2010; Saetang and Surachetpong 2020).

Oral administration of sildenafil produced dose-dependent decreases in MPAP and PVR in awake sheep with acute PH induced via a thromboxane A_2 analog infusion (Weimann et al. 2000). Maximum pulmonary vasodilation was achieved within 15 minutes of sildenafil treatment and maintained for the entire 90 minute observation period. The highest dose investigated (2.5 mg/kg PO) reduced MPAP by 43% and PVR by 45% without having any significant effects on SVR or CO. The same model of acute PH was also used to show that nebulized sildenafil was effective in producing selective pulmonary vasodilation without effecting CO, SVR, or MAP (Ichinose et al. 2001). Unfortunately, these reductions in PVR and MPAP were short lived with nebulization.

In exercising thoroughbreds sildenafil administration (5 mg/kg PO) had no effect on exercise-induced increases in MPAP or the occurrence of exercise-induced pulmonary hemorrhage (Colahan et al. 2010).

Sildenafil appears to cause minimal electrocardiogram (ECG) changes in most circumstances and may even be anti-arrhythmic under certain conditions. In conscious healthy dogs, oral sildenafil administration (3 mg/kg) did not produce any significant changes in PR interval, QRS duration, or QT interval (Kim et al. 2005). Long-term sildenafil therapy in dogs with naturally occurring MMVD also did not result in any significant ECG changes (Kijtawornrat et al. 2017). Sildenafil administration at up to 3 mg/kg IV did not significantly alter the PR interval, QRS width, QT interval, QTc, effective refractory period, or post-repolarization refractoriness in halothane-anesthetized dogs (Sugiyama et al. 2001). In chloralose urethane anesthetized dogs, sildenafil administration (2 mg/kg PO) 24 hours prior significantly prolonged the QT interval and reduced both number and severity of ischemia-induced ventricular arrhythmias (Nagy et al. 2004).

Respiratory System

Multiple inert gas analysis showed that sildenafil administration significantly altered respiratory function in propofol-anesthetized pigs that were mechanically ventilated with 21% oxygen (Kleinsasser et al. 2001). Approximately 30 minutes after sildenafil treatment (0.65, 1.3, or 2.6 mg/kg PO), there were significant alterations in V/Q matching in all treatment groups; blood flow to areas of normal V/Q decreased and intrapulmonary shunt flow increased. The alveolar-arterial oxygen gradient increased while $PaCO_2$ and arterial pH remained unchanged. There were no significant changes to dead-space ventilation, airway pressures, or compliance.

In a model of acute pulmonary embolism using xylazine-ketamine anesthetized dogs, sildenafil infusions did not significantly change PaO_2. However, sildenafil treatment had protective effects on the lung and was able to mitigate the amount of oxidative stress induced by the pulmonary embolism (Dias-Junior et al. 2005a). Lung protective effects of sildenafil have also been demonstrated in a saline lavage-induced model of acute lung injury (Kosutova et al. 2018). Lung injury was produced in tiletamine-zolazepam anesthetized rabbits by repetitive saline lavage until compliance was less than 30% of baseline and the PaO_2 was less than 200 mmHg, which corresponds to a PaO_2 to FiO_2 ratio of less than 200 and more than meets the criteria for acute lung injury (Bernard et al. 1994). Sildenafil treatment (1 mg/kg IV) significantly improved compliance and gas exchange resulting in increased PaO_2, decreased $PaCO_2$, and decreased shunt fraction. Sildenafil also attenuated lung injury by reducing neutrophil accumulation and decreasing pro-inflammatory cytokine production that resulted in decreased epithelial apoptosis, decreased alveolar-capillary membrane damage, and decreased edema.

Sildenafil nebulization did not significantly change PaO_2, $PaCO_2$, or shunt fraction in awake sheep spontaneously breathing 60–70% oxygen during acute PH induced by a thromboxane A_2 analog (Ichinose et al. 2001).

Central Nervous System

Several animal models have been used to investigate the central nervous system (CNS) effects of sildenafil. In rats subjected to cerebral ischemia, sildenafil enhanced neurogenesis and improved neurologic function (Zhang et al. 2002, 2006). Sildenafil also significantly improved neurologic recovery in a mouse model of subarachnoid hemorrhage (Han et al. 2012). Neuroprotective effects of sildenafil have also been observed with rabbits in the context of acute spinal cord injury (Kara et al. 2015). Animal models investigating its impact on the seizure threshold have yielded conflicting results, with sildenafil reported to have both pro-convulsant and anticonvulsant effects (Riazi et al. 2006; Nieoczym et al. 2018).

Other Effects

Phosphodiesterase plays a significant role in the regulation of cellular activity in a variety of cell types, thus the effects of PDE-5 inhibition with sildenafil have been investigated in several body systems. Animal models of ischemia and reperfusion injury have reported sildenafil to have cardioprotective and renoprotective effects (Ockaili et al. 2002; Choi et al. 2009; Zahran et al. 2019). Sildenafil has inhibitory effects on smooth muscle activity in the esophagus, the lower esophageal sphincter, the stomach, and the small intestine (Zhang et al. 2001; Zhu et al. 2007; Xu and Chen 2006). Immune function, both in health and disease, has also been shown to be altered by sildenafil in multiple animal models (Kniotek and Boguska 2017).

Contraindications

Sildenafil should not be administered to animals being treated with organic nitrates, as it may cause excessive decreases in MAP.

Drug Interactions

The hypotensive effects of SNP or NTG are markedly increased by the concurrent administration of sildenafil, thus sildenafil should not be administered with nitrates (Schwemmer et al. 2001; Yoo et al. 2002). Any drugs that inhibit cytochrome P450 enzyme system have the potential to decrease the clearance of sildenafil and increase the AUC as well as the potential for adverse effects (Kim et al. 2005; Bae et al. 2009).

Nitric Oxide

NO is a gas that can be inhaled in small concentrations to produce selective pulmonary vasodilation. The exogenous NO may be sourced from either a compressed gas cylinder containing a mix of NO and nitrogen or produced using special equipment that generates NO from air using pulsed electrical discharges (Yu et al. 2015).

Mechanism of Action

Inhaled NO serves as a direct source of NO that diffuses into the vascular smooth muscle cells and activates soluble guanylate cyclase. The resulting increase in intracellular levels of cGMP leads to smooth muscle relaxation (Ignarro and Gruetter 1980).

Pharmacokinetics

The uptake of NO from the alveoli is dependent on respiratory rate, tidal volume, deadspace volume, and pulsed vs. continuous administration (Heinonen et al. 2000; Martin et al. 2014). Fractional uptake of NO decreases and NO accumulation in the breathing circuit occurs with prolonged pulses, pulses in the later part of inspiration, or with continuous administration. Pulsed delivery during the first third of inspiration is the most efficient method of delivery, with uptake of NO being as high as 92% (Heinonen et al. 2002; Grubb et al. 2013). The disappearance of NO from plasma is then extremely rapid, if not instantaneous. Due to the challenges of direct NO measurement, investigations instead focus on downstream nitrogen oxide species (Viinikka 1996; Horton and Schiefer 2019). In rats, inhaled NO administration produced significant increases in plasma nitrate levels, with the majority being cleared in the urine during the first 24 hours after administration (Yoshida et al. 1980).

Metabolism

Once inhaled NO diffuses into the pulmonary vessels, it enters RBCs and interacts with oxyhemoglobin to yield nitrate and met-hemoglobin (Yoshida et al. 1980). The NO may also react with oxygen gas in the lung and form NO_2, which is extremely toxic to cells and can cause pulmonary edema and respiratory failure leading to death (Greenbaum et al. 1967). Given this information, there is concern for the potential of met-hemoglobinemia and NO_2 toxicity with prolonged inhaled NO administration or when administering high concentrations. Delivery of NO into the endotracheal tube (ET) vs. other parts of the breathing circuit and using pulsed as opposed to continuous administration will minimize NO_2 production (Breuer et al. 1997; Heinonen et al. 2002). Adverse effects have not been reported when using appropriate dosing and monitoring, even with long-term administration (Barst et al. 2012).

Clinical Use

Inhaled NO was FDA approved in 1999 for the treatment of hypoxic respiratory failure in neonates with evidence of PH. In veterinary medicine, inhaled NO is primarily used for treating hypoxemia in anesthetized horses. Inhaled NO has not yet found widespread clinical use in veterinary medicine due to the cost and availability of the specialized equipment required.

Effect on Patients Under General Anesthesia

Inhaled NO has been shown to improve oxygenation and V/Q matching in anesthetized animals without producing any significant effects on systemic hemodynamics

(Heinonen et al. 2001, 2002; Nyman et al. 2012; Wiklund et al. 2017, 2020). Inhaled delivery of NO produces selective vasodilation in the ventilated regions of lung, resulting in blood-flow redistribution with increased blood flow to these ventilated areas of lung and decreased right-to-left shunting. These changes in blood flow occur without any significant effects on PAP, CO, or SVR. The ability to improve oxygenation is affected by mode of ventilation, CO, and how NO is administered (Heinonen et al. 2002; Auckburally et al. 2019). Spontaneously breathing horses experienced significantly greater improvements in oxygenation compared to mechanically ventilated horses, and mechanically ventilated horses may only benefit from inhaled NO when MAP is maintained above 70 mmHg with dobutamine. Pulsed administration is also only efficacious when it occurs during the first half of the inspiratory phase. Any observed improvements in oxygenation will be maintained as long as the inhaled NO continues to be administered during anesthesia, as the beneficial effects quickly dissipate when it is discontinued (Nyman et al. 2012).

Effects on Organ Systems

Cardiovascular System

Once inhaled NO enters the blood, it is rapidly inactivated by its reaction with hemoglobin, thus limiting its cardiovascular effects to pulmonary circulation (Frostell et al. 1991). In the absence of elevated PVR, treatment with inhaled NO does not produce any significant changes in PVR or PAP (Frostell et al. 1991; Lester et al. 1999; Kästner et al. 2005). When inhaled NO is administered in the context of increased PVR, several animal models have demonstrated dose-dependent decreases in PVR and PAP. Inhaled NO significantly attenuated the increase in PVR and PAP caused by administration of a thromboxane analog to sheep and foals (Fratacci et al. 1991; Lester et al. 1999). In neonatal foals, inhaling 80 ppm NO was also able to reverse the PH produced by breathing a hypoxic gas mixture. The ability of inhaled NO to inhibit HPV has also been described in sheep, dogs, and pigs (Frostell et al. 1991; Romand et al. 1994; Emil et al. 1996). Tachyphylaxis has not been reported, even when used for long-term treatment of PH (Barst et al. 2012).

Respiratory System

In addition to the improvements in oxygenation and V/Q matching described above, inhaled NO has also been reported to have bronchodilating effects. Similar to its effects on lungs with normal PVR, inhaled NO does not significantly alter respiratory mechanics in animals without bronchoconstriction (Högman et al. 1993). In Guinea pigs, rabbits, and swine with methacholine-induced bronchoconstriction, inhaled NO acted as a potent bronchodilator and was able to markedly decrease airway resistance and improve compliance (Dupuy et al. 1992; Högman et al. 1993; Putensen et al. 1995).

Central Nervous System

Inhaled NO at 50 ppm does not alter cerebral blood flow, autoregulation, or ICP under normal conditions (Terpolilli et al. 2012, 2013). In an animal model investigating ischemic brain damage with mice and sheep, inhaled NO at 50 ppm acted as a selective vasodilator in areas of low perfusion and significantly increased blood flow to the ischemic area, reduced infarct size, and improved neurologic outcome (Terpolilli et al. 2012). Beneficial effects of inhaled NO were also observed in a model exploring traumatic brain injury (TBI) in mice, where inhaled NO for 24 hours was reported to reduce ICP, selectively increase blood flow to traumatized tissue, reduce lesion size, and improve neurologic outcome without any adverse effects (Terpolilli et al. 2013).

Other Effects

Breathing 20 ppm of NO during CPR may offer improved blood flow, increased survival rates, and improved neurologic outcomes in multiple animal models of cardiac arrest (Brücken et al. 2015; Derwall et al. 2015). Inhaled NO has also been reported to reduce the complications associated receiving RBCs after a prolonged period of storage (Baron et al. 2012, 2013). Platelet function and coagulation may be impaired by inhaled NO (Högman et al. 1994; Kermarrec et al. 1998).

Contraindications

In humans, inhaled NO is contraindicated in preterm neonates who are normally dependent on right-to-left shunting of blood (INOMAX 2013).

Drug Interactions

The bronchodilating effects of terbutaline and inhaled NO are additive (Dupuy et al. 1992). Nebulized sildenafil administration can potentiate the pulmonary vasodilating actions of inhaled NO (Ichinose et al. 2001).

Conclusions

Pharmacologic manipulation of blood pressure with an exogenous source of NO occurred 100 years before we knew about the role of NO in regulating vascular tone. Although NO was initially investigated for its role in the cardiovascular system, advances in technology are making inhaled NO delivery more feasible and its potential treatment for a variety of respiratory disorders is being explored. In addition, a more recent understanding of the importance of NO in immunity and neurologic function will likely provide new applications for therapeutics that manipulate the NO pathway. As drug development strategies shift to creating NO mimetic molecules and novel NO donors, we will surely see new vasodilating agents find their way into the clinic.

References

Achiel, R., Carver, A., and Sanders, R.A. (2020). Treatment of congestive heart failure with intravenous nitroglycerin in three dogs with degenerative valvular disease. *J. Am. Anim. Hosp. Assoc.* 56 (1): 37–41.

Akabane, R., Sato, T., Sakatani, A. et al. (2018). Pharmacokinetics of single-dose sildenafil administered orally in clinically healthy dogs: effect of feeding and dose proportionality. *J. Vet. Pharmacol. Ther.* 41 (3): 457–462.

Akabane, R., Sakatani, A., Ogawa, M. et al. (2020). The effect of sildenafil on pulmonary haemodynamics in a canine model of chronic embolic pulmonary hypertension. *Res. Vet. Sci.* 133: 106–110.

Arnold, W.P., Longnecker, D.E., and Epstein, R.M. (1984). Photodegradation of sodium nitroprusside: biologic activity and cyanide release. *Anesthesiology* 61 (3): 254–260.

Auckburally, A., Grubb, T.L., Wiklund, M., and Nyman, G. (2019). Effects of ventilation mode and blood flow on arterial oxygenation during pulse-delivered inhaled nitric oxide in anesthetized horses. *Am. J. Vet. Res.* 80 (3): 275–283.

Bach, J.F., Rozanski, E.A., MacGregor, J. et al. (2006). Retrospective evaluation of sildenafil citrate as a therapy for pulmonary hypertension in dogs. *J. Vet. Intern. Med.* 20: 1132–1135.

Bae, S.H., Bae, S.K., and Lee, M.G. (2009). Effect of hepatic CYP inhibitors on the metabolism of sildenafil and formation of its metabolite, N-desmethylsildenafil, in rats in vitro and in vivo. *J. Pharm. Pharmacol.* 61 (12): 1637–1642.

Baron, D.M., Yu, B., Lei, C. et al. (2012). Pulmonary hypertension in lambs transfused with stored blood is prevented by breathing nitric oxide. *Anesthesiology* 116 (3): 637–647.

Baron, D.M., Beloiartsev, A., Nakagawa, A. et al. (2013). Adverse effects of hemorrhagic shock resuscitation with stored blood are ameliorated by inhaled nitric oxide in lambs*. *Crit. Care Med.* 41 (11): 2492–2501.

Barst, R.J., Channick, R., Ivy, D., and Goldstein, B. (2012). Clinical perspectives with long-term pulsed inhaled nitric oxide for the treatment of pulmonary arterial hypertension. *Pulm. Circ.* 2 (2): 139–147.

Becker, R.C., Corrao, J.M., Bovill, E.G. et al. (1990). Intravenous nitroglycerin-induced heparin resistance: a qualitative antithrombin III abnormality. *Am. Heart J.* 119 (6): 1254–1261.

Bedford, R.F. (1978). Increasing halothane concentrations reduce nitroprusside dose requirement. *Anesth. Analg.* 57 (4): 457–462.

Bedford, R.F. (1979). Sodium nitroprusside: hemodynamic dose-response during enflurane and morphine anesthesia. *Anesth. Analg.* 58 (3): 174–178.

Behnia, R., Raymon, F., Cheng, S.C., and Sharmahd, S. (1978). Metabolism of sodium nitroprusside in dogs awake and anesthetized with halothane. *Anesthesiology* 48 (4): 260–262.

Bernard, G.R., Artigas, A., Brigham, K.L. et al. (1994). Report of the American-European consensus conference on acute respiratory distress syndrome: definitions, mechanisms, relevant outcomes, and clinical trial coordination. Consensus Committee. *J. Crit. Care* 9 (1): 72–81.

Bloor, B.C., Stead, S.W., Snipper, D.M., and Flacke, W.E. (1989). Effect of halothane concentration on tachyphylaxis to sodium nitroprusside. *J. Cardiovasc. Pharmacol.* 13 (3): 398–404.

Bogaert, M.G., Rosseel, M.T., and De Schaepdryver, A.F. (1969). Excretion in urine of metabolites of glyceryl trinitrate (trinitrin) in rabbits. *Arch. Int. Pharmacodyn. Ther.* 179 (2): 480–482.

Bower, E.A. and Law, A.C. (1993). The effects of N omega-nitro-L-arginine methyl ester, sodium nitroprusside and noradrenaline on venous return in the anaesthetized cat. *Br. J. Pharmacol.* 108 (4): 933–940.

Breuer, J., Waidelich, F., Irtel von Brenndorff, C. et al. (1997). Technical considerations for inhaled nitric oxide therapy: time response to nitric oxide dosing changes and formation of nitrogen dioxide. *Eur. J. Pediatr.* 156 (6): 460–462.

Brown, A., Davison, E., and Sleeper, M. (2010). Clinical efficacy of sildenafil in treatment of pulmonary arterial hypertension in dogs. *J. Vet. Intern. Med.* 24: 850–854.

Brücken, A., Derwall, M., Bleilevens, C. et al. (2015). Brief inhalation of nitric oxide increases resuscitation success and improves 7-day-survival after cardiac arrest in rats: a randomized controlled animal study. *Crit. Care* 17 (19): 408.

Chen, H.I., Chen, S.J., and Cheng, C.F. (1979). Direct and reflex effects of nitroglycerin on the blood volume distribution, evaluated by regional weighing in the cat. *J. Pharm. Pharmacol.* 31 (12): 810–813.

Choi, D.E., Jeong, J.Y., Lim, B.J. et al. (2009). Pretreatment of sildenafil attenuates ischemia-reperfusion renal injury in rats. *Am. J. Physiol. Renal Physiol.* 297 (2): F362–F370.

Chung, S.J. and Fung, H.L. (1990). Identification of the subcellular site for nitroglycerin metabolism to nitric oxide in bovine coronary smooth muscle cells. *J. Pharmacol. Exp. Ther.* 253 (2): 614–619.

Colahan, P.T., Jackson, C.A., Rice, B. et al. (2010). The effect of sildenafil citrate administration on selected physiological parameters of exercising thoroughbred horses. *Equine Vet. J. Suppl.* 42 (38): 606–612.

Colley, P.S. and Cheney, F.W. (1977). Sodium nitroprusside increases Qs/Qt in dogs with regional atelectasis. *Anesthesiology* 47 (4): 338–341.

Commarato, M.A., Winbury, M.M., and Kaplan, H.R. (1973). Glyceryl trinitrate and pentrinitrol (pentaerythritol trinitrate): comparative cardiovascular effects in dog, cat and rat by different routes of administration. *J. Pharmacol. Exp. Ther.* 187 (2): 300–307.

Corbin, J.D., Beasley, A., Blount, M.A., and Francis, S.H. (2005). High lung PDE5: a strong basis for treating pulmonary hypertension with PDE5 inhibitors. *Biochem. Biophys. Res. Commun.* 334 (3): 930–938.

Cossum, P.A., Roberts, M.S., Yong, A.C., and Kilpatrick, D. (1986). Distribution and metabolism of nitroglycerin and its metabolites in vascular beds of sheep. *J. Pharmacol. Exp. Ther.* 237 (3): 959–966.

Cottrell, J.E., Patel, K., Turndorf, H., and Ransohoff, J. (1978). Intracranial pressure changes induced by sodium nitroprusside in patients with intracranial mass lesions. *J. Neurosurg.* 48 (3): 329–331.

Crandall, L.A. (1933). The fate of glyceryl trinitrate in the tolerant and non-tolerant animal. *J. Pharmacol. Exp. Ther.* 48 (2): 127–140.

Derwall, M., Ebeling, A., Nolte, K.W. et al. (2015). Inhaled nitric oxide improves transpulmonary blood flow and clinical outcomes after prolonged cardiac arrest: a large animal study. *Crit. Care* 19 (1): 328.

Dias-Junior, C.A., Souza-Costa, D.C., Zerbini, T. et al. (2005a). The effect of sildenafil on pulmonary embolism-induced oxidative stress and pulmonary hypertension. *Anesth. Analg.* 101 (1): 115–120.

Dias-Junior, C.A., Vieira, T.F., Moreno, H. Jr. et al. (2005b). Sildenafil selectively inhibits acute pulmonary embolism-induced pulmonary hypertension. *Pulm. Pharmacol. Ther.* 18 (3): 181–186.

DiCarlo, F.J., Crew, M.C., Haynes, L.J. et al. (1968). The absorption and biotransformation of glyceryl trinitrate-1,3-14C by rats. *Biochem. Pharmacol.* 17 (10): 2179–2183.

D'Oliveira, M., Sykes, M.K., Chakrabarti, M.K. et al. (1981). Depression of hypoxic pulmonary vasoconstriction by sodium nitroprusside and nitroglycerine. *Br. J. Anaesth.* 53 (1): 11–18.

Dupuy, P.M., Shore, S.A., Drazen, J.M. et al. (1992). Bronchodilator action of inhaled nitric oxide in guinea pigs. *J. Clin. Invest.* 90 (2): 421–428.

Eades, S.C., Stokes, A.M., and Moore, R.M. (2006). Effects of an endothelin receptor antagonist and nitroglycerin on digital vascular function in horses during the prodromal stages of carbohydrate overload-induced laminitis. *Am. J. Vet. Res.* 67 (7): 1204–1211.

Emil, S., Kanno, S., Berkeland, J. et al. (1996). Sustained pulmonary vasodilation after inhaled nitric oxide for hypoxic pulmonary hypertension in swine. *J. Pediatr. Surg.* 31 (3): 389–393.

Fesler, P., Pagnamenta, A., Rondelet, B. et al. (2006). Effects of sildenafil on hypoxic pulmonary vascular function in dogs. *J. Appl. Phys.* 101 (4): 1085–1090.

Fratacci, M.D., Frostell, C.G., Chen, T.Y. et al. (1991). Inhaled nitric oxide. A selective pulmonary vasodilator of heparin-protamine vasoconstriction in sheep. *Anesthesiology* 75 (6): 990–999.

Friederich, J.A. and Butterworth, J.F. 4th (1995). Sodium nitroprusside: twenty years and counting. *Anesth. Analg.* 81 (1): 152–162.

Frostell, C., Fratacci, M.D., Wain, J.C. et al. (1991). Inhaled nitric oxide. A selective pulmonary vasodilator reversing hypoxic pulmonary vasoconstriction. *Circulation* 83 (6): 2038–2047.

Gilhooly, M.H., Eades, S.C., Stokes, A.M., and Moore, R.M. (2005). Effects of topical nitroglycerine patches and ointment on digital venous plasma nitric oxide concentrations and digital blood flow in healthy conscious horses. *Vet. Surg.* 34 (6): 604–609.

Goldstein, I., Burnett, A.L., Rosen, R.C. et al. (2019). The serendipitous story of sildenafil: an unexpected oral therapy for erectile dysfunction. *Sex. Med. Rev.* 7 (1): 115–128.

Gönczi, M., Papp, R., Kovács, M. et al. (2009). Modulation of gap junctions by nitric oxide contributes to the anti-arrhythmic effect of sodium nitroprusside? *Br. J. Pharmacol.* 156 (5): 786–793.

Greenbaum, R., Bay, J., Hargreaves, M.D. et al. (1967). Effects of higher oxides of nitrogen on the anaesthetized dog. *Br. J. Anaesth.* 39 (5): 393–404.

Grubb, T., Frendin, J.H., Edner, A. et al. (2013). The effects of pulse-delivered inhaled nitric oxide on arterial oxygenation, ventilation-perfusion distribution and plasma endothelin-1 concentration in laterally recumbent isoflurane-anaesthetized horses. *Vet. Anaesth. Analg.* 40 (6): e19–e30.

Hamaguchi, M., Ishibashi, T., Katsumata, N. et al. (1992). Effects of sodium nitroprusside (MR7S1) and nitroglycerin on the systemic, renal, cerebral, and coronary circulation of dogs anesthetized with enflurane. *Cardiovasc. Drugs Ther.* 6 (6): 611–622.

Han, B.H., Vellimana, A.K., Zhou, M.L. et al. (2012). Phosphodiesterase 5 inhibition attenuates cerebral vasospasm and improves functional recovery after experimental subarachnoid hemorrhage. *Neurosurgery* 70 (1): 178–187.

Harris, S.N., Rinder, C.S., Rinder, H.M. et al. (1995). Nitroprusside inhibition of platelet function is transient and reversible by catecholamine priming. *Anesthesiology* 83: 1145–1152.

Heinonen, E., Högman, M., and Meriläinen, P. (2000). Theoretical and experimental comparison of constant inspired concentration and pulsed delivery in NO therapy. *Intensive Care Med.* 26 (8): 1116–1123.

Heinonen, E., Hedenstierna, G., Meriläinen, P. et al. (2001). Pulsed delivery of nitric oxide counteracts hypoxaemia in the anaesthetized horse. *Vet. Anaesth. Analg.* 28 (1): 3–11.

Heinonen, E., Nyman, G., Meriläinen, P., and Högman, M. (2002). Effect of different pulses of nitric oxide on venous admixture in the anaesthetized horse. *Br. J. Anaesth.* 88 (3): 394–398.

Hill, A.B., Sykes, M.K., and Reyes, A. (1979). A hypoxic pulmonary vasoconstrictor response in dogs during and after infusion of sodium nitroprusside. *Anesthesiology* 50 (6): 484–488.

Hinckley, K.A., Fearn, S., Howard, B.R., and Henderson, I.W. (1996a). Nitric oxide donors as treatment for grass induced acute laminitis in ponies. *Equine Vet. J.* 28 (1): 17–28.

Hinckley, K.A., Fearn, S., Howard, B.R., and Henderson, I.W. (1996b). Glyceryl trinitrate enhances nitric oxide mediated perfusion within the equine hoof. *J. Endocrinol.* 151 (2): R1–R8.

Höbel, M. and Raithelhuber, A. (1976). Studies on the metabolism and distribution of 14C-sodium nitroprusside in rats (author's transl). *Arzneimittelforschung* 26 (11): 2015–2019.

Hoff, T.K., Hood, D.M., and Wagner, I.P. (2002). Effectiveness of glyceryl trinitrate for enhancing digital submural perfusion in horses. *Am. J. Vet. Res.* 63 (5): 648–652.

Högman, M., Frostell, C., Arnberg, H., and Hedenstierna, G. (1993). Inhalation of nitric oxide modulates methacholine-induced bronchoconstriction in the rabbit. *Eur. Respir. J.* 6 (2): 177–180.

Högman, M., Frostell, C., Arnberg, H. et al. (1994). Prolonged bleeding time during nitric oxide inhalation in the rabbit. *Acta Physiol. Scand.* 151 (1): 125–129.

Horton, A. and Schiefer, I.T. (2019). Pharmacokinetics and pharmacodynamics of nitric oxide mimetic agents. *Nitric Oxide* 1 (84): 69–78.

Ichinose, F., Erana-Garcia, J., Hromi, J. et al. (2001). Nebulized sildenafil is a selective pulmonary vasodilator in lambs with acute pulmonary hypertension. *Crit. Care Med.* 29 (5): 1000–1005.

Ignarro, L.J. and Gruetter, C.A. (1980). Requirement of thiols for activation of coronary arterial guanylate cyclase by glyceryl trinitrate and sodium nitrite. *Biochim. Biophys. Acta* 831: 221–231.

Ignarro, L.J., Buga, G.M., Wood, K.S. et al. (1987). Endothelium-derived relaxing factor produced and released from artery and vein is nitric oxide. *Proc. Natl. Acad. Sci. U.S.A.* 84 (24): 9265–9269.

INOMAX (2013). INOMAX- nitric oxide gas. INO Therapeutics. https://www.inomax.com/wp-content/themes/inomax-website/dist/downloads/Inomax-PI.pdf (accessed 30 June 2022).

Ioannides, C., Parke, D.V., and Taylor, I.W. (1982). Elimination of glyceryl trinitrate: effects of sex, age, species and route of administration. *Br. J. Pharmacol.* 77 (1): 83–88.

Ivankovich, A.D., Miletich, D.J., and Tinker, J.H. (1978). Sodium nitroprusside: metabolism and general considerations. *Int. Anesthesiol. Clin.* 16 (2): 1–29.

Johnson, E.M. Jr., Harkey, A.B., Blehm, D.J., and Needleman, P. (1972). Clearance and metabolism of organic nitrates. *J. Pharmacol. Exp. Ther.* 182 (1): 56–62.

Kadowitz, P.J., Nandiwada, P., Gruetter, C.A. et al. (1981). Pulmonary vasodilator responses to nitroprusside and nitroglycerin in the dog. *J. Clin. Invest.* 67 (3): 893–902.

Kamijo, T., Tomaru, T., Miwa, A.Y. et al. (1994). The effects of dobutamine, propranolol and nitroglycerin on an experimental canine model of congestive heart failure. *Jpn. J. Pharmacol.* 65 (3): 223–231.

Kara, H., Degirmenci, S., Ak, A. et al. (2015). Neuroprotective effects of sildenafil in experimental spinal cord injury in rabbits. *Bosn. J. Basic Med. Sci.* 15 (1): 38–44.

Kästner, S.B., Kull, S., Kutter, A.P. et al. (2005). Cardiopulmonary effects of dexmedetomidine in sevoflurane-anesthetized sheep with and without nitric oxide inhalation. *Am. J. Vet. Res.* 66 (9): 1496–1502.

Kato, R. and Yamazoe, Y. (1992). Sex-specific cytochrome P450 as a cause of sex- and species-related differences in drug toxicity. *Toxicol. Lett.* 64, 65: 661–667.

Keene, B.W., Atkins, C.E., Bonagura, J.D. et al. (2019). ACVIM consensus guidelines for the diagnosis and treatment of myxomatous mitral valve disease in dogs. *J. Vet. Intern. Med.* 33 (3): 1127–1140.

Kellum, H.B. and Stepien, R.L. (2007). Sildenafil citrate therapy in 22 dogs with pulmonary, hypertension. *J. Vet. Intern. Med.* 21: 1258–1264.

Kermarrec, N., Zunic, P., Beloucif, S. et al. (1998). Impact of inhaled nitric oxide on platelet aggregation and fibrinolysis in rats with endotoxic lung injury. Role of cyclic guanosine 5′-monophosphate. *Am. J. Respir. Crit. Care Med.* 158 (3): 833–839.

Kijtawornrat, A., Komolvanich, S., Saengklub, N. et al. (2017). Long-term effect of sildenafil on echocardiographic parameters in dogs with asymptomatic myxomatous mitral valve degeneration. *J. Vet. Med. Sci.* 79 (4): 788–794.

Kim, E.J., Seo, J.W., Hwang, J.Y., and Han, S.S. (2005). Effects of combined treatment with sildenafil and itraconazole on the cardiovascular system in telemetered conscious dogs. *Drug Chem. Toxicol.* 28 (2): 177–186.

Kleinsasser, A., Loeckinger, A., Hoermann, C. et al. (2001). Sildenafil modulates hemodynamics and pulmonary gas exchange. *Am. J. Respir. Crit. Care Med.* 163 (2): 339–343.

Kniotek, M. and Boguska, A. (2017). Sildenafil can affect innate and adaptive immune system in both experimental animals and patients. *J. Immunol. Res.* 2017: 4541958.

Kosutova, P., Mikolka, P., Balentova, S. et al. (2018). Effects of phosphodiesterase 5 inhibitor sildenafil on the respiratory parameters, inflammation and apoptosis in a saline lavage-induced model of acute lung injury. *J. Physiol. Pharmacol.* 69 (5): 815–826.

Lee, N.H. and Belpaire, F.M. (1972). Study of the increased glyceryl trinitrate metabolism after pretreatment with phenobarbital in rat liver. *Biochem. Pharmacol.* 21 (23): 3171–3177.

Lee, F.W., Salmonson, T., Metzler, C.H., and Benet, L.Z. (1990). Pharmacokinetics and pharmacodynamics of glyceryl trinitrate and its two dinitrate metabolites in conscious dogs. *J. Pharmacol. Exp. Ther.* 255 (3): 1222–1229.

Lee, F.W., Salmonson, T., and Benet, L.Z. (1993). Pharmacokinetics and pharmacodynamics of nitroglycerin and its dinitrate metabolites in conscious dogs: intravenous infusion studies. *J. Pharmacokinet. Biopharm.* 21 (5): 533–550.

Lester, G.D., DeMarco, V.G., and Norman, W.M. (1999). Effect of inhaled nitric oxide on experimentally induced pulmonary hypertension in neonatal foals. *Am. J. Vet. Res.* 60 (10): 1207–1212.

Luis Fuentes, V., Abbott, J., Chetboul, V. et al. (2020). ACVIM consensus statement guidelines for the classification, diagnosis, and management of cardiomyopathies in cats. *J. Vet. Intern. Med.* 34 (3): 1062–1077.

Manohar, M. (1995). Effects of glyceryl trinitrate (nitroglycerin) on pulmonary vascular pressures in standing thoroughbred horses. *Equine Vet. J.* 27 (4): 275–280.

Martin, A.R., Jackson, C., Katz, I.M., and Caillibotte, G. (2014). Variability in uptake efficiency for pulsed versus constant concentration delivery of inhaled nitric oxide. *Med. Gas Res.* 4 (1): 1.

Mehta, J. and Mehta, P. (1980). Comparative effects of nitroprusside and nitroglycerin on platelet aggregation in patients with heart failure. *J. Cardiovasc. Pharmacol.* 2 (1): 25–33.

Miyazaki, H., Ishibashi, M., Hashimoto, Y., Idzu, G., Furuta, Y. (1982). Simultaneous determination of glyceryl trinitrate and its principal metabolites, 1,2- and 1,3-glyceryl dinitrate, in plasma by gas chromatography-negative ion chemical ionization-selected ion monitoring. *J. Chromatogr.* 239: 277–286.

Moncada, S. and Higgs, A. (1993). The L-arginine-nitric oxide pathway. *N. Engl. J. Med.* 329 (27): 2002–2012.

Morris, P.J., Todd, M., and Philbin, D. (1982). Changes in canine intracranial pressure in response to infusions of sodium nitroprusside and trinitroglycerin. *Br. J. Anaesth.* 54 (9): 991–995.

Morris, A.A., Page, R.L. 2nd, Baumgartner, L.J. et al. (2017). Thiocyanate accumulation in critically ill patients receiving nitroprusside infusions. *J. Intensive Care Med.* 32 (9): 547–553.

Morse, M.A. and Rutlen, D.L. (1994). Influence of nitroglycerin on splanchnic capacity and splanchnic capacity-cardiac output relationship. *J. Appl. Phys.* 76 (1): 112–119.

Murrel, W. (1879). Nitro-glycerine as a remedy for angina pectoris. *Lancet* 1: 80–81. 113–115, 151–152, 225–227.

Nagy, O., Hajnal, A., Parratt, J.R., and Végh, A. (2004). Sildenafil (Viagra) reduces arrhythmia severity during ischaemia 24 h after oral administration in dogs. *Br. J. Pharmacol.* 141 (4): 549–551.

Needleman, P. (1970). Tolerance to the vascular effects of glyceryl trinitrate. *J. Pharmacol. Exp. Ther.* 171 (1): 98–102.

Needleman, P. and Hunter, F.E. Jr. (1965). The transformation of glyceryl trinitrate and other nitrates by glutathione-organic nitrate reductase. *Mol. Pharmacol.* 1 (1): 77–86.

Needleman, P., Blehm, D.J., Harkey, A.B. et al. (1971). The metabolic pathway in the degradation of glyceryl trinitrate. *J. Pharmacol. Exp. Ther.* 179 (2): 347–353.

Nieoczym, D., Socała, K., and Wlaź, P. (2018). Evaluation of the role of different neurotransmission systems in the anticonvulsant action of sildenafil in the 6 Hz-induced psychomotor seizure threshold test in mice. *Biomed. Pharmacother.* 107: 1674–1681.

Nyman, G., Grubb, T.L., Heinonen, E. et al. (2012). Pulsed delivery of inhaled nitric oxide counteracts hypoxaemia during 2.5 hours of inhalation anaesthesia in dorsally recumbent horses. *Vet. Anaesth. Analg.* 39 (5): 480–487.

Ockaili, R., Salloum, F., Hawkins, J., and Kukreja, R.C. (2002). Sildenafil (Viagra) induces powerful cardioprotective effect via opening of mitochondrial K(ATP) channels in rabbits. *Am. J. Physiol. Heart Circ. Physiol.* 283 (3): H1263–H1269.

Pagani, M., Vatner, S.F., and Braunwald, E. (1978). Hemodynamic effects of intravenous sodium nitroprusside in the conscious dog. *Circulation* 57 (1): 144–151.

Page, I.H., Corcoran, A.C., Dustan, H.P., and Koppanyi, T. (1955). Circulation cardiovascular actions of sodium nitroprusside in animals and hypertensive patients. *Circulation* 11 (2): 188–198.

Palmer, R.M., Ferrige, A.G., and Moncada, S. (1987). Nitric oxide release accounts for the biological activity of endothelium-derived relaxing factor. *Nature* 327 (6122): 524–526.

Parameswaran, N., Hamlin, R.L., Nakayama, T., and Rao, S.S. (1999). Increased splenic capacity in response to transdermal application of nitroglycerine in the dog. *J. Vet. Intern. Med.* 13 (1): 44–46.

Parsons, G.H., Leventhal, J.P., Hansen, M.M., and Goldstein, J.D. (1981). Effect of sodium nitroprusside on hypoxic pulmonary vasoconstriction in the dog. *J. Appl. Physiol. Respir. Environ. Exerc. Physiol.* 51 (2): 288–292.

Philbrick, D.J., Hopkins, J.B., Hill, D.C. et al. (1979). Effects of prolonged cyanide and thiocyanate feeding in rats. *J. Toxicol. Environ. Health Part A* 5 (4): 579–592.

Pirintr, P., Saengklub, N., Limprasutr, V. et al. (2017). Sildenafil improves heart rate variability in dogs with asymptomatic myxomatous mitral valve degeneration. *J. Vet. Med. Sci.* 79 (9): 1480–1488.

Pouleur, H., Covell, J.W., and Ross, J. Jr. (1980). Effects of nitroprusside on venous return and central blood volume in the absence and presence of acute heart failure. *Circulation* 61 (2): 328–337.

Putensen, C., Räsänen, J., and López, F.A. (1995). Improvement in VA/Q distributions during inhalation of nitric oxide in pigs with methacholine-induced bronchoconstriction. *Am. J. Respir. Crit. Care Med.* 151 (1): 116–122.

Quintavalla, F., Menozzi, A., Pozzoli, C. et al. (2017). Sildenafil improves clinical signs and radiographic features in dogs with congenital idiopathic megaoesophagus: a randomised controlled trial. *Vet. Rec.* 180 (16): 404.

Reade, M.C., Davies, S.R., Morley, P.T. et al. (2012). Australian resuscitation council. Review article: management of cyanide poisoning. *Emerg. Med. Australas.* 24: 225–238.

Riazi, K., Roshanpour, M., Rafiei-Tabatabaei, N. et al. (2006). The proconvulsant effect of sildenafil in mice: role of nitric oxide-cGMP pathway. *Br. J. Pharmacol.* 147 (8): 935–943.

Romand, J.A., Pinsky, M.R., Firestone, L. et al. (1994). Inhaled nitric oxide partially reverses hypoxic pulmonary vasoconstriction in the dog. *J. Appl. Phys.* 76 (3): 1350–1355.

Rovin, J.D., Stamler, J.S., Loscalzo, J., and Folts, J.D. (1993). Sodium nitroprusside, an endothelium-derived relaxing factor congener, increases platelet cyclic GMP levels and inhibits epinephrine-exacerbated in vivo platelet thrombus formation in stenosed canine coronary arteries. *J. Cardiovasc. Pharmacol.* 22 (4): 626–631.

Saetang, K. and Surachetpong, S.D. (2020). Short-term effects of sildenafil in the treatment of dogs with pulmonary hypertension secondary to degenerative mitral valve disease. *Vet. World* 13 (10): 2260–2268.

Saito, D., Ueda, M., Yoshida, H. et al. (1978). Comparative vasodilator effects of nitroprusside, phentolamine, and nitroglycerin on hemodynamics, regional myocardial function and epicardial electrogram in dogs with acute myocardial ischemia. *Jpn. Heart J.* 19 (6): 926–937.

Schultz, J., Segal, N., Kolbeck, J. et al. (2012). Sodium nitroprusside enhanced cardiopulmonary resuscitation (SNPeCPR) improves vital organ perfusion pressures and carotid blood flow in a porcine model of cardiac arrest. *Resuscitation* 83 (3): 374–377.

Schultz, J., Andersen, A., Gade, I.L. et al. (2020). Riociguat, sildenafil and inhaled nitric oxide reduces pulmonary vascular resistance and improves right ventricular function in a porcine model of acute pulmonary embolism. *Eur. Heart J. Acute Cardiovasc. Care* 9 (4): 293–301.

Schulz, V. (1984). Clinical pharmacokinetics of nitroprusside, cyanide, thiosulphate and thiocyanate. *Clin. Pharmacokinet.* 9 (3): 239–251.

Schulz, V., Bonn, R., and Kindler, J. (1979). Kinetics of elimination of thiocyanate in 7 healthy subjects and in 8 subjects with renal failure. *Klinische Wochenschrift* 57: 243–247.

Schwemmer, M., Bassenge, E., Stoeter, M. et al. (2001). Potentiation of sildenafil-induced hypotension is minimal with nitrates generating a radical intermediate. *J. Cardiovasc. Pharmacol.* 38 (1): 149–155.

Sobrero, M.A. (1847). Sur plusieurs composes detonants produits avec l'acide nitrique et de le sucre, la dextrin, la mannite et la glycerine. *CR Acad. Sci.* 25: 247–248.

Sugiyama, A., Satoh, Y., Shiina, H. et al. (2001). Cardiac electrophysiologic and hemodynamic effects of sildenafil, a PDE5 inhibitor, in anesthetized dogs. *J. Cardiovasc. Pharmacol.* 38 (6): 940–946.

Terpolilli, N.A., Kim, S.W., Thal, S.C. et al. (2012). Inhalation of nitric oxide prevents ischemic brain damage in experimental stroke by selective dilatation of collateral arterioles. *Circ. Res.* 110 (5): 727–738.

Terpolilli, N.A., Kim, S.W., Thal, S.C. et al. (2013). Inhaled nitric oxide reduces secondary brain damage after traumatic brain injury in mice. *J. Cereb. Blood Flow Metab.* 33 (2): 311–318.

Terrett, N.K., Bell, A.S., Brown, D., and Ellis, P. (1996). Sildenafil (Viagra), a potent and selective inhibitor of type 5 cGMP phosphodiesterase with utility for the treatment of male erectile dysfunction. *Bioorg. Med. Chem. Lett.* 6: 1819–1824.

Thiagarajah, S., Azar, I., Lear, E., and Albert, D. (1985). Intracranial pressure changes during infusions of verapamil as compared with sodium nitroprusside. *Bull. N. Y. Acad. Med.* 61 (7): 650–656.

Tinker, J.H. and Michenfelder, J.D. (1976). Sodium nitroprusside: pharmacology, toxicology and therapeutics. *Anesthesiology* 45 (3): 340–354.

Tjostheim, S.S., Kellihan, H.B., Grint, K.A., and Stepien, R.L. (2019). Effect of sildenafil and pimobendan on intracardiac heartworm infections in four dogs. *J. Vet. Cardiol.* 23: 96–103.

Toyoshima, Y., Kanemoto, I., Arai, S., and Toyoshima, H. (2007). A case of long-term sildenafil therapy in a young dog with pulmonary hypertension. *J. Vet. Med. Sci.* 69: 1073–1075.

Vatner, S.F., Higgins, C.B., Milland, R.W., and Franklin, D. (1972). Direct and reflex effects of nitroglycerin on coronary and left ventricular dynamics in conscious dogs. *J. Clin. Invest.* 51 (11): 2872–2882.

Vesey, C.J., Simpson, P.J., Adams, L., and Cole, P.V. (1979). Metabolism of sodium nitroprusside and cyanide in the dog. *Br. J. Anaesth.* 51 (2): 89–97.

Viinikka, L. (1996). Nitric oxide as a challenge for the clinical chemistry laboratory. *Scand. J. Clin. Lab. Invest.* 56 (7): 577–581.

Voss, G.I., Katona, P.G., and Dauchot, P.J. (1985). Effectiveness of sodium nitroprusside as a function of total peripheral resistance in the anesthetized dog. *Anesthesiology* 62 (2): 130–134.

Walker, D.K., Ackland, M.J., James, G.C. et al. (1999). Pharmacokinetics and metabolism of sildenafil in mouse, rat, rabbit, dog and man. *Xenobiotica* 29 (3): 297–310.

Weimann, J., Ullrich, R., Hromi, J. et al. (2000). Sildenafil is a pulmonary vasodilator in awake lambs with acute pulmonary hypertension. *Anesthesiology* 92 (6): 1702–1712.

Weiss, M.H., Spence, J., Apuzzo, M.L. et al. (1979). Influence of nitroprusside on cerebral pressure autoregulation. *Neurosurgery* 4: 56–59.

Wiklund, M., Granswed, I., and Nyman, G. (2017). Pulsed inhaled nitric oxide improves arterial oxygenation in colic horses undergoing abdominal surgery. *Vet. Anaesth. Analg.* 44 (5): 1139–1148.

Wiklund, M., Kellgren, M., Wulcan, S. et al. (2020). Effects of pulsed inhaled nitric oxide on arterial oxygenation during mechanical ventilation in anaesthetised horses undergoing elective arthroscopy or emergency colic surgery. *Equine Vet. J.* 52 (1): 76–82.

Xu, X. and Chen, J.D. (2006). Inhibitory effects of sildenafil on small intestinal motility and myoelectrical activity in dogs. *Dig. Dis. Sci.* 51 (4): 671–676.

Yang, H.J., Oh, Y.I., Jeong, J.W. et al. (2018). Comparative single-dose pharmacokinetics of sildenafil after oral and rectal administration in healthy beagle dogs. *BMC Vet. Res.* 14 (1): 291.

Yannopoulos, D., Matsuura, T., Schultz, J. et al. (2011). Sodium nitroprusside enhanced cardiopulmonary resuscitation improves survival with good neurological function in a porcine model of prolonged cardiac arrest. *Crit. Care Med.* 39 (6): 1269–1274.

Yannopoulos, D., Bartos, J.A., George, S.A. et al. (2017). Sodium nitroprusside enhanced cardiopulmonary resuscitation improves short term survival in a porcine model of ischemic refractory ventricular fibrillation. *Resuscitation* 110: 6–11.

Yoo, K.Y., Kim, H.S., Moon, J.D., and Lee, J. (2002). Sildenafil (Viagra) augments sodium nitroprusside-induced but not nitroglycerin-induced hypotension in dogs. *Anesth. Analg.* 94 (6): 1505–1509.

Yoshida, K., Kasama, K., Kitabatake, M. et al. (1980). Metabolic fate of nitric oxide. *Int. Arch. Occup. Environ. Health* 46 (1): 71–77.

Yu, B., Muenster, S., Blaesi, A.H. et al. (2015). Producing nitric oxide by pulsed electrical discharge in air for portable inhalation therapy. *Sci. Transl. Med.* 7 (294): 294ra107.

Yuen, P.H., Denman, S.L., Sokoloski, T.D., and Burkman, A.M. (1979). Loss of nitroglycerin from aqueous solution into plastic intravenous delivery systems. *J. Pharm. Sci.* 68 (9): 1163–1166.

Zahran, M.H., Barakat, N., Khater, S. et al. (2019). Renoprotective effect of local sildenafil administration in renal ischaemia-reperfusion injury: a randomised controlled canine study. *Arab. J. Urol.* 17 (2): 150–159.

Zhang, X., Tack, J., Janssens, J., and Sifrim, D.A. (2001). Effect of sildenafil, a phosphodiesterase-5 inhibitor, on oesophageal peristalsis and lower oesophageal sphincter function in cats. *Neurogastroenterol. Motil.* 13 (4): 325–331.

Zhang, R., Wang, Y., Zhang, L. et al. (2002). Sildenafil (Viagra) induces neurogenesis and promotes functional recovery after stroke in rats. *Stroke* 33 (11): 2675–2680.

Zhang, R.L., Zhang, Z., Zhang, L. et al. (2006). Delayed treatment with sildenafil enhances neurogenesis and improves functional recovery in aged rats after focal cerebral ischemia. *J. Neurosci. Res.* 83 (7): 1213–1219.

Zhao, G., Messina, E., Xu, X. et al. (2006). Ranolazine, a novel anti-anginal agent, does not alter isosorbide dinitrate- or sildenafil-induced changes in blood pressure in conscious dogs. *Eur. J. Pharmacol.* 541 (3): 171–176.

Zhu, H., Xu, X., and Chen, J.D. (2007). Inhibitory effects of sildenafil on gastric motility and gastric slow waves in dogs. *Neurogastroenterol. Motil.* 19 (3): 218–224.

22

Behavior Drugs

Erin Wendt-Hornickle

Introduction

Over 10 years ago, it was estimated that 40% of companion animals in the US had behavior disorders (Amat et al. 2009; Martinez et al. 2011). Aggression in dogs or inappropriate urination in cats, for example, are the most common reasons why adult animals are relinquished to animal shelters (Salman et al. 1998). Luckily, successful treatment of some behavior problems can occur with a combination of accurate diagnoses, behavior modification programs, environmental management and pharmacologic therapy.

Because of the prevalence of behavior problems, it is not unusual that patients presenting for anesthesia are receiving one or more behavior-modifying drugs. These patients may pose challenges related to the behavior disorder itself (e.g. separation anxiety, aggression) or co-morbidities associated with the condition requiring anesthesia and surgery (e.g. electrolyte abnormalities, hypovolemia). It is also important to understand the physiologic effects these drugs may have during the perianesthetic period to manage the anesthetists' expectations and preparations for potential complications during this time.

Selective Serotonin Reuptake Inhibitors (SSRIs)

Mechanism of Action

The effect of serotonin (5-hydroxytryptamine; 5HT) is determined by the amount available to bind to 5HT receptors on the post-synaptic membrane (Isbister and Buckley 2005) and autoreceptors on the pre-synaptic membrane which act as negative feedback to serotonin release (Mohammad-Zadeh et al. 2008). Serotonin that is not bound to 5HT receptors is removed from the synaptic cleft by binding to a selective serotonin transporter, which then moves it into the pre-synaptic cytosol where it is metabolized by monoamine oxidase (MAO) or repackaged into synaptic vesicles (Cerrito and Raiteri 1979). The mechanism of action of SSRIs is the pre-synaptic inhibition of the reuptake of synaptic serotonin within the central nervous system (CNS) allowing an increase in available serotonin for neurotransmission at $5HT_{1A}$ receptors.

Clinical Use

The most commonly used SSRIs in veterinary medicine are fluoxetine, paroxetine, sertraline and citalopram. Conditions treated include separation anxiety, compulsive disorders, phobias and fear- and anxiety-induced aggression in dogs and compulsive disorders, impulsive behaviors, aggression and urine marking in cats. In horses, fluoxetine has been used to decrease libido in breeding animals (Sherman and Papich 2009).

Metabolism

All SSRIs are metabolized in the liver to variably active metabolites and excreted through the kidneys or eliminated in bile (Crowell-Davis 2006a). Doses should be reduced in patients with hepatic and renal disease.

Fluoxetine is metabolized to an active metabolite, norfluoxetine. Citalopram is metabolized to less active metabolites, demethylcitalopram, di-demethylcitalopram, citalopram-N-oxide and an inactive deaminated proprionic acid. Evidence suggests that cats metabolize citalopram slower than other species (rats and dogs) (Lainesse et al. 2007). Some data suggests that dogs convert citalopram to its metabolites more than humans (Forest Laboratories, Inc. 2002). In humans, paroxetine is metabolized to many inactive metabolites (SmithKline Beecham Pharmaceuticals 2004). Sertraline is metabolized to a less active *N*-desmethylsertraline (Tremaine et al. 1989).

Pharmacology in Veterinary Anesthesia and Analgesia, First Edition. Edited by Turi Aarnes and Phillip Lerche.
© 2024 John Wiley & Sons, Inc. Published 2024 by John Wiley & Sons, Inc.

Pharmacokinetics

Pharmacokinetics differ with each SSRI and species examined. In dogs, fluoxetine has an elimination half-life of 3–13 hours; norfluoxetine has an elimination half-life of 33–64 hours. Cats have a longer reported half-life of 47 and 55 hours for fluoxetine and norfluoxetine respectively (Ciribassi et al. 2003). In humans, paroxetine has a long half-life of 10 days (SmithKline Beecham Pharmaceuticals 2004). The half-lives of citalopram, demethylcitalopram and didemethylcitalopram in humans are 1.5, 2, and 4 days respectively (Pollock 2001). Sertraline is extensively protein bound (97%). The clearance of sertraline is greater than 35 ml/min/kg in both rats and dogs (Tremaine et al. 1989).

Effects on Organ Systems

Serotonin is released from platelets in response to vascular injury. It causes platelet aggregation and local vasoconstriction to promote coagulation. Since platelets do not have the ability to synthesize serotonin, it can become depleted during surgical procedures, resulting in eventual impaired coagulation (McCloskey et al. 2008; Andrade et al. 2010). The degree of impairment seems to be correlated with the degree of serotonin reuptake inhibition in humans (Meijer et al. 2004). More research is required before determining the clinical relevance of SSRIs and intraoperative hemorrhage in veterinary species.

Patients receiving SSRIs most commonly experience sedation and decreased appetite. Other side effects include tremors, constipation, diarrhea, nausea, irritability or agitation, insomnia, hyponatremia and seizures (Fitzgerald and Bronstein 2013; Crowell-Davis 2006a). All SSRIs can potentially cause arrhythmias through inhibition of L-type Ca^{2+} currents and attenuation of outward K^+ currents (Park et al. 1999).

Other Effects

Paroxetine has mild anticholinergic effects and may induce stool and urine retention (Landsberg et al. 2013). In dogs receiving supra-clinical doses, mydriasis, elevations in liver enzymes, hindlimb weakness, hyperactivity and anorexia may occur (Davies and Kluwe 1998). A syndrome of inappropriate antidiuretic hormone release has been reported in humans with the use of SSRIs (Rosner 2004).

Serotonin Syndrome

Serotonin syndrome is a potentially fatal complication most commonly occurring from an overdose of an SSRI or from a drug interaction when two or more drugs that alter serotonin levels are combined. Symptoms most commonly include CNS depression, agitation, hyperreflexia, myoclonus, shivering, vomiting, diarrhea, incoordination, hyperthermia and tremors (Peck et al. 2010; Pugh et al. 2013). Serotonin syndrome may also cause cardiovascular effects such as bradycardia, tachycardia, arrhythmias and changes in blood pressure (Pugh et al. 2013). If not treated, serotonin syndrome can result in seizures, rhabdomyolysis, renal failure, coma and death.

Contraindications

Many SSRIs are excreted through milk. Some have been shown to decrease feeding in neonates and should only be used in lactating females when the benefits outweigh the risks. Caution should be used in diabetic patients, as administration and withdrawal of SSRIs can exacerbate glucose abnormalities (Sanders et al. 2008). Decreased libido is a side effect of fluoxetine and its use should be limited to non-breeding animals.

Drug Interactions

Drug interactions seen with administration of SSRIs are with drugs that also inhibit serotonin reuptake, for example, monoamine oxidase inhibitors (MAOIs; Gillman 2005). Avoid the use of SSRIs in patients receiving drugs that affect serotonin levels such as tramadol, meperidine, pethidine and other antidepressants (Peck et al. 2010). There is speculation that all phenylpiperidine opioids (fentanyl, meperidine, tramadol, alfentanil, sufentanil, remifentanil) can act as weak SSRIs (Greenier et al. 2014). Fluoxetine, paroxetine and sertraline competitively inhibit some cytochrome p450 enzymes (Crowell-Davis 2006a; Sherman and Papich 2009; Landsberg et al. 2013). Patients receiving fluoxetine or paroxetine may have the potential for increased plasma concentration of drugs highly dependent upon hepatic metabolism or drugs that also inhibit cytochrome p450 enzymes (CYP). Examples include benzodiazepines, beta blockers, ketoconazole, trazodone, warfarin, tricyclic antidepressants (TCAs) and MAO-Is as well as barbiturates, phenothiazines, tramadol, methadone, and codeine (Crowell-Davis 2006a; Landsberg et al. 2013). The interference with methadone results in a significant increase in the plasma levels of methadone in dogs (Kukanich and Cohen 2011). The interference with the normal metabolism of codeine to morphine by inhibiting the cytochrome p450 enzyme, CYP2D6, can result in inadequate analgesia (Becker 2008). Concurrent use of non-steroidal anti-inflammatory drugs (NSAIDs) or anticoagulants may increase the risk of bleeding in surgical patients due to the interference of platelet function seen with high doses of SSRIs (Bromhead and Feeney 2009; Peck et al. 2010).

Effects on Patients under General Anesthesia

Administration of SSRIs should never be discontinued abruptly. Since the risks of SSRIs to anesthetized patients are relatively low, their use should be continued through the perianesthetic period with special consideration given to potential drug interactions. It is not currently recommended to avoid the use of phenylpiperidine opioids in patients receiving SSRIs, but rather, increase awareness of the potential for serotonin syndrome. Recommendations on the use of methadone in patients receiving SSRIs requires further research.

Tricyclic Antidepressants

Mechanism of Action

The primary mechanism of the behavioral modification effects of TCAs is the inhibition of the pre-synaptic reuptake of serotonin and norepinephrine within the CNS. This is achieved by blocking transporters responsible for the reuptake of these neurotransmitters into the pre-synaptic cytosol, allowing for an increase in activity within the synapse. TCAs may also affect several other receptors. Some have antihistaminic, anticholinergic and anti-α1-adrenergic effects. These effects will vary, depending upon which TCA is being administered (Table 22.1).

Clinical Use

The most commonly used TCAs are amitriptyline and clomipramine. Doxepin and imipramine are also available, although their use among veterinary practitioners is less common. TCAs are used to treat separation anxiety, aggression, compulsive disorders and anxiety in dogs. In cats, they are used to treat aggression, psychogenic alopecia, anxiety and feline lower urinary tract disease (FLUTD). TCAs have also been used successfully in several cases as an adjunctive treatment for neuropathic pain (Cashmore et al. 2009; Micó et al. 2006).

TCAs are also used in other species. In one reported case, clomipramine was used, in combination with xylazine, to collect semen from a stallion with a radius fracture (Turner et al. 1995). More recently, a combination of imipramine and xylazine was successful at improving induced ejaculation rates in eight stallions (McDonnell 2001). There is a potential that TCAs are misused as doping agents in competition horses (Hagedorn et al. 2002). TCAs have also been used in birds for feather-picking disorders with little success (Seibert et al. 2004; Juarbe-Díaz 2000). Digging behavior and aggressive behaviors have been treated in rodents (Gao and Cutler 1994).

Metabolism

TCAs are metabolized via the liver's CYP pathway in demethylation, hydroxylation and glucuronide conjugation reactions. Metabolism of amitriptyline results in the formation of the active metabolite nortriptyline. Both amitriptyline and nortriptyline are excreted in the urine. Caution should be used in patients with renal disease or hepatic disease (Landsberg et al. 2013). Clomipramine is absorbed quickly from the gastrointestinal (GI) tract and has extensive first-pass metabolism (King et al. 2000a). It is metabolized to an active metabolite, desmethylclomipramine which has a half-life of approximately 2.4 hours (King et al. 2000a, 2000b; Hewson et al. 1998). In dogs and rats, the majority of excretion is through bile and the remainder is excreted by the kidneys (Crowell-Davis 2006b). Cats metabolize clomipramine at a much slower rate than both dogs and rats and may need lower doses (Lainesse et al. 2007).

Table 22.1 Tricyclic antidepressants work by inhibiting the presynaptic reuptake of serotonin and norepinephrine within the central nervous system (CNS). They also affect several other receptors. These effects will vary depending upon which drug is administered.

| | Receptors affected | | | | | |
Drug	NE	5-HT	Alpha 1	Alpha 2	H1	Cholinergic
Amitriptyline	±	++	+++	±	++++	++++
Clomipramine	+	+++	++	0	+	++
Doxepin	++	+	++	0	+++	++
Imipramine[a]	+	+	++	0	+	++

Potter (1984), Potter et al. (1995), Crowell-Davis (2006b), Horowitz and Mill (2010), Landsberg et al. (2013).

[a] In addition to these effects, imipramine also inhibits MAO activity (Egashira et al. 1999).

Pharmacokinetics

TCAs are highly protein bound (Bromhead and Feeney 2009). The pharmacokinetics of clomipramine and amitriptyline have been described in dogs. After oral doses, clomipramine is extensively protein bound (96%), and peak concentrations occur within 1–3 hours (King et al. 2000a; Crowell-Davis 2006b). The average plasma elimination half-life is reported to be between 2 and 21 hours depending upon whether the dog was fasted (King et al. 2000a, 2000b; Hewson et al. 1998). The terminal half-life becomes shorter with repeated doses (King et al. 2000b). Clearance of clomipramine is rapid at 23.3 ml/kg/min (Sherman and Papich 2009). After intravenous (IV) administration of clomipramine, elimination half-life is two hours and plasma clearance is 1.4 l/h/kg (King et al. 2000a).

The pharmacokinetics of oral amitriptyline has also been reported in the dog. After oral administration of amitriptyline in dogs, peak concentration is reached after two hours (Kukes et al. 2009). In dogs that receive an oral dose of 4 mg/kg, terminal half-life is four hours and the bioavailability only 6% (Norkus et al. 2015a). These results led to a follow-up study examining a higher dose (mean dose 8 mg/kg) and the effect of fasted versus non-fasted dogs. In that study, bioavailability in fasted dogs after receiving 8 mg/kg was extremely variable ranging from 58% to 91% (Norkus et al. 2015b).

Metabolism of imipramine results in two active metabolites, desipramine and norimipramine. In humans, it has a half-life of 5–30 hours (Potter et al. 1995; Nelson 2004). In cattle, imipramine has a terminal elimination half-life of approximately 140 minutes (Cordel et al. 2001).

Effects on Organ Systems

TCAs have a narrow therapeutic index and can activate many receptor types. Most notable adverse effects of TCAs are from the cardiovascular, adrenergic and CNS effects. TCAs can increase heart rate through their anticholinergic effects (Peck et al. 2010) or decrease heart rate through reflex responses secondary to their α-1 adrenergic effects as well as through the depletion of norepinephrine (Johnson 1990). These effects may also lead to orthostatic hypotension and hypotension while under general anesthesia. Healthy dogs receiving clinically relevant doses of TCAs will have normal electrocardiograms (ECGs) (Reich et al. 2000); however, more serious effects on the cardiovascular system can be seen in cases of accidental overdose. Excitation and agitation may occur, progressing to seizures, respiratory depression, coma, ventricular fibrillation and death (Johnson 1990). TCAs are thought to have membrane-stabilizing actions by disruption of the sodium/potassium pump leading to increases in the refractory period, decreases in conduction velocity and decreases in ventricular automaticity. The summation of these effects precludes the development of arrhythmias. Sinus tachycardia, atrioventricular block, widening of the QRS complex, QT prolongation and hypertension can occur, progressing to ventricular arrhythmias, and hypotension (Johnson 1990; Peck et al. 2010). A cardiac assessment is recommended prior to treatment with TCAs (Sherman and Papich 2009).

Other Effects

Side effects associated with TCAs may include sedation, vomiting, miosis, mydriasis, blurred vision, xerostomia and other anticholinergic effects such as urinary retention, delayed gastric emptying and decreased intestinal peristalsis and constipation (Johnson 1990; Crowell-Davis 2006b; Sherman and Papich 2009).

Contraindications

TCAs are contraindicated in patients with underlying cardiac disease, glaucoma and those unable to handle potential urinary retention. They should not be given to patients receiving an MAOI. Amitriptyline and clomipramine cross the placenta and are excreted in milk; they should not be used in pregnant or lactating patients.

Drug Interactions

Patients who have been treated with TCAs may have altered responses to several drugs given during anesthesia, including anticholinergics, catecholamines and anesthetic drugs. Because TCAs have anticholinergic effects, the use of drugs that also have anticholinergic effects (ketamine, meperidine, pancuronium) may be addictive (Hines and Marschall 2008; Bromhead and Feeney 2009). These potential adverse effects are most common during the beginning of treatment with TCAs. An increase in the likelihood of postoperative agitation is also possible; agitation is less likely to occur with glycopyrrolate as it does not cross the blood–brain barrier. Hypertension and arrhythmias may result from the use of indirect acting sympathomimetics (e.g. ephedrine) in conjunction with TCAs due to the elevated level of norepinephrine available to bind to postsynaptic adrenergic receptors (Hines and Marschall 2008; Peck et al. 2010). Ventricular arrhythmias can develop if hypercapnia occurs during inhalant anesthesia, particularly halothane (Bromhead and Feeney 2009). Patients may have increased anesthetic requirements secondary to increased neurotransmitter availability in the CNS (Hines and Marschall 2008). TCAs may augment the analgesic and respiratory depressant effects of opioids as well as the sedative and depressant effects of barbiturates and doses of these drugs may need to be decreased to avoid potential adverse effects (Stoelting and Hillier 2006a).

Effect on Patients under General Anesthesia

Administration of TCAs should not be discontinued abruptly. Since the risks of TCAs to anesthetized patients are relatively low, their use should be continued through the perianesthetic period with special consideration given to potential drug interactions. A treatment plan for hypotension, should it occur, is necessary.

Monoamine Oxidase Inhibitors (MAOIs)

Mechanism of Action

MAO are a group of enzymes responsible for the catabolism of several neurotransmitters within the CNS including dopamine, norepinephrine, epinephrine, serotonin, tyramine, phenylethylamine and exogenous amines from food or drugs. MAO-A is primarily responsible for the oxidative deamination of norepinephrine, epinephrine, dopamine and serotonin, while MAO-B catabolizes phenylethylamine, tyramine, dopamine and exogenous substances, although species differences do exist (Crowell-Davis 2006c; Peck et al. 2010). For example, dopamine is a substrate of both MAO-A and MAO-B in primates but not in rats (Glover et al. 1977; O'Carroll et al. 1983; Kato et al. 1986; Paterson et al. 1991).

Drugs that inhibit MAO, MAOIs, interfere with both MAO-A and MAO-B by irreversibly inactivating them. This leads to an increase in these neurotransmitters available for release. These effects are not limited to the CNS but increase in neurotransmitters (e.g. norepinephrine) and also in the peripheral autonomic nervous system (Stoelting and Hillier 2006a).

Selegiline (L-deprenyl) is the most common MAOI given to veterinary patients. At low doses, it is selective for the irreversible inhibition of MAO-B. Selegiline most likely works by increasing available dopamine due to inhibition of reuptake and metabolism and by increasing phenylethylamine (Sherman and Papich 2009; Landsberg et al. 2013). It also activates superoxide dismutase and catalase, which are responsible for removing free radicals (Landsberg et al. 2013). Selegiline also inhibits presynaptic catecholamine receptors, inhibits the uptake of catecholamines, induces release of catecholamines from their intraneuronal stores and stimulates action potential-transmitter release coupling (Knoll et al. 1996).

Clinical Use

Selegiline is administered to both dogs and cats with cognitive dysfunction (Landsberg 2006). Selegiline is also used in dogs to treat sleep conditions and pituitary-dependent hyperadrenocorticism, although consistent evidence regarding efficacy in the latter is lacking. Its use in other species in limited, however, it is considered to have a high abuse potential in race horses to increase their performance (Dirikolu et al. 2003).

Metabolism

Selegiline is metabolized to desmethylselegiline, levoamphetamine and levomethamphetamine. Desmethylselegiline is believed to possess some MAO-B inhibitory properties, although to a lesser extent than that of selegiline (Mahmood 1997). Excretion occurs through the kidneys.

Pharmacokinetics

In humans, the pharmacokinetics of selegiline have been reported (Mahmood 1997) and are extremely variable. Time-to-peak concentrations is less than one hour. The clearance of selegiline exceeds hepatic blood flow suggesting extrahepatic metabolism. The elimination half-life is approximately 1.5 hours. The pharmacokinetics of selegiline have also been reported in dogs (Mahmood et al. 1994). Terminal half-life, volume of distribution of the central compartment, and systemic clearance of selegiline were approximately 60 minutes, 6.5 l/kg, and 156 ml/min/kg, respectively. After oral administration, selegiline appeared to be absorbed rapidly with peak concentrations reached in 25 minutes. The absolute bioavailability of selegiline in the dog was approximately 8%. In mice, selegiline is well absorbed after oral administration; however, it has an extensive first-pass effect and had only 25% bioavailability (Magyar et al. 2007).

Effects on Organ Systems

Effects on most organ systems when used at clinically relevant doses are minimal. Patients may experience orthostatic hypotension. Adverse effects are notable with overdoses. Signs associated with overdose are caused by excessive sympathetic nervous system activity, such as tachycardia, mydriasis and hyperthermia. This can progress to seizures and coma.

Other Effects

Gastrointestinal (GI) upset, hyperactivity and restlessness can occasionally be a side effect of selegiline administration. Species differences exist in regard to the amount of MAO-A and MOA-B present, therefore, the efficacy and side-effect profile of MAOIs in one species may be very different from another.

Contraindications

Selegiline should not be administered to patients receiving other antidepressants (TCAs, SSRIs), ephedrine, phenyl-propanolamine, topical amitraz (potential MAO inhibitor) or other MAOIs.

In humans receiving MAO-A or mixed MAO inhibitors, eating foods that have high levels of tyramine in them (e.g. cheese, chicken liver, chocolate) can cause acute hypertension. At clinically relevant doses of selegiline in dogs, this does not occur, however, using cheese regularly as a treat for dogs is not recommended due to the potential for variation in enzymes (Crowell-Davis 2006c).

Drug Interactions

Serotonin syndrome may develop when combining this drug with various other drugs including TCAs, SSRIs and other MAOIs. Administration of meperidine, pethidine and dextromethorphan to humans and rats receiving MAOI therapy can result in an excitatory response (agitation, skeletal muscle rigidity) due to enhanced serotonin activity (Marley and Wozniak 1985; Bromhead and Feeney 2009). Administration of any opioid with MAOIs may result in a depressive response (hypotension, respiratory depression and coma) presumably due to slowed breakdown of opioids by N-demethylase inhibition (Bromhead and Feeney 2009). The incidence of other opioids causing adverse events in patients receiving MAOIs is less common (Insler et al. 1994). Similar to TCAs, a profound pressor effect may be seen after administration of both indirectly and directly acting sympathomimetics (Pavy et al. 1995; Peck et al. 2010). Concurrent use of acepromazine, α-2 adrenergic agonists and opioids with selegiline is discouraged (Crowell-Davis 2006c). Possible drug interactions have also been observed in dogs receiving metronidazole, prednisone, and trimethoprim sulfa (Crowell-Davis 2006c).

Effect on Patients under General Anesthesia

Due to the additional norepinephrine present, patients may have exaggerated response to drugs with sympathomimetic effects such as ketamine, meperidine, pancuronium and indirect acting vasopressors (e.g. ephedrine). If hypotension during anesthesia should occur, drugs with direct-acting effects (i.e. phenylephrine) as well as decreases in the dosage by 66% are recommended (Wells and Bjorksten 1989; Hines and Marschall 2008). Patients may have increased anesthetic requirements secondary to increased neurotransmitter availability in the CNS (Stoelting and Hillier 2006a). Ideally, selegiline administration should be slowly discontinued in patients requiring anesthesia.

Atypical Antidepressants and Miscellaneous Behavior-Modifying Drugs

Benzodiazepines

Mechanism of Action

Benzodiazepines exert their effects through actions on the gamma-aminobutyric-acid-A (GABAA) receptor, specifically, the α-subunits on the GABA$_A$ receptors. There, benzodiazepines enhance the affinity of the receptor for GABA, leading to an increase in chloride conductance and hyperpolarization of the post-synaptic cell membrane. This ultimately results in anxiolysis (α-2 subunits) and sedation (α-1 subunits) (McKernan et al. 2000). Midazolam and diazepam are two commonly used benzodiazepines administered during the perianesthetic period. Midazolam's chronic use for behavioral disorders in veterinary patients is limited, however, and the use of midazolam and diazepam in this context are covered elsewhere in this text. The benzodiazepines used for the chronic management of behavioral disorders include alprazolam, clonazepam, clorazepate, diazepam, flurazepam, lorazepam and oxazepam.

Clinical Use

The use of benzodiazepines in chronic behavioral therapy is considered for fear or anxiety disorders, including fear aggression, separation anxiety and noise phobias in dogs and some forms of feline inappropriate urination and predation behaviors in cats (Landsberg et al. 2013). Benzodiazepines are also used for feather-picking behaviors in birds, foal rejection due to fear in mares and inhibition of sexual behavior in stallions (McDonnell et al. 1987; Seibert 2007; Wong et al. 2015). Alprazolam has a fast onset, short duration of action (three hours) and high potency and is often the benzodiazepine chosen for acute fear and panic (Horwitz and Mill 2010; Landsberg et al. 2013).

Metabolism

Most benzodiazepines are metabolized by the liver and excreted mainly through the kidneys or secondarily in bile, although species variations exist. Clorazepate is metabolized to its active metabolite, nordiazepam, in the stomach prior to absorption (Ballenger 1998; Forrester et al. 1990). Diazepam is metabolized to the active metabolite, nordiazepam (Forrester et al. 1990; Ballenger 1998). Nordiazepam is further metabolized to oxazepam (3-hydroxynordiazepam) and *p*-hydroxynordiazepam (Ruelius et al. 1965). Alprazolam is metabolized to relatively inactive metabolites, 4-hydroxyalprazolam and α-hydroxyalprazolam. Oxazepam and lorazepam are metabolized directly via Phase II conjugation in the liver to inactive compounds; there are no active metabolites (Ballenger 1998).

Pharmacokinetics

The pharmacokinetics of diazepam in the dog and cat have been reported (Löscher and Frey 1981; Cotler et al. 1984). The half-life of diazepam in dogs is less than one hour and clearance is in excess of hepatic blood flow at 57–60 ml/min/kg after rectal administration (Papich and Alcorn 1995). The half-life of diazepam in cats is 5.5 hours and clearance is 4.7 ml/min/kg (Cotler et al. 1984). In both dogs and cats, the metabolites have much longer half-lives. Nordiazepam has a half-life of 2.2–2.8 hours and 21.3 hours for dogs and cats, respectively (Cotler et al. 1984; Papich and Alcorn 1995). In horses, the half-life of diazepam and nordiazepam are 7–22 and 18–28 hours, respectively (Crowell-Davis 2006d). In dogs receiving clorazepate, peak nordiazepam levels are reached within 98 minutes with a single dose and the elimination half-life is 6–9 hours minutes (Forrester et al. 1990; Brown and Forrester 1991). Lorazepam in dogs has a half-life of less than one hour and a systemic clearance of 19.3 ml/min/kg (Sherman and Papich 2009). The pharmacokinetics of a single dose of alprazolam has been evaluated in horses (Wong et al. 2015). Maximum concentrations were reached in three hours (range 1–12). Low levels of the metabolite, α-hydroxyalprazolam were also found.

Effects on Organ Systems

Benzodiazepines cause little change in cardiovascular parameters and have little effect on ventilation in most veterinary species. The exception is non-human primates, in which they can cause dose-dependent respiratory depression, especially when combined with opioids.

A decrease in inhalational anesthetic requirements is achieved with the use of benzodiazepines (Seddighi et al. 2011). Benzodiazepines produce decreases in the cerebral metabolic rate of oxygen consumption and cerebral blood flow. There is little to no change in intracranial pressure (ICP) with the use of these drugs.

Other Effects

Paradoxical excitement, transient agitation and disinhibition leading to increased aggression can occur. Oral administration of diazepam has been associated with idiopathic hepatic necrosis in cats (Levy et al. 1994; Center et al. 1996). Other side effects include ataxia, increased appetite and muscle relaxation (Crowell-Davis 2006d; Horwitz and Mill 2010). Patients requiring chronic benzodiazepine administration can become physically dependent and develop tolerance (Horwitz and Mill 2010).

Contraindications

Benzodiazepines are excreted through milk and pass through the placenta; these drugs are generally avoided in pregnant or lactating patients (Crowell-Davis 2006d). The use of benzodiazepines in patients with aggression is controversial because of the loss of inhibition of aggressive behavior and variability between patients. Caution should be used in patients with decreased hepatic or renal function.

Drug Interactions

Drugs also known to cause CNS depression may be addictive if given concurrently with benzodiazepines. Examples include other antidepressants, acepromazine, α-2 adrenergic agonists, opioids, induction agents and inhalant anesthetics (Hayashi et al. 1994; Seddighi et al. 2011; Monteiro et al. 2014).

Effect on Patients under General Anesthesia

In general, benzodiazepines should be continued through the perianesthetic period.

Trazodone

Mechanism of Action
Trazodone is classified as a serotonin ($5HT_{2A}$) antagonist at low doses and a weak serotonin reuptake inhibitor at higher doses (Stahl 2009). It also acts as an antagonist at histaminic and post-synaptic α-1 adrenergic receptors.

Clinical Use

Trazodone is used as an adjunct to treat generalized anxiety, separation anxiety, and phobias in dogs (Gruen and Sherman 2008). It has been used successfully to promote calming and reduce anxiety in hospitalized patients or those requiring postoperative confinement (Gruen and

Sherman 2008; Gruen et al. 2014; Gilbert-Gregory et al. 2016). Recently, researchers have begun to identify the feasibility of rectal administration of trazodone in dogs (O'Donnell et al. 2020). Anesthetists may consider this route during anesthesia to assist with hospital-induced stress and anxiety during the post-anesthetic time period. Trazodone has also been successfully used in cats in similar clinical scenarios (Stevens et al. 2016). The use of trazodone for sedation in equids has been reported with variable success (Knych et al. 2017; Davis et al. 2018; Moss et al. 2021). Finally, trazodone administration has been evaluated in healthy pigeons (Desmarchelier et al. 2019).

Metabolism

In species that have been studied, trazodone is metabolized by the liver via CYP to an active metabolite, meta-chlorophenyl piperazine (mCPP), which functions as a serotonin agonist. Its levels within the CNS are less than 10% of trazodone, itself, and antagonist actions overwhelm those of mCPP (Stahl 2009).

Pharmacokinetics

The pharmacokinetics of oral and IV trazodone has been reported in dogs (Jay et al. 2013). Bioavailability after oral administration is 85% and the mean elimination half-life is approximately 166 minutes. Maximum plasma concentrations were reached after 445 minutes. After IV administration, the elimination half-life is 169 minutes, volume of distribution is 2.5 l/kg and total body clearance is 11 ml/min/kg. The pharmacokinetics of rectal trazodone has also been reported (O'Donnell et al. 2020). When administered rectally in dogs, maximum plasma concentrations were reached in 15 minutes and were on average, 1 µg/ml. The volume of distribution and clearance corrected for bioavailability were 10.3 l/kg (7.37–14.4 l/kg), and 639 ml/kg/h (594–719 ml/kg/h), respectively. The elimination half-life was 12 hours. Sedation was common; the maximum extent of sedation was observed 30 minutes after trazodone administration.

In horses, the pharmacokinetics of trazodone has been reported for oral and IV routes (Knych et al. 2017; Davis et al. 2018). For oral dosages of 4, 7.5, and 10 mg/kg, terminal phase half-life was approximately seven hours (Knych et al. 2017; Davis et al. 2018). When given IV at 1.5 mg/kg, total clearance was 6.85 ± 2.80 ml/min/kg, volume of distribution at steady state was 1.06 ± 0.07 l/kg, and elimination half-life was 8.58 ± 1.88 hours (Knych et al. 2017).

In healthy pigeons, a much higher dose (30 mg/kg orally) is required to achieve the therapeutic levels described in humans (0.13–2.2 mcg/ml) (Desmarchelier et al. 2019).

At this dose, the time to maximum serum concentration or the maximum serum concentration could not be identified in this study because of rapid absorption in the first 30 minutes. The mean elimination half-life, however, is reported as approximately twice that of dogs (335 minutes).

Effects on Organ Systems

In humans, trazodone has a very low risk of significant adverse effects over a wide dose range. Less anticholinergic effects are seen than with TCA administration (Bryant and Ereshefsky 1982). Dogs may develop transient sinus tachycardia after IV administration of 8 mg/kg (Jay et al. 2013). Priapism is a rarely reported complication in dogs (Murphy et al. 2017). Some horses administered IV trazodone experience side effects such as sweating, aggression, excitation, ataxia and tremors that were plasma concentration dependent (Knych et al. 2017). Horses given oral trazodone may experience over-sedation, tremors and transient arrhythmias (Davis et al. 2018). Pigeons that receive 30 mg/kg orally do not experience any adverse effects nor do they become sedate (Desmarchelier et al. 2019).

Contraindications

Few contraindications exist to using trazodone at clinically relevant doses. Patients with a history of glaucoma or those receiving MAOIs should not receive trazodone. Horses undergoing general anesthesia should not receive trazodone at doses that cause ataxia, as it may impact recovery.

Drug Interactions

In humans, trazodone inhibits CYP2D6; caution should be used when given in combination with SSRIs that also inhibit CYP enzymes (fluoxetine, paroxetine) but their concurrent use has been used successfully, albeit cautiously, in dogs (Gruen and Sherman 2008). In addition, trazodone should be used with caution with other drugs that affect serotonin levels.

Effect on Patients under General Anesthesia

Administering trazodone in dogs two hours prior to anesthesia induction, reduces the mean alveolar concentration (MAC) of isoflurane by an average of 17% without impacting hemodynamic parameters (Hoffman et al. 2018). In dogs under anesthesia, trazodone at cumulative IV doses up to 44.3 mg/kg did not significantly depress any measured index of cardiac conduction but did decrease heart rate and prolong the Q-Tc interval (Byrne and Gomoll 1982), a measure of delayed ventricular repolarization, making them more susceptible to arrhythmias. Dogs may experience hypotension, to a similar degree as acepromazine, while under general anesthesia (Murphy et al. 2017). Aside from equid patients, trazodone administration at clinically relevant doses can be continued during the perianesthetic period.

Buspirone

Mechanism of Action

Buspirone is a full agonist at pre-synaptic serotonin receptors ($5HT_{1A}$) and a partial agonist at post-synaptic receptors. These effects result in decreased serotonin synthesis and inhibition of neuronal firing and a decreased serotonin turnover (Eison 1989). Buspirone also acts as a dopamine antagonist at dopamine D_2 receptors (Peroutka 1985) and as a partial agonist at α-1 adrenergic receptors (Howland 2015).

Clinical Use

Buspirone is considered a mild anxiolytic and is therefore most commonly used in conjunction with SSRIs and TCAs. It has been used in the treatment of mild chronic fears and anxieties as well as urine marking and increasing affiliative social behavior in cats (Horwitz and Mill 2010). It has been used in horses for the treatment of equine self-mutilation syndrome, however, must not be used in performance horses (Dodman et al. 2004).

Pharmacokinetics

The pharmacokinetics of buspirone have been described in humans (Gammans et al. 1986; Mahmood and Sahajwalla 1999). Buspirone given orally is well absorbed but undergoes first-pass metabolism. Bioavailability is low at just 4% (Mahmood and Sahajwalla 1999). The half-life varies considerably in healthy humans, from 2 to 33 hours. Clearance of buspirone is prolonged in humans with cirrhosis and renal disease. One veterinary source suggests that buspirone has a short elimination half-life and must be administered several times per day (Sherman and Papich 2009).

Metabolism

Buspirone is partially metabolized by CYP enzymes in the liver to the active metabolite, 1-pyrimidinylpiperazine as well as several inactive metabolites (Crowell-Davis 2006e). Metabolites are excreted in the urine. In horses, measurable amounts of the parent drug can also be found in urine (Stanley 2000).

Effects on Organ Systems

At clinically relevant doses, there are no cardiovascular or respiratory effects with buspirone administration (Hanson et al. 1986).

Other Effects

The most common side effects in humans are dizziness, headaches, nausea, insomnia, nervousness and fatigue (Newton et al. 1982).

Contraindications

In humans, buspirone is contraindicated in patients with severe renal or hepatic failure.

Drug Interactions

Buspirone should not be given with MAOIs (Crowell-Davis 2006e) or other drugs that affect serotonin levels. In humans, co-administration of buspirone with verapamil, diltiazem, erythromycin and itraconazole (drugs metabolized by CYP) results in elevated levels of buspirone (Mahmood and Sahajwalla 1999).

Effect on Patients under General Anesthesia

There are no known adverse effects on patients undergoing general anesthesia, although they may be possible given buspirone's similar mechanisms of action to other behavior-modifying drugs.

β-Adrenergic Antagonists

Mechanism of Action

β-adrenergic antagonists are uncommonly used as behavior-modifying drugs in veterinary patients. Their use in the management of heart disease and how this impacts anesthesia is covered elsewhere. Propranolol is a nonselective, competitive β-adrenergic receptor antagonist. It equally and reversibly antagonizes $β_1$ and $β_2$ receptors ameliorating the sympathetic symptoms of anxiety. Like many other drugs, propranolol is used as a racemic mixture. The pharmacodynamic effects of propranolol are mediated primarily by the (−) stereoisomer which is 100 times more potent than the (+) stereoisomer (Whelan et al. 1989). Pindolol is another β-adrenergic receptor antagonist used for behavior modification that may also have inhibitory actions on serotonin neurons (leading to disinhibition).

Clinical Use

Propranolol is used to decrease the physiologic signals of fear such as tachycardia, tachypnea and GI upset. It is usually used in combination with other psychotropic medications in the treatment of fear, anxiety and phobias. Pindolol is not used as a stand-alone therapeutic but administered with other antidepressant drugs (e.g. TCAs); however, evidence suggests it may not be effective for anxiety symptoms in humans (Stein et al. 2001).

Pharmacokinetics

In humans, there is considerable variation in the pharmacokinetics due to wide variations in the magnitude of hepatic first-pass metabolism (Shand 1976). It is extensively protein bound (90–95%) and the elimination half-life is 2–3 hours (Shand 1976; Frisk-Holmberg et al. 1981). The bioavailability of an oral dose of propranolol in the dog is reported to be approximately 27% (Tse et al. 1980). The time-to-peak concentration is 1.7 hours and the plasma elimination half-life is 2.7 hours (Tse et al. 1980). In the cat, propranolol clearance, volume of distribution and elimination half-life is 31 ml/min/kg, 1.6 l/kg, and 35 minutes, respectively (Weidler et al. 1979). In comparison to other species, cats are able to clear propranolol from the plasma faster than primates but slower than both rats and dogs (Weidler et al. 1979). In horses, propranolol is 70% bioavailable and has a plasma half-life of two hours (Aramaki et al. 2000).

Metabolism

Propranolol is metabolized in the liver via oxidation and conjugation reactions. One of the major metabolites, 4-hydroxypropranolol, has equal β-antagonist and membrane-stabilizing efficacy as the parent drug (Fitzgerald and O'Donnell 1971), but the elimination half-life is short.

Effects on Organ Systems

β-adrenergic antagonists cause bradycardia due to their effect on β_1 receptors. By the same mechanism, they decrease myocardial contractility resulting in decreased cardiac output. Antagonism of β_2 receptors causes increases in systemic vascular resistance, including coronary vascular resistance. Overall, there is a decrease in myocardial oxygen demand (Olson et al. 1976) such that the increase in resistance seen in coronary vessels is not detrimental to the patient. B-adrenergic antagonists will increase airway resistance due to actions on β_2 receptors (Macdonald et al. 1967). β-adrenergic antagonists cross the blood–brain barrier and can cause lethargy and fatigue with chronic therapy (Wilcox et al. 1984).

Other Effects

β antagonists prevent glucose recovery during periods of sustained hypoglycemia due to decreased hepatic and renal glucose production (Cersosimo et al. 1998). Because the distribution of potassium is influenced by sympathetic nervous system activity, the β-adrenergic antagonists will inhibit uptake of potassium into cells and may cause elevations in plasma potassium (Swenson 1986). Sodium retention may occur in patients receiving propranolol due to alterations in intra-renal hemodynamics secondary to decreased cardiac output. Thrombocytopenia has been associated with chronic β-adrenergic agonist treatment (Stoelting and Hillier 2006b).

Contraindications

Beta blockers are contraindicated in patients with existing bradycardia, congestive heart failure not caused by tachycardia, hypovolemia, diabetes or chronic obstructive airway disease (Stoelting and Hillier 2006b).

Drug Interactions

Propranolol will slow the clearance of amide local anesthetics (e.g. bupivacaine, mepivacaine, ropivacaine) by decreasing both hepatic blood flow and metabolism (Saranteas et al. 2003). Caution is recommended when using local anesthetics in patients receiving propranolol. Because propranolol and fentanyl are both basic lipophilic amines, pulmonary first-pass uptake of fentanyl in patients receiving propranolol may be decreased (Roerig et al. 1989). Halothane increases concentrations of (−) propranolol by stereoselective inhibition of metabolism (Whelan et al. 1989). Diltiazem administration increases the bioavailability of propranolol by approximately 50–60% (Lankford et al. 1994). Using propofol in patients that are receiving propranolol results in changes in propranolol clearance and protein binding; the end result is a 65% decrease in the clearance of propranolol (Perry et al. 1991). The administration of phenobarbital and phenytoin to dogs receiving propranolol will have a decrease in the unbound fraction of the drug due to elevated α-1 acid glycoprotein binding and an increase in the volume of distribution (Bai and Abramson 1982).

Effect on Patients under General Anesthesia

The clearance of propranolol is largely dependent on hepatic extraction and thus hepatic blood flow. Any circumstance that decreases blood flow to the liver will decrease clearance and prolong the elimination half-life of propranolol (Breckenridge et al. 1973). Excessive myocardial depression can occur if an overdose or relative overdose of β-adrenergic antagonists is given. Successful treatment of bradycardia may include administering atropine, isoproterenol, dobutamine, glucagon or calcium chloride (Stoelting and Hillier 2006b). The use of dopamine to treat hypotension caused by bradycardia is not universally recommended because α-adrenergic-induced vasoconstriction is likely with the doses required to overcome the beta blockade (Stoelting and Hillier 2006b). Current recommendations from the American Heart Association are to continue beta blockers for patients already receiving them as long-term therapy. If a patient is to begin treatment with a beta-blocker, this should begin well in advance of anesthesia to decrease adverse effects (Fleisher et al. 2014).

Clonidine

Mechanism of Action

Clonidine is a centrally acting partial α_2-adrenergic agonist ($220:1$ α_2 to α_1). Sedative effects of clonidine are due to actions on α_{2a} receptors in the CNS resulting in inhibition of norepinephrine release within the pontine locus ceruleus. Clonidine also exerts actions on the imidazoline receptor.

Clinical Use

Clonidine, an antihypertensive agent in humans, is used to block autonomic responses to anxiety in veterinary patients. It is also used in the treatment of fear and territorial aggression, noise and storm phobias and nocturnal barking. Doses are given 1/2–2 hours prior to the event, up to twice daily (Landsberg et al. 2013).

Metabolism

In humans, clonidine is metabolized by CYP enzymes with a majority of metabolism achieved via the CYP2D6 enzyme.

Pharmacokinetics

In humans, an oral dose of clonidine has a rapid distribution reaching peak concentrations in less than two hours (Lowenthal 1980). It has moderate bioavailability (75%) and long elimination half-life of 8–15 hours (Davies et al. 1977; Anavekar et al. 1982). The pharmacokinetics of oral clonidine in dogs differs slightly. When given a 225- mcg tablet, peak concentrations are reached in about

one hour with an elimination half-life around two hours (Xu et al. 2016). A sustained release (SR) mini-tablet has been designed and pharmacokinetics have also been reported for dogs. In this SR formulation, when given 225 mcg orally, the time-to-maximum concentration is 2.8 hours with an elimination half-life of 2.4 hours (Xu et al. 2016). Pharmacokinetics of IV clonidine have been reported in rats as well as cats, although this data has little clinical relevance with regard to behavior-modification therapy (Paalzow and Edlund 1979).

Effects on Organ Systems

Clonidine has effects on peripheral α_{2b} receptors that are responsible for mediating vasoconstriction. It also affects α_{2a} receptors within the CNS resulting in a decrease in sympathetic nervous system outflow (sympatholysis). The result of these effects is usually a period of hypertension and bradycardia with an overall decrease in cardiac output followed by peripheral vasodilation, hypotension, bradycardia and a continued decreased cardiac output. In patients treated chronically, cardiac output returns to pre-drug levels through homeostatic cardiovascular reflexes (Stoelting and Hillier 2006c). Clonidine has minimal respiratory effects. Patients treated chronically do not have increased ventilatory depression when opioids are given (Stoelting and Hillier 2006c). Clonidine will cause sedation through its effect on post-synaptic α_{2a} receptors within the CNS.

Other Effects

Renal function is preserved during clonidine therapy (Pichot et al. 2012). Urine flow increases with administration of α_2-adrenergic agonists in many species (Humphreys et al. 1975). Clonidine has analgesic effects through its actions on α_{2A} receptors within the substantia gelatinosa of the spinal cord that modulate pain.

Contraindications

Caution should be used in patients with existing heart disease.

Drug Interactions

Patients treated with clonidine will have a reduction in their anesthetic requirements by up to 50% (Khafagy et al. 2012). The cardiovascular effects of indirect sympathomimetics like ketamine may be attenuated by clonidine administration (Munro et al. 1993).

Effect on Patients under General Anesthesia

Clonidine has several potential effects on patients undergoing general anesthesia. Bradycardia, changes in systemic blood pressure and decreased anesthetic requirements are the most common. Lower plasma concentrations of catecholamines in response to surgical stimulation also occur. In humans, abrupt discontinuation of clonidine can result in hypertension (Karachalios et al. 2005); this is especially profound if patients are also receiving a TCA (Stiff and Harris 1983) or MAOI due to the effects of norepinephrine. For this reason, it is recommended that clonidine administration be continued throughout the perianesthetic period.

Gabapentin

Mechanism of Action

The mechanism of action of gabapentin is not entirely understood. Although structurally similar to GABA, Gabapentin does not bind to these receptors, but may increase neuronal GABA synthesis (Landsberg et al. 2013). Gabapentin also works through decreased excitatory neurotransmitter release as a result of modulation of voltage-gated calcium channels (Taylor 2009) as well as potassium channels (Stefan and Feuerstein 2007).

Clinical Use

Gabapentin is used for generalized anxiety disorders, compulsive disorders, phobias and conditions in which pain plays a role, such as self-mutilatory disorders, hyperesthesia and interstitial cystitis (Landsberg et al. 2013). It is also used as an adjunct in the management of chronic and neuropathic pain conditions. Its use had been reported in dogs, cats, horses and laboratory animals.

Metabolism

The metabolism of gabapentin differs by species. In dogs, approximately 40% is metabolized in the liver to N-methyl gabapentin (Vollmer et al. 1986). Both the parent drug and metabolite are excreted by the kidneys necessitating dose adjustments in patients with decreased kidney function. In rodents and primates, however, very little is metabolized in the liver (Radulovic et al. 1995).

Pharmacokinetics

Gabapentin is rapidly absorbed in the several species examined. The pharmacokinetics of oral gabapentin has been described in dogs (Kukanich et al. 2011). Peak concentrations are reached in 1.5 hours and terminal half-lives of 10 and 20 mg/kg doses are 3.3 and 3.4 hours, respectively.

The pharmacokinetics of IV, oral and transdermal gabapentin have been described in cats (Adrian et al. 2018). In cats receiving 10 mg/kg orally, bioavailability is over 94%, peak concentrations are reached in one hour and the half-life 3.5 hours. When given the transdermal route (10 mg/kg), most cats have plasma concentrations below the lower limit of quantification, therefore, this route is not recommended.

In horses, an oral dose of 5 mg/kg and 20 mg/kg reached maximum plasma concentrations by one hour and plasma elimination half-life was 3.4 and 7 hours, respectively (Dirikolu et al. 2008; Terry et al. 2010). When doses between 10 and 160 mg/kg are administered via a nasogastric tube, time-to-maximum plasma concentration is between 1.4 and 2.6 hours and elimination half-life is between 2 and 15.7 hours (Gold et al. 2020). Overall, the bioavailability of gabapentin is lower in horses (<20%) than other species (Terry et al. 2010).

In cattle, a 15 mg/kg oral dose of gabapentin has a half-life of approximately eight hours and plasma levels above that reported to be therapeutic in humans are maintained for up to 15 hours (Stock and Coetzee 2015).

In rats receiving an oral dose of 50 mg/kg, peak concentrations were reached in 1.7 hours and plasma elimination half-life was 1.7 hours (Radulovic et al. 1995). It is important to note that many species experience non-linear kinetics, therefore increasing the dose administered does not necessarily increase the effects.

Effects on Organ Systems

In healthy humans, gabapentin has no effect on cardiovascular conduction (Chen et al. 2012). At high doses (30 mg/kg) in healthy dogs, gabapentin has the potential to cause bradycardia and increased PR and RR intervals as well as second-degree atrioventricular block (Gharamaleki et al. 2011).

Other Effects

The most common side effects reported in humans are somnolence, ataxia and dizziness (Chen et al. 2012). Rare reports of hepatotoxicity and hepatocellular damage exist (Jackson et al. 2018). Gabapentin has an abuse potential in that up to 1% of the general population (15–22% in those with opioid addictions) have a history of overuse, abuse or diversion (Smith et al. 2016). In dogs, mild ataxia and sedation has been reported (Platt et al. 2006). Horses receiving up to 80 mg/kg experience no physiologic effects, including ataxia, however, higher doses cause sedation (Gold et al. 2020).

Drug Interactions

The renal clearance of gabapentin can be slowed by cimetidine (Lal et al. 2010). Other interactions with drugs do not seem to occur with gabapentin, most likely due to the absence of protein binding (Stoelting and Hillier 2006d).

Effect on Patients under General Anesthesia

To date, there is one study specifically examining the effects of gabapentin in anesthetized dogs (Johnson et al. 2019). Gabapentin has an isoflurane-sparing effect in dogs administered 20 mg/kg orally two hours prior to anesthesia. There are no hemodynamic or other physiologic variables effected in dogs anesthetized with isoflurane. In fact, extubation times are significantly faster (6 vs. 23 minutes) in dogs receiving gabapentin compared to those that are not (Johnson et al. 2019). In addition to inhalant sparing effects, gabapentin also prevents an increase in intraocular pressure in response to intubation in dogs (Trbolova et al. 2017).

Methylphenidate

Mechanism of Action

Methylphenidate is uncommonly used as a behavior-modifying drug in veterinary species. It is a CNS stimulant and is structurally similar to amphetamine (Stoelting and Hillier 2006e). It enhances the release of dopamine and blocks dopamine and norepinephrine reuptake.

Clinical Use

Methylphenidate is used to treat some cases of over-activity disorders, learning deficits and aggression in dogs. In these conditions, methylphenidate has a paradoxical calming effect. It is rarely used in race horses, although prohibited, to enhance performance.

Metabolism

Methylphenidate is rapidly metabolized to α-phenyl-2-piperidine acetic acid (ritalinic acid). In humans, half-life varies with age. In children, the half-life is approximately 2.5 hours; in adults it is 3.5 hours (Kimko et al. 1999).

Pharmacokinetics

The pharmacokinetics of an immediate-release (IR) and sustained-release (SR) preparation of methylphenidate have been described in healthy dogs (Lavy et al. 2011). Time-to-maximum plasma concentration in these dogs was 0.21 and 0.42 hours for IR and SR respectively. The plasma elimination half-lives were 0.22 hours for both preparations. In horses given IV methylphenidate, the apparent alpha half-life was 19 minutes and the beta half-life was 2.4 hours. If given by subcutaneous or IM injection, plasma concentrations peak in approximately one hour and are no longer detectable by six hours. Methylphenidate levels can be detected in the urine for much longer, between 12 and 24 hours (Shults et al. 1981). When rats receive oral methylphenidate, the plasma elimination rate is constant; however, the clearance decreases with increasing doses. The recovery of the parent drug and its metabolites is approximately 16–18% in 24 hours, suggesting that the dose-dependent characteristics may be due to pre-systemic elimination of the drug (Aoyama et al. 1990).

Effects on Organ Systems

In humans, bradycardia, hallucinations and growth suppression have been described (Hodgkins et al. 2012). In dogs, mild hyperkinesia is reported with immediate release preparations (Lavy et al. 2011).

Other Effects

Chronic administration of methylphenidate can result in dependence and tapering the dose is necessary prior to discontinuation (Guler et al. 2015; Pérez et al. 2016).

Contraindications

In some patients, CNS stimulants such as methylphenidate will have an activating effect and may aggravate the underlying condition. Their use in these patients is contraindicated.

Drug Interactions

CNS stimulants can interact with MAOIs and should not be used together. Methylphenidate can decrease the metabolism of coumarin anticoagulants, anticonvulsants, TCAs and phenylbutazone and these combinations are discouraged (Crowell-Davis 2006e).

Effect on Patients under General Anesthesia

Methylphenidate has more prominent effects on mental activities than motor activities within the CNS. It has been used to induce emergence from propofol anesthesia in rats (Chemali et al. 2012) and may have similar effects in other species.

Discontinuation Syndrome

Abrupt discontinuation of any antidepressant or behavior-modifying drug can be associated with the risk of negative effects; these effects are collectively known as the discontinuation syndrome (Bromhead and Feeney 2009). Signs may include nausea, abdominal pain, diarrhea, changes in sleep patterns, lethargy and headaches. In addition, patients may experience a relapse of their original behavior symptoms. With the exception of MAO-Is, most behavior-modifying drugs should be continued through the perianesthetic period. However, in all cases, it is recommended to weigh the risks versus benefits to each patient when deciding to continue or discontinue medications prior to anesthesia (Table 22.2).

Table 22.2 A summary of behavior-modifying medication administration recommendations prior to general anesthesia in veterinary patients.

Continue	Discontinue
Selective serotonin reuptake inhibitors	Monoamine oxidase inhibitors
Selective norepinephrine reuptake inhibitors	+/− Trazodone in equid patients
Tricyclic antidepressants	
Benzodiazepines	
Trazodone in most patients	
Buspirone	
Beta antagonists[a]	
Clonidine	

[a] If a patient is to begin treatment with a beta-blocker, this should begin well in advance of anesthesia to decrease adverse effects (Fleisher et al. 2014).

References

Adrian, D., Papich, M.G., Baynes, R. et al. (2018). The pharmacokinetics of gabapentin in cats. *J. Vet. Intern. Med.* 32 (6): 1996–2002.

Amat, M., Ruiz de la Torre, J.L., Fatjó, J. et al. (2009). Potential risk factors associated with feline behavior problems. *Appl. Anim. Behav. Sci.* 121: 134–139.

Anavekar, S.N., Jarrott, B., Toscano, M., and Louis, W.J. (1982). Pharmacokinetic and pharmacodynamic studies of oral clonidine in normotensive subjects. *Eur. J. Clin. Pharmacol.* 23 (1): 1–5.

Andrade, C., Sandarsh, S., Chethan, K.B., and Nagesh, K.S. (2010). Serotonin reuptake inhibitor antidepressants and abnormal bleeding: a review for clinicians and a reconsideration of mechanisms. *J. Clin. Psychiatry* 71 (12): 1565–1575.

Aoyama, T., Kotaki, H., and Iga, T. (1990). Dose-dependent kinetics of methylphenidate enantiomers after oral administration of racemic methylphenidate to rats. *J. Pharmacobiodyn.* 13 (10): 647–652.

Aramaki, S., Mori, M., Nakata, M. et al. (2000). Pharmacokinetics of propranolol and its metabolites in horses after intravenous or oral administration. *Biol. Pharm. Bull.* 23 (11): 1333–1340.

Bai, S.A. and Abramson, F.P. (1982). Interactions of phenobarbital with propranolol in the dog. 1. Plasma protein binding. *J. Pharmacol. Exp. Ther.* 222 (3): 589–594.

Ballenger, J.C. (1998). Benzodiazepines. In: *The American Psychiatric Press Textbook of Psychopharmacology*, 2e (ed. A.F. Schatzberg and C.B. Nemeroff), 271–286. Washington, DC: American Psychiatric Press.

Becker, D.E. (2008). Psychotropic drugs: implications for dental practice. *Anesth. Prog.* 55 (3): 89–99.

Breckenridge, A., Buranapong, P., Dollery, C.T. et al. (1973). Hepatic clearance of propranolol in dogs. *Br. J. Pharmacol.* 48 (2): 336–337.

Bromhead H. and Feeney A. (2009) Anaesthesia & psychiatric drugs part 1 – antidepressants. Anesthesia Tutorial of the Week [Online], Available: http://www.totw.anaesthesiologist.org [14 Dec 2009].

Brown, S.A. and Forrester, S.C.F. (1991). Serum disposition of oral clorazepate from regular-release and sustained delivery tablets in dogs. *J. Vet. Pharmacol. Ther.* 14 (4): 426–429.

Bryant, S.G. and Ereshefsky, L. (1982). Antidepressant properties of trazodone. *Clin. Pharm.* 1 (5): 406–417.

Byrne, J.E. and Gomoll, A.W. (1982). Differential effects of trazodone and imipramine on intracardiac conduction in the anesthetized dog. *Arch. Int. Pharmacodyn. Ther.* 259 (2): 259–270.

Cashmore, R.G., Harcourt-Brown, T.R., and Freeman, P.M. (2009). Clinical diagnosis and treatment of suspected neuropathic pain in three dogs. *Aust. Vet. J.* 87: 45–50.

Center, S.A., Elston, T.H., Rowland, P.H. et al. (1996). Fulminant hepatic failure associated with oral administration of diazepam in 11 cats. *J. Am. Vet. Med. Assoc.* 209 (3): 618–625.

Cerrito, F. and Raiteri, M. (1979). Serotonin release is modulated by presynaptic autoreceptors. *Eur. J. Pharmacol.* 57 (4): 427–430.

Cersosimo, E., Zaitseva, I.N., and Ajmal, M. (1998). Effects of beta-adrenergic blockade on hepatic and renal glucose production during hypoglycemia in conscious dogs. *Am. J. Physiol.* 275: 792–797.

Chemali, J.J., Van Dort, C.J., Brown, E.N., and Solt, K. (2012). Active emergence from propofol general anesthesia is induced by methylphenidate. *Anesthesiology* 116 (5): 998–1005.

Chen, D., Lal, R., Zomorodi, K. et al. (2012). Evaluation of gabapentin enacarbil on cardiac repolarization: a randomized, double-blind, placebo- and active-controlled, crossover thorough QT/QTc study in healthy adults. *Clin. Ther.* 34 (2): 351–362.

Ciribassi, J., Luescher, A., Pasloske, K.S. et al. (2003). Comparative bioavailability of fluoxetine after transdermal and oral administration to healthy cats. *Am. J. Vet. Res.* 64 (8): 994–998.

Cordel, C., Swan, G.E., Mülders, M.S., and Bertschinger, H.J. (2001). Pharmacokinetics of intravenous imipramine hydrochloride in cattle. *J. Vet. Pharmacol. Ther.* 24 (2): 143–145.

Cotler, S., Gustafson, J.H., and Colburn, W.A. (1984). Pharmacokinetics of diazepam and nordiazepam in the cat. *J. Pharm. Sci.* 73 (3): 348–351.

Crowell-Davis, S. (2006a). Selective serotonin reuptake inhibitors. In: *Veterinary Psychopharmacology* (ed. S. Crowell-Davis and T. Murray), 80–110. Wiley: Ames, IA, USA.

Crowell-Davis, S. (2006b). Tricyclic antidepressants. In: *Veterinary Psychopharmacology* (ed. S. Crowell-Davis and T. Murray), 79–206. Wiley: Ames, IA, USA.

Crowell-Davis, S. (2006c). Monoamine oxidase inhibitors. In: *Veterinary Psychopharmacology* (ed. S. Crowell-Davis and T. Murray), 134–147. Wiley: Ames, IA, USA.

Crowell-Davis, S. (2006d). Benzodiazepines. In: *Veterinary Psychopharmacology* (ed. S. Crowell-Davis and T. Murray), 34–71. Wiley: Ames, IA, USA.

Crowell-Davis, S. (2006e). Azapirones. In: *Veterinary Psychopharmacology* (ed. S. Crowell-Davis and T. Murray), 111–118. Wiley: Ames, IA, USA.

Crowell-Davis, S. (2006f). CNS stimulants. In: *Veterinary Psychopharmacology* (ed. S. Crowell-Davis and T. Murray), 166–178. Wiley: Ames, IA, USA.

Davies, T.S. and Kluwe, W.M. (1998). Preclinical toxicological evaluation of sertraline hydrochloride. *Drug Chem. Toxicol.* 21 (4): 521–537.

Davies, D.S., Wing, A.M., Reid, J.L. et al. (1977). Pharmacokinetics and concentration-effect relationships of intervenous and oral clonidine. *Clin. Pharmacol. Ther.* 21 (5): 593–601.

Davis, J.L., Schirmer, J., and Medlin, E. (2018). Pharmacokinetics, pharmacodynamics and clinical use of trazodone and its active metabolite m-chlorophenylpiperazine in the horse. *J. Vet. Pharmacol. Ther.* 41 (3): 393–401.

Desmarchelier, M.R., Beaudry, F., Ferrell, S.T., and Frank, D. (2019). Determination of the pharmacokinetics of a single oral dose of trazodone and its effect on the activity level of domestic pigeons (*Columba livia*). *Am. J. Vet. Res.* 80 (1): 102–109.

Dirikolu, L., Lehner, A.F., Karpiesiuk, W. et al. (2003). Detection, quantification, metabolism, and behavioral effects of selegiline in horses. *Vet. Ther.* 4 (3): 257–268.

Dirikolu, L., Dafalla, A., Ely, K.J. et al. (2008). Pharmacokinetics of gabapentin in horses. *J. Vet. Pharmacol. Ther.* 31 (2): 175–177.

Dodman, N., Shuster, L., Patronek, G.J., and Kinney, L. (2004). Pharmacologic treatment of equine self-mutilation. *Int. J. Appl. Res. Vet. Med.* 2: 90–98.

Egashira, T., Takayama, F., and Yamanaka, Y. (1999). The inhibition of monoamine oxidase activity by various antidepressants: differences found in various mammalian species. *Jpn. J. Pharmacol.* 81 (1): 115–121.

Eison, M.S. (1989). The new generation of serotonergic anxiolytics: possible clinical roles. *Psychopathology* 22 (1): 13–20.

Fitzgerald, K.T. and Bronstein, A.C. (2013). Selective serotonin reuptake inhibitor exposure. *Top Companion Anim. Med.* 28 (1): 13–17.

Fitzgerald, J.D. and O'Donnell, S.R. (1971). Pharmacology of 4-hydroxypropranolol, a metabolite of propranolol. *Br. J. Pharmacol.* 43 (1): 222–235.

Fleisher, L.A., Fleischmann, K.E., Auerbach, A.D. et al. (2014). ACC/AHA Guideline on Perioperative Cardiovascular Evaluation and Management of Patients Undergoing Noncardiac Surgery: Executive Summary a Report of the American College of Cardiology/American Heart Association Task Force on Practice Guidelines. *Circulation* 130 (24): 2215–2245.

Forest Laboratories (2002). *Celexa Product Information 2004 Physicians' Desk Reference*, 1292–1296. Montvale, New Jersey: Thomson PDR.

Forrester, S.D., Brown, S.A., Lees, G.E., and Hartsfield, S.M. (1990). Disposition of clorazepate in dogs after single- and multiple-dose oral administration. *Am. J. Vet. Res.* 51 (12): 2001–2005.

Frisk-Holmberg, M., Paalzow, L., and Edlund, P.O. (1981). Clonidine kinetics in man – evidence for dose dependency and changed pharmacokinetics during chronic therapy. *Br. J. Clin. Pharmacol.* 12 (5): 653–658.

Gammans, R.E., Mayol, R.F., and LaBudde, J.A. (1986). Metabolism and disposition of buspirone. *Am. J. Med.* 80 (3B): 41–51.

Gao, B. and Cutler, M.G. (1994). Effects of acute and chronic administration of the antidepressants, imipramine, phenelzine and mianserin, on the social behaviour of mice. *Neuropharmacology* 33 (6): 813–824.

Gharamaleki, N., Niazmand, F., and Safarmashaei, S. (2011). Study of the effect of Gabapentin oral administration on Lead II electrocardiogram changes in dog. *Ann. Biol. Res.* 2 (4): 301–305.

Gilbert-Gregory, S.E., Stull, J.W., Rice, M.R., and Herron, M.E. (2016). Effects of trazodone on behavioral signs of stress in hospitalized dogs. *J. Am. Vet. Med. Assoc.* 249 (11): 1281–1291.

Gillman, P.K. (2005). Monoamine oxidase inhibitors, opioid analgesics and serotonin toxicity. *Br. J. Anaesth.* 95 (4): 434–441.

Glover, V., Sandler, M., Owen, F., and Riley, G.J. (1977). Dopamine is a monoamine oxidase B substrate in man. *Nature* 265 (5589): 80–81.

Gold, J.R., Grubb, T.L., Green, S. et al. (2020). Plasma disposition of gabapentin after the intragastric administration of escalating doses to adult horses. *J. Vet. Intern. Med.* 34 (2): 933–940.

Greenier, E., Lukyanova, V., and Reede, L. (2014). Serotonin syndrome: fentanyl and selective serotonin reuptake inhibitor interactions. *AANA J.* 82 (5): 340–345. PMID: 25842648.

Gruen, M.E. and Sherman, B.L. (2008). Use of trazodone as an adjunctive agent in the treatment of canine anxiety disorders: 56 cases (1995–2007). *J. Am. Vet. Med. Assoc.* 233 (12): 1902–1907.

Gruen, M.E., Roe, S.C., Griffith, E. et al. (2014). Use of trazodone to facilitate postsurgical confinement in dogs. *J. Am. Vet. Med. Assoc.* 245 (3): 296–301.

Guler, G., Yildirim, V., Kutuk, M.O., and Toros, F. (2015). Dystonia in an adolescent on risperidone following the discontinuation of methylphenidate: a case report. *Clin. Psychopharmacol. Neurosci.* 13: 115–117.

Hagedorn, H.W., Meiser, H., Zankl, H., and Schulz, R. (2002). The isomeric metabolites of doxepin in equine serum and urine. *J. Pharm. Biomed. Anal.* 29 (1–2): 317–323.

Hanson, R.C., Braselton, J.P., Hayes, D.C. et al. (1986). Cardiovascular and renal effects of buspirone in several animal models. *Gen. Pharmacol.* 17 (3): 267–274.

Hayashi, K., Nishimura, R., Yamaki, A. et al. (1994). Comparison of sedative effects induced by medetomidine, medetomidine-midazolam and medetomidine-butorphanol in dogs. *J. Vet. Med. Sci.* 56 (5): 951–956.

Hewson, C.J., Conlon, P.D., Luescher, U.A., and Ball, R.O. (1998). The pharmacokinetics of clomipramine and desmethylclomipramine in dogs: parameter estimates following a single oral dose and 28 consecutive daily oral doses of clomipramine. *J. Vet. Pharmacol. Ther.* 21 (3): 214–222.

Hines, R.L. and Marschall, K.E. (2008). Psychiatric disease/substance abuse/drug overdose. In: *Stoelting's Anesthesia and Co-Existing Disease*, 5e (ed. R.L. Hines and K.E. Marschall), 533–556. Philadelphia, PA, USA: Churchill Livingstone.

Hodgkins, P., Shaw, M., Coghill, D., and Hechtman, L. (2012). Amfetamine and methylphenidate medications for attention-deficit/hyperactivity disorder: complementary treatment options. *Eur. Child Adolesc. Psychiatry* 21 (9): 477–492.

Hoffman, E.A., Aarnes, T.K., Ricco Pereira, C.H. et al. (2018). Effect of oral trazodone on the minimum alveolar concentration of isoflurane in dogs. *Ve.t Anaesth. Analg.* 45 (6): 754–759.

Horwitz, D. and Mill, D. (ed.) (2010). *BSAVA Manual of Canine and Feline Behavioural Medicine*. NJ, USA: Wiley.

Howland, R.H. (2015). Buspirone: back to the future. *J. Psychosoc. Nurs. Ment. Health Serv.* 53 (11): 21–24.

Humphreys, M.H., Reid, I.A., and Chou, L.Y. (1975). Suppression of antidiuretic hormone secretion by clonidine in the anesthetized dog. *Kidney Int.* 7 (6): 405–412.

Insler, S.R., Kraenzler, E.J., Licina, M.G. et al. (1994). Cardiac surgery in a patient taking monoamine oxidase inhibitors: an adverse fentanyl reaction. *Anesth. Analg.* 78 (3): 593–597.

Isbister, G.K. and Buckley, N.A. (2005). The pathophysiology of serotonin toxicity in animals and humans: implications for diagnosis and treatment. *Clin. Neuropharmacol.* 28 (5): 205–214.

Jackson, C.D., Clanahan, M.J., Joglekar, K., and Decha-Umphai, S.T. (2018). Hold the Gaba: a case of gabapentin-induced hepatotoxicity. *Cureus* 10 (3): e2269.

Jay, A.R., Krotscheck, U., Parsley, E. et al. (2013). Pharmacokinetics, bioavailability, and hemodynamic effects of trazodone after intravenous and oral administration of a single dose to dogs. *Am. J. Vet. Res.* 74 (11): 1450–1456.

Johnson, L.R. (1990). Tricyclic antidepressant toxicosis. *Vet. Clin. North Am. Small Anim. Pract.* 20 (2): 393–403.

Johnson, B.A., Aarnes, T.K., Wanstrath, A.W. et al. (2019). Effect of oral administration of gabapentin on the minimum alveolar concentration of isoflurane in dogs. *Am. J. Vet. Res.* 80 (11): 1007–1009.

Juarbe-Díaz, S.V. (2000). Animal behavior case of the month. Congo African Grey parrot examined because of feather picking and self-injurious behavior. *J. Am. Vet. Med. Assoc.* 216 (10): 1562–1564.

Karachalios, G.N., Charalabopoulos, A., Papalimneou, V. et al. (2005). Withdrawal syndrome following cessation of antihypertensive drug therapy. *Int. J. Clin. Pract.* 59 (5): 562–570.

Kato, T., Dong, B., Ishii, K., and Kinemuchi, H. (1986). Brain dialysis: in vivo metabolism of dopamine and serotonin by monoamine oxidase A but not B in the striatum of unrestrained rats. *J. Neurochem.* 46 (4): 1277–1282.

Khafagy, H.F., Ebied, R.S., Osman, E.S. et al. (2012). Perioperative effects of various anesthetic adjuvants with TIVA guided by bispectral index. *Korean J. Anesthesiol.* 63 (2): 113–119.

Kimko, H.C., Cross, J.T., and Abernethy, D.R. (1999). Pharmacokinetics and clinical effectiveness of methylphenidate. *Clin. Pharmacokinet.* 37 (6): 457–470.

King, J.N., Maurer, M.P., Hotz, R.P., and Fisch, R.D. (2000a). Pharmacokinetics of clomipramine in dogs following single-dose intravenous and oral administration. *Am. J. Vet. Res.* 61 (1): 74–79.

King, J.N., Maurer, M.P., Altmann, B.O., and Strehlau, G.A. (2000b). Pharmacokinetics of clomipramine in dogs following single-dose and repeated-dose oral administration. *Am. J. Vet. Res.* 61 (1): 80–85.

Knoll, J., Miklya, I., Knoll, B. et al. (1996). (−)Deprenyl and (−)1-phenyl-2-propylaminopentane, [(−)PPAP], act primarily as potent stimulants of action potential-transmitter release coupling in the catecholaminergic neurons. *Life Sci.* 58 (10): 817–827.

Knych, H.K., Mama, K.R., Steffey, E.P. et al. (2017). Pharmacokinetics and selected pharmacodynamics of trazodone following intravenous and oral administration to horses undergoing fitness training. *Am. J. Vet. Res.* 78 (10): 1182–1192.

Kukanich, B. and Cohen, R.L. (2011). Pharmacokinetics of oral gabapentin in Greyhound dogs. *Vet. J.* 187 (1): 133–135.

Kukanich, B., Kukanich, K.S., and Rodriguez, J.R. (2011). The effects of concurrent administration of cytochrome P-450 inhibitors on the pharmacokinetics of oral methadone in healthy dogs. *Vet. Anaesth. Analg.* 38 (3): 224–230.

Kukes, V.G., Kondratenko, S.N., Savelyeva, M.I. et al. (2009). Experimental and clinical pharmacokinetics of amitryptiline: comparative analysis. *Bull. Exp. Biol. Med.* 147 (4): 434–437.

Lainesse, G., Frank, D., Beaudry, F., and Doucet, M. (2007). Comparative oxidative metabolic profiles of clomipramine in cats, rats and dogs: preliminary results from an in vitro study. *J. Vet. Pharmacol. Ther.* 30 (5): 387–393.

Lal, R., Sukbuntherng, J., Luo, W. et al. (2010). Clinical pharmacokinetic drug interaction studies of gabapentin enacarbil, a novel transported prodrug of gabapentin, with naproxen and cimetidine. *Br. J. Clin. Pharmacol.* 69 (5): 498–507.

Landsberg, G. (2006). Therapeutic options for cognitive decline in senior pets. *J. Am. Anim. Hosp. Assoc.* 42 (6): 407–413.

Landsberg, G., Hunthausen, W., and Ackerman, L. (2013). Pharmacologic intervention in behavioral therapy. In: *Behavior Problems of the Dog and Cat*, 3e (ed. G. Landsberg, W. Hunghausen and L. Ackerman), 113–168. New York: Saunders Elsevier.

Lankford, S.M., Maskasame, C., and Bai, S.A. (1994). Effects of diltiazem on the disposition and metabolism of the enantiomers of propranolol in the dog during multiple oral dosing. *Drug Metab. Dispos.* 22 (5): 776–787.

Lavy, E., Prise, U., Soldani, G. et al. (2011). Pharmacokinetics of methylphenidate after oral administration of immediate and sustained-release preparations in Beagle dogs. *Vet. J.* 189 (3): 336–340.

Levy, J.K., Cullen, J.M., Bunch, S.E. et al. (1994). Adverse reaction to diazepam in cats. *J. Am. Vet. Med. Assoc.* 205 (2): 156–157.

Löscher, W. and Frey, H.H. (1981). Pharmacokinetics of diazepam in the dog. *Arch. Int. Pharmacodyn. Ther.* 254 (2): 180–195.

Lowenthal, D.T. (1980). Pharmacokinetics of clonidine. *J. Cardiovasc. Pharmacol.* 2 (1): 29–37.

Macdonald, A.G., Ingram, C.G., and McNeill, R.S. (1967). The effect of propranolol on airway resistance. *Br. J. Anaesth.* 39 (12): 919–926.

Magyar, K., Szatmáry, I., Szebeni, G., and Lengyel, J. (2007). Pharmacokinetic studies of (−)-deprenyl and some of its metabolites in mouse. *J. Neural Transm. Suppl.* 72: 165–173.

Mahmood, I. (1997). Clinical pharmacokinetics and pharmacodynamics of selegiline. An update. *Clin. Pharmacokinet.* 33 (2): 91–102.

Mahmood, I. and Sahajwalla, C. (1999). Clinical pharmacokinetics and pharmacodynamics of buspirone, an anxiolytic drug. *Clin. Pharmacokinet.* 36 (4): 277–287.

Mahmood, I., Peters, D.K., and Mason, W.D. (1994). The pharmacokinetics and absolute bioavailability of selegiline in the dog. *Biopharm. Drug Dispos.* 15 (8): 653–664.

Marley, E. and Wozniak, K.M. (1985). Interactions between relatively selective monoamine oxidase inhibitors and an inhibitor of 5-hydroxytryptamine re-uptake, clomipramine. *J. Psychiatr. Res.* 19 (4): 597–608.

Martinez, A.G., Pernas, G.S., Casalta, F.J.D. et al. (2011). Risk factors associated with behavioral problems in dogs. *J. Vet. Behav.* 6: 225–231.

McCloskey, D.J., Postolache, T.T., Vittone, B.J. et al. (2008). Selective serotonin reuptake inhibitors: measurement of effect on platelet function. *Transl. Res.* 151 (3): 168–172.

McDonnell, S.M. (2001). Oral imipramine and intravenous xylazine for pharmacologically-induced ex copula ejaculation in stallions. *Anim. Reprod. Sci.* 68 (3–4): 153–159.

McDonnell, S.M., Garcia, M.C., and Kenney, R.M. (1987). Pharmacological manipulation of sexual behaviour in stallions. *J. Reprod. Fertil. Suppl.* 35: 45–49.

McKernan, R.M., Rosahl, T.W., and Reynolds, D.S. (2000). Sedative but not anxiolytic properties of benzodiazepines are mediated by the Gaba A receptor alpha 1 subtype. *Nat. Neurosci.* 3: 587–592.

Meijer, W.E., Heerdink, E.R., Nolen, W.A. et al. (2004). Association of risk of abnormal bleeding with degree of serotonin reuptake inhibition by antidepressants. *Arch. Intern. Med.* 164 (21): 2367–2370.

Micó, J.A., Ardid, D., Berrocoso, E., and Eschalier, A. (2006). Antidepressants and pain. *Trends Pharmacol. Sci.* 27 (7): 348–354.

Mohammad-Zadeh, L.K.F., Moses, L., and Gwaltney-Brant, S.M. (2008). Serotonin: a review. *J. Vet. Pharmacol. Ther.* 31: 187–199.

Monteiro, E.R., Nunes-Junior, J.S., and Bressan, T.F. (2014). Randomized clinical trial of the effects of a combination of acepromazine with morphine and midazolam on sedation, cardiovascular variables and the propofol dose requirements for induction of anesthesia in dogs. *Vet. J.* 200 (1): 157–161.

Moss, A.L., Hritz, R.L., Hector, R.C., and Wotman, K.L. (2021). Investigation of the effects of orally administered trazodone on intraocular pressure, pupil diameter, physical examination variables, and sedation level in healthy equids. *Am. J. Vet. Res.* 82 (2): 138–143.

Munro, H.M., Sleigh, J.W., and Paxton, L.D. (1993). The cardiovascular response to ketamine: the effects of clonidine and lignocaine. *Acta Anaesthesiol. Scand.* 37 (1): 75–78.

Murphy, L.A., Barletta, M., Graham, L.F. et al. (2017). Effects of acepromazine and trazodone on anesthetic induction dose of propofol and cardiovascular variables in dogs undergoing general anesthesia for orthopedic surgery. *J. Am. Vet. Med. Assoc.* 250 (4): 408–416.

Nelson, J.C. (2004). Tricyclic and tetracyclic drugs. In: *Textbook of Psychopharmacology* (ed. A.F. Schatzberg and C.B. Nemeroff), 207–230. Washington, DC, USA: The American Psychiatric Press.

Newton, R.E., Casten, G.P., Alms, D.R. et al. (1982). The side effect profile of buspirone in comparison to active controls and placebo. *J. Clin. Psychiatry* 43 (12): 100–102.

Norkus, C., Rankin, D., and KuKanich, B. (2015a). Pharmacokinetics of intravenous and oral amitriptyline and its active metabolite nortriptyline in Greyhound dogs. *Vet. Anaesth. Analg.* 42 (6): 580–589.

Norkus, C., Rankin, D., and KuKanich, B. (2015b). Evaluation of the pharmacokinetics of oral amitriptyline and its active metabolite nortriptyline in fed and fasted Greyhound dogs. *J. Vet. Pharmacol. Ther.* 38 (6): 619–622.

O'Carroll, A.M., Fowler, C.J., Phillips, J.P. et al. (1983). The deamination of dopamine by human brain monoamine oxidase. Specificity for the two enzyme forms in seven brain regions. *Naunyn-Schmiedeberg's Arch. Pharmacol.* 322 (3): 198–202.

O'Donnell, E.M., Press, S.A., Karriker, M.J., and Istvan, S.A. (2020). Pharmacokinetics and efficacy of trazodone following rectal administration of a single dose to healthy dogs. *Am. J. Vet. Res.* 81 (9): 739–746.

Olson, E.G., Goodyer, A.V., Langou, R.A. et al. (1976). N-dimethylisopropyl propranolol. Effects on myocardial oxygen demands. *Circulation* 53 (3): 501–505.

Paalzow, L.K. and Edlund, P.O. (1979). Pharmacokinetics of clonidine in the rat and cat. *J. Pharmacokinet. Biopharm.* 7 (5): 481–494.

Papich, M.G. and Alcorn, J. (1995). Absorption of diazepam after its rectal administration in dogs. *Am. J. Vet. Res.* 56 (12): 1629–1636.

Park, K.S., Kong, I.D., Park, K.C., and Lee, J.W. (1999). Fluoxetine inhibits L-type Ca^{2+} and transient outward K^{+} currents in rat ventricular myocytes. *Yonsei Med. J.* 40 (2): 144–151.

Paterson, I.A., Juorio, A.V., Berry, M.D., and Zhu, M.Y. (1991). Inhibition of monoamine oxidase-B by (−)-deprenyl potentiates neuronal responses to dopamine agonists but does not inhibit dopamine catabolism in the rat striatum. *J. Pharmacol. Exp. Ther.* 258 (3): 1019–1026.

Pavy, T.J., Kliffer, A.P., and Douglas, M.J. (1995). Anaesthetic management of labour and delivery in a woman taking long-term MAOI. *Can. J. Anaesth.* 42 (7): 618–620.

Peck, T., Wong, A., and Norman, E. (2010). Anaesthetic implications of psychoactive drugs. *Continuing Educ. Anaesthesia Crit. Care Pain* 10: 177–181.

Pérez, C.A., Garcia Sean, S., and Yu, R.D. (2016). Extrapyramidal symptoms as a result of risperidone discontinuation during combination therapy with methylphenidate in a pediatric patient. *J. Child Adolesc. Psychopharmacol.* **26** (2): 182. E-pub.

Peroutka, S.J. (1985). Selective interaction of novel anxiolytics with 5-hydroxytryptamine1A receptors. *Biol. Psychiatry* 20 (9): 971–979.

Perry, S.M., Whelan, E., Shay, S. et al. (1991). Effect of i.v. anaesthesia with propofol on drug distribution and metabolism in the dog. *Br. J. Anaesth.* 66 (1): 66–72.

Pichot, C., Ghignone, M., and Quintin, L. (2012). Dexmedetomidine and clonidine: from second- to first-line sedative agents in the critical care setting? *J. Intensive Care Med.* 27 (4): 219–237.

Platt, S.R., Adams, V., Garosi, L.S. et al. (2006). Treatment with gabapentin of 11 dogs with refractory idiopathic epilepsy. *Vet. Rec.* 159 (26): 881–884.

Pollock, B.G. (2001). Citalopram: a comprehensive review. *Expert Opin. Pharmacother.* 2 (4): 681–698.

Potter, W.Z. (1984). Psychotherapeutic drugs and biogenic amines. Current concepts and therapeutic implications. *Drugs* 28 (2): 127–143.

Potter, W.Z., Manji, H.K., and Rudorfer, M.V. (1995). Tricyclics and tetracyclics. In: *Textbook of*

Psychopharmacology (ed. A.F. Schatzberg and C.B. Nemeroff), 141–160. Washington, DC, USA: The American Psychiatric Press.

Pugh, C.M., Sweeney, J.T., Bloch, C.P. et al. (2013). Selective serotonin reuptake inhibitor (SSRI) toxicosis in cats: 33 cases (2004–2010). *J. Vet. Emerg. Crit. Care* 23 (5): 565–570.

Radulovic, L.L., Türck, D., von Hodenberg, A. et al. (1995). Disposition of gabapentin (neurontin) in mice, rats, dogs, and monkeys. *Drug Metab. Dispos.* 23 (4): 441–448.

Reich, M.R., Ohad, D.G., Overall, K.L., and Dunham, A.E. (2000). Electrocardiographic assessment of antianxiety medication in dogs and correlation with serum drug concentration. *J. Am. Vet. Med. Assoc.* 216 (10): 1571–1575.

Roerig, D.L., Kotrly, K.J., Ahlf, S.B. et al. (1989). Effect of propranolol on the first pass uptake of fentanyl in the human and rat lung. *Anesthesiology* 71 (1): 62–68.

Rosner, M.H. (2004). Severe hyponatremia associated with the combined use of thiazide diuretics and selective serotonin reuptake inhibitors. *Am. J. Med. Sci.* 327 (2): 109–111.

Ruelius, H.W., Lee, J.M., and Alburn, H.E. (1965). Metabolism of diazepam in dogs: transformation to oxazepam. *Arch. Biochem. Biophys.* 111 (2): 376–380.

Salman, M.D., New, J.G. Jr., Scarlett, J.M. et al. (1998). Human and animal factors related to relinquishment of dogs and cats in 12 selected animal shelters in the United States. *J. Appl. Anim. Welf. Sci.* 1 (3): 207–226.

Sanders, N.M., Wilkinson, C.W., Taborsky, G.J. Jr. et al. (2008). The selective serotonin reuptake inhibitor sertraline enhances counterregulatory responses to hypoglycemia. *Am. J. Physiol. Endocrinol. Metab.* 294 (5): 853–860.

Saranteas, T., Mourouzis, C., Koumoura, F., and Tesseromatis, C. (2003). Effects of propranolol or paracetamol on lidocaine concentrations in serum and tissues. *J. Oral Maxillofac. Surg.* 61 (5): 604–607.

Seddighi, R., Egger, C.M., Rohrbach, B.W. et al. (2011). The effect of midazolam on the end-tidal concentration of isoflurane necessary to prevent movement in dogs. *Vet. Anaesth. Analg.* 38 (3): 195–202.

Seibert, L. (2007). Pharmacotherapy for behavioral disorders in pet birds. *J. Exot. Pet Med.* 6 (1): 30–37.

Seibert, L.M., Crowell-Davis, S.L., Wilson, G.H., and Ritchie, B.W. (2004). Placebo-controlled clomipramine trial for the treatment of feather picking disorder in cockatoos. *J. Am. Anim. Hosp. Assoc.* 40 (4): 261–269.

Shand, D.G. (1976). Pharmacokinetics of propranolol: a review. *Postgrad. Med. J.* 52 (4): 22–25.

Sherman, B.L. and Papich, M.G. (2009). Drugs affecting animal behavior. In: *Veterinary Pharmacology and Therapeutics*, 9e (ed. M.G. Papich and J.E. Riviere), 509–538. Ames, IA, USA: Wiley.

Shults, T., Kownacki, A.A., Woods, W.E. et al. (1981). Pharmacokinetics and behavioral effects of methylphenidate in Thoroughbred horses. *Am. J. Vet. Res.* 42 (5): 722–726.

Smith, R.V., Havens, J.R., and Walsh, S.L. (2016). Gabapentin misuse, abuse and diversion: a systematic review. *Addiction* 111 (7): 1160–1174.

SmithKline Beecham Pharmaceuticals (2004). *Paroxetine® Product Information. Physicians' Desk Reference*, 1590–1594. Montvale, New Jersey: Montvale PDR.

Stahl, S.M. (2009). Mechanism of action of trazodone: a multifunctional drug. *CNS Spectr.* 14: 536–546.

Stanley, S.M.R. (2000). Equine metabolism of buspirone studied by high-performance liquid chromatography/mass spectrometry. *J. Mass Spectrom.* 35: 402–407.

Stefan, H. and Feuerstein, T.J. (2007). Novel anticonvulsant drugs. *Pharmacol. Ther.* 113 (1): 165–183.

Stein, M.B., Sareen, J., Hami, S., and Chao, J. (2001). Pindolol potentiation of paroxetine for generalized social phobia: a double-blind, placebo-controlled, crossover study. *Am. J. Psychiatry* 158 (10): 1725–1727.

Stevens, B.J., Frantz, E.M., Orlando, J.M. et al. (2016). Efficacy of a single dose of trazodone hydrochloride given to cats prior to veterinary visits to reduce signs of transport- and examination-related anxiety. *J. Am. Vet. Med. Assoc.* 249 (2): 202–207.

Stiff, J.L. and Harris, D.B. (1983). Clonidine withdrawal complicated by amitriptyline therapy. *Anesthesiol.* 59 (1): 73–74.

Stock, M.L. and Coetzee, J.F. (2015). Clinical pharmacology of analgesic drugs in cattle. *Vet. Clin. North Am. Food Anim. Pract.* 1: 113–138.

Stoelting, R.K. and Hillier, S. (2006a). Drugs used for psychopharmacologic therapy. In: *Pharmacology & Physiology in Anesthetic Practice*, 4e (ed. R.K. Stoelting and S. Hillier), 398–419. Philadelphia, PA, USA: Lippincott Williams & Wilkins.

Stoelting, R.K. and Hillier, S. (2006b). Alpha- and beta-adrenergic receptor antagonists. In: *Pharmacology & Physiology in Anesthetic Practice*, 4e (ed. R.K. Stoelting and S. Hillier), 321–337. Philadelphia, PA, USA: Lippincott Williams & Wilkins.

Stoelting, R.K. and Hillier, S. (2006c). Antihypertensive drugs. In: *Pharmacology & Physiology in Anesthetic Practice*, 4e (ed. R.K. Stoelting and S. Hillier), 338–351. Philadelphia, PA, USA: Lippincott Williams & Wilkins.

Stoelting, R.K. and Hillier, S. (2006d). Antiepileptic drugs. In: *Pharmacology & Physiology in Anesthetic Practice*, 4e (ed. R.K. Stoelting and S. Hillier), 569–579. Philadelphia, PA, USA: Lippincott Williams & Wilkins.

Stoelting, R.K. and Hillier, S. (2006e). Central nervous system stimulants and muscle relaxants. In: *Pharmacology*

& *Physiology in Anesthetic Practice*, 4e (ed. R.K. Stoelting and S. Hillier), 591–598. Philadelphia, PA, USA: Lippincott Williams & Wilkins.

Swenson, E.R. (1986). Severe hyperkalemia as a complication of timolol, a topically applied beta-adrenergic antagonist. *Arch. Intern. Med.* 146 (6): 1220–1221.

Taylor, C.P. (2009). Mechanisms of analgesia by gabapentin and pregabalin – calcium channel alpha(2)-delta [Ca-v alpha(2)-delta] ligands. *Pain* 142: 13–16.

Terry, R.L., McDonnell, S.M., Van Eps, A.W. et al. (2010). Pharmacokinetic profile and behavioral effects of gabapentin in the horse. *J. Vet. Pharmacol. Ther.* 33 (5): 485–494.

Trbolova, A., Ghaffari, M.S., and Capik, I. (2017). Effects of premedication with oral gabapentin on intraocular pressure changes following tracheal intubation in clinically normal dogs. *BMC Vet. Res.* 13 (1): 288.

Tremaine, L.M., Welch, W.M., and Ronfeld, R.A. (1989). Metabolism and disposition of the 5-hydroxytryptamine uptake blocker sertraline in the rat and dog. *Drug Metab. Dispos.* 17 (5): 542–550.

Tse, F.L., Sanders, T.M., and Reo, J.P. (1980). Bioavailability of propranolol in the dog. *Arch. Int. Pharmacodyn. Ther.* 248 (2): 180–189.

Turner, R.M., McDonnell, S.M., and Hawkins, J.F. (1995). Use of pharmacologically induced ejaculation to obtain semen from a stallion with a fractured radius. *J. Am. Vet. Med. Assoc.* 206 (12): 1906–1908.

Vollmer, K.O., von Hodenberg, A., and Kölle, E.U. (1986). Pharmacokinetics and metabolism of gabapentin in rat, dog and man. *Arzneimittelforschung* 36 (5): 830–839.

Weidler, D.J., Jallad, N.S., Garg, D.C., and Wagner, J.G. (1979). Pharmacokinetics of propranolol in the cat and comparisons with humans and three other species. *Res. Commun. Chem. Pathol. Pharmacol.* 26 (1): 105–114.

Wells, D.G. and Bjorksten, A.R. (1989). Monoamine oxidase inhibitors revisited. *Can. J. Anaesth.* 36 (1): 64–74.

Whelan, E., Wood, A.J., Koshakji, R. et al. (1989). Halothane inhibition of propranolol metabolism is stereoselective. *Anesthesiol.* 71 (4): 561–564.

Wilcox, R.G., Bennett, T., Macdonald, I.A. et al. (1984). The effects of acute or chronic ingestion of propranolol or metoprolol on the physiological responses to prolonged, submaximal exercise in hypertensive men. *Br. J. Clin. Pharmacol.* 17 (3): 273–281.

Wong, D.M., Davis, J.L., Alcott, C.J. et al. (2015). Pharmacokinetics and physiologic effects of alprazolam after a single oral dose in healthy mares. *J. Vet. Pharmacol. Ther.* 38 (3): 301–304.

Xu, B., Wang, Y., and Zhu, H. (2016). Mini-tablet combination for sustained release of clonidine hydrochloride and hydrochlorothiazide: preparation and pharmacokinetics in beagle dogs. *Pharmazie* 71 (2): 76–83.

23

Adjunctive Analgesic Pharmaceuticals

Reza Seddighi

α-2 Adrenoceptor Agonists

α-2 agonists, such as dexmedetomidine, detomidine, and romifidine, are commonly used as part of anesthetic-sedative protocols in small and large animals (Seddighi 2014). Although sedation is considered a dominant clinical effect of these drugs, they also provide effective and dose-dependent analgesia and muscle relaxation. It is believed that activation of α-2 adrenoceptors in supraspinal and spinal sites produces antihyperalgesia, analgesia, and sedation (Yaksh and Reddy 1981; Pertovaara et al. 1991; Molina and Herrero 2006). α-2 adrenergic receptors comprise three distinct receptor subtypes (A, B, and C) (Bylund 1992), play a significant role in modulating pain pathways, and may share a common cyclic guanosine 3',5'-monophosphate (cGMP) pathway with the opioid receptors (Vulliemoz et al. 1998; Hellyer et al. 2003). Therefore, it is not surprising that the analgesic efficacy of α-2 agonists is enhanced by the concomitant use of opioids (Kuo and Keegan 2004). Activation of supraspinal α-2 receptors within the pons plays an important role in the descending noradrenergic–serotonergic modulation of nociceptive input, resulting in analgesic and antihyperalgesic effects (Guo et al. 1996; Hellyer et al. 2007). It has been proposed that α-2 agonists mediate their analgesic action not only via stimulation of the spinal α-2 receptors but also by directly suppressing the locus coeruleus which, in turn, increases spinal-cord norepinephrine concentrations. This increase in spinal norepinephrine concentration activates spinal α-2 receptors, which results in antinociception (Guo et al. 1996).

In the spinal region, α-2 adrenergic receptors are present in high density in the substantia gelatinosa, in the intermediolateral cell columns of the spinal cord, and on primary afferent terminals, indicating their direct involvement in antinociception (Yaksh 1985; Yaksh et al. 1995). Stimulation of α-2 adrenergic receptors suppresses nociceptive signals at various points in the pain pathway via inhibition of neurotransmitter release from the primary afferent fibers in the dorsal horn. This neurotransmitter inhibition affects pre- and post-synaptic modulation of nociceptive signals, influences descending modulatory systems from the brainstem, inhibits the release of substance P, and alters ascending modulation of nociceptive signals in the diencephalon and limbic areas (Kuraishi et al. 1985; Murrell and Hellebrekers 2005).

The analgesic effect of α-2 agonists may have an added benefit in controlling chronic pain as α-2 agonists may also attenuate or reverse allodynia in states of chronic pain via a spinally mediated antinociceptive effect (Molina and Herrero 2006).

Clinical Application of α-2 Agonists

Clinically, the degree of sedation and analgesia produced by an α-2 agonist is related not only to the density, location, and type of α-2 adrenoceptors but also to the individual selectivity and affinity of the specific drug molecule for the α-1 and α-2 receptor binding sites (Sinclair 2003). α-2 agonists are not only used as part of anesthetic protocols but are also used in the form of a single dose or continuous rate infusion (CRI) during the recovery period to provide analgesia (Valtolina et al. 2009; van Oostrom et al. 2011), especially in combination with opioids to provide a synergistic analgesic effect (Ambrisko et al. 2005).

Epidural administration of α-2 agonists blocks nociceptive pathways at the level of the spinal cord (primarily mediated via α-2A subunits) and has synergistic analgesic effects with epidural opioids (Branson et al. 1993). Following epidural administration, dexmedetomidine, due to high lipophilicity, is rapidly absorbed into the cerebrospinal fluid (CSF) and binds to α-2 receptors in the spinal cord to provide analgesia (Schnaider et al. 2005). However, epidural and spinal administration of α-2 agonists results in systemic absorption, which often causes dose-dependent, adverse cardiovascular and respiratory effects (Vesal et al. 1996; Seddighi 2003); the onset and the extent of the adverse effects are primarily influenced by the lipid solubility of the drug. For instance, dexmedetomidine is more rapidly absorbed than medetomidine; thus, the systemic effects of dexmedetomidine can occur sooner after epidural or spinal administration than those of medetomidine (Kallio et al. 1989). In dogs, however, epidural administration of dexmedetomidine caused adequate neuraxial analgesia with minimal adverse cardiovascular and respiratory effects (Sabbe et al. 1994). In this author's opinion, the extent of the cardiorespiratory effects of α-2 agonists are dose-dependent, and severe adverse effects can be prevented by administration of lower doses.

α-2 agonists can be used for peripheral nerve blocks or IV regional anesthesia, alone or in combination with local anesthetics, to improve analgesia and/or prolong the duration of peripheral nerve conduction blockade (Singelyn et al. 1996; Madan et al. 2001; Memis et al. 2004). In peripheral nerve blockade, dexmedetomidine is more effective than clonidine, lidocaine, and cocaine and has similar efficacy to ropivacaine (Kosugi et al. 2010).

Binding to α-2A receptors is listed as one of the mechanisms for peripheral neural blockade of dexmedetomidine (Yoshitomi et al. 2008). Another mechanism may include blockade of other receptors (i.e. tetrodotoxin-sensitive, voltage-gated Na^+ channels and/or tetraethylammonium-sensitive [delayed-rectifier] K^+ channels). An inhibitory effect of dexmedetomidine on voltage-gated Na^+ channels in rat spinal nerves has also been reported (Oda et al. 2007); this effect was not reversible by yohimbine, indicating that the effect was not due to α-2 receptor action. The addition of dexmedetomidine to levobupivacaine for axillary brachial plexus block in human subjects shortened the onset and prolonged the duration of the block (Esmaoglu et al. 2010). In dogs, radial perineural infiltration using medetomidine and mepivacaine significantly prolonged the duration of peak motor block, peak sensory block, and residual sensory block compared with control (mepivacaine only) (Lamont and Lemke 2008). This author believes that including a low-dose α-2 adrenoceptor agonist (e.g. dexmedetomidine, 1–2 mcg/mL) in a peripheral nerve blockade is useful in prolonging the analgesic effect and may provide a multimodal approach to blocking nociceptive transmission.

Anticonvulsant Medications

Gabapentin and pregabalin are among several anticonvulsant medications being used more commonly to control pain in animals and people (Procopio 2010; Aghighi et al. 2012; Crociolli et al. 2015; Love and Thompson 2014).

By binding to the α2δ subunit of voltage-gated calcium channels, these drugs disrupt calcium influx and thus result in analgesia via a decrease in associated cellular activities, including neurotransmitter release, excitability, and gene expression (Cao 2006; Tran-Van-Minh and Dolphin 2010). Another mechanism involved in the analgesic activity of these drugs is upregulation of descending noradrenergic inhibitory pathways (Hayashida et al. 2008), the same mechanism involved in the analgesic activity of α-2 agonists. Gabapentin is a structural analog of the inhibitory neurotransmitter gamma-aminobutyric acid (GABA), and its use is associated with an increase in the brain's concentration of GABA (KuKanich 2013).

Clinical Application of Gabapentin and Pregabalin

Although these drugs are primarily used in the management of chronic and neuropathic pain, their use in the control of acute pain has also been reported. For instance, in a controlled study in 60 human patients undergoing hysterectomy, preoperative oral gabapentin (1.2 g) decreased pain scores and morphine consumption in the first 24 hours postoperatively but was also associated with a lower incidence of chronic incisional pain at 1, 3, and six months postoperatively (Sen et al. 2009). In veterinary patients, some studies have failed to demonstrate gabapentin's efficacy in the control of acute pain associated with thermal stimulation in awake cats (Pypendop et al. 2010), and in dogs undergoing forelimb amputation (Wagner et al. 2010). However, in a study in dogs undergoing mastectomy, administration of gabapentin (10 mg/kg PO) perioperatively was associated with a significant decrease in the dose of rescue analgesia with morphine during the first 72 hours postoperatively (Crociolli et al. 2015).

In human medicine, the overall efficacy of these drugs in the management of chronic neuropathic pain (e.g. diabetic neuropathy and post-herpetic neuralgia) is promising (Dworkin et al. 2010; Ko et al. 2010). In contrast, in veterinary medicine, the available information on the efficacy of these drugs in the control of chronic pain is limited, and the results are conflicting. For instance, in dogs undergoing hemilaminectomy, perioperative gabapentin (10 mg/kg, PO q 12 hours) did not reduce the pain score compared to a placebo group (Aghighi et al. 2012). In that study, gabapentin plasma concentrations at 24 and 72 hours were lower than 1 μg/ml, and although analgesic concentrations of gabapentin have not been determined in dogs, a plasma concentration of ≥2 μg/ml is necessary for gabapentin to be efficacious in humans (KuKanich 2013).

Gabapentin is currently available in the form of capsules (100 and 300 mg) and tablets (600 and 800 mg). An important consideration for gabapentin use in dogs and cats is the difference in its disposition in these species compared with humans. The terminal half-life of gabapentin in dogs (3–4 hours) and cats (3 hours) is shorter than in humans. The difference in the metabolism rate of gabapentin in dogs and cats necessitates doses of 10–20 mg/kg q 8 hours to maintain therapeutic concentrations (KuKanich 2013). Therefore, the lack of sufficient analgesic efficacy of gabapentin in some veterinary reports may be the result of inappropriate administration intervals and doses.

Pregabalin is less commonly used in veterinary patients, primarily due to its expense compared with gabapentin; nevertheless, its pharmacokinetics have been described in dogs. Based on the available data, an oral dosage of 4 mg/kg q 12 hours is recommended for dogs (KuKanich 2013). Although the pharmacokinetics of this drug in cats has not been extensively evaluated, based on a report, oral administration of pregabalin (4 mg/kg) in cats resulted in moderate sedation in 4/6 cats and the achieved blood concentrations were within the range considered efficacious for human seizure control (2.8–8.2 µg/ml) (Cautela et al. 2010). Based on that report, doses of 1–2 mg/kg, BID, is considered reasonable in cats; however, further studies are recommended.

Similarly, in dogs, sedation and ataxia are occasional adverse effects of gabapentin, and these are more common when higher doses are used; therefore, dose adjustment may be necessary for individual animals, especially when gabapentin is used in combination with other drugs. In addition, abrupt discontinuation of gabapentin after chronic administration may result in withdrawal syndrome and seizure activity. Therefore, in chronic use, tapering the dose over the course of one week is recommended (KuKanich 2013).

In summary, despite the limited number of placebo-controlled studies and conflicting reports on the efficacy of gabapentin in veterinary patients, particularly for treatment of chronic pain, the author frequently considers gabapentin administration (10–20 mg/kg q 8 hours) as part of a multimodal analgesic combination in clinical practice.

NMDA Antagonists

N-methyl-D-aspartate (NMDA) receptors (NMDARs) are amino-acid receptors predominantly located in the central nervous system (CNS) and are involved in perception and transmission of noxious stimuli mediated by the excitatory neurotransmitter glutamate (Muir 2010). Multiple variants of NMDARs are required for normal brain function, and they play a central role in learning, memory, and the development of the CNS in hyperactive states (Petrenko et al. 2003). NMDARs contribute to the pathogenesis of wind-up in chronic pain and the development of primary and secondary hyperalgesia and allodynia. These manifestations commonly occur following a severe or chronic nerve or tissue injury in which stimulus-independent firing of the second-order neurons and increased production of glutamate receptors occur (Love and Thompson 2014). Therefore, blockade of NMDARs can enhance analgesia and produce antihyperalgesic effects, particularly in subjects suffering from chronic pain.

Multiple drugs with nonselective NMDAR antagonism are available, and those most commonly used in veterinary medicine include amantadine and ketamine. Methadone, a pure opioid agonist, has some NMDA antagonistic effects and is also discussed briefly later.

Amantadine

Amantadine is primarily known as an antiviral medication; however, the NMDA-antagonistic properties of this drug have expanded its use to control pain, particularly for treatment of central sensitization. In humans, amantadine has been reported as efficacious in decreasing pain in the postoperative period (Fisher et al. 2000) and in postherpetic neuralgia (Buerkle and Yaksh 1998). In veterinary medicine, there are anecdotal reports of the efficacy of amantadine in treating chronic pain in cats (Robertson 2005). However, the general consensus is that amantadine is best used in combination with analgesics such as non-steroidal anti-inflammatory drugs (NSAIDs), opioids, or gabapentin (KuKanich 2013). For instance, in osteoarthritic dogs refractory to NSAID therapy, amantadine combined with meloxicam significantly improved activity over meloxicam alone (Lascelles et al. 2008).

Clinical Application of Amantadine

The pharmacokinetics of amantadine in dogs are not fully understood, nevertheless, administration of 3–5 mg/kg q 24 hours is recommended for cats and dogs (Love and Thompson 2014; Robertson 2005). In dogs, the limited data indicate a short half-life of 5 hours after a 30 mg/kg dose (Bleidner et al. 1965). In cats, amantadine has a high oral bioavailability, yet a similarly short half-life (5.5 hours) is reported after a 5 mg/kg dose (Siao et al. 2011). In contrast, the half-life in humans is 15 hours (Aoki and Sitar 1992); thus, a dose interval adjustment to q 12 hours is recommended by others (KuKanich 2013). Amantadine is primarily excreted in the urine and its accumulation may result in subsequent neuropsychiatric toxic effects in humans with renal impairment and geriatrics (Ing et al. 1979; Miller and Miller 1994). To this author's knowledge, such adverse effects are not reported in animals receiving amantadine; however, it is reasonable to assume that the same dose adjustment and caution in the administration of amantadine in geriatrics and animals with renal disease would be warranted.

Ketamine

Ketamine is primarily considered a dissociative anesthetic that is most commonly used for induction of anesthesia. In hemodynamically unstable human trauma patients, ketamine is considered as a preferred anesthetic induction agent due to its indirect sympathomimetic effects that typically result in increased blood pressure, pulse rate, and cardiac output. In addition, ketamine has amnestic, analgesic, and anxiolytic activities (Green et al. 2011).

In addition to its anesthetic effects, ketamine's use as an analgesic and in the treatment of hyperalgesia has gained significant interest. In humans, ketamine improves perioperative opioid efficacy (Suzuki et al. 1999) and decreases opioid-induced hyperalgesia (Minville et al. 2010). In a literature review of analgesic effects of ketamine in people, a mean reduction of 40% in opioid consumption was reported when low-dose infusion of ketamine (infusion rates of less than 1.2 mg/kg/h) was used perioperatively (Jouguelet-Lacoste et al. 2015). Controlled studies investigating the analgesic effects of ketamine in veterinary patients are limited. In a prospective randomized study in conscious cats, low-dose ketamine (5–23 μg/kg/min) resulted in mild sedation but did not affect thermal and mechanical antinociception (Ambros and Duke 2013). In contrast, in a clinical study in dogs undergoing forelimb amputation, perioperative low-dose ketamine infusion (0.12–0.6 mg/kg/h) reduced pain scores and ketamine-treated dogs were more active on day three compared with the control group (Wagner et al. 2002). In ponies, low-dose ketamine infusion (20 μg/kg/min) reduced the withdrawal response to an electrical nociceptive stimulation (Peterbauer et al. 2008), but lower dose rates (approximately 0.6–1.3 μg/kg/min) did not affect responses to mechanical stimulation induced by a hoof tester applied to the withers and radius areas (Fielding et al. 2006). Therefore, based on the available literature, it seems that ketamine's effect in preventing acute pain is variable, and differences among studies may be the result of variabilities in the nature of the noxious stimulation, dose rates, and the methodology used.

In contrast, the results of studies on the antihyperalgesic effects of ketamine and its beneficial use in chronic and neuropathic pain are more consistent. For instance, in people, topical ketamine (combined with amitriptyline) (AmiKet®) is recommended as the potential first-line treatment option for post-herpetic neuralgia and neuropathic conditions (Sawynok and Zinger 2016). The role of ketamine in controlling cancer pain nonresponsive to conventional opioids has also been advocated (Zgaia et al. 2015). Ketamine administration is reportedly effective in decreasing pain and discomfort in humans suffering from complex regional pain syndrome (Sigtermans et al. 2009). Nevertheless, there are reports of cognitive function impairment in patients who were treated long-term with ketamine infusion to control complex regional pain syndrome (Kim et al. 2016).

There is no multi-case report or controlled study on the use of ketamine in controlling chronic and neuropathic pain in veterinary medicine, but it is likely that ketamine would have the same beneficial effects as in humans and can be considered for controlling pain in animals with different forms of chronic pain.

Clinical Application of Ketamine

For animals undergoing surgical procedures using general anesthesia, particularly those with chronic inflammation and pain, ketamine may be incorporated in the anesthetic protocol for induction of anesthesia, as well as used as a CRI intra- and postoperatively. In the author's practice, ketamine is commonly used in combination with benzodiazepines for induction of anesthesia and is used in the form of a CRI (1–3 mg/kg/h) intraoperatively for its analgesic and particularly antihyperalgesic properties. Additionally, the author recommends administration of a ketamine CRI (0.5–1 mg/kg/h) in awake animals as a component of multimodal analgesia in animals that suffer from chronic pain, refractory to the traditional opioid-NSAID analgesic therapy.

Methadone

As an opioid, methadone is discussed in detail in another chapter; however, some of its effects are discussed here with an emphasis on its use in the management of chronic pain. Methadone is available as a racemic mixture and although the L-enantiomer is primarily responsible for the opioid activity, both enantiomers are capable of binding to the NMDA receptor (KuKanich and Papich 2009). Due to NMDA antagonistic effect and inhibition of norepinephrine and serotonin reuptake, methadone is used in neuropathic pain and is considered a suitable agent to treat painful conditions poorly controlled with other opioids. Typical examples of such conditions include chronic and neuropathic pain (Foley 2003; Morley et al. 2003). Based on a clinical report, switching from morphine to methadone in human cancer patients with uncontrolled pain or significant adverse effects from opioid treatment resulted in the reduction of pain and adverse effects in the majority (80%) of the patients (Mercadante et al. 2001).

In veterinary clinical practice, the main limitation in oral administration of methadone is the low bioavailability of the drugs as demonstrated in a study where detectable plasma concentrations were not achieved after oral administration of methadone in dogs (Kukanich et al. 2005).

Serotonin and Norepinephrine-Modulating Agents

The monoamine neurotransmitters serotonin and norepinephrine are among the most important neurotransmitters in the CNS and are vital for normal activities such as mood, vigilance, and modulation of nociception. Several groups of drugs, primarily antidepressants and mood modifiers, have been developed to control the synaptic concentration of these transmitters. In addition, as serotonin and norepinephrine have been implicated as principal mediators of endogenous analgesic mechanisms in the descending pain pathways, clinical use of many serotonin- and norepinephrine-modulating drugs have been recommended for providing analgesia, particularly in controlling chronic pain (Lamont et al. 2000; Marks et al. 2009).

Membrane proteins known as serotonin and norepinephrine transporters are responsible for the reuptake of these neurotransmitters. Therefore, chemicals that inhibit this reuptake cause an increase in the synaptic concentration of these neurotransmitters, resulting in more profound and sustained effects. Tricyclic antidepressants (TCAs), such as amitriptyline and amoxapine, non-selectively inhibit the reuptake transporters at presynaptic terminals and, thereby, increase their availability.

Due to the potential for significant adverse effects, such as inhibitory effects on muscarinic, α-adrenergic, and H_1 receptors, TCAs have been predominantly replaced by newer generations of antidepressants, such as selective serotonin reuptake inhibitors (SSRIs), norepinephrine reuptake inhibitors, and dual serotonin and norepinephrine reuptake inhibitors (SNRIs) (Marks et al. 2009). In this section, amitriptyline, a TCA, followed by tramadol and tapentadol (TAP), which employ their effect via modulation of the same neurotransmitters, will be discussed.

Amitriptyline

Amitriptyline was originally known as an antiviral medication. It is currently known for its efficacy in the treatment of neuropathic pain and has been evaluated in many placebo-controlled human trials. Amitriptyline improved pain and sleep disorders in fibromyalgia (Goldenberg et al. 1996) and was found superior in improving pain, fatigue, and quality of life compared to duloxetine, an SSNRI (Hauser et al. 2011).

Placebo-controlled studies on the efficacy of amitriptyline for treatment of neuropathic pain in veterinary patients are lacking. Nevertheless, in a study of 15 cats with idiopathic cystitis non-responsive to other treatments, amitriptyline administration (10 mg daily PO) for 12 months, decreased clinical signs in nine cats (Chew et al. 1998). In a case report of three dogs with a history of chronic behavioral or locomotor disorders unresponsive to conventional analgesics (NSAIDs, corticosteroids, and opioids), amitriptyline administration (1.1–1.4 mg/kg, PO q 12 hours) resulted in dramatic improvement or full resolution of clinical signs (Cashmore et al. 2009).

Clinical Application of Amitriptyline

Amitriptyline is available in tablet and injectable form and the common dose used in humans is 10–15 mg q 24 hours (Chinn et al. 2016), but the daily dose to achieve results may vary from 75 to 150 mg (Gupta et al. 1999). In dogs, doses of 1–2 mg/kg q 12 hours are recommended (KuKanich 2013); however, in a pharmacokinetic study in dogs, an oral dose of 3–4 mg/kg was associated with a short half-life of 5 hours (Kukes et al. 2009). The latter results, therefore, may suggest the need for higher dose (3–4 mg/kg q 12 hours) recommendation for clinical cases. In cats, the currently used dose of amitriptyline (1–2.2 mg/kg q 12 hours) may also require adjustment, as these doses are associated with a short half-life and low plasma concentrations (KuKanich 2013). Nonetheless, to prevent adverse effects and reduce the risk of development of serotonin syndrome, gradual dose escalation is recommended, especially when mood-modifying drugs from different classes are co-administered (e.g. tramadol, amitriptyline, dextromethorphan, etc.) (Love and Thompson 2014).

Tramadol

Tramadol is a synthetic codeine analog and is classified as an atypical opioid with weak opioid agonistic activity. In addition, tramadol has some similarities to TCAs in that it inhibits serotonin and norepinephrine reuptake and may also facilitate 5-hydroxytryptamine release (Desmeules et al. 1996). Tramadol, after gabapentinoids and TCAs, is recommended as the second line of treatment for moderate and severe neuropathic pain in people (Moulin et al. 2014). In the US, tramadol was not a controlled substance until recently (2014), when it was upgraded to a class-IV controlled substance. Metabolism of tramadol results in several metabolites, but only O-desmethyltramadol (ODM) (also known as M1 metabolite), and N,O-desmethyl tramadol (DDM) have been associated with pharmacologic effects (Grond and Sablotzki 2004). The ODM metabolite shows a higher affinity for opioid receptors than the parent drug and is responsible for the mu-opioid-derived analgesic activity. Nevertheless, this affinity for mu receptors of the CNS remains low, and approximately 6000 times lower than that of morphine (Gillen et al. 2000; Dayer et al. 1994). Additionally, there are differences between species in relation to tramadol metabolism. For instance, because ODM is not an important metabolite in dogs, tramadol is not expected to exert a substantial opioid effect in this species. Cats, in contrast, produce significant concentrations of ODM; thus, an important opioid effect is expected in cats (Pypendop and Ilkiw 2008). Nevertheless, the DDM metabolite may also be associated with some opioid effects, at least in greyhounds (KuKanich and Papich 2011). Tramadol has a shorter elimination half-life in dogs (1.1 hours) compared with humans (5.6 hours) (KuKanich 2013).

IV tramadol significantly reduced the minimum alveolar concentration of sevoflurane in dogs (Seddighi et al. 2009) but when used to control acute pain in veterinary studies, the results have been very variable. In a study in dogs undergoing tibial plateau-leveling osteotomy, hydrocodone-acetaminophen and tramadol failed to control postoperative pain (Benitez et al. 2015). Similarly, in dogs undergoing cutaneous tumor removal, preoperative administration of tramadol did not affect the requirement for rescue analgesia (Karrasch et al. 2015).

In cats undergoing ovariohysterectomy, tramadol (2, 4 mg/kg) administered intramuscularly (IM) at the preoperative period was superior to pethidine (6 mg/kg IM), but only the higher dose of tramadol (4 mg/kg) eliminated the need for rescue analgesia during the first 6 hours postextubation (Evangelista et al. 2014). In cats, thermal thresholds increased proportionally with increasing doses of tramadol (Pypendop et al. 2009).

In contrast, veterinary studies on the efficacy of tramadol for the control of chronic pain are limited; in a clinical study on 69 dogs with multiple forms of cancer and moderate to severe pain, tramadol (combined with metamizole) was well tolerated and improved pain scores and quality of life in those animals (Flor et al. 2013). In another clinical study in dogs with osteoarthritis, compared with the placebo group, pain significantly improved in the animals that received carprofen (2.2 mg/kg q 12 hours) or tramadol (4 mg/kg q 8 hours) (Malek et al. 2012).

Clinical Application of Tramadol

Based on the literature, and the author's clinical experience, it seems that tramadol has a limited efficacy, if any, in controlling acute pain. However, the use of tramadol, particularly if combined with other analgesics (e.g. opioids and NSAIDs), can provide an additional benefit in animals with chronic painful conditions.

Based on a pharmacokinetic study in dogs, doses of 5 mg/kg q 6 hours or 2.5 mg/kg q 4 hours predicted tramadol and ODM plasma concentrations consistent with analgesia in humans (KuKanich and Papich 2004). Under clinical conditions, doses of 4–10 mg/kg PO q 8 hours are recommended for dogs (KuKanich 2013). But when tramadol was used for several days (20 mg/kg PO for eight days), the achieved plasma concentrations were reduced by 60–70% (Matthiesen et al. 1998). The latter may be due to either decreased drug absorption or enhanced systemic metabolism. Nevertheless, this may dictate a need for dose adjustment in the longer-term use of tramadol in dogs. Doses of 2–4 mg/kg PO q 12 hours are recommended for cats (KuKanich 2013).

The main adverse effects of tramadol may include sedation and dysphoria, especially in cats (Lamont 2008). Tramadol tablets have a bitter taste and can result in profuse salivation and retching in dogs and cats. Other adverse effects of tramadol overdose include restlessness, difficulty walking, salivation, vomiting, tremors, and convulsions. These excitatory effects are more likely if tramadol is co-administered with other serotonin and norepinephrine reuptake and monoamine oxidase inhibitors, such as selegiline (Lamont 2008). Diazepam may be effective in controlling tramadol-induced convulsions (KuKanich 2013). Higher risk of gastrointestinal (GI) adverse effects was reported in three dogs that received a combination of tramadol with deracoxib (Case et al. 2010). In humans, tramadol co-administration increases the potential for NSAID-associated GI adverse effects, and this is thought to be primarily due to serotonin-enhanced gastric acid secretion and decreased platelet aggregation (Torring et al. 2008). Therefore, concurrent administration of acid-suppressing agents (e.g. H_2 blockers or proton pump inhibitors) with tramadol may be beneficial in preventing adverse GI effects (KuKanich 2013).

Tapentadol

TAP is a novel opioid pain reliever with a dual mechanism of action: mu opioid receptor agonist and noradrenaline reuptake inhibitor. TAP lacks some of the inherent limitations of tramadol, such as the need for an active metabolite for opioid activity (Tzschentke et al. 2007). This drug is currently approved by the US Food and Drug Administration (FDA) for the control of moderate to severe pain, and its analgesic potency is considered to be between tramadol and morphine. TAP does not seem to cause the confusional (and excitatory) states associated with tramadol (Power 2011). Veterinary reports evaluating the efficacy of TAP in dogs are few. In pre-clinical research in a tail-flick test model of acute nociception in 15 dogs,

TAP and morphine, but not tramadol, induced dose-dependent antinociception (Kogel et al. 2014).

Overall, the limited information on this drug indicates favorable pharmacokinetics and clinical efficacy, and it is likely that TAP may be used in the near future as an alternative to tramadol in veterinary patients.

Prostaglandin Receptor Antagonists

Prostaglandin E2 (PGE2) is an important prostanoid with roles in homeostasis, pain, and inflammation. PGE2 binds to several receptors, of which, the EP4 receptor is responsible for mediating inflammation and pain in osteoarthritis. It is proposed that selective inhibition of EP4 receptors would maintain a more favorable homeostasis compared with nonselective PG inhibitors, and this is achieved by using a new class of drugs known as piprants (Shaw et al. 2015). Piprants were developed for the control of pain and inflammation associated with osteoarthritis in dogs and cats. The safety of long-term oral administration of the newly developed drug grapiprant has been reported in 36 beagles (Rausch-Derra et al. 2015). In early 2016, in the US, galliprant (grapiprant tablets – Aratana Therapeutics) received approval from FDA as a new analgesic and anti-inflammatory medication for osteoarthritis (OA) in dogs. To evaluate the effectiveness of grapiprant in alleviating pain in dogs with OA, 285 client-owned dogs with OA were enrolled in a study and treated with either grapiprant (2 mg/kg) per OS or placebo (Rausch-Derra et al. 2016). Grapiprant treatment improved the pain interference and pain severity score in the grapiprant group compared to placebo. Grapiprant was generally well tolerated, but a higher percentage of treated dogs (17.02%) had occasional vomiting as compared to the placebo group (6.25%).

Based on these preliminary clinical reports, and in view of FDA approval, grapiprant may be considered a valuable addition to multimodal approach to management of pain in dogs with osteoarthritis.

Future Adjunctive Analgesic Pharmaceuticals

With simultaneous advancement in pain research and pharmaceutical technology, many other new analgesics have been developed, but yet require further research to prove their efficacy and potentially refine their pharmacologic properties. In this section, some of these new drugs with potential for use as analgesics in future, are briefly discussed.

Anti-Glial Medications

The crucial role of glial cells, astrocytes, and microglia in the maintenance of neuronal homeostasis in the CNS is well known. Upon activation, these cells release a number of signaling molecules with protective or pathologic effects on the nervous system. The role of microglia in nociception and development of neuropathic pain via the release of pro-inflammatory immune factors in the spinal cord and dorsal root ganglia has been reported (Milligan and Watkins 2009). Glial activation opposes opioid-induced analgesia, reduces opioid efficacy, and creates dependence (Vallejo et al. 2010; Mika et al. 2013). Therefore, it has been proposed that pharmacologic attenuation of glial-cell activation would have a therapeutic effect in the treatment of chronic and neuropathic pain. Ibudilast (development codes AV-411 or MN-166), an inhibitor of glial activation and cyclic nucleotide phosphodiesterases, is in clinical use in Asia as a bronchodilator for the treatment of asthma. However, with its anti-glial activity, this drug has a potential for treatment of neuropathic pain and opioid withdrawal. *In vitro*, ibudilast suppresses glial lipopolysaccharide-induced production of inflammatory mediators, such as tumor necrosis factor α, nitric oxide, IL-1, and IL-6, and increases the production of anti-inflammatory cytokines, such as IL-10 (Kawanokuchi et al. 2004; Mizuno et al. 2004). In a study on rats, ibudilast had an additive antinociceptive effect when combined with morphine and partly restored morphine-induced antinociception in morphine-tolerant rats but did not attenuate the development of morphine tolerance (Lilius et al. 2009).

Overall, based on the available information, it seems there is potential for future clinical application of anti-glial medications; however, further research is necessary to determine their efficacy in a clinical setting.

TRPV1 Receptor Antagonists

The analgesic efficacy of capsaicin, the active gradient in chili pepper, has been known for many years; but its mechanism of action has only been recently recognized. Capsaicin exerts its effects via the vanilloid receptor-1 (VR1), a nonselective cation calcium channel, and a member of the ligand-gated ion channel receptors called transient receptor potential channel (TRP). These receptors are primarily located on small myelinated and medium unmyelinated sensory fibers in different areas of the brain and spinal cord; their activation results in calcium and sodium influx and thus, membrane depolarization and transduction (Gunthorpe and Szallasi 2008; Kym et al. 2009). In neurogenic inflammation, transient receptor potential cation channel subfamily V member (TRPV1) receptors are triggered by inflammatory mediators and have a pivotal role in intracellular signaling and peripheral and central sensitization (Cui et al. 2006).

TRPV1 agonists result in an initial excitatory effect, but prolonged stimulation will result in receptor desensitization. To avoid the excitatory effects, considerable interest has been focused on the development of TPRV1 antagonists (Norman et al. 2007). Efficacy of some TPRV1 antagonists in laboratory conditions have been investigated and resulted in favorable preliminary findings (Hodgetts et al. 2010; Voight et al. 2014). In contrast, in a randomized placebo-controlled study in dogs with hip arthritis, an experimental TRPV1 antagonist (ABT-116) was inferior to carprofen or tramadol (Malek et al. 2012).

More recently, resiniferatoxin (RTX), a TRPV1 agonist with a greater potency compared to capsaicin, has been investigated for its analgesic activity. RTX can be administered spinally (intrathecal), or locally into the surrounding areas of nerve terminals, or directly into a nerve trunk or a dorsal root ganglion (Iadarola and Gonnella 2013).

Intrathecal administration of RTX results in prolonged calcium influx and subsequent cytotoxicity and death of only those sensory neurons that express the TRPV1 ion channel. This mechanism selectively targets and permanently deletes TRPV1-expressing C-fiber neuronal cell bodies in the dorsal root ganglia. In a clinical study on 72 companion dogs with bone cancer, animals received either standard of care analgesic therapy (control, n = 36) or intrathecal administration of RTX (1.2 µg/kg) in addition to standard-of-care analgesic therapy. Significantly more dogs in the control group (78%) required unblinding and adjustment in the analgesic protocol or euthanasia within six weeks of randomization, than dogs that received RTX (50%) (Brown et al. 2015).

In summary, based on the available information, TRPV1 modulators such as RTX, may be considered valid options in animals with chronic pain; however, further evaluations are warranted to determine their role in the multimodal analgesic treatment of complex, painful conditions that are nonresponsive to conventional therapies.

References

Aghighi, S.A., Tipold, A., Piechotta, M. et al. (2012). Assessment of the effects of adjunctive gabapentin on postoperative pain after intervertebral disc surgery in dogs. *Vet. Anaesth. Analg.* 39: 636–646.

Ambrisko, T.D., Hikasa, Y., and Sato, K. (2005). Influence of medetomidine on stress-related neurohormonal and metabolic effects caused by butorphanol, fentanyl, and ketamine administration in dogs. *Am. J. Vet. Res.* 66: 406–412.

Ambros, B. and Duke, T. (2013). Effect of low dose rate ketamine infusions on thermal and mechanical thresholds in conscious cats. *Vet. Anaesth. Analg.* 40: e76–e82.

Aoki, F.Y. and Sitar, D.S. (1992). Effects of chronic amantadine hydrochloride ingestion on its and acetaminophen pharmacokinetics in young adults. *J. Clin. Pharmacol.* 32: 24–27.

Benitez, M.E., Roush, J.K., Mcmurphy, R. et al. (2015). Clinical efficacy of hydrocodone-acetaminophen and tramadol for control of postoperative pain in dogs following tibial plateau leveling osteotomy. *Am. J. Vet. Res.* 76: 755–762.

Bleidner, W.E., Harmon, J.B., Hewes, W.E. et al. (1965). Absorption, distribution and excretion of amantadine hydrochloride. *J. Pharmacol. Exp. Ther.* 150: 484–490.

Branson, K.R., Ko, J.C., Tranquilli, W.J. et al. (1993). Duration of analgesia induced by epidurally administered morphine and medetomidine in dogs. *J. Vet. Pharmacol. Ther.* 16: 369–372.

Brown, D.C., Agnello, K., and Iadarola, M.J. (2015). Intrathecal resiniferatoxin in a dog model: efficacy in bone cancer pain. *Pain* 156: 1018–1024.

Buerkle, H. and Yaksh, T.L. (1998). Pharmacological evidence for different alpha 2-adrenergic receptor sites mediating analgesia and sedation in the rat. *Br. J. Anaesth.* 81: 208–215.

Bylund, D.B. (1992). Subtypes of alpha 1- and alpha 2-adrenergic receptors. *FASEB J.* 6: 832–839.

Cao, Y.Q. (2006). Voltage-gated calcium channels and pain. *Pain* 126: 5–9.

Case, J.B., Fick, J.L., and Rooney, M.B. (2010). Proximal duodenal perforation in three dogs following deracoxib administration. *J. Am.Anim. Hosp. Assoc.* 46: 255–258.

Cashmore, R.G., Harcourt-Brown, T.R., Freeman, P.M. et al. (2009). Clinical diagnosis and treatment of suspected neuropathic pain in three dogs. *Aust. Vet. J.* 87: 45–50.

Cautela, M.A., Dewey, C.W., Schwark, W.S. et al. (2010). Pharmacokinetics of oral pregabalin in cats after single dose administration. Proceedings of ACVIM Annual Forum, USA.

Chew, D.J., Buffington, C.A., Kendall, M.S. et al. (1998). Amitriptyline treatment for severe recurrent idiopathic cystitis in cats. *J. Am. Vet. Med. Assoc.* 213: 1282–1286.

Chinn, S., Caldwell, W., and Gritsenko, K. (2016). Fibromyalgia pathogenesis and treatment options update. *Curr. Pain Headache Rep.* 20: 25.

Crociolli, G.C., Cassu, R.N., Barbero, R.C. et al. (2015). Gabapentin as an adjuvant for postoperative pain management in dogs undergoing mastectomy. *J. Vet. Med. Sci.* 77: 1011–1015.

Cui, M., Honore, P., Zhong, C. et al. (2006). TRPV1 receptors in the CNS play a key role in broad-spectrum analgesia of TRPV1 antagonists. *J. Neurosci.* 26: 9385–9393.

Dayer, P., Collart, L., and Desmeules, J. (1994). The pharmacology of tramadol. *Drugs* 47 (Suppl 1): 3–7.

Desmeules, J.A., Piguet, V., Collart, L., and Dayer, P. (1996). Contribution of monoaminergic modulation to the analgesic effect of tramadol. *Br. J. Clin. Pharmacol.* 41: 7–12.

Dworkin, R.H., O'connor, A.B., Audette, J. et al. (2010). Recommendations for the pharmacological management of neuropathic pain: an overview and literature update. *Mayo Clin. Proc.* 85: S3–S14.

Esmaoglu, A., Yegenoglu, F., Akin, A., and Turk, C.Y. (2010). Dexmedetomidine added to levobupivacaine prolongs axillary brachial plexus block. *Anesth. Analg.* 111: 1548–1551.

Evangelista, M.C., Silva, R.A., Cardozo, L.B. et al. (2014). Comparison of preoperative tramadol and pethidine on postoperative pain in cats undergoing ovariohysterectomy. *BMC Vet. Res.* 10: 252.

Fielding, C.L., Brumbaugh, G.W., Matthews, N.S. et al. (2006). Pharmacokinetics and clinical effects of a subanesthetic continuous rate infusion of ketamine in awake horses. *Am. J. Vet. Res.* 67: 1484–1490.

Fisher, K., Coderre, T.J., and Hagen, N.A. (2000). Targeting the N-methyl-D-aspartate receptor for chronic pain management. Preclinical animal studies, recent clinical experience and future research directions. *J. Pain Symp. Manag.* 20: 358–373.

Flor, P.B., Yazbek, K.V., Ida, K.K., and Fantoni, D.T. (2013). Tramadol plus metamizole combined or not with anti-inflammatory drugs is clinically effective for moderate to severe chronic pain treatment in cancer patients. *Vet. Anaesth. Analg.* 40: 316–327.

Foley, K.M. (2003). Opioids and chronic neuropathic pain. *N. Engl. J. Med.* 348: 1279–1281.

Gillen, C., Haurand, M., Kobelt, D.J., and Wnendt, S. (2000). Affinity, potency and efficacy of tramadol and its metabolites at the cloned human mu-opioid receptor. *Naunyn-Schmiedeberg's Arch. Pharmacol.* 362: 116–121.

Goldenberg, D., Mayskiy, M., Mossey, C. et al. (1996). A randomized, double-blind crossover trial of fluoxetine and amitriptyline in the treatment of fibromyalgia. *Arth. Rheumatol.* 39: 1852–1859.

Green, S.M., Roback, M.G., Kennedy, R.M., and Krauss, B. (2011). Clinical practice guideline for emergency department ketamine dissociative sedation: 2011 update. *Ann. Emerg. Med.* 57: 449–461.

Grond, S. and Sablotzki, A. (2004). Clinical pharmacology of tramadol. *Clin. Pharmacokinet.* 43: 879–923.

Gunthorpe, M.J. and Szallasi, A. (2008). Peripheral TRPV1 receptors as targets for drug development: new molecules and mechanisms. *Curr. Pharm. Des.* 14: 32–41.

Guo, T.Z., Jiang, J.Y., Buttermann, A.E., and Maze, M. (1996). Dexmedetomidine injection into the locus ceruleus produces antinociception. *Anesthesiology* 84: 873–881.

Gupta, S.K., Shah, J.C., and Hwang, S.S. (1999). Pharmacokinetic and pharmacodynamic characterization of OROS and immediate-release amitriptyline. *Br. J. Clin. Pharmacol.* 48: 71–78.

Hauser, W., Petzke, F., Uceyler, N., and Sommer, C. (2011). Comparative efficacy and acceptability of amitriptyline, duloxetine and milnacipran in fibromyalgia syndrome: a systematic review with meta-analysis. *Rheumatology (Oxford)* 50: 532–543.

Hayashida, K., Obata, H., Nakajima, K., and Eisenach, J.C. (2008). Gabapentin acts within the locus coeruleus to alleviate neuropathic pain. *Anesthesiology* 109: 1077–1084.

Hellyer, P.W., Bai, L., Supon, J. et al. (2003). Comparison of opioid and alpha-2 adrenergic receptor binding in horse and dog brain using radioligand autoradiography. *Vet. Anaesth. Analg.* 30: 172–182.

Hellyer, P.W., Robertson, S.A., and Fails, A.D. (2007). Pain and its management. In: *Lumb & Jones' Veterinary Anesthesia and Analgesia*, 4e (ed. W.J. Tranquilli, J.C. Thurman and K.A. Grimm), 31–60. Ames, IA: Blackwell Publishing.

Hodgetts, K.J., Blum, C.A., Caldwell, T. et al. (2010). Pyrido[2,3-b]pyrazines, discovery of TRPV1 antagonists with reduced potential for the formation of reactive metabolites. *Bioorg. Med. Chem. Lett.* 20: 4359–4363.

Iadarola, M.J. and Gonnella, G.L. (2013). Resiniferatoxin for pain treatment: an interventional approach to personalized pain medicine. *Open Pain J.* 6: 95–107.

Ing, T.S., Daugirdas, J.T., Soung, L.S. et al. (1979). Toxic effects of amantadine in patients with renal failure. *Can. Med. Assoc. J.* 120: 695–698.

Jouguelet-Lacoste, J., La Colla, L., Schilling, D., and Chelly, J.E. (2015). The use of intravenous infusion or single dose of low-dose ketamine for postoperative analgesia: a review of the current literature. *Pain Med.* 16: 383–403.

Kallio, A., Scheinin, M., Koulu, M. et al. (1989). Effects of dexmedetomidine, a selective alpha 2-adrenoceptor agonist, on hemodynamic control mechanisms. *Clin. Pharmacol. Ther.* 46: 33–42.

Karrasch, N.M., Lerche, P., Aarnes, T.K. et al. (2015). The effects of preoperative oral administration of carprofen or tramadol on postoperative analgesia in dogs undergoing cutaneous tumor removal. *Can. Vet. J.* 56: 817–822.

Kawanokuchi, J., Mizuno, T., Kato, H. et al. (2004). Effects of interferon-beta on microglial functions as inflammatory and antigen presenting cells in the central nervous system. *Neuropharmacology* 46: 734–742.

Kim, M., Cho, S., and Lee, J.H. (2016). The effects of long-term ketamine treatment on cognitive function in complex regional pain syndrome: a preliminary study. *Pain Med.* pii: pnv112.

Ko, S.H., Kwon, H.S., Yu, J.M. et al. (2010). Comparison of the efficacy and safety of tramadol/acetaminophen combination therapy and gabapentin in the treatment of painful diabetic neuropathy. *Diab. Med.* 27: 1033–1040.

Kogel, B., Terlinden, R., and Schneider, J. (2014). Characterisation of tramadol, morphine and tapentadol in an acute pain model in Beagle dogs. *Vet. Anaesth. Analg.* 41: 297–304.

Kosugi, T., Mizuta, K., Fujita, T. et al. (2010). High concentrations of dexmedetomidine inhibit compound action potentials in frog sciatic nerves without alpha(2) adrenoceptor activation. *Br. J. Pharmacol.* 160: 1662–1676.

KuKanich, B. (2013). Outpatient oral analgesics in dogs and cats beyond nonsteroidal antiinflammatory drugs: an evidence-based approach. *Vet. Clin. N. Am. Small Anim. Pract.* 43: 1109–1125.

KuKanich, B. and Papich, M.G. (2004). Pharmacokinetics of tramadol and the metabolite O-desmethyltramadol in dogs. *J. Vet. Pharmacol. Ther.* 27: 239–246.

KuKanich, B. and Papich, M.G. (2009). Opioid analgesic drugs. In: *Veterinary Pharmacology and Therapeutics*, 9e (ed. J.E. Riviere, M.G. Papich and H.R. Adams), 302–329. Ames, Iowa: Wiley.

KuKanich, B. and Papich, M.G. (2011). Pharmacokinetics and antinociceptive effects of oral tramadol hydrochloride administration in Greyhounds. *Am. J. Vet. Res.* 72: 256–262.

Kukanich, B., Lascelles, B.D., Aman, A.M. et al. (2005). The effects of inhibiting cytochrome P450 3A, p-glycoprotein, and gastric acid secretion on the oral bioavailability of methadone in dogs. *J. Vet. Pharmacol. Ther.* 28: 461–466.

Kukes, V.G., Kondratenko, S.N., Savelyeva, M.I. et al. (2009). Experimental and clinical pharmacokinetics of amitryptiline: comparative analysis. *Bull. Exp. Biol. Med.* 147: 434–437.

Kuo, W.C. and Keegan, R.D. (2004). Comparative cardiovascular, analgesic, and sedative effects of medetomidine, medetomidine-hydromorphone, and medetomidine-butorphanol in dogs. *Am. J. Vet. Res.* 65: 931–937.

Kuraishi, Y., Hirota, N., Sato, Y. et al. (1985). Noradrenergic inhibition of the release of substance P from the primary afferents in the rabbit spinal dorsal horn. *Brain Res.* 359: 177–182.

Kym, P.R., Kort, M.E., and Hutchins, C.W. (2009). Analgesic potential of TRPV1 antagonists. *Biochem. Pharmacol.* 78: 211–216.

Lamont, L.A. (2008). Adjunctive analgesic therapy in veterinary medicine. *Vet. Clin. N. Am. Small Anim. Pract.* 38: 1187–1203.

Lamont, L.A. and Lemke, K.A. (2008). The effects of medetomidine on radial nerve blockade with mepivacaine in dogs. *Vet. Anaesth. Analg.* 35: 62–68.

Lamont, L.A., Tranquilli, W.J., and Grimm, K.A. (2000). Physiology of pain. *Vet. Clin. N. Am. Small Anim. Pract.* 30: 703–728.

Lascelles, B.D., Gaynor, J.S., Smith, E.S. et al. (2008). Amantadine in a multimodal analgesic regimen for alleviation of refractory osteoarthritis pain in dogs. *J. Vet. Intern. Med.* 22: 53–59.

Lilius, T.O., Rauhala, P.V., Kambur, O., and Kalso, E.A. (2009). Modulation of morphine-induced antinociception in acute and chronic opioid treatment by ibudilast. *Anesthesiology* 111: 1356–1364.

Love, L. and Thompson, D. (2014). Nontraditional analgesic agents. In: *Pain Management in Veterinary Practice* (ed. C.M. Egger, L. Love and T.J. Doherty), 105–114. Wiley: Ames, IA.

Madan, R., Bharti, N., Shende, D. et al. (2001). A dose response study of clonidine with local anesthetic mixture for peribulbar block: a comparison of three doses. *Anesth. Analg.* 93: 1593–1597.

Malek, S., Sample, S.J., Schwartz, Z. et al. (2012). Effect of analgesic therapy on clinical outcome measures in a randomized controlled trial using client-owned dogs with hip osteoarthritis. *BMC Vet. Res.* 8: 185.

Marks, D.M., Shah, M.J., Patkar, A.A. et al. (2009). Serotonin-norepinephrine reuptake inhibitors for pain control: premise and promise. *Curr. Neuropharmacol.* 7: 331–336.

Matthiesen, T., Wohrmann, T., Coogan, T.P., and Uragg, H. (1998). The experimental toxicology of tramadol: an overview. *Toxicol. Lett.* 95: 63–71.

Memis, D., Turan, A., Karamanlioglu, B. et al. (2004). Adding dexmedetomidine to lidocaine for intravenous regional anesthesia. *Anesth. Analg.* 98: 835–840.

Mercadante, S., Casuccio, A.F., Fulfaro, L. et al. (2001). Switching from morphine to methadone to improve analgesia and tolerability in cancer patients: a prospective study. *J. Clin. Oncol.* 19: 2898–2904.

Mika, J., Zychowska, M., Popiolek-Barczyk, K. et al. (2013). Importance of glial activation in neuropathic pain. *Eur. J. Pharmacol.* 716: 106–119.

Miller, K.S. and Miller, J.M. (1994). Toxic effects of amantadine in patients with renal failure. *Chest* 105: 1630.

Milligan, E.D. and Watkins, L.R. (2009). Pathological and protective roles of glia in chronic pain. *Nat. Rev. Neurosci.* 10: 23–36.

Minville, V., Fourcade, O., Girolami, J.P., and Tack, I. (2010). Opioid-induced hyperalgesia in a mice model of orthopaedic pain: preventive effect of ketamine. *Br. J. Anaesth.* 104: 231–238.

Mizuno, T., Kurotani, T., Komatsu, Y. et al. (2004). Neuroprotective role of phosphodiesterase inhibitor ibudilast on neuronal cell death induced by activated microglia. *Neuropharmacology* 46: 404–411.

Molina, C. and Herrero, J.F. (2006). The influence of the time course of inflammation and spinalization on the antinociceptive activity of the alpha2-adrenoceptor agonist medetomidine. *Eur. J. Pharmacol.* 532: 50–60.

Morley, J.S., Bridson, J., Nash, T.P. et al. (2003). Low-dose methadone has an analgesic effect in neuropathic pain: a double-blind randomized controlled crossover trial. *Palliat. Med.* 17: 576–587.

Moulin, D., Boulanger, A., Clark, A.J. et al. (2014). Pharmacological management of chronic neuropathic pain: revised consensus statement from the Canadian Pain Society. *Pain Res. Manag.* 19: 328–335.

Muir, W.W. (2010). NMDA receptor antagonists and pain: ketamine. *Vet. Clin. N. Am. Equine Pract.* 26: 565–578.

Murrell, J.C. and Hellebrekers, L.J. (2005). Medetomidine and dexmedetomidine: a review of cardiovascular effects and antinociceptive properties in the dog. *Vet. Anaesth. Analg.* 32: 117–127.

Norman, M.H., Zhu, J., Fotsch, C. et al. (2007). Novel vanilloid receptor-1 antagonists: 1. Conformationally restricted analogues of trans-cinnamides. *J. Med. Chem.* 50: 3497–3514.

Oda, A., Iida, H., Tanahashi, S. et al. (2007). Effects of alpha2-adrenoceptor agonists on tetrodotoxin-resistant Na^+ channels in rat dorsal root ganglion neurons. *Eur. J. Anaesthesiol.* 24: 934–941.

Pertovaara, A., Kauppila, T., Jyvasjarvi, E., and Kalso, E. (1991). Involvement of supraspinal and spinal segmental alpha-2-adrenergic mechanisms in the medetomidine-induced antinociception. *Neuroscience* 44: 705–714.

Peterbauer, C., Larenza, P.M., Knobloch, M. et al. (2008). Effects of a low dose infusion of racemic and S-ketamine on the nociceptive withdrawal reflex in standing ponies. *Vet. Anaesth. Analg.* 35: 414–423.

Petrenko, A.B., Yamakura, T., Baba, H., and Shimoji, K. (2003). The role of N-methyl-D-aspartate (NMDA) receptors in pain: a review. *Anesth. Analg.* 97: 1108–1116.

Power, I. (2011). An update on analgesics. *Br. J. Anaesth.* 107: 19–24.

Procopio, M. (2010). New users of the anticonvulsants gabapentin, lamotrigine, oxcarbazepine or tiagabine are at increased risk of suicidal acts compared with new users of topiramate. *Evid.-Based Ment. Health* 13: 102.

Pypendop, B.H. and Ilkiw, J.E. (2008). Pharmacokinetics of tramadol, and its metabolite O-desmethyl-tramadol, in cats. *J. Vet. Pharmacol. Ther.* 31: 52–59.

Pypendop, B.H., Siao, K.T., and Ilkiw, J.E. (2009). Effects of tramadol hydrochloride on the thermal threshold in cats. *Am. J. Vet. Res.* 70: 1465–1470.

Pypendop, B.H., Siao, K.T., and Ilkiw, J.E. (2010). Thermal antinociceptive effect of orally administered gabapentin in healthy cats. *Am. J. Vet. Res.* 71: 1027–1032.

Rausch-Derra, L.C., Huebner, M., and Rhodes, L. (2015). Evaluation of the safety of long-term, daily oral administration of grapiprant, a novel drug for treatment of osteoarthritic pain and inflammation, in healthy dogs. *Am. J. Vet. Res.* 76: 853–859.

Rausch-Derra, L., Huebner, M., Wofford, J., and Rhodes, L. (2016). A prospective, randomized, masked, placebo-controlled multisite clinical study of Grapiprant, an EP4 prostaglandin receptor antagonist (PRA), in dogs with osteoarthritis. *J. Vet. Intern. Med.* 30: 756–763.

Robertson, S.A. (2005). Managing pain in feline patients. *Vet. Clin. N. Am. Small Anim. Pract.* 35: 129–146.

Sabbe, M.B., Penning, J.P., Ozaki, G.T., and Yaksh, T.L. (1994). Spinal and systemic action of the alpha 2 receptor agonist dexmedetomidine in dogs. Antinociception and carbon dioxide response. *Anesthesiology* 80: 1057–1072.

Sawynok, J. and Zinger, C. (2016). Topical amitriptyline and ketamine for post-herpetic neuralgia and other forms of neuropathic pain. *Expert Opin. Pharmacother.* 17: 601–609.

Schnaider, T.B., Vieira, A.M., Brandao, A.C., and Lobo, M.V. (2005). Intraoperative analgesic effect of epidural ketamine, clonidine or dexmedetomidine for upper abdominal surgery. *Rev. Bras. Anestesiol.* 55: 525–531.

Seddighi, M. (2003). A comparison of the hemodynamic effects of epidurally administered medetomidine and xylazine in dogs [abstract]. *Vet. Anaesth. Analg.* 30: 98.

Seddighi, R. (2014). α-2 adrenoceptor agonists. In: *Pain Management in Veterinary Practice* (ed. C.M. Egger, L. Love and T.J. Doherty), 93–104. Wiley: Ames, IA.

Seddighi, M.R., Egger, C.M., Rohrbach, B.W. et al. (2009). Effects of tramadol on the minimum alveolar concentration of sevoflurane in dogs. *Vet. Anaesth. Analg.* 36: 334–340.

Sen, H., Sizlan, A., Yanarates, O. et al. (2009). A comparison of gabapentin and ketamine in acute and chronic pain after hysterectomy. *Anesth. Analg.* 109: 1645–1650.

Shaw, K.K., Rausch-Derra, L.C., and Rhodes, L. (2015). Grapiprant: an EP4 prostaglandin receptor antagonist and novel therapy for pain and inflammation. *Vet. Med. Sci.* 2: 3–9.

Siao, K.T., Pypendop, B.H., Stanley, S.D., and Ilkiw, J.E. (2011). Pharmacokinetics of amantadine in cats. *J. Vet. Pharmacol. Ther.* 34: 599–604.

Sigtermans, M.J., Van Hilten, J.J., Bauer, M.C. et al. (2009). Ketamine produces effective and long-term pain relief in patients with complex regional pain syndrome type 1. *Pain* 145: 304–311.

Sinclair, M.D. (2003). A review of the physiological effects of alpha2-agonists related to the clinical use of medetomidine in small animal practice. *Can. Vet. J.* 44: 885–897.

Singelyn, F.J., Gouverneur, J.M., and Robert, A. (1996). A minimum dose of clonidine added to mepivacaine prolongs the duration of anesthesia and analgesia after axillary brachial plexus block. *Anesth. Analg.* 83: 1046–1050.

Suzuki, M., Tsueda, K., Lansing, P.S. et al. (1999). Small-dose ketamine enhances morphine-induced analgesia after outpatient surgery. *Anesth. Analg.* 89: 98–103.

Torring, M.L., Riis, A., Christensen, S. et al. (2008). Perforated peptic ulcer and short-term mortality among tramadol users. *Br. J. Clin. Pharmacol.* 65: 565–572.

Tran-Van-Minh, A. and Dolphin, A.C. (2010). The alpha2delta ligand gabapentin inhibits the Rab11-dependent recycling of the calcium channel subunit alpha2delta-2. *J. Neurosci.* 30: 12856–12867.

Tzschentke, T.M., Christoph, T., Kogel, B. et al. (2007). (−)-(1R,2R)-3-(3-dimethylamino-1-ethyl-2-methyl-propyl)-phenol hydrochloride (tapentadol HCl): a novel mu-opioid receptor agonist/norepinephrine reuptake inhibitor with broad-spectrum analgesic properties. *J. Pharmacol. Exp. Ther.* 323: 265–276.

Vallejo, R., Tilley, D.M., Vogel, L., and Benyamin, R. (2010). The role of glia and the immune system in the development and maintenance of neuropathic pain. *Pain Pract.* 10: 167–184.

Valtolina, C., Robben, J.H., Uilenreef, J. et al. (2009). Clinical evaluation of the efficacy and safety of a constant rate infusion of dexmedetomidine for postoperative pain management in dogs. *Vet. Anaesth. Analg.* 36: 369–383.

Van Oostrom, H., Doornenbal, A., Schot, A. et al. (2011). Neurophysiological assessment of the sedative and analgesic effects of a constant rate infusion of dexmedetomidine in the dog. *Vet. J.* 190: 338–344.

Vesal, N., Cribb, P.H., and Frketic, M. (1996). Postoperative analgesic and cardiopulmonary effects in dogs of oxymorphone administered epidurally and intramuscularly, and medetomidine administered epidurally: a comparative clinical study. *Vet. Surg.* 25: 361–369.

Voight, E.A., Gomtsyan, A.R., Daanen, J.F. et al. (2014). Discovery of (R)-1-(7-chloro-2,2-bis(fluoromethyl) chroman-4-yl)-3-(3-methylisoquinolin-5-yl)urea (A-1165442): a temperature-neutral transient receptor potential vanilloid-1 (TRPV1) antagonist with analgesic efficacy. *J. Med. Chem.* 57: 7412–7424.

Vulliemoz, Y., Virag, L., and Whittington, R.A. (1998). Interaction of the alpha-2 adrenergic- and opioid receptor with the cGMP system in the mouse cerebellum. *Brain Res.* 813: 26–31.

Wagner, A.E., Walton, J.A., Hellyer, P.W. et al. (2002). Use of low doses of ketamine administered by constant rate infusion as an adjunct for postoperative analgesia in dogs. *J. Am. Vet. Med. Assoc.* 221: 72–75.

Wagner, A.E., Mich, P.M., Uhrig, S.R., and Hellyer, P.W. (2010). Clinical evaluation of perioperative administration of gabapentin as an adjunct for postoperative analgesia in dogs undergoing amputation of a forelimb. *J. Am. Vet. Med. Assoc.* 236: 751–756.

Yaksh, T.L. (1985). Pharmacology of spinal adrenergic systems which modulate spinal nociceptive processing. *Pharmacol. Biochem. Behav.* 22: 845–858.

Yaksh, T.L. and Reddy, S.V. (1981). Studies in the primate on the analgetic effects associated with intrathecal actions of opiates, alpha-adrenergic agonists and baclofen. *Anesthesiology* 54: 451–467.

Yaksh, T.L., Pogrel, J.W., Lee, Y.W., and Chaplan, S.R. (1995). Reversal of nerve ligation-induced allodynia by spinal alpha-2 adrenoceptor agonists. *J. Pharmacol. Exp. Ther.* 272: 207–214.

Yoshitomi, T., Kohjitani, A., Maeda, S. et al. (2008). Dexmedetomidine enhances the local anesthetic action of lidocaine via an alpha-2A adrenoceptor. *Anesth. Analg.* 107: 96–101.

Zgaia, A.O., Irimie, A., Sandesc, D. et al. (2015). The role of ketamine in the treatment of chronic cancer pain. *Clujul Med.* 88: 457–461.

24

Diuretics
Andrew Claude

Introduction

It is important to have a thorough understanding of diuretic pharmaceuticals when contemplating certain anesthetic protocols. Although diuretics are not considered anesthetic drugs, it is not unusual to employ them pre- and peri-operatively during specific disease processes in patients needing anesthesia. In both human and veterinary medicine, diuretics are commonly used when treating patient hypertension, heart and renal failure, increased intracranial and intraocular pressures, and edema. Different diuretic drugs vary in their pharmacology, however, the prominent feature for most diuretics is an increased urine output by interrupting sodium ion (Na^+) and water reabsorption in various locations of the nephron. Although the method of action of most diuretics is relatively well understood in human medicine, their efficacy, safety, and optimal doses are based on underpowered research trials (Svensen 2013). Unfortunately, for common veterinary species (dogs, cats, horses, and cattle), the pharmacology of diuretics is far less understood and derived chiefly from human applications. For other species (rodents, rabbits, birds, and other exotic animals), diuretic pharmacology is largely speculative. There are few, if any, studies that specifically investigate the physiologic and pharmacologic influences of diuretics on the renal function of canine, feline, or other animal species, with or without anesthesia.

Diuretics affect specific areas of the renal tubular network (Figure 24.1); thus, understanding diuretic drug pharmacokinetics requires an understanding of renal tubular physiology. The basic structure and functional unit of the kidney is the nephron. The primary function of the renal nephron is to regulate the concentration of water and solutes by filtering the blood, reabsorbing what is needed, and excreting the rest as urine. Renal nephrons consist of the corpuscle (Bowman's capsule and glomerular tuft), associated extension of tubules, and supporting vasculature. The afferent renal arterioles supply the glomerulus with blood. Cellular components and medium-to-high molecular weight proteins are retained in the blood, while fluid nearly identical to plasma is extruded through the glomerulus into Bowman's space. There are numerous characteristics of segmental tubular reabsorption and specific details of transport mechanisms of each segment are beyond the scope of this chapter. Some transport mechanisms will be highlighted here, however, the reader is encouraged to research veterinary physiology textbooks in order to further review the intricate details of transport and co-transport mechanisms within the renal tubules.

The majority of diuretic pharmaceuticals exert their effects in four primary areas of the renal tubular network: the proximal convoluted tubules, the ascending limb of the loop of Henle, the distal convoluted tubules, and the collecting ducts. The proximal convoluted tubule is the segment where the majority of water and solutes are isotonically reabsorbed. In the proximal tubule, most solute reabsorption is driven by the active transport of Na^+ via the Na^+/K^+-ATPase pump located on the basolateral plasma membrane. Active transport of Na^+ out and K^+ into the proximal tubular cell creates an electrochemical gradient favoring Na^+ and Cl^- uptake from the tubular fluid in conjunction with a slightly hypotonic state within the tubular lumen, which in turn, favors water reabsorption.

The thick ascending loops of Henle and distal convoluted tubular segments are effectively impermeable to water. These segments reabsorb Na^+, K^+, Ca^{2+}, and Mg^{2+} ions against a concentration gradient. Tubular fluid leaving the distal convoluted tubule is nearly void of ionic solutes, with an osmolality of approximately $100 \, mOsm/kg \, H_2O$, compared to fluid entering the distal convoluted tubules, with an osmolality of approximately $300 \, mOsm/kg \, H_2O$. As in the proximal tubule, salt reabsorption in the thick ascending loops of Henle and distal convoluted tubules is driven by the basolateral Na^+/K^+-ATPase pumps (Valender 2000).

Pharmacology in Veterinary Anesthesia and Analgesia, First Edition. Edited by Turi Aarnes and Phillip Lerche.
© 2024 John Wiley & Sons, Inc. Published 2024 by John Wiley & Sons, Inc.

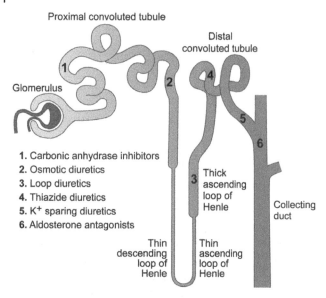

Proximal convoluted tubule

Distal convoluted tubule

Glomerulus

1. Carbonic anhydrase inhibitors
2. Osmotic diuretics
3. Loop diuretics
4. Thiazide diuretics
5. K⁺ sparing diuretics
6. Aldosterone antagonists

Thick ascending loop of Henle

Collecting duct

Thin descending loop of Henle

Thin ascending loop of Henle

Figure 24.1 Diagram of the renal nephron showing the primary areas for which common diuretics exert their effects (Kochevar 2009).

The collecting duct tubules are lined by two cell types: principal cells, which are the primary cell type, and intercalated cells. NaCl reabsorption within the collecting duct is primarily performed by the principal cells, utilizing basolateral Na^+/K^+-ATPase pumps. Similar to the proximal tubules, movement of Na^+ ions from the luminal space creates an electrochemical gradient that drives Cl^- into the cell. Aldosterone, a mineralocorticoid secreted by the adrenal cortex during periods of hypotension/hypovolemia, acts on principal cells by enhancing Na^+ reabsorption, which, in turn, enhances water reabsorption. Aldosterone release is also stimulated by hyperkalemia, which then causes increased principal cell K^+ excretion into the tubular lumen. Vasopressin controls water reabsorption in the distal collecting ducts by regulating water channel (aquaporin – 2) location in the intercalated cells. Under basal physiologic conditions, vasopressin determines final urine osmolality. Nearly 99% of the ultrafiltrate is reabsorbed in the tubular network (Kochevar 2009, Valender 2000).

Proximal Convoluted Tubules

Carbonic Anhydrase Inhibiting Diuretics

Method of Action

Acetazolamide, methazolamide, and dorzolamide are sulfanilamide carbonic anhydrase inhibiting diuretics. Carbonic anhydrase (CA) is an enzyme found throughout the body that catalyzes the formation of carbonic acid from CO_2 and H_2O. Carbonic anhydrase increases the hydration of CO_2 several hundredfold and is vital for HCO_3^-, Na^+, and Cl^- reabsorption in the proximal convoluted tubular cells. Under normal circumstances, Na^+ ions are exchanged for H^+ ions via the Na^+/H^+ exchange pump, maintaining cellular electrochemical neutrality and driving renal Cl^- reabsorption (Valender 2000). Acetazolamide causes several key changes in proximal convoluted renal tubular cell homeostasis. It binds to CA resulting in a noncompetitive inhibition of carbonic acid production, leading to a reduction of H^+ and HCO_3^- concentrations in the renal tubular fluid and a decrease in Na^+ reabsorption. Due to changes in the cellular electrochemical gradient, Cl^- is retained to offset the net loss of HCO_3^- into the tubular fluid, and potassium ions are substituted for the lost H^+, resulting in potassium wasting. Sodium and HCO_3^- retention in the renal lumen forms $NaHCO_3$ which, in turn, leads to a decreased reabsorption of water. Acetazolamide is considered a weak diuretic because most excess tubular fluid retention is reclaimed in more distal tubular segments, resulting in minimal gross renal water loss.

Pharmacokinetics

There is little to no information regarding the pharmacokinetics of acetazolamide in animals. One report states that the onset of action is 30 minutes, maximal effects is two to four hours, and the duration of action is approximately four to six hours in small animals (Roberts 1985). In humans, oral absorption is good, with onset of action approximately 30 minutes and maximum effects at two to four hours after administration. The duration of action of acetazolamide is four to six hours, and drug elimination occurs primarily via the kidneys (Kochevar 2009).

Therapeutic Uses

Acetazolamide has limited diuretic use in veterinary and human medicine due to its weak diuretic effect and rapid development of drug tolerance. The most common application for acetazolamide in veterinary medicine is in patients with glaucoma, as acetazolamide decreases intra-ocular pressures via a reduction in aqueous humor production. Acetazolamide also decreases the production of cerebral spinal fluid (CSF) and is occasionally used in patients with increased intracranial pressures (ICPs); however, osmotic and loop diuretics are preferable (Hastie and Shanewise 2015).

Prior to anesthesia, acetazolamide is used to decrease serum potassium concentration in horses that have a genetic predisposition for hyperkalemic periodic paralysis.

Adverse Effects and Other Considerations

Carbonic anhydrase inhibiting diuretics can result in electrolyte and pH disturbances. Loss of HCO_3^- in the renal tubular fluid causes a risk of hyperchloremic metabolic acidosis with paradoxical alkaluria. In addition, renal tubular cells will substitute K^+ excretion for H^+ in the Na^+/H^+ exchange step, resulting in K^+ wasting and hypokalemia. The degree of K^+ wasting in the urine is directly proportional to the concentration of Na^+ in the renal tubular fluid. Furthermore, ammonium excretion is inhibited, leading to an increased risk of encephalopathy in patients with liver insufficiencies (Hastie and Shanewise 2015).

Acetazolamide should be avoided in patients with pre-existing metabolic or respiratory acidosis or those who cannot mount respiratory compensation. In one study conducted on anesthetized dogs, acetazolamide increased ventilation-perfusion mismatching and reduced arterial PO_2 when compared to a control group (Swenson et al. 1993). Acetazolamide also decreased the CO_2 sensitivity of the peripheral and central chemoreceptor groups and the hypoxic sensitivity effect of the carotid bodies in anesthetized cats (Teppema and Dahan 2004). Anesthetized patients that are currently receiving acetazolamide should be artificially ventilated.

Carbonic anhydrase inhibiting diuretics are self-limiting, as an increased concentration of H^+ associated with metabolic acidosis tends to offset Na^+ loss in the nephron, which inhibits the effects of the drug on CA.

Sulfanilamide derivative side effects include: central nervous system (CNS) disorientation, drowsiness, and systemic hypersensitivities.

Proximal Convoluted Tubules

Osmotic Diuretics

Method of Action

Mannitol is an inert, sugar-alcohol compound that inhibits water reabsorption in the proximal convoluted tubules and thin segments of the ascending loop of Henle. Mannitol is not absorbed from the gastrointestinal (GI) tract when given orally and results in profound osmotic diarrhea; therefore, mannitol is administered intravenously (IV). When administered IV, mannitol is not metabolized, does not undergo biodegradation, and is freely filtered by the glomerulus. Within the renal nephron, mannitol undergoes limited to no reabsorption from the renal tubules, increases glomerular filtration rate, and alters plasma and renal tubular osmolarity with increased renal water losses. Ions, such as Na^+, Cl^-, and HCO_3^-, are diluted in the renal tubules, resulting in a net decrease in their reabsorption. Mannitol also increases plasma osmolarity, leading to an acute expansion of intravascular volume at the expense of interstitial hydration and parenchymal volume.

The presence of mannitol in blood circulation stimulates the release of atrial natriuretic peptide and vasodilatory prostaglandins in response to an acute increased blood volume (Kochevar 2009).

Mannitol has actions beyond renal effects: it improves blood flow by decreasing blood viscosity via hemodilution, it augments cardiac output by increasing blood volume, it causes vasodilation and has mild positive inotropic effects, and it has oxygen free radical scavenging effects (Hastie and Shanewise 2015).

Pharmacokinetics

In humans and veterinary patients, mannitol undergoes two-compartment distribution and elimination and is excreted unchanged in the urine (Rudehill et al. 1993). Distribution and elimination half-lives are dose-dependent and occur within minutes after administration in patients with normal renal function. Mannitol penetration into tissues is limited due to rapid decline of plasma levels. In patients with impaired renal function, mannitol distribution, and elimination can be delayed (Kochevar 2009).

Therapeutic Uses

In veterinary medicine, mannitol is primarily used to acutely decrease intracranial or intraocular pressures. The effects of mannitol on ICP and cerebral perfusion occur rapidly after administration, with maximum effects occurring within one hour. The mechanics of brain parenchymal reduction following IV mannitol therapy are governed by the osmotic, hemodynamic, and diuretic theories. The osmotic theory states that brain shrinkage is due to the osmotically driven movement of water from the parenchyma into the vascular space. The hemodynamic theory states that cerebral blood volume decreases as a result of decreased blood viscosity, improved cardiac output, and a transient increase in cerebral perfusion pressure. These hemodynamic effects thereby enhance oxygenation of the brain, resulting in compensatory cerebral vasoconstriction and secondary reduction in brain volume. Finally, the diuretic theory states that intracranial volume reduction results from an acute decrease in central venous pressure (CVP), resulting in a decrease in cerebral blood and brain volume (Kochevar 2009). Realistically, all three mechanisms likely play roles in acute reduction in ICP; however, the diuretic mechanism would provide a sustained effect compared to the other two mechanisms (Paczynski 1997). Mannitol may also decrease ICP by decreasing CSF volume via decreased production.

Acute reduction in intraocular pressure is due to the loss of water content in the eye. Vitreous shrinkage from fluid loss causes the lens to displace posteriorly, which improves intraocular pressures by allowing the drainage angle to increase.

Mannitol can be useful to differentiate acute oliguria as a function of prerenal versus renal insufficiency. In the presence of prerenal azotemia, mannitol administration will increase urine output, while in patients in renal failure, mannitol therapy will not affect urine production (Hastie and Shanewise 2015).

Mannitol can be used prior to anesthesia to help improve renal blood flow and GFR in patients who are at risk of acute tubular necrosis and/or renal failure (Behnia et al. 1996). Mannitol should not be administered to anuric patients; however, a test dose (0.25 g–0.5 g/kg) may be used to attempt diuresis. In human medicine, mannitol has been shown to preserve renal function for kidney transplants, and it has decreased the incidence of post-transplant acute renal failure.

Adverse Effects and Other Considerations

Although mean arterial pressures (MAPs) increase after IV administration of mannitol, rapid injections (especially in dehydrated patients) can lead to acute hypotension, possibly from Na^+ displacement; therefore, slow IV administration (20–30 minutes) is recommended. In patients with impaired renal function, pulmonary edema could develop. Patients with compensatory congestive heart failure (CHF) can decompensate due to an acute increase in blood volume. Hypertonic dehydration and electrolyte imbalances (Na^+, K^+, Mg^{2+}, and PO_4^{-3}) can develop, leading to exacerbated disease processes, malaise, and cardiac arrhythmias.

Chronic mannitol administration can result in a hyperosmolar state (plasma osmolarity increases by 25 mOsm/l or greater) and subsequent osmotic compensation. During osmotic compensation, fluid volume and electrolyte concentrations shift intracellularly due to the production of idiogenic osmoles. In order to counteract the chronic dehydrating effect of hyperosmotic plasma, cells respond by generating newly osmotically active intracellular particles. Cellular osmotic compensation decreases the osmotic gradient from tissue to plasma, thus limiting mannitol's therapeutic effectiveness. This state may also promote conditions where iatrogenic edema may occur, especially in the brain. The risk of edema formation is greatest when chronic mannitol administration is suddenly stopped, leaving the intracellular osmoles as the most active osmotic site. To prevent this condition, the return-to-normal plasma osmolarity should occur slowly, with a duration approximately equal to the time the patient spent in the hyperosmotic state.

For patients in which the blood–brain barrier integrity may be disrupted (trauma, vascular diseases, etc.), mannitol leakage into the brain parenchyma will exacerbate cerebral edema.

Mannitol should not be used in patients with ongoing intracranial hemorrhage, anuric renal failure, severe dehydration, CHF, or a predisposition to pulmonary edema (Kochevar 2009).

Ascending Loops of Henle and Distal Convoluted Tubules

Loop Diuretics

Mechanism of Action

Loop diuretics include furosemide, ethacrynic acid, bumetanide, and torsemide. All are sulfonamides except ethacrynic acid. The following discussion will be limited to furosemide as the prototypical loop diuretic. Unlike other diuretics that gain access to sites of action via glomerular filtration, furosemide must be actively secreted into the tubular lumen via an organic acid transport pathway in order to bind to the luminal symport system. Furosemide is highly protein bound, rendering it too large to be filtered at the glomerulus; therefore, active secretion is necessary. Furosemide blocks the Na^+, K^+, and Cl^- symporter in the thick ascending loops of Henle and the early segment of the distal convoluted tubules by binding to Cl^- sites of the transporter protein. The transmembrane Na^+ gradient generated by ATPase drives the Na-K-Cl symporter at the luminal tubular cell membrane. Furosemide blocks the Na-K-Cl symporter, causing the Cl^- concentration in the cell to decrease, which leads to cellular hyperpolarization and transcellular ion transport inactivation. Furosemide also enhances the production of renal prostaglandins, which further inhibit the reabsorption of Na^+ and Cl^- at the ascending limb of the loops of Henle. The overall effects of furosemide on the nephron result in decreased Na^+ reabsorption and increased water retention in the tubular lumen. Furosemide is considered a potent diuretic for several reasons: it produces a large volume of retained water in the tubular lumen, its primary sites of action are where water resorption is virtually nonexistent (the ascending loops of Henle and distal convoluted tubules), and the segments that reabsorb water distal to the effects of furosemide are overwhelmed, resulting in large volumes of fluid loss. Inhibition of the Na-K-Cl symporter also inhibits the reabsorption of Ca^{2+}, Mg^{2+}, K^+, and H^+ from the tubular fluid (Svensen 2013). Furosemide has numerous extra-renal effects, including decreases in: systemic and pulmonary blood volume, CVPs, pulmonary wedge pressure, venous compliance, and right atrial pressure. All effects of furosemide depend on functional kidneys and normal production of prostaglandins.

Pharmacokinetics

Injectable furosemide is approved for use in dogs, cats, horses, and in cattle not intended for food. In the dog, IV furosemide has approximately 77% bioavailability, with a terminal half-life of one hour and peak effects 30 minutes after administration. Oral administration results in variable bioavailability and rapid elimination, which has led to investigations into a sustained release formula. In most species, 50–60% of the drug is eliminated unchanged in the urine or is conjugated to glucuronic acid and excreted in bile. In the dog, the rate of urinary excretion of furosemide is correlated with its diuretic effects. Similar to humans, the natriuretic response and concentration of diuretic in the urine can be represented by a sigmoid curve (Figure 24.2). Based on the shape of the curve, in order to elicit a diuretic response, a maximum concentration of furosemide must be reached at the site of action (Kochevar 2009). The curve plateaus above the maximum urinary concentration, which demonstrates that greater dosing does not provide additional benefits. Intermittent furosemide doses provide brief effects, and higher doses do not translate to longer effect times; consequently, constant rate infusions (CRIs) have been used as a long-term diuretic therapy in dogs.

In horses, the terminal half-life of furosemide is similar to other species (approximately one hour after IV administration), and it is eliminated primarily through the kidneys. Studies comparing oral versus IV administration of furosemide in horses have demonstrated that systemic bioavailability after oral dosing is poor and highly variable (Johansson et al. 2000). Like dogs, CRI of furosemide in the horse provides more uniform plasma levels and urine flow compared to intermittent regimens.

In patients with renal insufficiency, plasma half-life is prolonged. Protein-losing nephropathies will decrease the diuretic effect of furosemide due to the active drug binding to excessive albumin in the urine.

Therapeutic Uses

In small animals, furosemide is primarily used for diseases involving renal, cardiac, or hepatic origins. For patients in anuric renal failure, furosemide has been used to re-establish diuresis and to promote excretion of elevated electrolytes in the blood. As stated above, furosemide dosing in renal patients may have to be adjusted more frequently due to a longer half-life and the potential for increased renal drug loss. Furosemide is considered one of the primary drugs to help relieve and control systemic and pulmonary edema associated with CHF. Although furosemide decreases cardiac preload and plasma volume, when used alone, it can activate the renin-angiotensin-aldosterone system, which can lead to long-term treatment failure. For this reason, it is recommended furosemide be combined with an angiotensin converting enzyme inhibitor when treating chronic CHF. Furosemide is also used to help control edema associated with liver insufficiencies and intracranial pathology (i.e. trauma or neoplasia). Furosemide decreases brain volume by shifting fluid from the cerebral parenchyma into plasma and by inhibiting CSF production by inhibiting Na^+ transport in the glial tissues. The effect of furosemide on ICP is synergistic with mannitol. In a study performed on rats, the combination of furosemide and mannitol resulted in a greater reduction of brain water when compared to mannitol alone (Thenuwara et al. 2002). Because Ca^{2+} and Mg^{2+} follow the $Na^+/K^+/Cl^-$ co-transport, these ions are also lost in the urine; therefore, furosemide can be used to treat conditions involving hypercalcemia (Svensen 2013).

A novel loop diuretic, torsemide, has been shown to produce a higher level of urinary Na^+/K^+ ratio in comparison to furosemide when administered to anesthetized dogs (Uchida et al. 1991).

In horses, furosemide is commonly used for exercise-induced pulmonary edema and hemorrhage, which is seen especially in racing Thoroughbreds. Furosemide reduces atrial, pulmonary arterial, and pulmonary wedge pressures via decreased plasma volume in horses. In the horseracing industry, furosemide has been used extensively as a performances enhancing drug. Controlled treadmill studies have not shown reproducible advantages (i.e. enhanced oxygen consumption or increased time to fatigue) of diuretic use in exercising horses (Hinchcliff et al. 1993). In fact, studies involving furosemide in racehorses suffering from exercise-induced pulmonary edema demonstrated that any

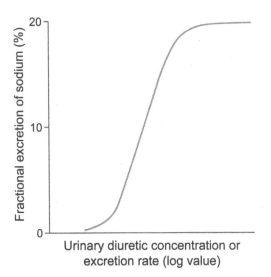

Figure 24.2 Pharmacodynamics of loop diuretic. The relation between the natriuretic response and the amount of diuretic reaching the site of action is represented by a sigmoid curve (Kochevar 2009).

performance benefits of furosemide were more likely due to decreases in body weight related to water loss (Soma et al. 1998).

Adverse Effects and Other Considerations

In almost all veterinary species, the majority of adverse effects regarding furosemide involve global fluid-volume loss (dehydration) and electrolyte abnormalities. The most common electrolyte abnormalities associated with furosemide therapy are hyponatremia, hypokalemia (with or without an associated metabolic acidosis), and hypochloremia. Other electrolyte disturbances include hypocalcemia and hypomagnesemia. Patients with renal, cardiac, or hepatic disease have increased risks of adverse effects from furosemide therapy. Chronic and/or high doses of furosemide can cause ototoxicity in dogs and cats and can result in depletion of water-soluble vitamins (B-complex vitamins). Common drug interactions with furosemide include: aminoglycosides (may result in enhanced ototoxicity), NSAIDs, anti-insulin effect due to decreased plasma K^+ concentration, and synergistic effects with other classes of diuretics.

By competitively binding to the organic transport site within the renal tubular cells and inhibiting the production of renal prostaglandins, NSAIDs decrease furosemide uptake and consequently inhibit its natriuretic, chloriuretic, and diuretic effects. Another possible mechanism that may explain the inhibitory effects that NSAIDs have on loop (other) diuretics is both drugs compete for the organic acid transport system (Kochevar 2009).

Furosemide therapy is contraindicated in dehydrated patients, anuric patients that do not respond to test-doses of furosemide, or those suffering from electrolyte abnormalities.

Distal Convoluted Tubules

Thiazide and Thiazide-like Diuretics

Method of Action

Thiazide diuretics are benzothiadiazide analogs and are derivatives of carbonic anhydrase inhibiting sulfonamides. There are two primary examples of this diuretic class of drugs used in veterinary medicine: chorothiazide and hydrochlorothiazide. Hydrochlorothiazide is the only product approved in veterinary medicine for use in cattle (Kochevar 2009). Newer products include cyclothiazide and methycyclothiazide; however, there is minimal research that supports clinical applications of these diuretics in veterinary medicine. Non-benzothiadiazine derivatives behave similarly but are not classified as thiazides. Examples of these drugs include: metolazone and

chlorthalidon; again, these drugs have limited, if any, use in veterinary medicine. The primary mechanism of action of thiazide diuretics is via Na^+ loss in the distal convoluted tubules and possibly some secondary effects in the proximal convoluted tubules as a carbonic anhydrase inhibitor. In the distal convoluted tubules, NaCl reabsorption is mediated through an electroneutral cotransport (symport) system on the basolateral membrane of the renal tubular cell. The primary influence of Cl^- reabsorption is the transmembrane Na^+ gradient established by the activity of the basolateral Na^+/K^+ ATPase cotransport (Na-K-Cl symport system). The NaCl cotransport is reversibly inhibited by thiazide diuretics, causing a decrease in Na^+, Cl^-, HCO_3^-, K^+, and water reabsorption from the tubular lumen. Because the majority (90%) of the Na^+ is reabsorbed prior to the distal convoluted tubules, the peak diuretic effects of thiazides are moderate compared to loop diuretics. Thiazide diuretics enhance Ca^{2+} reabsorption; the exact mechanism is poorly understood, but it may be related to an increase in Ca^{2+} binding proteins.

Pharmacokinetics

The pharmacokinetics of thiazide diuretics have not been established in domestic animals. In humans, thiazide diuretics absorb slowly and incompletely from the GI tract, they are highly protein bound, and they are excreted almost exclusively through the kidneys. Peak effects of hydrochlorothiazide occur in 4 hours and last up to 12 hours (Kochevar 2009). Thiazide diuretics gain access to the basolateral membranes via the renal tubular organic acid secretion pathway; therefore, their effectiveness is a function of renal blood flow rather than glomerular filtration.

Therapeutic Uses

In dogs and cats, thiazide diuretics are used for edema associated with cardiac, hepatic, and renal diseases. These drugs have also been used to reduce the amount of urine volume in patients with nephrogenic diabetes insipidus. Most commonly, thiazide drugs are used as an adjunct therapy with loop diuretics. In cattle, thiazide diuretics have been used primarily for edema associated with the udder.

Adverse Effects and Other Considerations

The primary concerns with thiazide diuretics are related to fluid and electrolyte disturbances. Because thiazides can mobilize a moderate amount of fluid from the kidneys (interfering with ion transfer in the renal tubular cells), hypovolemia, hyponatremia, hypokalemia, hypochloremia, hypercalcemia, and pH abnormalities can all occur (especially in patients with underlying renal disease).

Drug interactions with thiazide diuretics include: decreased effectiveness of anticoagulants and insulin, increased effects of some anesthetics (opioids, dexmedetomidine, and neuromuscular blocking drugs), loop diuretics, digitalis glycosides, and vitamin D. Similar to loop diuretics, the effects of thiazide diuretics may be reduced with concurrent NSAID administration.

Distal Convoluted Tubules and Collecting Ducts

Potassium-Sparing Diuretics

Method of Action

Potassium-sparing diuretics are cyclic amidine drugs and include amiloride and triamterene. Triamterene is the most commonly used amidine diuretic in veterinary medicine. Both drugs are organic bases that are secreted into the proximal tubule by the organic base transport system. The unique feature of these diuretics is the renal loss of NaCl and water with concurrent K^+ retention. Principal cells of the late distal convoluted tubules and the collecting ducts contain Na^+/K^+ ATPase channels in the luminal membrane. These channels provide a pathway for Na^+ reabsorption, which results in a negative, transepithelial voltage potential on the luminal side. The transepithelial voltage potential drives K^+ out of the principal cell into the tubular lumen thereby maintaining cellular electrochemical neutrality. Potassium-sparing diuretics block the Na^+/K^+ ATPase channel, causing Na^+ and water retention in the luminal space and preservation of K^+, H^+, Ca^{2+}, and Mg^{2+} within the principal cell. Apart from its renal effects, triamterene can cause a prolongation of the cardiac action potential duration and functional refractory period, which could result in a decreased heart rate and increased myocardial contractile force.

Pharmacokinetics

Pharmacokinetic information for triamterene in veterinary patients is unknown. In humans, both triamterene and amidine are orally administered, with triamterene reaching up to 70% bioavailability and excretion being primarily renal. The peak onset of action of triamterene is 6–8 hours and duration of action is 12–16 hours. The parent drug is biodegraded in the liver to an active metabolite, 4-hydroxytriamterene sulfate, which is actively secreted into the renal tubules. Renal and/or hepatic disease could impair the elimination of triamterene (Kochevar 2009).

Therapeutic Uses

The clinical importance of triamterene is its K+ sparing effects. Because the sites of action are the distal tubular segments, triamterene has relatively weak diuretic effects; therefore, triamterene is primarily used in combination with loop and thiazide diuretics. Both triamterene and amidine have been used for the treatment of edema associated with CHF, liver disease, renal disease, steroid-induced edema, and idiopathic edema.

Adverse Effects and Other Considerations

The most common adverse effect related to these diuretics is hyperkalemia. Concurrent administration of drugs such as NSAIDs, ACE inhibitors, and beta-blockers can increase the risk of hyperkalemia. Both triamterene and amidine can cause GI upset, and it is recommended to administer with food. These diuretics are contraindicated in patients with advanced renal or hepatic disease.

Collecting Ducts

Mineralocorticoid Antagonists

Method of Action

Spironolactone is a four-ring, steroid hormone, chemically similar to aldosterone, and is the only mineralocorticoid antagonist approved in the US. Under normal circumstances, HSP90, which is a protective chaperone protein, is incapable of binding to target DNA within the collecting duct epithelial cells. The HSP90 protein is activated by aldosterone, allowing it to move into cell nuclei and bind to the target DNA. The aldosterone-protein-DNA sequencing complex is responsible for mineralocorticoid response elements that regulate aldosterone-induced protein production, resulting in Na^+ reabsorption (plus water) and K^+/H^+ excretion in the collecting ducts. Aldosterone-induced proteins are believed to have multiple effects, including synthesis, activation, and distribution of Na^+ channels and Na^+/K^+ ATPase, changes in the permeability of tight junctions, and increased ATP production. The net result of aldosterone's influence on HSP90 and target DNA is an increased permeability to Na^+, water reabsorption, and augmented loss of K^+ and H^+ into the collecting duct lumens. Spironolactone blocks the effects of aldosterone by binding to the mineralocorticoid receptor and facilitating the inactivity of HSP90 protective chaperone protein. The net result of spironolactone within the collecting ducts is an increased loss of Na^+ and water into the tubular fluid, corresponding to an increased retention of K^+ and H^+ within the epithelial cells. In addition to its aldosterone antagonist effects, spironolactone also behaves like a Ca^{2+} channel blocker, resulting in direct vasodilation. Spironolactone can also result in an increased release of atrial natriuretic proteins.

Pharmacokinetics

In humans, spironolactone is moderately absorbed in the GI, with 60–90% bioavailability and has extensive hepatic metabolism during the first pass-effect. Canrenone is the active metabolite, with a longer half-life than the parent drug; this extends the biological effects of spironolactone up to 16 hours. Peak diuresis occurs in one to three hours.

In dogs, oral spironolactone provides 50% bioavailability on an empty stomach, but increases to 90% when administered with food. Approximately 70% of the drug is excreted in feces and 18% in the urine (Kochevar 2009).

Both spironolactone and its metabolites are highly protein-bound. Spironolactone and canrenone can cross the placenta, and canrenone has been detected in human breast milk.

Therapeutic Uses

In dogs and cats, spironolactone is used primarily as an adjunct therapy with loop or thiazide diuretics to reduce K^+ loss in the urine. In addition to alleviating edema, spironolactone also counteracts the hyperaldosteronism associated with congestive heart disease, ascites, renal failure, and hypertension. Human studies have shown that spironolactone blocks aldosterone's effects, thus blocking the ventricular myocardial deterioration accompanying CHF. There is no comprehensive evidence that supports similar findings in veterinary patients; however, the diuretic benefits of spironolactone were not demonstrated in a study involving greyhound dogs (Riordan et al. 2005).

Adverse Effects and Other Considerations

Adverse effects associated with spironolactone are considered mild and are reversible upon discontinuation of the drug. GI upset, anorexia, electrolyte abnormalities (hyperkalemia and hyponatremia), and dehydration are the most likely adverse side effects.

In dogs, electrolyte disturbances and other adverse effects do not appear to be of great concern. A study of halothane-anesthetized dogs demonstrated that high concentrations of canrenone can cause bradycardia, reduced myocardial contractility, and hypotension via calcium channel current blockade. (Sugiyama et al. 2004). In cats, hyperkalemia and azotemia can occur in patients with renal insufficiency and/or advanced heart disease.

Aspirin inhibits the natriuretic effects of spironolactone. When administered together, spironolactone can prolong the half-life of digoxin; therefore, it is imperative that enhanced monitoring of digoxin serum levels and clinical effects are performed (Kochevar 2009).

Miscellaneous and Experimental Diuretics

Dopamine Receptor Agonists

Dopamine receptors (DA-1 and DA-2) have been considered potential targets for low-dose dopamine therapy to manage low-output renal failure in dogs, cats, and humans. At low doses (<5 mcg/kg/min), dopamine is a mixed DA-1 and DA-2 receptor agonist, facilitating renal perfusion, urine output, and natriuresis. However, the degree of increased urine production and creatinine clearance are not sufficient to be considered therapeutic for patients in renal failure. Low-dose dopamine does not significantly affect urine output, Na^+ excretion, glomerular filtration, or fractional sodium excretion in cats (Wohl et al. 2000). In contrast to mixed DA-1/DA-2 agonists, DA-1 selective agonists may increase renal blood flow and diuresis, especially in cats. A study using fenoldopam, a selective DA-1 agonist with no α- or β-adrenergic effects, induced diuresis with Na^+ excretion for up to six hours in cats (Simmons et al. 2006). The pharmacokinetics of fenoldopam in dogs and cats are similar to that in humans (O'Neill et al. 2016); plasma clearance is rapid and a CRI is necessary to reach and maintain effective plasma levels. Unfortunately, the diuretic effects of fenoldopam for dogs and cats with low-output renal disease is still controversial. A retrospective study of 62 critically ill dogs and cats with acute kidney injury showed that, although fenoldopam appeared relatively safe, it was not associated with improved survival, shorter duration of hospital stay, or renal biochemistry parameters when compared to patients not receiving fenoldopam (Nielsen et al. 2015).

Aquaretics

Arginine vasopressin promotes solute and water reabsorption via V2 receptor activation on the principal cells in the collecting ducts. Anti-V2 agents (aquaretics) promote solute and water excretion by interfering with the effects of arginine vasopressin on the principal cells in the collecting ducts. In dogs, tolvaptan (a V2 antagonist) has been shown to elicit a potent aquaretic response, reducing cardiac preload without unfavorable effects on systemic or renal hemodynamics, the renin-angiotensin-aldosterone system, or the sympathetic nervous system in dogs with CHF (Onogawa et al. 2011). Tolvaptan binds extensively to plasma proteins (>97%) in mice, rats, dogs, and humans and is excreted into the feces via the biliary route (Furukawa et al. 2011). Aquaretics show promise for being effective and safe diuretics; however, current scientific evidence and application in veterinary patients is lacking.

References

Behnia, R., Koushanpour, E., Brunner, E.A. et al. (1996). Effects of hyperosmotic mannitol infusion on hemodynamics of dog kidney. *Anesth. Analg.* 82: 902–908.

Furukawa, M., Umehara, K., Kashiyama, E. et al. (2011). Nonclinical pharmacokinetics of a new nonpeptide V2 receptor antagonist, tolvaptan. *Cardiovasc. Drugs Therap.* 1: S83–S89.

Hastie, M. and Shanewise, J. (2015). Diuretics. In: *Stoelting's Pharmacology and Physiology in Anesthesia Practice*, 5e (ed. P. Flood, J. Rathmell and S. Shafer), 533–541. Philadelphia PA: Wolters Kluwer Health.

Hinchcliffe, K.W., McKeever, K.H., Muir, W.W. 3rd et al. (1993). Effect if furosemide and weight carriage on energetic responses of horses to incremental exertion. *Am. J. Vet. Res.* 54: 1500–1504.

Johansson, A.M., Gardner, S.Y., Levine, J.F. et al. (2000). Pharmacokinetics and pharmacodynamics of furosemide after oral administration to horses. *J. Vet. Intern. Med.* 17: 887–895.

Kochevar, D. (2009). Diuretics. In: *Veterinary Pharmacology & Therapeutics*, 9e (ed. J. Riviere and M. Papich), 647–669. Ames, IA: Blackwell Publishing.

Nielsen, L.K., Bracker, K., Price, L.L. et al. (2015). Administration of fenoldopam in critically ill small animal patients with acute kidney injury: 28 dogs and 34 cats (2008-2012). *J. Vet. Emerg. Crit. Care* 25: 396–404.

O'Neill, K.E., Labato, M.A., Court, M.H. et al. (2016). The pharmacokinetics of intravenous fenoldopam in healthy, awake cats. *J. Vet. Pharmacol. Therap.* 39: 202–204.

Onogawa, T., Sakamoto, Y., Nakamura, S. et al. (2011). Effects of tolvaptan on systemic and renal hemodynamic function in dogs with congestive heart failure. *Cardiovasc. Drugs Therap.* 1: S67–S76.

Paczynski, R. (1997). Osmotherapy: basic concepts and controversies. *Crit. Care Clin.* 13: 105–123.

Riordan, L. et al. (2005). Diuretic efficacy of oral spironolactone when used in conjunction with furosemide in healthy adult greyhounds. *J. Vet. Res.* 58: 632–635.

Roberts, S. (1985). Assessment and management of the ophthalmic emergency. *Compend. Contin. Educ.* 7: 739–752.

Rudehill, A., Gordon, E., Ohman, G. et al. (1993). Pharmakoinetics and effects of mannitol on hemodynamics, blood and cerebrospinal fluid electrolytes, and osmolality during intracranial surgery. *J. Neurosurg. Anesthesiol.* 5: 4–12.

Simmons, J.P., Wohl, J.S., Schwartz, D.D. et al. (2006). Diuretic effects of fenoldopam in healthy cats. *J. Vet. Emerg. Crit. Care* 16: 96–103.

Soma, L.R., Uboh, C.E. et al. (1998). Review of furosemide in horse racing: its effects and regulation. *J. Vet. Pharmacol. Therap.* 21: 228–240.

Sugiyama, A., Satoh, Y., Takalara, A. et al. (2004). Electropharmacological effects of a spironolactone derivative, potassium canrenoate, assessed in the halothane-anesthetized canine model. *J. Pharm. Sci.* 96: 436–443.

Svensen, C. (2013). Electrolyte and diuretics. In: *Pharmacology and Physiology for Anesthesia, Foundations and Clinical Application* (ed. H. Hemmings and D. Talmage), 608–614. Philadelphia, PA: Elsevier-Saunders.

Swenson, E.R., Robertson, H.T., Hlastala, M.P. et al. (1993). Effects of carbonic anhydrase inhibition on ventilation-perfusion matching in the dog lung. *J. Clin. Investig.* 92: 702–709.

Teppema, L.J. and Dahan, A. (2004). Low-dose acetazolamide reduces the hypoxic ventilator response in the anesthetized cat. *Respir. Physiol. Neurobiol.* 140: 43–51.

Thenuwara, K., Todd, M.M., Brian, J.E. Jr. et al. (2002). Effect of mannitol and furosemide on plasma osmolality and brain water. *Anesthesiology* 96: 416–421.

Uchida, T., Ohtaki, Y., Kido, H. et al. (1991). Diuretic profile of a novel loop diuretic torasemide in rats and dogs. *Drugs Exp. Clin. Res.* 17: 293–298.

Valender, J. (2000). Renal physiology. In: *Cunningham's Textbook of Veterinary Physiology*, 5e (ed. G. Bradley), 460–494. St. Louis, MO: Elsevier Saunders.

Wohl, J. Schwartz, D.D., Flournoy, W.S. et al. (2000). Renal hemodynamics and diuretic effects of low-dose dopamine in the cat. *Seventh International Veterinary Emergency and Critical Care Symposium*, Orlando, USA (6–10 September 2000). American College of Veterinary Emergency and Critical Care.

25

Antiepileptics

Laurie Cook and Ashley C. Hechler

Introduction

Seizures are one of the most common neurologic problems encountered in dogs and cats. Idiopathic epilepsy is the most common cause of seizures in dogs and is also reported in cats, horses, and rodents (Aleman et al. 2006; Thomas 2010; Boothe et al. 2012; Munana 2013; Pakozdy et al. 2013; Charalambous et al. 2014; Pakozdy et al. 2014). This disease is analogous to genetic epilepsy in humans and is an inherent tendency toward seizures in an otherwise healthy patient (Munana 2013). Epilepsy can also be secondary to extracranial and intracranial diseases that lead to seizures.

Idiopathic epilepsy is generally treated with maintenance anti-epileptic medications with a goal of reducing the frequency and severity of the seizures, but usually not eliminating seizures. Seizure control is balanced with the side effects of the medications to improve the patient's overall quality of life. Treatment of other diseases that cause seizures usually center on treatment of the underlying disease process as well as anti-epileptic medications while attempting to minimize side effects (Dewey 2006; Munana 2013). There are many anti-epileptic medications used in veterinary patients. Some of these medications may be more effective for a particular patient, and trials of different medications may be needed to find what works best for the patient. Factors to consider when choosing an anti-epileptic medication include efficacy, side effects, cost and frequency of administration (Munana 2013).

Patients may also present on an emergency basis having cluster seizures or status epilepticus. Cluster seizures are multiple seizures that happen within a short period of time with only a brief period of recovery. Status epilepticus is a prolonged seizure greater than five minutes. Both situations run the risk of injury to the brain, metabolic derangements or death if left untreated. Different medications are needed in an emergency setting to stop such seizure activity and keep seizures controlled in the short term.

Patients can also have seizures during anesthesia. This usually appears as involuntary eye and facial muscle twitching in an anesthetized patient.

With advances in drug therapy within the last few years, there are more drugs available to try to reduce seizures while minimizing side effects. However, patients on anti-epileptic medications may pose unique challenges to the anesthetist. Anti-epileptics may alter metabolism or disposition of other medications. In addition, many anti-epileptics have sedative effects that can magnify the sedative effects of anesthetic medications. Generally, it is recommended that epileptic patients do not miss doses of their maintenance anti-epileptic medication prior to anesthesia (Perks et al. 2012). Additional concerns for the anesthetist are patients that have seizures during anesthesia or in the peri-operative periods. This chapter will focus on the most commonly currently used anti-epileptic medications including mechanisms of action, pharmacokinetics, clinical use, efficacy data when available, dosing and side effects (Table 25.1) and how these medications may impact anesthetic decision making.

Anti-Epileptic Medications

Phenobarbital

Phenobarbital (PB) is a phenyl barbiturate and is one of the oldest anti-epileptics in human and veterinary patients. It was designed in the late 1800's with its first medicinal use in the early 1900's in humans as a sedative-hypnotic. The use of PB as an anti-epileptic drug (AED) was discovered somewhat serendipitously. In 1912, Alfred Hauptmann was a young scientist who slept above a ward of human epileptic patients. Disturbed by the noise of patients who had seizures at night, he began treating them with PB to sedate them, and subsequently noted that it also suppressed their seizure activity (Yasiry and Shorvon 2012).

Pharmacology in Veterinary Anesthesia and Analgesia, First Edition. Edited by Turi Aarnes and Phillip Lerche.
© 2024 John Wiley & Sons, Inc. Published 2024 by John Wiley & Sons, Inc.

Table 25.1 Maintenance anticonvulsants.

Drug	Maintenance dose	Loading dose	Time to steady state concentration (days)	Metabolism	Side effects	Potential Toxicities
Phenobarbital	2–3 mg/kg q 12 h (D) 1.5–2.5 mg/kg q 12 h (C) 5 mg/kg q 12 h (H)	12–24 mg/kg IV/24 h divided or single dose	10–14 (D) 16 (C)	Hepatic	Sedation Ataxia Polyuria/Polydipsia Polyphagia Weight gain Facial pruritus (C)	Hepatotoxicity Myelo-suppression Superficial necrolytic dermatitis
Potassium bromide	30 mg/kg q 24 h (D) 90 mg/kg q 24 h (H) [a]not recommended for use in cats	90–120 mg/kg/day for 5 d (D) 120 mg/kg/d for 5 d	100–200	Renal	Sedation Ataxia Polyuria/Polydipsia Polyphagia Hyperactivity Nausea Diarrhea	Pancreatitis (D) Pulmonary toxicity (C) Death (C)
Levetiracetam	20–60 mg/kg q 8 h	60 mg/kg IV once	1	Renal	Sedation (Mild) Ataxia Vomiting Restlessness	
Zonisamide	5–10 mg/kg q 12 h (D) 5 mg/kg q 12–24 h (C)		3-4 (D) 7 (C)	Hepatic and renal	Sedation (mild) Inappetence	Autoimmune reactions Idiosyncratic hepatotoxicity
Topiramate	5–10 mg/kg (D) 12.5–25 mg/CAT*		<1	Hepatic	Anorexia Sedation	
Gabapentin	10–30 m/kg q 8 h (D) 5–30 mg/kg q 8 h (C)			Renal	Sedation Ataxia Somnolence Vomiting	
Pregabalin	3–4 mg/kg q 8 h (D) 1–2 mg/kg q 12 h (C)			Renal	Sedation Ataxia	

(D) = Dogs; (C) = Cats; (H) = Horses
[a] No controlled clinical studies have been reported in cats. Anecdotally suggested dose for cats.
Source: Andrews and Hilary (2004), Lester (2015), and Plumb (2015).

Advances in AEDs with fewer side effects have led to a decline in its use in people but is still widely utilized in veterinary patients. For many years, it was the medication of choice in veterinary patients because it was inexpensive and relatively safe. Due to the increasing costs of PB, and the decreasing cost and availability of other medications with fewer side effects, a wider variety of AEDs are now used in veterinary patients. Proposed mechanism of action of PB includes enhanced inhibition at the postsynaptic GABA$_A$ receptor to gamma aminobutyric acid (GABA) by enhancing chloride influx into the neuron and subsequent

hyperpolarization (Twyman et al. 1989; Munana 2013), inhibiting the action of glutamate, and decreasing calcium influx into neurons (Dewey 2006).

Pharmacokinetics

PB can be administered orally, intravenously (IV), or injected into the corpus cavernosum of dogs with Tmax and serum levels similar to IV administration (Degim et al. 2002; Plumb 2015). In dogs, orally administered PB is rapidly absorbed within two hours with a bioavailability of 90% and peak plasma concentrations reached in 4–8 hours

(Al-Tahan and Frey 1985; Frey and Loscher 1985, Pedersoli et al. 1987, Cochrane et al. 1990a, 1990b; Ravis et al. 1989). The elimination half-life in dogs has a wide range from 37 to 74 hours (Ravis et al. 1984, Al-Tahan and Frey 1985, Frey 1985). Approximately 50% of PB is protein bound, and the majority is metabolized by the liver via microsomal enzyme activity including the cytochrome p450 pathway as well as glucuronosyl transferases and glutathione-S-transferases (Gaskill et al. 2005). Autoinduction occurs over time in dogs with chronic administration, due to microsomal enzyme induction resulting in more rapid metabolism. In one pharmacokinetic study, after 90 days of oral administration of PB, half-life decreased from 89 to 47 hours (Ravis et al. 1984). In cats, IV dosing has an elimination half-life of 58.8 ± 4.21 hours.

Recommended maintenance doses for Phenobarbital start at 2–3 mg/kg q 12 hours for dogs and 1.5–2.5 mg/kg q 12 hours for cats (Dewey 2006). Starting at oral maintenance doses, it generally takes 14 days in dogs and 10 days in cats to reach steady state concentrations. PB can be loaded with oral or IV doses of 12–25 mg/kg divided over 24 hours or in a single dose in dogs. Loading doses can also be calculated using the following equations:

- In PB naïve patients, Loading dose PB (mg) = BW (kg) × 0.8 × desired serum concentration (μg/ml).
- Patients on maintenance PB, Loading dose PB (mg) = BW (kg) × 0.8 × (desired serum concentration – current serum concentration (μg/ml)) (Smith 2005).

The half-life in horses is shorter than that in dogs, with a harmonic mean of 11.35 hours (range 6.5–17.3 hours) following a single IV dose and 9.9 hours following oral administration for 17 days (Reimer and Sweeney 1992).

The bioavailability of oral phenobarbital in goats is poor and it also has a very short half-life due to high clearance. One study found the bioavailability to be 24.9% after oral and IV administration of PB at 10 mg/kg. The half-life of oral administration (3.8 ± 0.826 hours) was similar to IV administration (4.0 ± 0.619 hours). Oral dosing of PB in goats has a Tmax of 1.75 ± 0.46 ng/l, a Cmax of 4478.7 ± 962.4 ng/l, and a clearance of 152.5 ± 102.7 ml/ hours/kg (Yates et al. 2020).

There is little information in the literature on use of phenobarbital in birds. One report on pharmacokinetics of orally administered phenobarbital to African gray parrots showed a short half life (1.43–1.66 hours) and rapid Tmax (2.05–2.41 hours) suggesting it may not have good clinical efficacy in birds. The cause of shorter Tmax and T1/2 were not known but may be due to differences in protein binding, drug distribution or clearance. Site of barbiturate metabolism in birds is not known but is presumed to be hepatic (Powers and Papich 2011).

Clinical Use and Efficacy

PB remains a popular AED in dogs and cats, and can also be used in horses, cattle, ferrets, guinea pigs, other rodents and birds (Reimer and Sweeney 1992; Aleman et al. 2006; Oglesbee 2011; Powers and Papich 2011; Plumb 2015). It has the most efficacy data in dogs and has been shown to be effective in reducing seizures by >50% in 60–80% of dogs with serum levels >20 μg/ml (Schwartz-Porsche et al. 1985; Dewey 2006; Boothe et al. 2012; Munana 2013). However, PB can result in no improvement in seizure frequency in 15% of patients based on cumulative data from these studies. It has also been shown to be superior to Potassium bromide (KBr) as a sole AED where 85% of dogs treated with PB became seizure free compared to 52% of dogs treated with KBr (Boothe et al. 2012). PB has good to moderate efficacy in 60–80% of cats with primary epilepsy (Pakozdy et al. 2013).

There is little information in the literature on efficacy of phenobarbital in horses, presumably because epilepsy is less commonly diagnosed and treated in horses compared with dogs and cats. It was reported to be effective in treating epilepsy in Arabian foals, but the dosage was not consistently reported (Aleman et al. 2006). There is scant to no information in the literature on use in other large animals.

Serum Biochemical Parameter Changes

Chronic treatment with PB causes increases in serum alkaline phosphatase (ALP) and alanine aminotransferase (ALT) in dogs without clinical signs of liver disease and these changes have long been attributed to hepatic microsomal enzyme induction (Gieger et al. 2000; Müller et al. 2000a; Hojo et al. 2002; Dewey 2006; Munana 2013). Increases in ALP, ALT, aspartate aminotransferase (AST), and gamma glutamyl transferase (GGT), due to enzyme induction, have been recognized in dogs, rats and humans. However, these changes vary between species (Ennulat et al. 2010). Cats appear more refractory than dogs, but occasionally increases in ALP and ALT may be noted (Pakozdy et al. 2013; Plumb 2015). An increase in total ALP due to enzyme induction appears to be primarily due to corticosteroid-induced ALP (C-ALP), although liver-ALP (L-ALP) and bone-ALP (B-ALP) may also be increased (Gaskill et al. 2004, 2005). This finding supports enzyme induction as the primary cause of increased serum ALP with chronic PB administration in dogs, however other factors may also influence this.

Whether the increase in ALT is due to hepatic enzyme induction or an indicator of hepatocellular injury is still uncertain. In one study comparing enzyme levels in the serum with those in the liver itself, serum ALT was elevated in PB treated dogs, but ALT in the liver was lower in PB treated dogs than control dogs. If enzyme induction was the cause of elevated serum ALT, one would also expect the ALT in the liver to be elevated. This study's finding did not support induction of hepatic ALT activity as the cause of elevated serum ALT (Gaskill et al. 2005).

Most commonly, enzyme induction is thought to be adaptive to exposure to a drug/toxin and not pathologic. However, prolonged exposure may overwhelm this adaptive process and hepatocellular injury may occur including degeneration, necrosis, or proliferation (Ennulat et al. 2010). One study that evaluated ALT, ALP, and liver histopathology found changes indicative of liver injury were more pronounced and more frequent in PB treated dogs than in control dogs. Varying degrees of inflammation, necrosis, and vascular changes were noted to be more significant in PB treated dogs compared with control dogs. However, there were no histopathologic changes specific to PB treatment (Gaskill et al. 2005). Changes in ALT and ALP resolved within 3–5 weeks after discontinuation of PB (Gieger et al. 2000).

Long-term treatment with phenobarbital alone or in combination with potassium bromide may cause hypertriglyceridemia (Kluger et al. 2008). Hypertriglyceridemia is a risk factor for pancreatitis which has been reported in dogs with chronic phenobarbital treatment. However, one study found a low prevalence (0.6%) of clinical acute pancreatitis in dogs treated with phenobarbital, potassium bromide, or both, despite 6.8% of the animals having increased canine pancreas-specific lipase (cPLI) values (Albarracin et al. 2015).

Serum thyroxine levels including total T4 (TT4) and free T4 (fT4) may be decreased in animals on chronic PB treatment. This may be due to increased hepatic clearance. It is unknown whether these patients are clinically affected by the reduced thyroxine levels. Some practitioners recommend thyroid supplementation when signs relatable to hypothyroidism are present (Gieger et al. 2000; Müller et al. 2000b; Daminet and Ferguson 2003; Dewey 2006).

Side Effects and Toxicity

Side effects include sedation, ataxia, polyuria and polydipsia (PU/PD), polyphagia (PG), and weight gain. These side effects are usually more profound at the beginning of treatment and will often subside within a few weeks to tolerable levels. For some patients, these side effects are intolerable and another anti-epileptic drug with fewer side effects may be chosen. Potential toxicities include hepatotoxicity (dogs), myelosuppression (cats and dogs), pseudolymphoma/anticonvulsant hypersensitivity syndrome (cats and dogs), and superficial necrolytic dermatitis (dogs). All of these are uncommon toxicities but can be serious (Pakozdy et al. 2013).

Hepatotoxicity in dogs is the most well-known and widely recognized toxicity, although it appears to occur uncommonly (Dayrell-Hart 1991; Dewey 2006). In one report of 18 dogs with hepatic failure due to PB treatment, common presenting clinical signs included sedation, lethargy, and ataxia. Most dogs had been on PB for a minimum of one year with a mean duration of 39 months, although one dog had only been treated with PB for five months. High serum PB levels were a significant risk factor for hepatotoxicity in these dogs. Seven of the affected dogs had serum PB levels ≥40 mcg/ml for six months to four years (median two years). Clinicopathologic changes in affected dogs included increases in ALP and ALT values, decreased serum albumin levels, increased total bilirubin, and increased pre and postprandial bile acids. Two dogs had elevated serum ammonia and two had a coagulopathy with elevated prothrombin and partial thromboplastin times. Liver histopathology of affected dogs revealed chronic hepatic fibrosis and cirrhosis. While many affected dogs died due to liver failure, approximately 50% of the dogs recovered with PB dosage reduction or switching to a different anticonvulsant (Dayrell-Hart 1991). Cats appear refractory to phenobarbital-induced hepatotoxicity but coagulopathies have been seen at high doses (10–40 mg/kg/day). Facial pruritus has also been noted in cats (Plumb 2015). In horses, PB has been shown to pass through the milk to nursing foals (Wong et al. 2008).

Drug Interactions

Phenobarbital has numerous drug interactions due to alterations in metabolism and cumulative side effects. Phenobarbital causes sedation in many patients, therefore, other drugs causing sedation may have additive effects when used concurrently.

One study showed patients administered phenobarbital 96 hours prior to anesthesia ultimately showed a longer duration of anesthesia when induced with xylazine–ketamine combination (Nossaman et al. 1990).

Phenobarbital is an inducer of hepatic microsomal enzymes including cytochrome P's and UDP-glucuronosyltransferase pathways in dogs. Therefore, it is known to reduce the effects of many drugs by lowering their serum concentrations due to increased hepatic clearance. Those of particular importance to anesthesia may include clonazepam, beta-blockers, methadone, quinidine, paroxetine and phenothiazines (Plumb 2015). It has also been shown to increase elimination of thiopental in greyhounds, as well as reducing time to recovery from anesthesia (Sams 1988). However, another report showed that the induction dose of thiopental required is not affected by prior treatment with phenobarbital (Dugdale et al. 2001). Chronic phenobarbital use can reduce serum levels of diazepam when administered IV and rectally in dogs. Despite lowered serum diazepam levels in these dogs, many still achieved therapeutic serum levels of diazepam (150 ng/ml)

(Wagner et al. 1998). This may be of clinical importance when treating an epileptic patient on chronic phenobarbital therapy with diazepam to stop a seizure, as higher doses could be needed. Due to hepatic enzyme induction, pretreatment with phenobarbital results in a fivefold increase in serum fluoride concentrations following an anesthetic event using sevoflurane (Martis et al. 1981). Halothane minimum alveolar concentration (MAC) in dogs was not significantly changed by phenobarbital (Viegas and Stoelting 1976).

Phenobarbital also induces UDP-glucuronosyltransferase in dogs. A threefold increase in morphine glucuronidation in hepatic microsomes was noted in dogs treated with phenobarbital thereby increasing clearance of morphine. Nonsteroidal anti-inflammatory drugs (NSAIDs) are also eliminated via glucuronidation, and total body clearance of carprofen increased more than twofold in phenobarbital treated dogs. Other drugs eliminated via glucuronidation could be affected similarly (Sasaki and Shimoda 2015). An increase in Cytosolic enzyme induction in dogs has been shown to last up to four weeks following discontinuation of phenobarbital (Fukunaga et al. 2009). Phenobarbital causes minimal to no hepatic microsomal enzyme induction, so drug interactions in cats are probably less important (Sasaki and Shimoda 2015). PB use in dogs has been shown to increase plasma levels of α-acid glycoprotein (AGP), a major binder of circulating drugs. Therefore, PB may influence the circulating levels of certain drugs given concurrently (Hojo et al. 2002; Dewey 2006). AGP is a plasma protein produced by hepatocytes and in humans, mainly binds basic and neutral drugs including propranolol, heparin, lidocaine and endogenous and exogenous steroids (Fournier et al. 2000; Bailey and Briggs 2004).

Potassium Bromide

Potassium bromide (KBr) is a halide salt that was initially used as an anti-epileptic medication in humans in the mid 1800's. Bromide's use in humans fell out of favor in the early 1900's with the advent of less sedating anti-epileptics, but has been used in dogs since the mid 1980's (Podell and Fenner 1993; Trepanier 1995; Dewey 2006; Boothe et al. 2012; Munana 2013; Charalambous et al. 2014). Bromide crosses the GABA gated chloride channels in the postsynaptic membranes and accumulates within neurons causing hyperpolarization and increasing the seizure threshold (Munana 2013).

Pharmacokinetics

Oral bioavailability of KBr in dogs is approximately 46% (Trepanier and Babish 1995). It is non-protein bound, diffuses easily across cell membranes and is eliminated unchanged through the kidneys. Bromide is reabsorbed in the renal tubules in competition with chloride. Therefore, maintaining a consistent dietary salt content is important. Increased dietary chloride levels will increase bromide elimination and reduce serum levels of bromide. Decreased dietary chloride levels will decrease bromide elimination and increase serum levels of bromide (Podell and Fenner 1993; Munana 2013). Elimination half-life ranges from 15 to 46 days in dogs. The total body clearance is 16.4 ml/kg/day and the volume of distribution is 0.4 l/kg (March et al. 2002). Therefore, if KBr is started at a maintenance dose, it can take months to achieve steady state concentrations (Munana 2013). For this reason, loading doses are often used to achieve therapeutic levels more quickly. A loading dose of 450–600 mg/kg divided over five days was established by Boothe (1998), but other loading protocols are used by various practitioners. If more rapid loading is desired, the 450–600 mg/kg dose can be divided over 24 hours orally or rectally in emergency situations (Munana 2013). Patients should be hospitalized if a 24-hour loading protocol is used to monitor for excessive sedation. Maintenance dose is approximately 30–40 mg/kg every 24 hours but higher doses may be needed to achieve therapeutic levels in some dogs (Munana 2013).

Potassium bromide can also be administered in horses with a loading dose of 120 mg/kg/day for one week, followed by a maintenance dose of 90 mg/kg/day have been suggested and result in serum bromide concentrations (approximately 1000 mcg/ml) consistent with therapeutic levels in dogs (MacKay 2015; Raidal and Edwards 2008). Pharmacokinetic studies in horses have shown elimination half-life of approximately 75 hours (Raidal and Edwards 2008). In sheep, sodium bromide can be administered IV at a dose of 154.6 mg/kg or potassium bromide can be given PO at 178.8 mg/kg. Following IV administration in sheep, the Cmax was 822.11 ± 93.61 mg/l with a clearance of 0.836 ± 0.255 ml/hours/kg. After oral administration, the bioavailability was 92%, the Cmax was 453.86 ± 43.37 mg/l and the Tmax was 108 ± 125 hours. The terminal half-life after IV and oral dosing was 387.93 ± 115.35 and 346.72 ± 94.05 hours, respectively (Quast et al. 2015).

Clinical Use and Efficacy

The use of KBr was initially described as an add-on anti-epileptic in dogs that were refractory to treatment with PB alone and was reported to increase efficacy from 53% to 76% (Podell and Fenner 1993; Trepanier 1995; Trepanier and Babish 1995; Munana 2013). It is now often used as a sole anticonvulsant. It remains a good choice particularly in patients that do not tolerate PB or in those with liver disease, because it is not metabolized through the liver. It can be administered orally or per rectum and is readily absorbed. Potassium containing products should not be administered intravenously. Sodium bromide can potentially be administered IV as a 3% solution in sterile water infused over at least eight hours (Plumb 2015).

Potassium bromide is moderately effective as a sole anticonvulsant with 52% of dogs becoming seizure free and 73.9% of dogs having a >50% reduction in seizures on bromide alone in one study (Boothe et al. 2012). Its efficacy, however, was less than treatment with PB alone where 82% of patients became seizure free. PB also was more effective than KBr at reducing seizure duration: 88% vs. 49%, respectively (Boothe et al. 2012).

Because KBr is eliminated through the kidneys, saline diuresis can increase elimination of bromide resulting in reduced serum bromide levels. Therefore, patients on IV fluid therapy should be watched for breakthrough seizures (Trepanier 1995; Rossmeisl and Inzana 2009; Plumb 2015).

Drug Interactions

There are very few drug interactions with bromides. Diuretics such as furosemide or thiazides may enhance elimination of bromides through the kidneys lowering serum bromide levels. Sodium containing fluids may also lower serum bromide levels. Since bromides can cause sedation, other medications causing sedation may have additive effects (Plumb 2015).

The effects of fluids with different chloride concentrations on serum bromide concentrations is of particular importance to anesthesia. One study found, after five hours of administration of saline (Na^+ 154 mmol/l; Cl^- 154 mmol/l) and lactated Ringer's solutions (Na^+ 131 mmol/l; Cl^- 110 mmol/l) at 10 ml/kg/hr, serum bromide concentrations were reduced by 17.6% and 14.2%, respectively. Saline and lactated Ringer's solutions did not lower bromide concentrations at a fluid rate of 2 ml/kg/hr. The maintenance solution (Na^+ 35 mmol/l; Cl^- 35 mmol/l), administered at 2 ml/kg/hr and 10 ml/kg/hr, did not reduce the serum bromide concentrations. Therefore, fluids with the lowest chloride concentration should be selected for patients on KBr, when utilizing high fluid rates (Fukunaga et al. 2018).

Following anesthesia with halothane, the serum concentration of bromide in dogs was significantly increased, peaking one day following anesthesia in 50% of dogs (Pedersoli 1980).

Side Effects and Toxicity

Side effects in dogs include sedation, lethargy, ataxia, PU/PD, polyphagia, nausea, diarrhea, and hyperactivity. Nausea and diarrhea are thought to occur due to gastrointestinal (GI) irritation from the bromide salt and is usually seen early in the course of treatment often subsiding as the dog adjusts to the drug. Additionally, dosing the drug with food will often eliminate the GI irritation (Munana 2013). Toxicities at therapeutic levels are uncommon, although pancreatitis was more common in dogs on KBr than dogs on PB in one study. The relationship between KBr and pancreatitis is still not known (Gaskill and Cribb 2000; Munana 2013).

Bromide toxicity, or bromism, is dose dependent and occurs in dogs with serum levels at or above the upper end of the therapeutic range. Signs of toxicity include excessive sedation, ataxia and paresis. With serum concentrations >3000 mg/l patients can become stuporous. Toxicity is easily treated with reduction or discontinuation of KBr and saline diuresis (Rossmeisl and Inzana 2009; Munana 2013).

KBr has many side effects in cats including PD, GI upset, weight gain, excessive sedation, and an asthma-like condition thought to be an allergic pulmonary toxicity. This pulmonary toxicity has proved fatal in some instances and consequently KBr is not routinely recommended for use in cats (Boothe et al. 2002; Munana 2013).

Levetiracetam

Levetiracetam (LV) was first used for the treatment of refractory focal seizures in adults in 1999. Its use in veterinary patients has grown in recent years for patients with refractory epilepsy and as a sole AED in dogs and cats (Munana et al. 2012). While the mechanism of action is not completely understood, LV inhibits the release of neurotransmitters by binding to a protein called SVA on presynaptic membranes. It also reduces the current through voltage-gated calcium channels, inhibits the release of intracellular calcium stores, and inhibits burst firing of neurons. It is believed that through these mechanisms it inhibits hypersynchronization and propagation of seizure activity (Munana 2013; Surges et al. 2008).

Pharmacokinetics

Bioavailability after oral administration of LV in dogs is 100%. Peak serum levels are achieved in 2 hours and elimination half-life in dogs is 3–6 hours. It is excreted largely unchanged in the urine (Isoherranen et al. 2001; Dewey et al. 2008; Patterson et al. 2008; Moore et al. 2010). LV is not metabolized through the liver, but a pharmacokinetic study of LV in dogs concurrently on PB showed increased clearance of LV possibly by increased oxidative metabolism in extrahepatic tissues (Moore et al. 2011). Bioavailability in cats is also 100% with peak serum levels achieved in 1.7 hours, and elimination half-life is three hours (Carnes et al. 2011).

The recommended dose in dogs and cats is 20 mg/kg q 8 hours. An extended-release formulation is available and a pharmacokinetic study showed that dogs dosed at approximately 30 mg/kg of extended release LV (KeppraXR[*]) achieved target therapeutic serum levels within 100–200 minutes and stayed at that level for 19.8–20.7 hours in fasted and fed animals, respectively. These data support its use in dogs (Beasley and Boothe 2012). Since it is dosed twice daily, it may be an easier option for many owners. Due to the limited extended-release product sizes available, pharmacokinetic studies evaluating once daily administration of levetiracetam in cats have been performed. Following oral administration with a median dose of 94.3 mg/kg PO q24 hours, the median Tmax was 5.2 hours and the median trough level was 7 mcg/ml (Barnes et al. 2018). Transdermal LV applied to the pinna of cats at 60 mg/kg q8 hours resulted in median serum concentrations between 14.8–17.4 mcg/ml during the sampling period (0.5–4 hours after administration) (Smith et al. 2019).

The pharmacokinetics of oral and IV administration of levetiracetam have been investigated in healthy foals using a dose of 32 mg/kg. Following IV administration the mean elimination half-life was 7.76 ± 0.51 hours, a mean clearance of 61.67 ± 10.96 ml/h/kg, and a mean apparent volume of distribution of 0.67 ± 0.124 l/kg. After intragastric administration, the peak concentration was 38.34 ± 7.42 mg/l and time to peak concentration was 0.875 (0.5–1.5) hours. The intragastric mean bioavailability was 103.04 (MacDonald 2018). In the adult horse, the bioavailability of orally administered immediate release LV was 96 ± 10% and 98 ± 13% for extended release when dosed at 30 mg/kg. The terminal half-life ranged from 6.2–7.07 hours for IV and both oral formulations (Cesar et al. 2018).

Clinical Use and Efficacy

LV is used commonly as a sole or add-on maintenance antiepileptic. It is also a good option in emergency situations such as status epilepticus or severe cluster seizures because of its availability in IV formulation. The IV formulation has been shown to be safe and potentially effective at doses of 30–60 mg/kg IV (Hardy et al. 2012). LVs efficacy as an add-on anti-epileptic has been shown to be effective in a group of dogs currently on PB and KBr with a 57% reduction in seizures (Volk et al. 2008). Its efficacy was evaluated in another group of dogs with refractory epilepsy as an add-on anti-epileptic and although there was a reduction in seizure frequency appreciated in LV treated dogs there was no clinically significant difference between LV and a placebo (Munana et al. 2012). Another study showed a reduction in seizures in 50% of dogs. Those dogs that responded to LV had a reduction in their seizure frequency of 75% and a decrease in seizure days per month of 68% (Volk et al. 2008). LV also reduced seizures in 7 out of 10 cats with epilepsy (Bailey et al. 2008).

Side Effects and Toxicity

Levetiracetam is well tolerated in dogs and cats. Side effects are limited to mild sedation and ataxia in some animals, but, in one study, these side effects reported by owners were not significantly different between LV and placebo groups (Volk et al. 2008; Munana et al. 2012). There are no common toxicities reported in dogs and cats, and no changes in laboratory parameters have been identified (Bailey et al. 2008; Volk et al. 2008; Hardy et al. 2012; Munana et al. 2012).

Zonisamide

Zonisamide (ZN) is a sulfonamide anti-epileptic drug. Its mechanism of action is also not completely understood, but the following actions may contribute to antiseizure activity: blockage of T-type calcium channels, inhibition of voltage-gated sodium channels, enhanced GABA release and inhibition of glutamate release (Munana 2013).

Pharmacokinetics

ZN is well absorbed in dogs with bioavailability of 68% and achieves peak plasma concentrations within three hours. Elimination half life is approximately 17 hours (Boothe and Perkins 2008). ZN is metabolized by the liver, likely through microsomal enzyme induction and then excreted in the urine. At steady state, the peak and trough concentrations of serum ZN only fluctuate by 10% (Boothe and Perkins 2008). In cats, peak plasma concentrations were achieved in four hours with an elimination half life of 33 hours (Hasegawa et al. 2008). Recommended dose in dogs is 5–10 mg/kg q 12 hours. Dogs that are also on PB may need the higher dose due to decreased bioavailability, Cmax, elimination half-life, and increased hepatic clearance (Orito et al. 2008). Anecdotally doses of 5 mg/kg q 12–24 hours have been used in cats (Orito et al. 2008; Munana 2013).

Rectal administration of 20–30 mg/kg zonisamide, suspended in sterile water or polyethylene glycol failed to achieve target plasma concentrations (Michaels et al. 2016).

One pharmacokinetic study found the Cmax in chickens, receiving 20 mg/kg orally was 15 ± 3 mcg/ml with a Tmax of 2 ± 1 hour. The half life was 6.5 ± 1 hour and the mean plasma concentration remained above 10 mcg/ml for at least six hours (de Matos et al. 2021). In Hispaniolan Amazon parrots, mean maximum plasma concentration following a dose of 20 mg/kg PO q12 hours was 25.11 ± 1.81 mcg/ml at 2.25 hours after administration. The mean plasma elimination half-life was 9.76 ± 0.93 hours (Keller et al. 2019).

Clinical Use and Efficacy

Zonisamide is used in dogs and cats as a sole or add-on maintenance anti-epileptic drug. There is no parenteral formulation for use in an emergency setting. Efficacy data for use as monotherapy showed a response rate of 60% (Chung et al. 2012). Efficacy as an add-on anti-epileptic drug showed response rates of 58–82% with a reduction in seizure frequency of 70–81% (Dewey et al. 2004; Von Klopmann et al. 2007). There is no efficacy data for ZN use in cats.

Side Effects and Toxicity

ZN appears to be well tolerated in dogs and cats. Side effects include sedation, ataxia, vomiting and loss of appetite in anywhere from 10% to 55% dogs (Dewey et al. 2004; Von Klopmann et al. 2007; Chung et al. 2012). Ataxia and sedation are usually more profound at the beginning of treatment and will often subside within a few weeks, however, dose reductions may be necessary if these side effects persist. Patients with historical allergic reactions to sulfonamide medications are predisposed to similar reactions with zonisamide. Rarely, a potentially life-threatening idiosyncratic hepatotoxicity (Miller et al. 2011; Schwartz et al. 2011) and renal tubular acidosis have been reported in dogs (Cook et al. 2011). A toxicity study in cats showed that daily doses of 20 mg/kg produced anorexia, diarrhea, vomiting, lethargy and ataxia in about 50% of cats (Hasegawa et al. 2008).

Serum Biochemical Parameter Changes

Serum thyroxine levels including total T4 (TT4) may be decreased in animals on chronic ZN treatment. One pharmacokinetic study found patients had decreased serum TT4 concentrations, but fT4 and TSH values were within the reference range. Despite remaining within the reference range, increased serum ALP and calcium values, and decreases in serum albumin concentrations, when compared to the patients' baseline values, were reported with chronic zonisamide use (Boothe and Perkins 2008).

Topiramate

Topiramate is a derivative of the monosaccharide D-fructose with a sulfamate functionality (Ziółkowski et al. 2012). It is used in humans for seizures as well as migraines and various psychiatric disorders. It has the potential to be useful in veterinary patients with refractory seizures and has been used infrequently in dogs and cats. Little information currently exists in the veterinary literature. Its mechanism of action is not fully understood, but it blocks action potentials elicited by sustained depolarization of neurons. It also increases the receptivity of $GABA_A$ receptors and antagonizes kainite/AMPA receptors (Ziółkowski et al. 2012).

Pharmacokinetics

Topiramate is rapidly absorbed after oral administration in dogs with a bioavailability ranging of 62–102% (Vuu et al. 2016). Bioavailability was approximately 50% higher when it was dosed in aqueous form compared with dry capsules (Streeter et al. 1995). Half-life is two to four hours in dogs (Streeter et al. 1995; Caldwell et al. 2005). It is largely non-protein bound but can bind to erythrocytes. 90% of the drug is eliminated in the urine and 6% in feces. However, dogs only excrete 28% unchanged in the urine, compared to 82% in people (Caldwell et al. 2005). Anecdotally, the dosage described for dogs ranges from 2 to 10 mg/kg q 8–12 hours, and the dose described for cats is 12.5–25 mg/cat q 12 hours (Grant and Rusbridge 2014; Plumb 2015). Co-administration of phenobarbital results in a 5.6-fold greater clearance and fourfold shorter elimination half-life than when given as a sole agent (Vuu et al. 2016).

Clinical Use and Efficacy

Topiramate has been used on a limited basis thus far by veterinary practitioners and usually as an add-on anti-epileptic for refractory seizure patients. There is little efficacy data in veterinary patients. However, one study exists looking at efficacy in 10 dogs. Fifty percent of dogs showed a response with a 66% reduction in seizure frequency (Kiviranta et al. 2013). One study safely administered topiramate to dogs with epilepsy at 10 and 20 m/kg IV over five minutes (Vuu et al. 2016).

Side Effects and Toxicity

Topiramate appears well tolerated in dogs and cats overall. The most common side effects reported in dogs include GI distress, sedation, ataxia, inappetence and irritability (Kiviranta et al. 2013). In cats, sedation and inappetence have been noted. There are no recognized toxicities in veterinary patients, but in humans, it may increase incidence of kidney stones and can cause a hyperchloremic metabolic acidosis (Plumb 2015).

Gabapentin

Gabapentin was developed as an anti-convulsant, however, is used more frequently as an analgesic in veterinary medicine. The mechanism of action is not fully understood but is believed to exert anticonvulsant properties by binding the α 2 delta-1 subunit of the voltage-gated calcium channels and inhibiting the release of neurotransmitters (Plumb 2015).

Pharmacokinetics

Gabapentin has an oral bioavailability of 80% in dogs when dosed at 50 mg/kg. Peak plasma concentrations occur two hours following administration. Gabapentin is partially metabolized and then eliminated renally. The elimination half-life is 2–4 hours in dogs (Plumb 2015). Cats have a wider range of bioavailability, ranging from 50% to 120%, with an average of 90%. Peak concentrations occur at 100 minutes after administration. Clearance was found to be 3 ml/min/kg with a mean elimination half-life of 2.8 hours (Siao et al. 2010). The Cmax in cats is reported to be 7.982 ± 1.053 mcg/ml. The same study found inadequate absorption of gabapentin when applied transdermally in cats (Adrian et al. 2018).

Clinical Use and Efficacy

Two studies investigated the efficacy of gabapentin as an adjunct for seizure management and found some improvement in seizure frequency (Govendir et al. 2005; Platt et al. 2006). However, controversy remains over the utility of gabapentin in seizure management. The recommended oral dose in dogs is 10–20 mg/kg orally q 8 hours (Plumb 2015). However, the dose can be gradually increased up to 60 mg/kg q 8 hours. The dose for cats ranges from 5 to 30 mg/kg orally q 8 hours (Plumb 2015).

Side Effects and Toxicity

Sedation and ataxia are the most common side effects reported, so other sedating drugs may have additive effects. Less commonly, somnolence and vomiting can be seen.

Drug Interactions

When given concurrently with antacids, the bioavailability of gabapentin decreases by 20%. Co-administration of gabapentin and hydrocodone may increase the area under the curve (AUC) resulting in increased efficacy and/or adverse effects. Gabapentin, in-turn, can reduce the AUC of hydrocodone (Plumb 2015). One study found oral administration of gabapentin to dogs, 2 hours prior to anesthesia, reduced the minimum alveolar concentration (MAC) of isoflurane by 20%. The time to extubation was also significantly shorter in patients receiving gabapentin and isoflurane (6 minutes) when compared to isoflurane alone (23 minutes) (Johnson et al. 2019). Another study in cats found gabapentin did not have any detectable effect on the MAC of isoflurane in cats (Reid et al. 2010).

Pregabalin

Pregabalin is a newer generation drug in the same class as gabapentin that has been used in dogs primarily as an add-on anti-epileptic in refractory seizure patients. Mechanism of action is not completely understood but may bind to a receptor protein on voltage-gated calcium channels and reduce neurotransmitter release (Sills 2006; Munana 2013).

Pharmacokinetics

There is little pharmacokinetic data on pregabalin in dogs and none in cats. One pharmacokinetic study showed that oral dosing of pregabalin in dogs achieved peak serum concentrations at 1.5 hours, and elimination half-life was approximately seven hours (Salazar et al. 2009). Elimination half-life is 10.4 hours in cats (Plumb 2015). Pregabalin is eliminated unchanged by the kidneys. Dosing recommendation for dogs is 3–4 mg/kg q 8–12 hours. To minimize side effects, some practitioners start at 1–2 mg/kg q 8 hours and then gradually increase the dose by 1 mg/kg each week until target dose is reached. Anecdotally, pregabalin has been used in cats at doses of 1–2 mg/kg q 12 hours (Munana 2013). Pregabalin clearance is correlated with renal function, requiring a dose reduction in patients with reduced renal function (Bockbrader et al. 2010).

Clinical Use and Efficacy

Pregabalin has been used primarily as an add-on anti-epileptic for refractory seizure patients. Little efficacy data exists, but one report showed that 57% of nine dogs had improved seizure control. Dogs that responded had a mean reduction in seizure frequency of 64% (Dewey et al. 2009).

Side Effects and Toxicity

Sedation and ataxia are the most common side effects reported, so other sedating drugs may have additive effects. There is no known toxicity in dogs and cats (Munana 2013).

Benzodiazepines

Benzodiazepine (BZ) drugs have anti-epileptic, sedative, anxiolytic and muscle relaxant effects. In dogs and cats, benzodiazepines are largely used in an emergency setting to stop seizure activity or for management of cluster seizures in the acute setting. Benzodiazepines used in dogs and cats include diazepam, midazolam, clonazepam, clorazepate, lorazepam and midazolam. BZs act on the $GABA_A$ receptor increasing chloride influx into neurons causing hyperpolarization (Muñana 1989, Dewey 2006).

Pharmacokinetics

See Table 25.2 under emergency control of seizures for information on half-life of the benzodiazepines. The BZ are metabolized by the liver via glucuronidation in dogs and then eliminated in the urine. Chronic dosing with PB increases clearance of diazepam after IV and rectal administration presumably due to rapid hepatic clearance. Therefore, patients on chronic PB therapy may require higher doses of diazepam (Wagner et al. 1998; Plumb 2015).

Clinical Use and Efficacy

The half-life of diazepam in dogs is too short for it to be effective as a maintenance anti-epileptic. In addition, tolerance to diazepam and other BZ may develop in dogs that are

Table 25.2 Half-lives, dosage and route of administration of benzodiazepines in emergency seizure management.

Drug	Elimination Half-life	Dosage/route of administration
Diazepam	1–3 hr (D) 5.5h (C) 7–22h (H)	0.5–1 mg/kg IV, rectal, intranasal (D,C)
Midazolam	77 min (D) 3.5–6.5h (H) 98 min (A)	0.1–0.5 mg/kg IV, IM, intranasal (D,C) 0.04–0.1 mg/kg IV, IM (H)
Lorazepam	1 hr (D)	0.2 mg/kg IV; intranasal

(D) = Dogs; (C) = Cats; (H) = Horses; (A) = Alpacas
Source: Lester (2015) and Plumb (2015).

being chronically treated (Dewey 2006). However, diazepam and midazolam are the drugs of choice for stopping seizure activity in an emergency setting in dogs, cats, horses, ruminants, and exotic animal species. The BZ may also be administered by owners, to patients with cluster seizures, with a goal of shortening the cluster seizure event. Diazepam can be dosed by rectal or intranasal administration to dogs and cats during a cluster seizure event. Oral administration of diazepam should be used with extreme caution in cats as a severe fulminant hepatic failure has been reported following oral administration (Center et al. 1996). This hepatic failure generally carries a very poor prognosis. However, there is at least one report of a cat surviving following intensive supportive care (Park 2012).

Midazolam can be dosed by intranasal administration or (IM) injection. It does not appear to be bioavailable in dogs following rectal administration likely due to extensive first pass metabolism. Pharmacokinetic studies have shown undetectable to low plasma concentrations following rectal administration (Court and Creenblatt 1992; Eagleson et al. 2012; Schwartz et al. 2013).

Lorazepam is also not bioavailable by rectal administration but is absorbed by intranasal administration in dogs (Podell et al. 1998). Clorazepate or lorazepam can be administered orally during a cluster seizure event (Plumb 2015). Further discussion of diazepam and midazolam are continued in the next section, Emergency control of seizures.

Acepromazine

Although not typically considered an AED, a brief discussion of acepromazine is warranted as it is frequently used in anesthetic protocols. There has historically been a belief that acepromazine was pro-convulsant and should be avoided in patients prone to seizures. However, the author's clinical experience does not support this. In addition, a study looking at use of acepromazine in epileptic dogs showed that treated dogs were not at risk for increased seizures, and actually abated seizure activity in a small number of dogs (Tobias et al. 2006). Another study did not show increased seizure activity following myelography in dogs premedicated with acepromazine (Drynan et al. 2012).

Ketamine

Ketamine, an N-methyl-D-aspartate (NMDA) receptor antagonist hypnotic agent, is a generally safe drug used for anesthetic induction and pain control in veterinary patients. Historically, ketamine has shown proconvulsant properties and the general recommendation has been to avoid its use in epileptic patients (Plumb 2015). However, there is increasing experimental evidence that NMDA receptor antagonists may have an effect against status epilepticus (De Sarro and De Sarro 1993). It has been shown to be effective at stopping refractory status epilepticus in children (Hofler et al. 2016). There is at least one case report documenting use of ketamine for management of status epilepticus in a dog. The dog was treated with a 5 mg/kg ketamine bolus followed by a constant rate of infusion (CRI) of 5 mg/kg/hr (Serrano et al. 2006).

Emergency Control of Seizures

Benzodiazepines are the preferred drugs for stopping active seizures. Diazepam may be dosed at 0.5–1 mg/kg IV and doses may be repeated 1–2 times if needed to stop a seizure (Smith 2005). If seizure activity is abated with diazepam boluses, a CRI 0.5–2 mg/kg/hr may be used in the clinic setting. If IV access cannot be achieved, diazepam can be given at 0.5 mg/kg intranasally or 1–2 mg/kg rectally (Podell 1995; Dewey 2006). Midazolam may be used in lieu of diazepam dosed at 0.2–0.5 mg/kg IV, () (IM) or intranasally (Plumb 2015). Midazolam may be safer and more effective than diazepam (Dewey 2006). Midazolam may also be continued as a CRI at 0.1–2.5 mg/kg/hr in the clinic setting. A recent study found seizure control was achieved in 77.4% of dogs presenting with cluster seizures or status epilepticus at a median dose of 0.3 mg/kg/hr (Bray et al. 2021). Midazolam is not bioavailable when dosed rectally (Court and Creenblatt 1992). Lorazepam may also be dosed IV or intranasally in dogs. Repeated high doses or CRI's should be used with caution as the injection contains propylene glycol and benzyl alcohol and could result in toxicity (Plumb 2015).

If seizures persist despite 1–2 mg/kg cumulative dose of diazepam and midazolam, PB may be given IV. In PB naïve patients, a cumulative dose up to 20–25 mg/kg may be given in 5 mg/kg increments with 15–30 minutes between (Smith 2005).

If seizures still cannot be stopped, induction of general anesthesia with propofol or pentobarbital is warranted. Propofol is given at 2–8 mg/kg IV cumulative dose to effect. If this is effective, a CRI of 0.1–0.6 mg/kg/min may be continued. The use of propofol to stop seizure activity is controversial as there are reports of epileptiform discharges noted on electroencephalogram (EEG) of epileptic dogs and humans anesthetized with propofol (Akos et al. 2012; Jaggy and Bernardini 1998; Loscher 2009; Brauer et al. 2012). Therefore, although the motor manifestations of seizures are stopped, seizure activity could be continual in the brain (non-convulsive status epilepticus). Alfaxalone, a neurosteroid anesthetic induction agent, has not been widely used to treat seizure activity, and one study in rats did not show efficacy for stopping seizure activity (Borowicz et al. 2002). Pentobarbital may be used at 3–15 mg/kg IV cumulative dose to effect. Isoflurane may also be used to maintain anesthesia (Smith 2005).

References

Adrian, D., Papich, M.G., Baynes, R. et al. (2018). The pharmacokinetics of gabapentin in cats. *J. Vet. Intern. Med.* 32 (6): 1996–2002:https://doi.org/10.1111/jvim.15313.

Akos, P., Thalhammer, J.G., Leschnik, M., and Halasz, P. (2012). Electroencephalographic examination of epileptic dogs under propofol restraint. *Acta Vet. Hung.* 60 (3): 309–324.

Albarracin, V., Teles, M., Melendez-Lazo, A. et al. (2015). Canine Pancreas-specific lipase and C-reactive protein in dogs treated with anticonvulsants (phenobarbital and potassium bromide). *Top. Companion Anim. Med.* 30 (2): 57–61.

Aleman, M., Gray, L.C., Williams, D.C. et al. (2006). Juvenile idiopathic epilepsy in Egyptian Arabian foals: 22 cases (1985–2005). *J. Vet. Intern. Med.* 20 (6): 1443–1449.

Al-Tahan, F. and Frey, H.H. (1985). Absorption kinetics and bioavailability of phenobarbital after oral administration to dogs. *J. Vet. Pharmacol. Ther.* 8 (2): 205–207.

Andrews, F.M.M. and Hilary, K. (2004). *Equine Internal Medicine.* St. Louis, MO: Saunders.

Bailey, D.N. and Briggs, J.R. (2004). The binding of selected therapeutic drugs to human serum alpha-1 acid glycoprotein and to human serum albumin in vitro. *Ther. Drug Monit.* 26 (1): 40–43.

Bailey, K.S., Dewey, C.W., Boothe, D.M. et al. (2008). Levetiracetam as an adjunct to phenobarbital treatment in cats with suspected idiopathic epilepsy. *J. Am. Vet. Med. Assoc.* 232 (6): 867–872.

Barnes, H.H., Martin, G., Van Hesteren, M., and Boothe, D.M. (2018). Serum levetiracetam concentrations and adverse events after multiple dose extended release levetiracetam administration to healthy cats. *J. Vet. Intern. Med.* 32 (3): 1145–1148.

Beasley, M.J. and Boothe, D. (2012). The pharmacokinetics of single dose extended release Keppra (R) with and without food in healthy adult dogs [abstract]. *J. Vet. Intern. Med.* 26: 819.

Bockbrader, H.N., Wesche, D., Miller, R. et al. (2010). A comparison of the pharmacokinetics and pharmacodynamics of pregabalin and gabapentin. *Clin. Pharmacokinet.* 49 (10): 661–669. https://doi.org/10.2165/11536200-000000000-00000. PMID: 20818832.

Boothe, D.M. (1998). Anticonvulsant therapy in small animals. *Vet. Clin. N. Am. Small Anim. Pract.* 28 (2): 411–448.

Boothe, D.M. and Perkins, J. (2008). Disposition and safety of zonisamide after intravenous and oral single dose and oral multiple dosing in normal hound dogs. *J. Vet. Pharmacol. Ther.* 31 (6): 544–553.

Boothe, D.M., George, K.L., and Couch, P. (2002). Disposition and clinical use of bromide in cats. *J. Am. Vet. Med. Assoc.* 221 (8): 1131–1135.

Boothe, D.M., Dewey, C., and Carpenter, D.M. (2012). Comparison of phenobarbital with bromide as a first-choice antiepileptic drug for treatment of epilepsy in dogs. *J. Am. Vet. Med. Assoc.* 240 (9): 1073–1083.

Borowicz, K.K., Zadrozniak, M., Swiader, M. et al. (2002). Interaction of the neurosteroid alphaxalone with conventional antiepileptic drugs in different types of experimental seizures. *Eur. J. Pharmacol.* 449 (1–2): 85–90.

Brauer, C., Kastner, S.B., Rohn, K. et al. (2012). Electroencephalographic recordings in dogs suffering from idiopathic and symptomatic epilepsy: diagnostic value of interictal short time EEG protocols supplemented by two activation techniques. *Vet. J.* 193 (1): 185–192.

Bray, K.Y., Mariani, C.L., Early, P.J. et al. (2021). Continuous rate infusion of midazolam as emergent treatment for seizures in dogs. *J. Vet. Intern. Med.* 35 (1): 388–396. https://doi.org/10.1111/jvim.15993. Epub 2020 Dec 16. PMID: 33325618; PMCID: PMC7848341.

Caldwell, G.W., Wu, W.N., Masucci, J.A. et al. (2005). Metabolism and excretion of the antiepileptic/antimigraine drug, topiramate in animals and humans. *Eur. J. Drug Metab. Pharmacokinet.* 30 (3): 151–164.

Carnes, M.B., Axlund, T.W., and Boothe, D.M. (2011). Pharmacokinetics of levetiracetam after oral and intravenous administration of a single dose to clinically normal cats. *Am. J. Vet. Res.* 72 (9): 1247–1252.

Center, S.A., Elston, T.H., Rowland, P.H. et al. (1996). Fulminant hepatic failure associated with oral administration of diazepam in 11 cats. *J. Am. Vet. Med. Assoc.* 209 (3): 618–625.

Cesar, F.B., Steward, A.J., Boothe, D.M. et al. (2018). Disposition of levetiracetam in healthy adult horses. *J. Vet. Pharmacol. Ther.* 41 (1): 92–97.

Charalambous, M., Brodbelt, D., and Volk, H.A. (2014). Treatment in canine epilepsy – a systematic review. *BMC Vet. Res.* 10: 257.

Chung, J.Y., Hwang, C.Y., Chae, J.S. et al. (2012). Zonisamide monotherapy for idiopathic epilepsy in dogs. *N. Z. Vet. J.* 60 (6): 357–359.

Cochrane, S.M., Black, W.D., Parent, J.M. et al. (1990a). Pharmacokinetics of phenobarbital in the cat following intravenous and oral administration. *Can. J. Vet. Res.* 54 (1): 132–138.

Cochrane, S.M., Parent, J.M., Black, W.D. et al. (1990b). Pharmacokinetics of phenobarbital in the cat following multiple oral administration. *Can. J. Vet. Res.* 54 (3): 309–312.

Cook, A.K., Allen, A.K., Espinosa, D., and Barr, J. (2011). Renal tubular acidosis associated with Zonisamide therapy in a dog. *J. Vet. Intern. Med.* 25 (6): 1454–1457.

Court, M.H. and Creenblatt, D.J. (1992). Pharmacokinetics and preliminary observations of behavioral changes following administration of midazolam to dogs. *J. Vet. Pharmacol. Ther.* 15 (4): 343–350.

Daminet, S. and Ferguson, D.C. (2003). Influence of drugs on thyroid function in dogs. *J. Vet. Intern. Med.* 17 (4): 463–472.

Dayrell-Hart, B. (1991). Hepatotoxicity of phenobarbital in dogs: 18 cases (1985–1989). *J. Am. Vet. Med. Assoc.* 199 (8): 1060–1066.

De Sarro, G.B. and De Sarro, A. (1993). Anticonvulsant properties of non-competitive antagonists of the N-methyl-D-aspartate receptor in genetically epilepsy-prone rats: comparison with CPPene. *Neuropharmacology* 32 (1): 51–58.

Degim, T., Dundaroz, R., Sizlan, A. et al. (2002). The use of the corpus cavernosum for the administration of phenobarbital: an experimental study in dogs. *Int. J. Pharm.* 246 (1–2): 105–109.

Dewey, C.W. (2006). Anticonvulsant therapy in dogs and cats. *Vet. Clin. N. Am. Small Anim. Pract.* 36 (5): 1107–1127. vii.

Dewey, C.W., Guiliano, R., Boothe, D.M. et al. (2004). Zonisamide therapy for refractory idiopathic epilepsy in dogs. *J. Am. Anim. Hosp. Assoc.* 40 (4): 285–291.

Dewey, C.W., Bailey, K.S., Boothe, D.M. et al. (2008). Pharmacokinetics of single-dose intravenous levetiracetam administration in normal dogs. *J. Vet. Emerg. Crit. Care* 18 (2): 153–157.

Dewey, C.W., Cerda-Gonzalez, S., Levine, J.M. et al. (2009). Pregabalin as an adjunct to phenobarbital, potassium bromide, or a combination of phenobarbital and potassium bromide for treatment of dogs with suspected idiopathic epilepsy. *J. Am. Vet. Med. Assoc.* 235 (12): 1442–1449.

Drynan, E.A., Gray, P., and Raisis, A.L. (2012). Incidence of seizures associated with the use of acepromazine in dogs undergoing myelography. *J. Vet. Emerg. Crit. Care (San Antonio)* 22 (2): 262–266.

Dugdale, A.H., Lakhani, K.H., and Brearley, J.C. (2001). Thiopentone induction dose requirement in dogs is little influenced by co-administration of diazepam or prior treatment with phenobarbitone or corticosteroids, but is reduced in the presence of brain pathology. *Vet. J.* 161 (1): 93–97.

Eagleson, J.S., Platt, S.R., Strong, D.L. et al. (2012). Bioavailability of a novel midazolam gel after intranasal administration in dogs. *Am. J. Vet. Res.* 73 (4): 539–545.

Ennulat, D., Walker, D., Clemo, F. et al. (2010). Effects of hepatic drug-metabolizing enzyme induction on clinical pathology parameters in animals and man. *Toxicol. Pathol.* 38 (5): 810–828.

Fournier, T., Medjoubi-N, N., and Porquet, D. (2000). Alpha-1-acid glycoprotein. *Biochim. Biophys. Acta Protein Struct. Mol. Enzymol.* 1482 (1–2): 157–171.

Frey, H.H. and Loscher, W. (1985). Pharmacokinetics of anti-epileptic drugs in the dog: a review. *J. Vet. Pharmacol. Ther.* 8: 219–233.

Fukunaga, K., Saito, M., Matsuo, E. et al. (2009). Long-lasting enhancement of CYP activity after discontinuation of repeated administration of phenobarbital in dogs. *Res. Vet. Sci.* 87 (3): 455–457.

Fukunaga, K., Matsumoto, H., Wate, M. et al. (2018). Effects of three infusion fluids with different sodium chloride contents on stead-state serum concentrations of bromide in dogs. *J. Vet. Pharmacol. Ther.* 41 (5): 684–690.

Gaskill, C.L. and Cribb, A.E. (2000). Pancreatitis associated with potassium bromide/phenobarbital combination therapy in epileptic dogs. *Can. Vet. J.* 41 (7): 555–558.

Gaskill, C.L., Hoffmann, W.E., and Cribb, A.E. (2004). Serum alkaline phosphatase isoenzyme profiles in phenobarbital-treated epileptic dogs. *Vet. Clin. Pathol.* 33 (4): 215–222.

Gaskill, C.L., Miller, L.M., Mattoon, J.S. et al. (2005). Liver histopathology and liver and serum alanine aminotransferase and alkaline phosphatase activities in epileptic dogs receiving phenobarbital. *Vet. Pathol.* 42: 147–160.

Gieger, T.L., Hosgood, G., Taboada, J. et al. (2000). Thyroid function and serum hepatic enzyme activity in dogs after phenobarbital administration. *J. Vet. Intern. Med.* 14 (3): 277–281.

Govendir, M., Perkins, M., and Malik, R. (2005). Improving seizure control in dogs with refractory epilepsy using gabapentin as an adjunctive agent. *Aust. Vet. J.* 83 (10): 602–608. https://doi.org/10.1111/j.1751-0813.2005. tb13269.x. PMID: 16255282.

Grant, D. and Rusbridge, C. (2014). Topiramate in the management of feline idiopathic ulcerative dermatitis in a two-year-old cat. *Vet. Dermatol.* 25 (3): 226–e260.

Hardy, B.T., Patterson, E.E., Cloyd, J.M. et al. (2012). Double-masked, placebo-controlled study of intravenous levetiracetam for the treatment of status epilepticus and acute repetitive seizures in dogs. *J. Vet. Intern. Med.* 26 (2): 334–340.

Hasegawa, D., Kobayashi, M., Kuwabara, T. et al. (2008). Pharmacokinetics and toxicity of zonisamide in cats. *J. Feline Med. Surg.* 10 (4): 418–421.

Hofler, J., Rohracher, A., Kalss, G. et al. (2016). (S)-ketamine in refractory and super-refractory status epilepticus: a retrospective study. *CNS Drugs* 30 (9): 869–876.

Hojo, T., Ohno, R., Shimoda, M., and Kokue, E. (2002). Enzyme and plasma protein induction by multiple oral administrations of phenobarbital at a therapeutic dosage regimen in dogs. *J. Vet. Pharmacol. Ther.* 25 (2): 121–127.

Isoherranen, N., Yagen, B., Soback, S. et al. (2001). Pharmacokinetics of levetiracetam and its enantiomer (R)-α-ethyl-2-oxo-pyrrolidine acetamide in dogs. *Epilepsia* 42 (7): 825–830.

Jaggy, A. and Bernardini, M. (1998). Idiopathic epilepsy in 125 dogs: a long-term study. Clinical and electroencephalographic findings. *J. Small Anim. Pract.* 39 (1): 23–29.

Johnson, B.A., Aarnes, T.K., Wanstrath, A.W. et al. (2019 Nov). Effect of oral administration of gabapentin on the minimum alveolar concentration of isoflurane in dogs. *Am. J. Vet. Res.* 80 (11): 1007–1009. https://doi.org/10.2460/ ajvr.80.11.1007. PMID: 31644338.

Keller, K.A., Guzman, D.S., Boothe, D.M. et al. (2019). Pharmacokinetics and safety of zonisamide after oral administration of single and multiple doses to Hispaniolan Amazon parrots (Amazona ventralis). *Am. J. Vet. Res.* 80 (2): 195–200.

Kiviranta, A.M., Laitinen-Vapaavuori, O., Hielm-Björkman, A., and Jokinen, T. (2013). Topiramate as an add-on antiepileptic drug in treating refractory canine idiopathic epilepsy. *J. Small Anim. Pract.* 54 (10): 512–520.

Kluger, E.K., Malik, R., Ilkin, W.J. et al. (2008). Serum triglyceride concentration in dogs with epilepsy treated with phenobarbital or with phenobarbital and bromide. *J. Am. Vet. Med. Assoc.* 233 (8): 1270–1277.

Lester, G.D. (2015). *Large Animal Internal Medicine.* St. Louis, MO: Elsevier.

Loscher, W. (2009). Preclinical assessment of proconvulsant drug activity and its relevance for predicting adverse events in humans. *Eur. J. Pharmacol.* 610 (1–3): 1–11.

MacDonald, K.D., Hart, K.A., Davis, J.L. et al. (2018). Pharmacokinetics of the anticonvulsant levetiracetam in neonatal foals. *Equine Vet. J.* 50 (4): 532–536.

MacKay, R.J. (2015). *Large Animal Internal Medicine.* St. Louis, MO: Elsevier.

March, P.A., Podell, M., and Sams, R.A. (2002). Pharmacokinetics and toxicity of bromide following high-dose oral potassium bromide administration in healthy beagles. *J. Vet. Pharmacol. Ther.* 25 (6): 425–432.

Martis, L., Lynch, S., Napoli, M.D., and Woods, E.F. (1981 Apr). Biotransformation of sevoflurane in dogs and rats. *Anesth. Analg.* 60 (4): 186–191. PMID: 6782910.

de Matos, R., Noonan, B.P., Schaefer, D.M.W. et al. (2021). Pharmacokinetics of zonisamide after oral single dosing and multiple-dose escalation administration in domestic chickens (Gallus gallus). *Vet. Med. Sci.* https://doi. org/10.1002/vms3.512. Epub ahead of print. PMID: 34004072.

Michaels, J.R., Hodshon, A.J., Thomas, W.B. et al. (2016). Pharmacokinetics of zonisamide following rectal administration to healthy dogs. *Am. J. Vet. Res.* 77 (12): 1374–1380.

Miller, M.L., Center, S.A., Randolph, J.F. et al. (2011). Apparent acute idiosyncratic hepatic necrosis associated with Zonisamide Administration in a dog. *J. Vet. Intern. Med.* 25 (5): 1156–1160.

Moore, S.A., Muñana, K.R., Papich, M.G., and Nettifee-Osborne, J. (2010). Levetiracetam pharmacokinetics in healthy dogs following oral administration of single and multiple doses. *Am. J. Vet. Res.* 71 (3): 337–341.

Moore, S.A., Munana, K.R., Papich, M.G., and Nettifee-Osborne, J.A. (2011). The pharmacokinetics of levetiracetam in healthy dogs concurrently receiving phenobarbital. *J. Vet. Pharmacol. Ther.* 34 (1): 31–34.

Müller, P.B., Taboada, J., Hosgood, G. et al. (2000a). Effects of long-term phenobarbital treatment on the liver in dogs. *J. Vet. Intern. Med.* 14 (2): 165–171.

Müller, P.B., Wolfsheimer, K.J., Taboada, J. et al. (2000b). Effects of long-term phenobarbital treatment on the thyroid and adrenal axis and adrenal function tests in dogs. *J. Vet. Intern. Med.* 14 (2): 157–164.

Muñana, K.R. (1989). Management of refractory epilepsy. *Top. Comp. Anim. Med.* **28** (2): 67–71.

Munana, K.R. (2013). Update: seizure management in small animal practice. *Vet. Clin. N. Am. Small Anim. Pract.* 43 (5): 1127–1147.

Munana, K.R., Thomas, W.B., Inzana, K.D. et al. (2012). Evaluation of levetiracetam as an adjunctive treatment for refractory epilepsy: a randomized, placebo-controlled, crossover trial. *J. Vet. Intern. Med.* 26: 341–348.

Nossaman, B.C., Amouzadeh, H.R., and Sangiah, S. (1990). Effects of chloramphenicol, cimetidine and phenobarbital on and tolerance to xylazine-ketamine anesthesia in dogs. *Vet. Hum. Toxicol.* 32 (3): 216–219.

Oglesbee, B. (2011). *Blackwell's Five Minute Veterinary Consult: Small Mammal.* Wiley: Ames, IA.

Orito, K., Saito, M., Fukunaga, K. et al. (2008). Pharmacokinetics of zonisamide and drug interaction with phenobarbital in dogs. *J. Vet. Pharmacol. Ther.* 31 (3): 259–264.

Pakozdy, A., Sarchahi, A.A., Leschnik, M. et al. (2013). Treatment and long-term follow-up of cats with suspected primary epilepsy. *J. Feline Med. Surg.* 15 (4): 267–273.

Pakozdy, A., Halasz, P., and Klang, A. (2014). Epilepsy in cats: theory and practice. *J. Vet. Intern. Med.* 28 (2): 255–263.

Park, F.M. (2012). Successful treatment of hepatic failure secondary to diazepam administration in a cat. *J. Feline Med. Surg.* 14 (2): 158–160.

Patterson, E.E., Goel, V., Cloyd, J.C. et al. (2008). Intramuscular, intravenous and oral levetiracetam in dogs: safety and pharmacokinetics. *J. Vet. Pharmacol. Ther.* 31 (3): 253–258.

Pedersoli, W.M. (1980 Jan). Serum bromide concentrations during and after halothane anesthesia in dogs. *Am. J. Vet. Res.* 41 (1): 77–80. PMID: 7362126.

Pedersoli, W.M., Wike, J.S., and Ravis, W.R. (1987). Pharmacokinetics of single doses of phenobarbital given intravenously and orally to dogs. *Am. J. Vet. Res.* 48 (4): 679–683.

Perks, A., Cheema, S., and Mohanraj, R. (2012). Anaesthesia and epilepsy. *Br. J. Anaesth.* 108 (4): 562–571.

Platt, S.R., Adams, V., Garosi, L.S. et al. (2006). Treatment with gabapentin of 11 dogs with refractory idiopathic epilepsy. *Vet. Rec.* 159 (26): 881–884. PMID: 17189599.

Plumb, D.C. (2015). *Veterinary Drug Handbook.* Ames, IA: Iowa State University Press.

Podell, M. (1995). The use of diazepam per rectum at home for the acute Management of Cluster Seizures in dogs. *J. Vet. Intern. Med.* 9 (2): 68–74.

Podell, M. and Fenner, W.R. (1993). Bromide therapy in refractory canine idiopathic epilepsy. *J. Vet. Intern. Med.* 7 (5): 318–327.

Podell, M., Wagner, S.O., and Sams, R.A. (1998). Lorazepam concentrations in plasma following its intravenous and rectal administration in dogs. *J. Vet. Pharmacol. Ther.* 21 (2): 158–160.

Powers, L.V. and Papich, M.G. (2011). Pharmacokinetics of orally administered phenobarbital in African grey parrots (*Psittacus erithacus erithacus*). *J. Vet. Pharmacol. Ther.* 34 (6): 615–617.

Quast, T.A., Combs, M.D., and Edwards, S.H. (2015). Pharmacokinetics of bromide in adult sheep following oral and intravenous administration. *Aust. Vet. J.* 93 (1-2): 20–25.

Raidal, S.L. and Edwards, S. (2008). Pharmacokinetics of potassium bromide in adult horses. *Aust. Vet. J.* 86 (5): 187–193.

Ravis, W.R., Nachreiner, R.F., Pedersoli, W.M., and Houghton, N.S. (1984). Pharmacokinetics of phenobarbital in dogs after multiple oral administration. *Am. J. Vet. Res.* 45 (7): 1283–1286.

Ravis, W.R., Pedersoli, W.M., and Wike, J.S. (1989). Pharmacokinetics of phenobarbital in dogs given multiple doses. *Am. J. Vet. Res.* 50 (8): 1343–1347.

Reid, P., Pypendop, B.H., and Ilkiw, J.E. (2010 Sep). The effects of intravenous gabapentin administration on the minimum alveolar concentration of isoflurane in cats. *Anesth. Analg.* 111 (3): 633–637. https://doi.org/10.1213/ANE.0b013e3181e51245. Epub 2010 Jun 14. PMID: 20547821.

Reimer, J.M. and Sweeney, R.W. (1992). Pharmacokinetics of phenobarbital after repeated oral administration in normal horses. *J. Vet. Pharmacol. Ther.* 15 (3): 301–304.

Rossmeisl, J.H. and Inzana, K.D. (2009). Clinical signs, risk factors, and outcomes associated with bromide toxicosis (bromism) in dogs with idiopathic epilepsy. *J. Am. Vet. Med. Assoc.* 234 (11): 1425–1431.

Salazar, V., Dewey, C.W., Schwark, W. et al. (2009). Pharmacokinetics of single-dose oral pregabalin administration in normal dogs. *Vet. Anaesth. Analg.* 36 (6): 574–580.

Sams, R.W.M. (1988). Effects of phenobarbital on thiopental pharmacokinetics in Greyhounds. *Am. J. Vet. Res.* 49 (2): 245–249.

Sasaki, K. and Shimoda, M. (2015). Possible drug–drug interaction in dogs and cats resulted from alteration in drug metabolism: a mini review. *J. Adv. Res.* 6 (3): 383–392.

Schwartz, M., Munana, K.R., and Olby, N.J. (2011). Possible drug-induced hepatopathy in a dog receiving zonisamide monotherapy for treatment of cryptogenic epilepsy. *J. Vet. Med. Sci.* 73 (11): 1505–1508.

Schwartz, M., Munana, K.R., Nettifee-Osborne, J.A. et al. (2013). The pharmacokinetics of midazolam after intravenous, intramuscular, and rectal administration in healthy dogs. *J. Vet. Pharmacol. Ther.* 36 (5): 471–477.

Schwartz-Porsche, D., Loscher, W., and Frey, H.H. (1985). Therapeutic efficacy of phenobarbital and primidone in canine epilepsy: a comparison. *J. Vet. Pharmacol. Ther.* 8 (2): 113–119.

Serrano, S., Hughes, D., and Chandler, K. (2006). Use of ketamine for the management of refractory status epilepticus in a dog. *J. Vet. Intern. Med.* 20 (1): 194–197.

Siao, K.T., Pypendop, B.H., and Ilkiw, J.E. (2010). Pharmacokinetics of gabapentin in cats. *Am. J. Vet. Res.* 71 (7): 817–821. https://doi.org/10.2460/ajvr.71.7.817. PMID: 20594085.

Sills, G.J. (2006). The mechanisms of action of gabapentin and pregabalin. *Curr. Opin. Pharmacol.* 6 (1): 108–113.

Smith, J.D. (2005). Status epilepticus in dogs. *Stand. Care Emerg. Crit. Care Med.* 7 (9): 1–6.

Smith, C., Barnes Heller, H.L., Reif, N. et al. (2019). Serum levetiracetam concentrations after transdermal levetiracetam administration, 3 times daily, to healthy cats. *J. Vet. Intern. Med.* 33 (2): 827–830.

Streeter, A.J., Stahle, P.L., Holland, M.L. et al. (1995). Pharmacokinetics and bioavailability of topiramate in the beagle dog. *Drug Metab. Dispos.* 23 (1): 90–93.

Surges, R., Volynski, K.E., and Walker, M.C. (2008). Review: Is levetiracetam different from other antiepileptic drugs? Levetiracetam and its cellular mechanism of action in epilepsy revisited. *Ther. Adv. Neurol. Disord.* 1 (1): 13–24.

Thomas, W.B. (2010). Idiopathic epilepsy in dogs and cats. *Vet. Clin. N. Am. Small Anim. Pract.* 40 (1): 161–179.

Tobias, K.M., Marioni-Henry, K., and Wagner, R. (2006). A retrospective study on the use of acepromazine maleate in dogs with seizures. *J. Am. Anim. Hosp. Assoc.* 42 (4): 283–289.

Trepanier, L.A. (1995). Use of bromide as an anticonvulsant for dogs with epilepsy. *J. Am. Vet. Med. Assoc.* 207 (2): 163–166.

Trepanier, L.A. and Babish, J.G. (1995). Pharmacokinetic properties of bromide in dogs after the intravenous and oral administration of single doses. *Res. Vet. Sci.* 58 (3): 248–251.

Twyman, R.E., Rogers, C.J., and Macdonald, R.L. (1989). Differential regulation of Gaba-aminobutyric acid receptor channels by diazepam and phenobarbital. *Ann. Neurol.* 25: 213–220.

Viegas, O. and Stoelting, R.K. (1976). Halothane MAC in dogs unchanged by phenobarbital. *Anesth. Analg.* 55 (5): 677–679. https://doi.org/10.1213/00000539-197609000-00013. PMID: 987722.

Volk, H.A., Matiasek, L.A., Luján Feliu-Pascual, A. et al. (2008). The efficacy and tolerability of levetiracetam in pharmacoresistant epileptic dogs. *Vet. J.* 176 (3): 310–319.

Von Klopmann, T., Rambeck, B., and Tipold, A. (2007). Prospective study of zonisamide therapy for refractory idiopathic epilepsy in dogs. *J. Small Anim. Pract.* 48 (3): 134–138.

Vuu, I., Coles, L.D., Maglalang, P. et al. (2016 Dec). Intravenous topiramate: pharmacokinetics in dogs with naturally occurring epilepsy. *Front. Vet. Sci.* 5 (3): 107. https://doi.org/10.3389/fvets.2016.00107. PMID: 27995128; PMCID: PMC5136567.

Wagner, S.O., Sams, R.A., and Podell, M. (1998). Chronic phenobarbital therapy reduces plasma benzodiazepine concentrations after intravenous and rectal administration of diazepam in the dog. *J. Vet. Pharmacol. Ther.* 21 (5): 335–341.

Wong, D.M., Papich, M.G., and Davis, J.L. (2008). Exposure to phenobarbital in a foal after nursing a mare treated with phenobarbital. *J. Vet. Intern. Med.* 22 (1): 227–230.

Yasiry, Z. and Shorvon, S.D. (2012). How phenobarbital revolutionized epilepsy therapy: the story of phenobarbital therapy in epilepsy in the last 100 years. *Epilepsia* 53 (Suppl 8): 26–39.

Yates, L.M., Leman, M., Knych, H.K. et al. (2020). Pharmacokinetics of intravenous and oral phenobarbital sodium in healthy goats. *Front. Vet Sci.* 21 (7): 86. https://doi.org/10.3389/fvets.2020.00086. PMCID: PMC7046625; PMCID: PMC7046625.

Ziółkowski, H., Jaroszewski, J.J., Ziółkowska, N., and Jasiecka, A. (2012). Characteristics of selected second-generation antiepileptic drugs used in dogs. *Polish J. Vet. Sci.* 15 (3): 571–582.

26

Antihistamines

S. Bryce Dooley

Introduction

The physiologic effects of histamine were first demonstrated in 1907 when an unknown amino acid extracted from mold ergot was applied experimentally to intestines and the horn of a cat's uterus. In 1910, histamine – an already known substance – was intentionally isolated and identified as the biologically active element seen in the 1907 experiment (Riley 1965). During the early twentieth century, histamine was also isolated as a naturally occurring substance in mammalian tissues, especially the liver, lungs, and skin. Since then, histamine has been intensely studied for its multiple effects on many body systems. It was histamine's direct connection to anaphylaxis and a shock-like syndrome characterized by bronchoconstriction, vasodilation, and increased cardiac contractility that led to investigation of drugs that could counteract these effects.

Histamine, its receptors, and its antagonists continue to be studied in order to understand exactly how histamine functions in different body systems. To date, a total of four different histamine receptors, H1, H2, H3, and H4, have been identified and gene sequenced in humans and other species (Yamashita et al. 1991; Fukui et al. 1994; Gantz et al. 1991, Lovenberg et al. 1999; Nguyen et al. 2001). The receptors do not share a great deal of genetic homology and, despite the existence of multiple receptor types expressed on shared locations, each histamine receptor has a particular set of physiologic consequences when activated.

Mechanism of Action

Histamine itself is an endogenous amine, produced from decarboxylation of L-histadine. It has far-reaching effects on the body given the multitude of locations and the increasing specificity of its different receptors.

Each histamine receptor belongs to the parent group of G protein coupled receptors (GPCRs). They exist simultaneously in an inactive and active form, even in the absence of histamine. This ability to independently cause cellular signaling even in the absence of its ligand is known as the receptor's constitutive activity. All four known histamine receptors have demonstrated constitutive activity (Wieland et al. 2001). While the receptors exist in equilibrium of active and inactive states, this can be disrupted via the binding of histamine or an antihistamine. With a similar structure to histamine, antihistamines have the ability to bind to the receptor site to not only prevent histamine from doing so but furthermore stabilize the receptor to its inactive state (Leurs et al. 2002; Bakker et al. 2000). In both instances, the effects mediated by histamine are diminished. While drugs used to antagonize histamine's effects are traditionally referred to as antihistamines, they may in fact be better categorized as histamine inverse agonists. For the sake of simplicity, however, the drugs will be referred to as antihistamines in this chapter. An understanding of the locations and effects of the different histamine receptors is essential to understanding how the commercially available antihistamines exert their effects.

H1 Receptor

H1 receptors reside in the respiratory tract, mast cells, smooth and cardiac muscle, conjunctiva, the adrenal medulla, and in many areas of the brain. Given the location of these receptors, activation of the H1 receptor is responsible for the clinical signs of allergic reaction and anaphylaxis such as sneezing, epiphora, bronchoconstriction, immediate vasodilation, and edema formation (Oda et al. 2000). These effects were responsible for the initial investigation into antihistamines.

When the H1 G_q receptor is activated, the intracellular messenger inositol triphosphate activates the endoplasmic or sarcoplasmic reticulum to release stores of ionized calcium, thus rapidly increasing the intracellular calcium concentration. As a result, both smooth muscle cells lining the airways and vasculature endothelial cells contract, resulting in bronchoconstriction and increased vascular permeability, respectively. Vasoconstriction of the coronary artery, pulmonary arteries and veins and hepatic presinusoidal vessels are all seen as H1-mediated responses (Felix et al. 1988; Mikkelsen et al. 1984; Shi et al. 1998; Shibamoto et al. 2005). Peripherally, histamine-induced nitric oxide production dilates vessels to such a degree that there is a systemic hypotension with extravasation of plasma and macromolecules (Mayhan 1994).

In the brain, H1 receptors are located postsynaptically in many areas. When activated, there is an excitation of the neurons via increased intracellular calcium and opening of the calcium-dependent potassium channels (Jahn et al. 1995; Brown et al. 2001). This plays a very strong role in the sleep–wake cycle of mammals and is implicated in learning and memory (Passani et al. 2007).

It was not until the 1940s that antihistamines safe enough for human use were developed. In experimental settings, they could effectively prevent histamine-induced vasodilation and small-intestinal contraction, both signs of preventing H1-receptor activation. Despite this, there was no effect seen on histamine-induced gastric-acid secretion, which led researchers to search for a second histamine receptor (Loew 1947).

H2 Receptor

In 1966, the H2 receptor was officially recognized as a separate receptor, causing histamine-induced gastric-acid secretion that would persist in the face of H1 antagonists (Ash and Schild 1966). H2 receptors exist on parietal cells, and H2 antihistamines work to prevent the binding of histamine at this level.

In spite of its many locations, the H2 receptor's largest role currently appreciated in physiology remains its direct effect on gastric-acid release. As a predominantly G_s-coupled receptor, activation of histamine receptors on parietal cells cause the release of hydrochloric acid and is mediated by an increase in intracellular ionized calcium concentration as well as by an intracellular increase in cAMP through adenylate cyclase coupling (Chew et al. 1980; Soll and Wollin 1979).

H2 receptors are also found in the cardiovascular and respiratory systems. In these locations, histamine's effects differ from those mediated by H1 receptors. In the cardiovascular system, H2 receptors are responsible for sustained vasodilation, increased myocardial contractility, and bronchodilation (Felix et al. 1988; Eyre 1969; Parsons and Ganellin 2006). Like H1 receptors, H2 receptors are also present throughout the brain facilitating an excitatory reaction (Brown et al. 2001). Recently, H2 receptors have been located on human T cells, indicating they may also play a role in the inflammatory cascade (Jutel et al. 2001; Lippert et al. 2004).

H3 Receptor

The third histamine receptor was described in 1983, at which time, it was determined to be located almost exclusively in the nervous system. An incredible amount of research has gone into discovering how this receptor intricately mediates its many psychological and physiologic effects. The H3 receptor is found throughout the brain as an autoinhibitory pre-synaptic receptor, receiving signals from histaminergic neurons localized in the tubaromammilary nucleus of the hypothalamus (Ireland-Denny et al. 2001).

In contrast to H1 receptors in the brain, H3 receptors act in an inhibitory manner. The H3 receptor inhibits the release of endogenous histamine, norepinephrine, serotonin, dopamine, and acetylcholine when activated (Arrang et al. 1983; Schlicker et al. 1988, 1993; Fink et al. 1990). This is caused by coupling of the $G_{i/o}$ protein which, when activated, leads to a decrease in intracellular calcium influx and a resulting decrease in depolarization frequency and histamine release (Arrang et al. 1985; Takeshita et al. 1998).

The H3 receptor may also play a role in other functions outside the central nervous system (CNS). H3 receptors have been identified in cardiac muscle and in the vascular system where they also appear to have inhibitory effects by decreasing release of norepinephrine (Luo et al. 1991; Xiao-Xing et al. 1991; Endou et al. 1994, Koyama et al. 2003). The H3 receptors outside the CNS do not appear to respond equally to antagonists determined to inhibit neuronal H3 receptors. This suggests that H3 receptors may have multiple subtypes (Taylor and Kilpatrick 1992).

Antagonizing this receptor leads to an increase in awareness and has improved memory and learning in experimental animals (Passani et al. 2007). As one of the newer receptors identified and cloned, targeted therapy for the H3 receptor is being developed for neurologic and psychological disorders.

H4 Receptor

Since its discovery in 2000, the H4 receptor has been shown to exist on the endothelium of the small intestine, respiratory tract, in bone marrow, and on hematopoietic cells, specifically immunologically active ones such as mast cells, eosinophils, and T cells (Liu et al. 2001; Schneider et al. 2002; Lippert et al. 2004). Although most closely related to the H3 receptor, they share only 37% genetic homology (Nakamura e al. 2000; Oda et al. 2000).

This receptor is coupled to a pertussis toxin sensitive $G_{i/o}$ protein. When activated, mast cells migrate toward a histamine gradient in epithelial tissue, eosinophils undergo a conformational change and express adhesion molecules necessary for chemotaxis, and pro-inflammatory cytokines are upregulated (Hofstra et al. 2003; Ling et al. 2004). This suggests an integral role in the inflammatory and immune system. Research is ongoing, but an in-depth understanding of the biological function of histamine at the H4 receptor remains to be elucidated.

Pharmacokinetics

In-depth pharmacokinetic data for antihistamines in veterinary species is lacking, and treatment is largely empirically based. Antihistamines share a similar biochemical structure with different substitution groups determining their class. Generally, antihistamines are highly protein-bound, distribute rapidly into tissues, and plasma clearance tends to occur in a biphasic manner. Bioavailability after oral administration varies widely as does clearance of the drugs across species (Bizikova et al. 2008; Hansson et al. 2004; Kuroda et al. 2013; Olsén et al. 2006). Current developments on H3 and H4 receptor antagonists are focused on efficacy and are not yet clinically applicable.

H1 Antihistamines

Due to their lipophilic nature, first-generation H1 antihistamines easily cross the blood–brain barrier and exert a sedating effect due to receptor binding in the brain. The chemical structure of second-generation H1 antagonists limits the ability to cross the blood–brain barrier and, as such, they are referred to as non-sedating antihistamines.

Detailed diphenhydramine studies in dogs and cats are sparse despite it being one of the most commonly used antihistamines. In large animals, diphenhydramine and antihistamines as a general drug class may not be of great use. The drug is rapidly distributed into tissues with a half-life of approximately 1.5 hours in the rabbit, 1 hour in the rat, monkey, dog, and sheep (Yoo et al. 1990). Although diphenhydramine distributes similarly in these species, the pharmacokinetics of diphenhydramine have been studied in horses, camels, and sheep to determine differing drug distribution and metabolism. Sheep rapidly clear the drug six times faster than horses while camels clear the drug twice as fast as horses (Wasfi et al. 2003).

Hydroxyzine, a first-generation compound, is commonly used successfully as an antipruritic agent in domestic species. It is the rapid conversion to the active metabolite cetirizine, a second-generation compound, which is responsible for the therapeutic effects. In one study in dogs, cetirizine plasma levels following hydroxyzine administration rapidly reached therapeutic concentrations with a half-life of approximately 10 hours regardless of IV or oral administration (Bizikova et al. 2008). This appears to be similar to cats where oral cetirizine administration resulted in high plasma concentrations and a half-life of 10 hours (Papich et al. 2008).

Clemastine is a highly protein bound weak base with low bioavailability in the dog (1–6%). Following oral administration in experimental healthy dogs, maximum concentration reached only 1 ng/ml with no inhibitory effect on histamine-induced wheals and erythema (Hansson et al. 2004). Likewise, chlorpheniramine undergoes rapid tissue distribution but the bioavailability is low in dogs and rabbits likely due to a first-pass metabolism (Athanikar and Chiou 1979; Huang and Chiou 1981).

In large animals, tripelennamine is one of the only antihistamines licensed for use in cattle and horses. *In vitro*, triepelennamine has been shown to inhibit histamine induced bovine pulmonary vein constriction, but clinical use *in vivo* is at best equivocal (Eyre 1971). One study showed that horses and camels distribute and clear the drug similarly with an average half-life of two hours (Wasfi et al. 2000). In large animals, chlorpheniramine has such poor potency that it is considered ineffective (Kuroda et al. 2013). Both clemastine and fexofenadine have high potency but very low bioavailability (3–4% in the horse for clemastine), which renders them useless (Törneke et al. 2003; Olsén et al. 2006).

H2-Receptor Antagonists

Cimetidine produces unusual biphasic plasma peak concentrations when administered orally to fasted dogs. This is also seen in laboratory animals, horses, and humans. Despite not being absorbed directly from the stomach, a low stomach pH of 3 increases the half-life from 24 minutes (with a stomach pH of 5) to 78 minutes (Mummaneni et al. 1995). In fasted dogs, orally administered cimetidine reaches Tmax in 30 minutes with good bioavailability of 75%. Administering cimetidine with food drastically reduces the bioavailability (Le Traon et al. 2009).

Ranitidine is approximately five times more potent than cimetidine and, in the rat, can decrease acid secretion for four hours (Scarpignato et al. 1987). In dogs, ranitidine has good bioavailability following oral administration with a half-life of four hours regardless of IV or oral dosing although its ability to significantly reduce stomach-acid secretion is under contention (Bersenas et al. 2005). Famotidine is a far more potent antagonist, approximately 50 times as potent as cimetidine. This is evidenced by a greater reduction in acid secretion in cats, rats and dogs (Coruzzi et al. 1986; Bersenas et al. 2005; Scarpignato et al. 1987).

In horses, the bioavailability of cimetidine varies widely but is generally much less than 50%, and a very large dose (48 mg/kg/day) is needed to reach therapeutic plasma levels (Smyth et al. 1990). Following oral administration, biphasic peak plasma concentrations are seen, but this does not occur following intragastric administration (Smyth et al. 1990; Sams et al. 1997).

Metabolism

Although an in-depth understanding of the metabolism and excretion of antihistamines in veterinary species is lacking, some research efforts have been successful in elucidating specific pathways. The major routes of metabolism and elimination are through the liver and kidney, respectively, although there is great variation in the degree of metabolism of different classes of antihistamines.

First-generation H1 antagonists are understood to undergo extensive hepatic metabolism. The predominant mechanism is via the cytochrome p450 enzyme CYP2D6 with a small degree of renal clearance. This metabolism becomes important in patients with hepatic insufficiency or concurrent administration of drugs that inhibit the cytochrome p450 pathway.

Despite sharing a common metabolic pathway, different species can eliminate the same drug in different fashions. For example, while camels largely eliminate diphenhydramine in its conjugated form with no hydroxy-metabolites detectable in urine, the major metabolite detected from horses is in fact hydroxy-diphenhydramine (Wasfi et al. 2003; Wynne et al. 1996). It is possible that not all first-generation H1 antagonists are excreted the same even within the same species. Although tripelennamine is also a first-generation H1 antihistamine, unlike diphenhydramine, it is largely excreted in camels via a hydroxylated metabolite (Wasfi et al. 2000). In sheep, in addition to hepatic metabolism, the intestinal tract is responsible for nearly 50% of the clearance of diphenhydramine (Kumar et al. 1999).

Second-generation H1 antagonists do not appear to entirely share the same route of metabolism. Ceterizine is one of the few second-generation H1 antagonists that does not get transformed into an active metabolite. Instead, it is largely eliminated via the kidneys via active tubular secretion and glomerular filtration. Ceterizine in horses undergoes very little biotransformation, which is consistent with studies performed in humans. Approximately 60–80% of cetirizine is eliminated in urine unchanged. Metabolites present are due to O-dealkylation by cytochrome p450 CYP3A4 (Olsén et al. 2008).

H2 antagonists, however, appear to be largely eliminated via the kidney, although a degree of hepatic metabolism does occur. Approximately 66% of an absorbed dose of ranitidine is eliminated unchanged in the urine of both dogs and rats. The metabolism that does occur plays a greater role at lower doses. Hepatic cytochrome p450 and the flavin-containing mono-oxygenase pathways are responsible for S-oxidation, N-oxidation, and N-demethylation of ranitidine (Eddershaw et al. 1996).

Renal clearance occurs by active tubular secretion as evidenced by the excretion of famotidine, cimetidine, and ranitidine in the dog and rat kidney (Boom et al. 1998). Although the process can be saturable, at therapeutic doses it is not (Muirhead and Somogyi 1991; Boom et al. 1997). This demonstrated ability for saturation is important when considering patients with compromised kidney function. In human subjects with impaired kidney function, famotidine total body clearance and renal clearance were significantly reduced (Takabatake et al. 1985).

Clinical Use

The most common clinical use for antihistamines remains in the treatment of pruritus for companion animals, especially dogs. In such a setting, both H1 and H2 antagonists may be employed in trial experiments given their range of efficacy (Scott and Miller 1999; Cook et al. 2004). It appears as if H2 blockers alone are not sufficient (Scott and Miller 1999) and may, in fact, not offer any relief to pruritic dogs on their own or in addition to H1 blockers (Scott et al. 1994). H2 blockers can be used to suppress gastric-acid secretion in companion animals which becomes clinically useful in the treatment of gastric or duodenal ulceration or in the event of regurgitation under general anesthesia. Famotidine can significantly raise gastric pH in dogs (Bersenas et al. 2005) and also reduces gastric volume in humans pre-anesthestically, suggesting prophylaxis potential against Mendelson's syndrome (Okuda et al. 1988). Famotidine is also beneficial in the treatment of stress and exercise-induced gastric lesions (Williamson et al. 2007), while cimetidine prevents sepsis-induced gastric ulcers (Odonkor et al. 1981).

Overall, clinical efficacy of antihistamines in large animals is equivocal. Arguably hydroxyzine, although not approved for use in large animals, shows promise as a component of treating equine urticaria (Rees 2001). Ceterizine can be a suitable component of treating allergies in horses based on its wheal formation inhibition and favorable pharmacokinetic profile (Olsén et al. 2008). Cyproheptadine has been reported as a potential treatment for photic headshaking in horses, but its successful outcomes, however, may be due more to its anti-serotonergic properties (Madigan et al. 1995). Antihistamines can also be used as an adjunct to treating respiratory disease in horses and cattle. In outbreaks of bovine respiratory syncytial virus, adding antihistamines to traditional therapies have helped return cattle to a state of health more quickly (Heckert and Hofmann 1993).

Previously H2 blockers may have been of use in the treatment of equine ulcers (Furr and Murray 1989), but the commonplace use of proton pump inhibitors for long-term ulcer prevention has rendered the H2 blockers unnecessary (Doucet et al. 2003). While cimetidine may play no role in healing or preventing equine gastric ulcers, it has been used as a treatment for equine melanoma (Nieto et al. 2001; Goetz et al. 1990).

First-generation antihistamines have been successfully used in the treatment of extrapyramidal signs induced by some common anesthetics such as propofol and alfaxalone (Sherer et al. 2017; Frias et al. 2020). The extrapyramidal signs manifest as myoclonus, dystonia, and ballismus that can be unresponsive to benzodiazepines and anticonvulsants. The antihistamines work in this situation via their anticholinergic properties that reset the balance between the dopaminergic and cholinergic influences in the nigrostriatal pathway (Glazer 2000).

Regarding the routine use of diphenhydramine in veterinary patients undergoing mast-cell tumor removal, there are limited sources identifying a specific benefit. In one paper assessing pre-treatment with diphenhydramine vs. placebo in canine patients undergoing mast-cell tumor removal, there was no statistically significant difference in plasma histamine levels between the two groups (Sanchez et al. 2017). Regardless, the safety profile of the medication and the slight reduction in histamine levels during mast-cell tumor manipulation can be supportive of veterinary practitioners choosing to use the medication preemptively.

Antihistamines may also be used in the event of an allergic reaction either in awake animals or those under general anesthesia. It is important to keep in mind that the drugs cannot reverse the action of histamine but instead prevent further activation of histamine receptors. In the event of an allergic reaction, however, more immunologically active substances than just histamine are at play. While histamine plays a large role in allergic reactions, in the event of true anaphylaxis, antihistamines alone are not enough to combat the cardiopulmonary effects (Silverman et al. 1988). The recently discovered H4 receptor may prove to have a large role in the inflammatory cascade.

Side Effects

Because of the inherent safety of antihistamines at therapeutic doses, reported drug interactions are rarely reported. Since their development in the mid-twentieth century, there has been the question of whether or not antihistamines are appropriate to be given prophylactically in the perioperative period.

CNS Effects

The most common side effect of antihistamines is sedation, more commonly seen with first-generation H1 antagonists that cross the blood–brain barrier. Under anesthesia, the administration of diphenhydramine has been shown to significantly increase sleeping time indicating an additive effect of the antihistamine-induced CNS depression (Winter and Flataker 1952). Despite this, when diphenhydramine is administered to awake dogs at clinically appropriate doses, appreciable sedation is not observed (Hoffmeister and Egger 2005; Sanchez et al. 2016). Also, in large animals, sedative side effects are not seen, potentially due to the metabolism in such species (Olsén et al. 2008).

First-generation antihistamines have low specificity and can cross react with other receptors. The older first-generation antihistamines especially have the potential to inhibit cholinergic, dopaminergic, and serotonin receptors. The dangers of toxicity of early antihistamines are associated with this lack of selectivity and their ability to cause an anticholinergic-like toxicity (Worth et al. 2016; Tanaka et al. 2011). In dogs, clinical signs of toxicity are dose related; very high doses of diphenhydramine lead to excitement, seizures, tremors, tachycardia, and hypertension whereas lower overdoses tend to result in milder clinical signs such as lethargy, nausea, and mydriasis (Worth et al. 2016). While the therapeutic margin of diphenhydramine is large, there is the probability that younger animals may be more sensitive to toxicity at lower doses (Lee 1966).

In the event of a serotonin syndrome event, cyproheptadine's anti-serotonergic properties have allowed for rapid control and treatment of a mild-to-moderate crisis (McDaniel 2001; Lappin and Auchincloss 1994).

Some of the later H1 antagonists have fewer side effects due to their lipophobic nature. Ceterizine, mizolastine, and terfenadine, for example, are far more selective for the H1 receptor with less binding to other receptors (Baroody and Naclerio 2000). Ceterizine at least has not been shown to cause anticholinergic side effects when administered to horses (Olsén et al. 2008).

Currently, H3 antagonists have yet to reach a clinically applicable stage in their development, although one would expect them to have substantial CNS effects regarding circadian rhythm and alertness.

Pulmonary Effects

In the lung, the actions of histamine at different receptors are opposing as are the actions of different antagonist classes. Histamine infusion causes a biphasic response in the pulmonary vasculature. An initial transient rise in pulmonary perfusion pressure with a correlating decrease in pulmonary vascular resistance is followed by a normalization of perfusion pressure and an increased pulmonary vascular resistance. When administered an H1 blocker, pulmonary vascular resistance is normalized. When administered an H2 antihistamine, the elevation of the pulmonary perfusion pressure was sustained with a marked increase in pulmonary vascular resistance. However, administering both an H1 and H2 blocker prevents changes in pulmonary pressure and vascular resistance. (Tucker et al. 1975). Via the H1 receptor, antihistamines can also lessen the severity of vascular permeability and pulmonary edema (Brigham et al. 1976).

Cardiovascular Effects

As a result of histamine release, H2 receptors facilitate an increase in heart rate and cardiac output while H1 receptors do the opposite. There is also a marked hypotension induced via both receptors and a decrease in total systemic resistance (Silverman et al. 1988; Wolff and Levi 1986). Although an initial tachycardia usually accompanies a drop in mean arterial pressure (MAP), the increase in cardiac output is transient and returns to baseline value within a few minutes. The arterial hypotension can be somewhat alleviated with administration of either an H1 or H2 blocker. If used individually, neither an H1 nor H2 blocker can completely abate the hypotension but, if given in combination, the arterial hypotension is prevented (Tucker et al. 1975). These findings have been repeatable *in vivo* and *in vitro* (Silverman et al. 1988).

When high doses of cimetidine are rapidly administered IV, there have been reports of peripheral hypotension, potentially due to histamine release. Unfortunately, combating this effect with a first-generation H1 antihistamine does not attenuate the hypotension (Paakhari et al. 1982).

Two notable antihistamines, terfenadine and astemizole, have been implicated in cardiac arrhythmias both in awake and anesthetized cats and dogs (Kii et al. 2003; Sugiyama 1997). These drugs cause bradycardia specifically by prolonging the QT interval, potentially leading to torsades des pointes and subsequent ventricular tachycardia (Usui et al. 1998). It appears that cats may be more sensitive to developing tachyarrythmias in response to terfenadine than are dogs.

In healthy human patients, ranitidine, but not loratidine, was found to decrease baroreceptor reflex and increase sympathetic predominance over heart rate (Nault et al. 2002).

On an anecdotal level, IV administration of famotidine to cats has been linked to hemolysis (Plumb 4th ed). However, when studied experimentally in over 140 hospitalized feline patients, no difference in hematocrit concentration over time or signs of hemolysis was found between feline patients that received famotidine by the IV or SC route (De Brito Galvao and Trepanier 2008).

Other Side Effects

As far as drug interactions are concerned, the greatest is the potential for increased sedation and respiratory depression when combined with opioids (Anwari and Iqbal 2003). There is evidence to suggest that H1 antihistamines and cimetidine can actually reduce emesis and potentiate opioid-induced analgesia when combined with fentanyl, morphine or nalbuphine (Sun et al. 1985; Bluhm et al. 1982; Lin et al. 2005). Moreover, H1 antagonists and famotidine when administered alone in mice can also produce antinociception (Sun et al. 1985; Abacıoğlu et al. 1993; Galeotti et al. 2002).

Beyond the risk for summation effect when administered with other anticholinergics or serotonin-reuptake inhibitors, antihistamines can potentially interfere with the metabolism of other drugs. Due to its imidazole ride, cimetidine has been proven to be an inhibitor of the p450 pathway, specifically CYP2D6 and CYP3A4 (Tanaka 1998; Somogyi and Gugler 1982). This clinically leads to prolonged half-lives and greater AUC for coadministered drugs that require the substrates for oxidative metabolism. Cimetidine significantly increases the Cmax of midazolam administered to human patients and significantly prolonged the duration of xylazine-ketamine anesthesia when tested in both rats and chickens (Klotz et al. 1985; Roder et al. 1993; Amouzadeh et al. 1989).

If using an H2 blocker such as famotidine for gastric-acid secretion prophylaxis in the perioperative period, it is essential to know if the patient has already received a proton pump inhibitor. In healthy dogs, administered both famotidine and pantoprazole, the intragastric pH was actually lower than if administered pantoprazole alone (Tolbert et al. 2015).

Contraindications

Overall, antihistamines are considered a reasonably safe group of drugs with most available over the counter. Given the lack of specificity of older generation antihistamines, certain conditions may require closer monitoring when considering the prolonged use of antihistamines. For example, given the anticholinergic side effects of first-generation H1 blockers, human literature reports iatrogenic increased intraocular pressures due to diphenhydramine administration. In healthy canine patients, however, pupil size did not significantly change following administration of diphenhydramine, although significant corneal dryness did result (Evans et al. 2012).

Although special consideration always needs to be given to pregnant or lactating animals, diphenhydramine, cimetidine, and ranitidine at high doses administered to rat dams has been shown not to have an effect on lactation composition. While the drugs were all detectable in the milk – cimetidine at a higher level than expected – they only caused very low plasma levels in nursing offspring with no deleterious effects in the offspring noted (Dostal and Schwetz 1989; Dostal et al. 1990).

References

Abacioğlu, N., Bediz, A., Çakici, İ. et al. (1993). Antinociceptive effects of H1-and H2-antihistaminics in mice. *Gen. Pharmacol. Vasc. Syst.* 24 (5): 1173–1176.

Amouzadeh, H.R., Sangiah, S., and Qualls, C.W., Jr (1989). Effects of some hepatic microsomal enzyme inducers and inhibitors on xylazine-ketamine anesthesia. *Vet. Hum. Toxicol.* 31 (6): 532–534.

Anwari, J.S., and Iqbal, S. (2003). Antihistamines and potentiation of opioid induced sedation and respiratory depression. *Anaesthesia* 58 (5): 494–495.

Arrang, J.M., Garbarg, M., and Schwartz, J.C. (1983). Auto-inhibition of brain histamine release mediated by a novel class (H3) of histamine receptor. *Nature* 302: 832–837.

Arrang, J.M., Garbarg, M., and Schwartz, J.C. (1985). Autoregulation of histamine release in brain by presynaptic H3-receptors. *Neuroscience* 15 (2): 553–562.

Ash, A.S.F. and Schild, H.O. (1966). Receptors mediating some actions of histamine. *Br. J. Pharmacol. Chemotherap.* 27 (2): 427–439.

Athanikar, N. and Chiou, W. (1979). Chlorpheniramine: effect of the first-pass metabolism on the oral bioavailability in dogs. *J. Pharmacokinet. Biopharm.* 7 (4): 383–396.

Bakker, R.A., Wieland, K., Timmerman, H., and Leurs, R. (2000). Constitutive activity of the histamine H1 receptor reveals inverse agonism of histamine H1 receptor antagonists. *Eur. J. Pharmacol.* 387 (1): 5–7.

Baroody, F. and Naclerio, R. (2000). Antiallergic effects of H1-receptor antagonists. *Allergy* 55 (64): 17–27.

Bersenas, A., Mathews, K., Allen, D., and Conlon, P. (2005). Effects of ranitidine, famotidine, pantoprazole, and omeprazole on intragastric pH in dogs. *Am. J. Vet. Res.* 66 (3): 425–431.

Bizikova, P., Papich, M., and Olivry, T. (2008). Hydroxyzine and cetirizine pharmacokinetics and pharmacodynamics after oral and intravenous administration of hydroxyzine to healthy dogs. *Vet. Dermatol.* 19 (6): 348–357.

Bluhm, R., Zsigmond, E., and Winnie, A. (1982). Potentiation of opioid analgesia by H1 and H2 antagonists. *Life Sci.* 31 (12, 13): 1229–1232.

Boom, S., Hoet, S., and Russel, F. (1997). Saturable urinary excretion kinetics of famotidine in the dog. *J. Pharm. Pharmacol.* 49 (3): 288–292.

Boom, S., Meyer, I., Wouterse, A., and Russel, F. (1998). A physiologically based kidney model for the renal clearance of ranitidine and the interaction with cimetidine and probenecid in the dog. *Biopharm. Drug Dispos.* 19 (3): 199–208.

Brigham, K., Bowers, R., and Owen, P. (1976). Effects of antihistamines on the lung vascular response to histamine in unanesthetized sheep. Diphenhydramine prevention of pulmonary edema and increased permeability. *J. Clin. Investig.* 58 (2): 391.

Brown, R., Stevens, D., and Haas, H. (2001). The physiology of brain histamine. *Prog. Neurobiol.* 63 (6): 637–672.

Chew, C., Hersey, S., Sachs, G., and Berglindh, T. (1980). Histamine responsiveness of isolated gastric glands. *Am. J. Physiol.* 238 (4): 312–320.

Cook, C., Scott, D., Miller, W. et al. (2004). Treatment of canine atopic dermatitis with cetirizine, a second generation antihistamine: a single-blinded, placebo-controlled study. *Can. Vet. J.* 45 (5): 414.

Coruzzi, G., Bertaccini, G., Noci, M., and Dobrilla, G. (1986). Inhibitory effect of famotidine on cat gastric secretion. *Agents Actions* 19 (3, 4): 188–193.

De Brito Galvao, J. and Trepanier, L. (2008). Risk of hemolytic anemia with intravenous administration of famotidine to hospitalized cats. *J. Vet. Intern. Med.* 22 (2): 325–329.

Dostal, L. and Schwetz, B. (1989). Determination of diphenhydramine in rat milk and plasma and its effects on milk composition and mammary gland nucleic acids. *J. Pharm. Sci.* 78 (5): 423–426.

Dostal, L., Weaver, R., and Schwetz, B. (1990). Excretion of high concentrations of cimetidine and ranitidine into rat milk and their effects on milk composition and mammary gland nucleic acid content. *Toxicol. Appl. Pharmacol.* 102 (3): 430–442.

Doucet, M.Y., Vrins, A.A., Dionne, R. et al. (2003). Efficacy of a paste formulation of omeprazole for the treatment of naturally occurring gastric ulcers in training standardbred racehorses in Canada. *Can. Vet. J.* 44 (7): 581–585.

Eddershaw, P., Chadwick, A., Higton, D. et al. (1996). Absorption and disposition of ranitidine hydrochloride in rat and dog. *Xenobiotica* 26 (9): 947–956.

Endou, M., Poli, E., and Levi, R. (1994). Histamine H3-receptor signaling in the heart: possible involvement of Gi/Go proteins and N-type Ca^{++} channels. *J. Pharmacol. Exp. Ther.* 269 (1): 221–229.

Evans, P., Lynch, G., and Labelle, P. (2012). Effects of oral administration of diphenhydramine on pupil diameter, intraocular pressure, tear production, tear film quality, conjunctival goblet cell density, and corneal sensitivity of clinically normal adult dogs. *Am. J. Vet. Res.* 73 (12): 1983–1986.

Eyre, P. (1969). The pharmacology of sheep tracheobronchial muscle: a relaxant effect of histamine on the isolated bronchi. *Br. J. Pharmacol.* 36 (3): 409–417.

Eyre, P. (1971). Pharmacology of bovine pulmonary vein anaphylaxis in vitro. *Br. J. Pharmacol.* 43 (2): 302–311.

Felix, S., Baumann, G., Helmus, S., and Sattelberger, U. (1988). The role of histamine in cardiac anaphylaxis; characerization of the histaminergic H1 and H2 receptor effects. *Basic Res. Cardiol.* 83 (5): 531–539.

Fink, K., Schlicker, E., Neise, A., and Göthert, M. (1990). Involvement of presynaptic H3 receptors in the inhibitory effect of histamine on serotonin release in the rat brain cortex. *Naunyn-Schmiedeberg's Arch. Pharmacol.* 342 (5): 513–519.

Frias, J., Michou, J., and Fadda, A. (2020). Chlorphenamine for prolonged drug-induced extrapyramidal side effects in a dog. *Vet. Rec.* 8 (4): 1136.

Fukui, H., Fujimoto, K., Mizuguchi, H. et al. (1994). Molecular cloning of the human histamine H1 receptor gene. *Biochem. Biophys. Res. Commun.* 201 (2): 894–901.

Furr, M.O., and Murray, M.J. (1989). Treatment of gastric ulcers in horses with histamine type 2 receptor antagonists. *Equine Vet. J. Suppl.* (7): 77–79.

Galeotti, N., Ghelardini, C., and Bartonlini, A. (2002). Antihistamine antinociception is mediated by Gi-protein activation. *Neuroscience* 109 (4): 811–818.

Gantz, I., Munzert, G., Tashiro, T. et al. (1991). Molecular cloning of the human histamine H2 receptor. *Biochem. Biophys. Res. Commun.* 178 (3): 1386–1392.

Glazer, W.M. (2000). Extrapyramidal side effects, tardive dyskinesia, and the concept of atypicality. *J. Clin. Psychiat.* 61 (3): 16–21.

Goetz, T., Ogilvie, G., Keegan, K., and Johnson, P. (1990). Cimetidine for treatment of melanomas in three horses. *J. Am. Vet. Med. Assoc.* 196 (3): 449–452.

Hansson, H., Bergvall, K., Bondesson, U. et al. (2004). Clinical pharmacology of clemastine in healthy dogs. *Vet. Dermatol.* 15 (3): 152–158.

Heckert, H. and Hofmann, W. (1993). Clinical indications of an auxiliary effect of antihistamines (parenteral benadryl) in the treatment of RSV infections of cattle. *Berl. Munch. Tierarztl. Wochenschr.* 106 (7): 230–235.

Hofmeister, E. and Egger, C. (2005). Evaluation of diphenhydramine as a sedative for dogs. *J. Am. Vet. Med. Assoc.* 226 (7): 1092–1094.

Hofstra, C., Desai, P., Thurmond, R., and Fung-Leung, W. (2003). Histamine H4 receptor mediates chemotaxis and calcium mobilization of mast cells. *J. Pharmacol. Exp. Ther.* 305 (3): 1212–1221.

Huang, S. and Chiou, W. (1981). Pharmacokinetics and tissue distribution of chlorpheniramine in rabbits after intravenous administration. *J. Pharmacokinet. Biopharm.* 9 (6): 711–723.

Ireland-Denny, L., Parihar, A., Miller, T. et al. (2001). Species-related pharmacological heterogeneity of histamine H3 receptors. *Eur. J. Pharmacol.* 433 (2): 141–150.

Jahn, K., Haas, H., and Hatt, H. (1995). Patch clamp study of histamine activated potassium currents on rabbit olfactory bulb neurons. *Naunyn-Schmiedeberg's Arch. Pharmacol.* 352 (4): 386–393.

Jutel, M., Watanabe, T., Klunker, S. et al. (2001). Histamine regulates T-cell and antibody responses by differential expression of H1 and H2 receptors. *Nature* 413 (6854): 420–425.

Kii, Y., Nakatsuji, K., Nose, I. et al. (2003). Effects of antihistamines, ebastine and terfenadine, on electrocardiogram in conscious dogs and cats. *Drug Dev. Res.* 58 (2): 209–217.

Klotz, U., Arvela, P., and Rosenkranz, B. (1985). Effect of single doses of cimetidine and ranitidine on the steady-state plasma levels of midazolam. *Clin. Pharmacol. Ther.* 38 (6): 652–655.

Koyama, M., Seyedi, N., Fung-Leung, W. et al. (2003). Norepinephrine release from the ischemic heart is greatly enhanced in mice lacking histamine H3 receptors. *Mol. Pharmacol.* 63 (2): 378–382.

Kumar, S., Riggs, K., and Rurak, D. (1999). Role of the liver and gut in systemic diphenhydramine clearance in adult nonpregnant sheep. *Drug Metab. Dispos.* 27 (2): 297–302.

Kuroda, T., Nagata, S., Takizawa, Y. et al. (2013). Pharmacokinetics and pharmacodynamics of d-chlorpheniramine following intravenous and oral administration in healthy Thoroughbred horses. *Vet. J.* 197 (2): 433–437.

Lappin, R. and Auchincloss, E. (1994). Treatment of the serotonin syndrome with cyproheptadine. *N. Engl. J. Med.* 331 (15): 1021–1022.

Lee, C. (1966). Comparative pharmacologic responses to antihistamines in newborn and young rats. *Toxicol. Appl. Pharmacol.* 8 (2): 210–217.

Le Traon, G., Burgaud, S., and Horspool, L.J. (2009). Pharmacokinetics of cimetidine in dogs after oral administration of cimetidine tablets. *J. Vet. Pharm. Therap.* 32 (3): 213–218.

Leurs, R., Church, M., and Taglialatela, M. (2002). H1-antihistamines: inverse agonism, anti-inflammatory actions and cardiac effects. *Clin. Exp. Allergy* 32 (4): 489–498.

Lin, T.F., Yeh, Y.C., Yen, Y.H. et al. (2005). Antiemetic and analgesic-sparing effects of diphenhydramine added to morphine intravenous patient-controlled analgesia. *Br. J. Anaesth.* 94 (6): 835–839.

Ling, P., Ngo, K., Nguyen, S. et al. (2004). Histamine H4 receptor mediates eosinophil chemotaxis with cell shape change and adhesion molecule upregulation. *Br. J. Pharmacol.* 142 (1): 161–171.

Lippert, U., Artuc, M., Grützkau, A. et al. (2004). Human skin mast cells express H2 and H4, but not H3 receptors. *J. Investig. Dermatol.* 123 (1): 116–123.

Liu, C., Ma, X.J., Jiang, X. et al. (2001). Cloning and pharmacological characterization of a fourth histamine receptor (H4) expressed in bone marrow. *Mol. Pharmacol.* 59 (3): 420–426.

Loew, E. (1947). Pharmacology of antihistamine compounds. *Physiol. Rev.* 27 (4): 542–573.

Lovenberg, T., Roland, B., Wilson, S. et al. (1999). Cloning and functional expression of the human histamine H3 receptor. *Mol. Pharmacol.* 55 (6): 1101–1107.

Luo, X.X., et al. (1991). Histamine H3-receptors inhibit sympathetic neurotransmission in guinea pig myocardium. *Eur. J. Pharmacol.* 204 (3): 311–314.

Madigan, J., Kortz, G., Murphy, C., and Rodger, L. (1995). Photic headshaking in the horse: 7 cases. *Equine Vet. J.* 27 (4): 306–311.

Mayhan, W. (1994). Nitric oxide accounts for histamine-induced increases in macromolecular extravasation. *Am. J. Physiol. Heart Circul. Physiol.* 266 (6): 2369–2373.

McDaniel, W. (2001). Serotonin syndrome: early management with cyproheptadine. *Ann. Pharmacotherap.* 35 (7, 8): 870–873.

Mikkelsen, E., Sakr, A., and Jesperson, L. (1984). Studies on the effect of histamine in isolated human pulmonary arteries and veins. *Acta Pharmacol. Toxicol.* 54 (2): 86–93.

Muirhead, M. and Somogyi, A. (1991). Effect of H2 antagonists on the differential secretion of triamterene and its sulfate conjugate metabolite by the isolated perfused rat kidney. *Drug Metab. Dispos.* 19 (2): 312–316.

Mummaneni, V., Amidon, G., and Dressman, J. (1995). Gastric pH influences the appearance of double peaks in the plasma concentration-time profiles of cimetidine after oral administration in dogs. *Pharm. Res.* 12 (5): 780–786.

Nakamura, T., Itadani, H., Hidaka, Y. et al. (2000). Molecular cloning and characterization of a new human histamine receptor, HH4R. *Biochem. Biophys. Res. Commun.* 279 (2): 615–620.

Nault, M.A., Milne, B., and Parlow, J. (2002). Effects of the selective H1 and H2 histamine receptor antagonists loratadine and ranitidine on autonomic control of the heart. *Anesthesiology* 96 (2): 336–341.

Nguyen, T., Shapiro, D., George, S. et al. (2001). Discovery of a novel member of the histamine receptor family. *Mol. Pharmacol.* 59 (3): 427–433.

Nieto, J., Spier, S., Hoogmoed, L. et al. (2001). Comparison of omeprazole and cimetidine in healing of gastric ulcers and prevention of recurrence in horses. *Equine Vet. Educ.* 13 (5): 260–264.

Oda, T., Morikawa, N., Saito, Y. et al. (2000). Molecular cloning and characterization of a novel type of histamine receptor preferentially expressed in leukocytes. *J. Biol. Chem.* 275 (47): 36781–36786.

Odonkor, P., Mowat, C., and Himal, H. (1981). Prevention of sepsis-induced gastric lesions in dogs by cimetidine via inhibition of gastric secretion and by prostaglandin via cytoprotection. *Gastroenterology* 80 (2): 375–379.

Okuda, T., Takatsu, T., Kumode, O. et al. (1988). Effect of preanesthetic famotidine on gastric volume and pH. *J. Anesth.* 2 (1): 17–21.

Olsén, L., Ingvast-Larsson, C., Larsson, P. et al. (2006). Fexofenadine in horses: pharmacokinetics, pharmacodynamics and effect of ivermectin pretreatment. *J. Vet. Pharmacol. Therap.* 29 (2): 129–135.

Olsén, L., Bondesson, U., Broström, H. et al. (2008). Cetirizine in horses: pharmacokinetics and pharmacodynamics following repeated oral administration. *Vet. J.* 177 (2): 242–249.

Paakkari, I., Tötterman, K., Kupari, M. et al. (1982). Peripheral hypotensive and central hypertensive effects of cimetidine. *Agents Actions* 12 (1, 2): 152–155.

Papich, M., Schooley, E., and Reinero, C. (2008). Pharmacokinetics of cetirizine in healthy cats. *Am. J. Vet. Res.* 69 (5): 670–674.

Parsons, M. and Ganellin, C. (2006). Histamine and its receptors. *Br. J. Pharmacol.* 147 (1): 127–135.

Passani, M.B., Giannoni, P., Bucherelli, C. et al. (2007). Histamine in the brain: beyond sleep and memory. *Biochem. Pharmacol.* 73 (8): 1113–1122.

Rees, C. (2001). Response to immunotherapy in six related horses with urticaria secondary to atopy. *J. Am. Vet. Med. Assoc.* 218 (5): 753–755.

Riley, J. (1965). Histamine and Sir Henry Dale. *Br. Med. J.* 1 (5448): 1488–1490.

Roder, J., Akkaya, R., Amouzadeh, H. et al. (1993). Effects of hepatic P-450 enzyme inhibitors and inducers on the duration of xylazine+ ketamine anesthesia in broiler chickens and mice. *Vet. Hum. Toxicol.* 35 (2): 116–118.

Sams, R., Gerken, D., Dyke, T. et al. (1997). Pharmacokinetics of intravenous and intragastric cimetidine in horses I. Effects of intravenous cimetidine on pharmacokinetics of intravenous phenylbutazone. *J. Vet. Pharmacol. Therap.* 20 (5): 355–361.

Sanchez, A., Valverde, A., Sinclair, M. et al. (2016). The pharmacokinetics of DPH after the administration of a single intravenous or intramuscular dose in healthy dogs. *J. Vet. Pharmacol. Therap.* 30: 452–459.

Sanchez, A., Valverde, A., Sinclair, M. et al. (2017). Antihistaminic and cardiorespiratory effects of diphenhydramine hydrochloride in anesthetized dogs undergoing excision of mast cell tumors. *J. Am. Vet. Med. Assoc.* 251 (7): 804–813.

Scarpignato, C., Tramacere, R., and Zappia, L. (1987). Antisecretory and antiulcer effect of the H2-receptor antagonist famotidine in the rat: comparison with ranitidine. *Br. J. Pharmacol.* 92 (1): 153–159.

Schlicker, E., Betz, R., and Göthert, M. (1988). Histamine H3 receptor-mediated inhibition of serotonin release in the rat brain cortex. *Naunyn-Schmiedeberg's Arch. Pharmacol.* 337 (5): 588–590.

Schlicker, E., Fink, K., Detzner, M., and Göthert, M. (1993). Histamine inhibits dopamine release in the mouse striatum via presynaptic H3 receptors. *J. Neural Transm. Gen. Sect.* 93 (1): 1–10.

Schneider, E., Rolli-Derkinderen, M., Arock, M., and Dy, M. (2002). Trends in histamine research: new functions during immune responses and hematopoiesis. *Trends Immunol.* 23 (5): 255–263.

Scott, D. and Miller, W. (1999). Antihistamines in the management of allergic pruritus in dogs and cats. *J. Small Anim.Pract.* 40 (8): 359–364.

Scott, D., Miller, W., Cayatte, S., and Decker, G. (1994). Failure of terfenadine as an antipruritic agent in atopic dogs: results of a double-blinded, placebo-controlled study. *Can. Vet. J.* 35 (5): 286.

Sherer, J., Salazar, T., Schesin, K. et al. (2017). Diphenhydramine for acute extrapyramidal symptoms after propofol administration. *Pediatrics* 139 (2): 1135.

Shi, W., Wang, C., Dandurand, R. et al. (1998). Differential responses of pulmonary arteries and veins to histamine and 5-HAT in lung explants of guinea-pigs. *Br. J. Pharmacol.* 123: 1525–1532.

Shibamoto, T., Cui, S., Ruan, Z., and Kurata, Y. (2005). Effects of norepinephrine and histamine on vascular resistance in isolated perfused mouse liver. *Jpn. J. Physiol.* 55: 143–148.

Silverman, H., Taylor, W., Smith, P. et al. (1988). Effects of antihistamines on the cardiopulmonary changes due to canine anaphylaxis. *J. Appl. Phys.* 64 (1): 210–217.

Smyth, G., Duran, S., Ravis, W., and Clark, C. (1990). Pharmacokinetic studies of cimetidine hydrochloride in adult horses. *Equine Vet. J.* 22 (1): 48–50.

Soll, A. and Wollin, A. (1979). Histamine and cyclic AMP in isolated canine parietal cells. *Am. J. Physiol.* 237 (5): 444–450.

Somogyi, A. and Gugler, R. (1982). Drug interactions with cimetidine. *Clin. Pharmacokinet.* 7 (1): 23–41.

Sugiyama, A., Aye, N.N., Katahira, S. et al. (1997). Effects of nonsedating antihistamine, astemizole, on the in situ canine heart assessed by cardiohemodynamic and monophasic action potential monitoring. *Toxicol. Appl. Pharmacol.* 143 (1): 89–95.

Sun, C., Hui, F., and Hanig, J. (1985). Effect of H1 blockers alone and in combination with morphine to produce antinociception in mice. *Neuropharmacology* 24 (1): 1–4.

Takabatake, T., Ohta, H., Maekawa, M. et al. (1985). Pharmacokinetics of famotidine, a new H2-receptor antagonist, in relation to renal function. *Eur. J. Clin. Pharmacol.* 28 (3): 327–331.

Takeshita, Y., Watanabe, T., Sakata, T. et al. (1998). Histamine modulates high-voltage-activated calcium channels in neurons dissociated from the rat tuberomammillary nucleus. *Neuroscience* 87 (4): 797–805.

Tanaka, E. (1998). Clinically important pharmacokinetic drug–drug interactions: role of cytochrome P450 enzymes. *J. Clin. Pharm. Therap.* 23 (6): 403–416.

Tanaka, T., Takasu, A., Yoshino, A. et al. (2011). Diphenhydramine overdose mimicking serotonin syndrome. *Psychiat. Clin. Neurosci.* 65 (5): 534.

Taylor, S.J., and Kilpatrick, G.J. (1992). Characterization of histamine-H3 receptors controlling non-adrenergic non-cholinergic contractions of the guinea-pig isolated ileum. *Br. J. Pharm.* 105 (3): 667–674.

Tolbert, M., Odunayo, A., Howell, R. et al. (2015). Efficacy of intravenous administration of combined acid suppressants in healthy dogs. *J. Vet. Intern. Med.* 29 (2): 556–560.

Törneke, K., Ingvast-Larsson, C., Pettersson, K. et al. (2003). Pharmacokinetics and pharmacodynamics of clemastine in healthy horses. *J. Vet. Pharmacol. Therap.* 26 (2): 151–157.

Tucker, A., Weir, E., Reeves, J., and Grover, R. (1975). Histamine H1-and H2-receptors in pulmonary and systemic vasculature of the dog. *Am. J. Phys.* 229 (4): 1008–1013.

Usui, T., Sugiyama, A., Ishida, Y. et al. (1998). Simultaneous assessment of the hemodynamic, cardiomechanical, and electrophysiological effects of terfenadine on the in vivo canine model. *Heart Vessels* 13 (2): 49–57.

Wasfi, I., Boni, N., Elghazali, M. et al. (2000). Lack of effect of repeated administration of tripelennamine on antipyrine disposition in camels. *J. Vet. Pharmacol. Therap.* 23 (6): 409–412.

Wasfi, I., Hadi, A., Elghazali, M. et al. (2003). Comparative pharmacokinetics of diphenhydramine in camels and horses after intravenous administration. *Vet. Res. Commun.* 27 (6): 463–473.

Wieland, K., Bongers, G., Yamamoto, Y. et al. (2001). Constitutive activity of histamine H3 receptors stably expressed in SK-N-MC cells: display of agonism and inverse agonism by H3 antagonists. *J. Pharmacol. Exp. Ther.* 299 (3): 908–914.

Williamson, K., Willard, M., McKenzie, E. et al. (2007). Efficacy of famotidine for the prevention of exercise-induced gastritis in racing Alaskan sled dogs. *J. Vet. Intern. Med.* 21 (5): 924–927.

Winter, C. and Flataker, L. (1952). The effect of cortisone, desoxycorticosterone, adrenocorticotrophic hormone and diphenhydramine upon the responses of albino mice to general anesthetics. *J. Pharmacol. Exp. Ther.* 105 (3): 358–364.

Wolff, A. and Levi, R. (1986). Histamine and cardiac arrhythmias. *Circul. Res.* 58 (1): 1–16.

Worth, A., Wismer, T., and Dorman, D. (2016). Diphenhydramine exposure in dogs: 621 cases (2008–2013). *J. Am. Vet. Med. Assoc.* 249 (1): 77–82.

Wynne P., Vine J., and Batty D. (1996). Diphenhydramine metabolism and excretion in the horse. *Proceedings of the 11th International Conference of Racing Analysts and Veterinarians*, Queensland, Australia. R&W Publications.

Xiao-Xing, L., Yue-Hua, T., and Bao-Hen, S. (1991). Histamine H3-receptors inhibit sympathetic neurotransmission in guinea pig myocardium. *Eur. J. Pharmacol.* 204 (3): 311–314.

Yamashita, M., Fukui, H., Sugama, K. et al. (1991). Expression cloning of a cDNA encoding the bovine histamine H1 receptor. *Proc. Natl. Acad.Sci. U.S.A.* 88 (24): 11515–11519.

Yoo, S., Axelson, J., Kwan, E., and Rurak, D. (1990). Pharmacokinetics of diphenhydramine after dose ranging in nonpregnant ewes. *J. Pharm. Sci.* 79 (2): 106–110.

27

Anti-nausea, Antacid, and Prokinetic Drugs

Phillip Lerche

Introduction

Peri-anesthetic vomiting, regurgitation and gastro-esophageal reflux (GER) are undesirable due to the risk for aspiration pneumonia, esophagitis, and development of esophageal stricture, all of which increase morbidity and mortality. Multiple factors contribute to peri-anesthetic vomiting and regurgitation in cats and dogs, including pre-anesthetic fasting time, patient factors, anesthetic drugs, and surgical procedure, position during, and duration of surgery (Figueiredo 2022). The AHAA Anesthesia and Monitoring Guidelines for Dogs and Cats recommend using such drugs only in patients with a history or increased risk of regurgitation (Grubb 2020). The use of medications with anti-emetic and/or antacid effects is common in clinical practice despite the absence of clear evidence that they effectively decrease the incidence of aspiration pneumonia or esophageal injury in healthy animals. This is likely due to the low incidence of side effects, the goal of decreasing patient discomfort (anti-emetic), and the desire to make gastric pH less acidic (antacids), which reduces tissue damage should reflux or aspiration of gastric contents occur. Many of these medications have also been evaluated in large animal species as they are used to treat gastrointestinal (GI) ulceration, however, as these species are not typically at risk for peri-anesthetic vomiting, regurgitation, or GER that leads to serious complications, the focus of this chapter will be largely on small animal.

Antiemetics

Maropitant

Injectable maropitant is licensed for use in cats and dogs to treat and prevent acute vomiting. Maropitant is also available in tablet form to treat and prevent vomiting associated with motion sickness.

Mechanism of Action

Neurokinin-1 (NK-1) receptors are present in many body systems, including both the vomiting center and the chemoreceptor trigger zone (CTZ), which are located inside and outside the blood–brain barrier respectively. Substance P is the primary ligand for the NK-1 receptor and has an emetic effect in these locations. Maropitant is an NK-1 receptor antagonist that acts by preventing substance P from binding to the NK-1 receptor, resulting in an anti-emetic effect.

Pharmacokinetics

Maropitant has a rapid onset when given IV to dogs (1.8 minutes), and a slower onset when given by the SC route to dogs (45 minutes) and cats (30–120 minutes) (Benchaoui 2007; Hickman 2008). If administered SC, it should be given one hour prior to a drug which is known to cause vomiting, e.g. opioids (Kraus 2017). Injection pain has been observed after administration of maropitant and is thought to be associated with the amount of unbound drug present. At lower temperatures, more maropitant is bound to cyclodextrin, and administering refrigerated maropitant to dogs resulted in a decrease in pain on injection compared to injecting room temperature or warmed drug (Narishetty 2009). Following parenteral administration, maropitant undergoes hepatic metabolism via cytochrome P450 enzymes. In dogs, the primary route of excretion is hepatic, with less than 1% excreted in urine (Benchaoui 2007). The pharmacokinetics of maropitant administered IV and via nasogastric tube have been evaluated in horses (Berryhill 2019). Selected pharmacokinetic data are compared in Table 27.1 (Benchaoui 2007; Hickman 2008; Berryhill 2019).

Pharmacodynamics

Anti-emetic Effect When Given Prior to an Emetigen   In dogs, maropitant 1 mg/kg administered SC one hour prior to hydromorphone eliminated nausea and vomiting

Table 27.1 Comparison of selected pharmacokinetic data for maropitant.

Species	Pharmacokinetic parameter	Maropitant 1 mg/kg IV	Maropitant 1 mg/kg SC	Maropitant 1 mg/kg PO (cat) 2 mg/kg PO/IG (dog/horse)
Cat	C_{max}	998^a	269	156
	T_{max}	NA	0.5–2.0	2–3
	$T_{1/2}$	4.9^a	6.6^a	NA
Dog	C_{max}	1920	92	81
	T_{max}	0.03	0.75	1.9
	$T_{1/2}$	6.25	7.75	4.0
Horse	C_{max}	814	NA	80
	T_{max}	NA	NA	1.5
	$T_{1/2}$	10.4	NA	11.6

IV, intravenous; SC, subcutaneous; PO, per os; IG, intragastric; C_{max}, peak plasma concentration (ng/mL); T_{max}, time to peak plasma concentration (h); $T_{1/2}$, half life (h); NA, data not available.
[a] Data from package insert, Cerenia, Zoetis, Inc., 2015.

compared to saline prior to hydromorphone, where all dogs experienced nausea, vomiting or retching (Kraus 2013). Kraus also showed that vomiting after hydromorphone can be prevented in dogs by administering maropitant 30 minutes before the opioid injection. However, in order to eliminate signs of both vomiting and nausea, maropitant needs to be given one hour before (Kraus 2014). Maropitant administered SC to dogs 45 minutes before morphine significantly reduced vomiting compared to metaclopromide and saline (Lorenzutti 2017).

In cats, maropitant 1 mg/kg administered SC two hours prior to xylazine significantly reduced the incidence of vomiting (Hickman 2008). Maropitant given SC 20 hours prior to premedication with dexmedetomidine and morphine significantly decreased nausea, retching and vomiting compared to saline (Martin-Flores 2016).

Impact on Gastro-esophageal Reflux Maropitant given prior to anesthesia did not decrease the incidence of GER and did not decrease the number of reflux events recorded by esophageal pH probe compared to saline control, despite maropitant effectively preventing vomiting (Johnson 2014). Dogs that were given maropitant (1 mg/kg SC) 45 minutes prior to anesthesia and then received an infusion of metoclopramide (2 mg/kg/d IV) for 24 hours did not have a decreased incidence of regurgitation (Jones 2019).

Impact on Inhalant Anesthetic Requirement, and Antinociceptive Effect Maropitant has been shown to reduce the MAC of sevoflurane in dogs between 16% (mechanical noxious stimulus) and 24% (visceral noxious stimulus) (Boscan 2011; Marquez 2015). MAC-BAR (MAC required to blunt autonomic response) of sevoflurane was reduced by 15% in dogs given maropitant (Fukui 2017). Maropitant reduced sevoflurane MAC in cats by 15% (Niyom 2013). MAC reduction by maropitant is likely due to antagonism of NK-1 receptors in the central nervous system (CNS), resulting in anti-nociception (Niyom 2013). In rats, more than 80% of visceral nociceptive afferent fibers have been shown to express substance P compared to about 21% of cutaneous afferents (Perry 1998). This likely explains differences in MAC reduction, based on whether a somatic or a visceral model of noxious stimulus is investigated.

Cardiovascular Effects Maropitant caused a decrease in arterial blood pressure when given IV to awake and anesthetized dogs, with significant hypotension (mean arterial BP < 60 mmHg) observed in the anesthetized dogs (Chi 2020).

Post-anesthetic Effects Dogs given maropitant prior to anesthesia had better recovery scores, faster return to eating, and better appetites compared to a control group (Ramsey 2014).

Ondansetron

Ondansetron is available in oral and injectable forms and is most commonly used off label as an anti-nausea drug in chemotherapy patients. It is also effective in decreasing nausea in dogs with acute vestibular syndrome, (Henze 2022), and as a general anti-emetic in cats (Trepanier 2010).

Mechanism of Action

Ondansetron is an antagonist of central and peripheral 5-hydroxytryptamine$_3$ (5-HT$_3$) receptors.

Pharmacokinetics

In dogs, ondansetron has a low oral bioavailability (<10%) due to first pass metabolism, is cleared via hepatic metabolism and largely excreted in bile (Saynor and Dixon 1989).

In cats, oral and subcutaneous bioavailability are 32% and 75%, respectively, with a half-life range of 1.5–3 hours (Quimby 2014). Clearance was reduced in cats with hepatic, but not renal disease (Fitzpatrick 2016).

Pharmacodynamics

Anti-emetic Effect When Given Prior to an Emetigen Ondansetron was comparable to maropitant in significantly decreasing nausea in dogs in a low-dose cisplatin nausea and vomiting model, compared to maropitant which did not decrease nausea and vomiting (Kenward 2017). In ferrets, ondansetron at 3 mg/kg IV and 10 mg/kg IV decreased morphine-induced vomiting by 47% and 70%, respectively (Wynn 1993). Ondansetron 0.22 mg/kg IM given to cats decreased the incidence of vomiting by 45% when administered together with dexmedetomidine and buprenorphine compared to a control group (Santos 2011).

Antacids

Antacids are frequently administered to cats and dogs that are at risk of GER in the peri-operative period to increase gastric pH, based on the theory that if regurgitation of stomach contents into the esophagus occurs, it will cause less mucosal irritation at a higher pH. The two main classes of antacids used in the preoperative period are proton pump inhibitors (PPIs) and histamine$_2$ receptor antagonists (H$_2$RAs), with the former being far more effective at changing gastric pH (Marks 2018).

Proton Pump Inhibitors

Mechanism of Action

PPIs act by irreversibly binding to and inhibiting the hydrogen-potassium-ATPase enzyme which exchanges intracellular hydrogen with extracellular potassium and contributes to secretion of hydrochloric acid by gastric parietal cells (Wallmark 1989). In other words, the stomach must produce new proton pumps in order for acid production to return to normal following administration of a PPI. Omeprazole is a prodrug that is converted to its active form within gastric parietal cells (Oosterhuis 1989).

Esomeprazole is the levorotatory isomer of omeprazole (S-omeprazole) (Hultman 2007). Like omeprazole, pantoprazole is also a prodrug (Beil 1999). Omeprazole, esomeprazole, and pantoprazole have all been studied in domestic animals.

Pharmacokinetics

Metabolism of omeprazole in dogs occurs in the liver via cytochrome P450 enzymes (CYP2C21, CYP2C41, CYP2C94) (Uno 2023). In dogs, rats and mice, omeprazole is metabolized extensively to multiple metabolites that are rapidly eliminated via the feces (approximately two thirds) and urine (one third) (Regårdh 1985; Hoffmann 1986). Omeprazole is relatively highly protein bound in dogs (90%).

Pharmacokinetics of esomeprazole have been studied in conscious dogs, goats and sheep. Esomeprazole (1 mg/kg IV) is rapidly metabolized in all three species, with a half-life of 6 minutes in goats, 12 minutes in sheep, and 42 minutes in dogs (Seo et al. 2019; Fladung 2022; Smith 2023).

Pantoprazole pharmacokinetics have been reported in neonatal calves (1 mg/kg IV), alpacas (1 mg/kg), and foals (1.5 mg/kg IV). Elimination half-life was 0.47, 1.43, and 2.81 hours in alpacas, foals and calves, respectively (Smith 2010; Ryan 2005; Olivarez 2020).

Pharmacodynamics

Impact on Gastric pH and Gastro-esophageal Reflux Omeprazole (1.45 mg/kg and 2.2 mg/kg PO) given to cats 18–24 hours and 4 hours prior to anesthesia showed a significant increase in gastric pH (range of pH was 6.6–7.8) compared to placebo (range of pH was 1.3–4.1). Esophageal pH was also higher in the treatment groups compared to placebo. Cats that received placebo were 2.75 times more likely to have an episode of GER compared to those receiving omeprazole (Garcia 2017).

Gastric pH was increased in dogs given omeprazole 1 mg/kg PO the evening before and 1 mg/kg PO three hours prior to anesthesia compared to a control group, as well as in dogs receiving a single omeprazole dose the evening before (Lotti 2021). GER was not different among groups in that study, and 7% of GER was strongly acidic in the dogs that received two doses of omeprazole compared to those receiving a single or no dose. In another study, when omeprazole (1 mg/kg PO) was given four hours prior to anesthesia, the incidence of GER was 4.7 times more likely to occur in the control group (Panti 2009). Esomeprazole (1 mg/kg IV) given 12–18 hours and 1–1.5 hours prior to anesthetic induction increased gastric and esophageal pH, however, it did not affect the incidence of GER compared to a control group (Zacuto 2012).

As an antacid, pantoprazole is as efficacious as omeprazole, however to the author's knowledge, its impact on GER during general anesthesia has not been evaluated.

Drug Interactions Omeprazole (1 mg/kg PO twice daily) and carprofen (4 mg/kg PO once daily) given to dogs for seven days has been shown to cause an increase in intestinal inflammatory markers, and dysbiosis (imbalance of gut bacteria) (Jones 2020).

Other PPIs

Long-acting Omeprazole
A long-acting form of omeprazole for IM administration has been evaluated in conscious dogs and horses (Odunayo 2022; Sykes 2017). Gastric pH was increased for five days in dogs following a dose of 4 mg/kg; side effects included vomiting and inappetence. In horses, gastric pH was increased 66% of the time for one to seven days after administration.

Histamine₂ Receptor Antagonists
Histamine subtype 2 (H_2) receptors in the gastric parietal cells result in increased acid (hydrogen) production in the stomach when stimulated. This group of drugs includes cimetidine, ranitidine, and famotidine.

Mechanism of Action
H_2RAs act by reversibly antagonizing H_2 receptors in gastric parietal cells. This results in lower concentrations of intracellular cAMP, which causes a decrease in hydrogen-potassium-ATPase activity, and therefore less hydrogen ion (acid) secretion into the lumen of the stomach.

Pharmacokinetics
Approximately 70% of ranitidine is eliminated via urinary excretion, with oxidation accounting for about 30% in dogs (Eddershaw 1996).

Pharmacodynamics
Impact on Gastric pH and Gastro-esophageal Reflux There are relatively few studies examining the effect of H2As on GER in the perianesthetic period. Ranitidine (2 mg/kg IV) given six hours prior to anesthesia did not significantly increase esophageal pH or reduce the incidence of GER in dogs (Favarato 2012). Famotidine administration twice daily in dogs has been shown to be better at increasing gastric pH compared to once daily dosing, and compared to ranitidine (Bersenas 2005).

Cardiovascular System Cimetidine (200 mg IV) caused vasodilation and decreased blood pressure in anesthetized dogs, whereas this did not occur when ranitidine (50 mg IV)
was given (Breuer 1984). Heart rate and cardiac output were not significantly different for either drug in that study. In another experimental study in anesthetized dogs, cimetidine resulted in dose-dependent decreases in heart rate and blood pressure at doses greater than 3 mg/kg IV, with decreases in cardiac output at doses greater than 30 mg/kg. This is in contrast to famotidine, which did not cause cardiovascular changes when given up to 30 mg/kg IV (Miyata 1990).

Cimetidine, ranitidine and famotidine have all been shown to blunt the cranial blood flow response to hypoxemia in awake dogs (Audibert 1991).

Prokinetics

Metoclopromide

Metoclopromide is available in injectable and oral formulations and is used off-label in veterinary medicine as it is not approved for use in animals. It has anti-emetic and pro-kinetic properties. There is limited data available concerning pharmacokinetics of metoclopramide in animals.

Mechanism of Action
Metoclopromide exerts its anti-emetic action via dopaminergic receptor antagonism, acting as an antagonist on the D_2 dopamine receptor subtype in the CTZ. Its prokinetic properties are mediated via dopamine D_2 antagonism, muscarinic receptor inhibition, $5HT_3$ receptor antagonism and $5HT_4$ receptor agonist activity. This results in increased lower esophageal sphincter and gastric wall tone, which promotes gastric emptying (Al-Saffar 2019).

Pharmacodynamics
Anti-emetic Effect When Given Prior to an Emetigen Metoclopromide 0.2 mg/kg given IM decreased the incidence of vomiting in dogs compared to saline (38% vs 71% respectively) when given prior to morphine and acepromazine (Lorenzutti 2017).

Impact on Gastro-esophageal Reflux In a study of dogs premedicated with acepromazine and morphine, where anesthesia was induced with thiopental and maintained with isoflurane, metoclopramide 1 mg/kg IV followed by an infusion of 1 mg/kg/h decreased GER by 54% (Wilson 2006). In the same study, lower doses of metoclopramide (0.4 mg/kg IV followed by 0.3 mg/kg/h) did not reduce the incidence of GER.

CNS Effects Metoclopramide given IV has been associated with development of extrapyramidal signs in dogs (Francesco 2021).

Cisapride

Cisapride is a prokinetic agent for use in cats and dogs that increases lower esophageal sphincter tone and increases intestinal motility.

Mechanism of Action

Cisapride is a 5-hydroxytryptamine$_4$ (5-HT$_4$) agonist, and partial 5-HT$_3$ antagonist, resulting in acetyl choline release from cholinergic nerves in the GI tract.

Pharmacokinetics

Limited pharmacokinetic data in animals is available. Cisapride is metabolized via hepatic cytochrome P450 enzymes in people (Desta 2001). In dogs bioavailability after oral dosing was 53%, and plasma half-life was 4–10 hours (Michiels 1987).

Pharmacodynamics

Effect on Gastro-esophageal Reflux When cisapride and esomeprazole were administered to dogs, GER events under anesthesia occurred in 11% of dogs compared to 38% of dogs in the control group, and 36% of dogs receiving esomeprazole alone (Zacuto 2012).

Cardiovascular System Heart rate, cardiac output, and mean arterial blood pressure decreased when cisapride (1 and 10 mg/kg) was administered to dogs anesthetized with thiopental and halothane (Sugiyama 1998).

Cisapride prolongs the QT interval of the electrocardiogram in people and dogs (Ollerstam 2007). Prolonged QT interval is correlated with development of potentially fatal arrhythmias (torsades des pointes) in people, and cisapride was withdrawn from use in human medicine in 2000. Anesthetized dogs given clinical and relatively high doses of cisapride (2–8 mg/kg) had prolonged QT intervals, and no evidence of spontaneous arrhythmias (Al-Wabel 2002). In that study, hemodynamics were not different regardless of cisapride dose, and heart rate increased. The authors speculate that differences in anesthetic protocol and fluid administration may explain the results compared to similar studies where heart rate tended to decrease.

Combinations

No single drug or combination of drugs is able to completely eliminate nausea, vomiting and GER in the perianesthetic period. Several combinations of drugs with differing mechanisms of action have been evaluated.

Postoperative regurgitation decreased from 35% to 9% in brachycephalic breeds that received a combination of metoclopramide (0.5 mg/kg SC) and famotidine 1 mg/kg SC or IV immediately prior to anesthesia (Costa 2020). This drug combination was used in conjunction with other strategies to reduce regurgitation and undesirable sequelae, e.g. reducing opioid usage and instituting intensive monitoring during recovery from anesthesia.

Administration of esomeprazole (1 mg/kg) and cisapride (1 mg/kg) 12–18 hours and 1–1.5 hours before anesthesia, respectively, resulted in 11% of dogs having GER events during anesthesia compared to 38% in the control group (Zacuto 2012).

Currently the recommendation when anesthetizing small animals is to avoid indiscriminate administration of antacids, instead reserving their use for patients with known history of, and predisposition to, GER; for example, those with esophageal inflammation or altered motility, and brachycephalic breeds (Grubb 2020).

References

Al-Saffar, A., Lennernäs, H., and Hellström, P.M. (2019). Gastroparesis, metoclopramide, and tardive dyskinesia: risk revisited. *Neurogastroenterol. Motil.* 31: e13617.

Al-Wabel, N.A., Strauch, S.M., et al. (2002). Electrocardiographic and hemodynamic effects of cisapride alone and combined with erythromycin in anesthetized dogs. *Cardiovasc. Toxicol.* 2: 195–208.

Audibert, G., Saunier, C., et al. (1991). Effects of H2-receptor blockers on response of cerebral blood flow to normocapnic hypoxia. *Anesth. Analg.* 72: 532–537.

Beil, W., Sewing, K.F., and Kromer, W. (1999). Basic aspects of selectivity of pantoprazole and its pharmacological actions. *Drugs Today* 35: 753–764.

Benchaoui, H.A., Cox, S.R, et al. (2007). The pharmacokinetics of maropitant, a novel neurokinin type-1 receptor antagonist, in dogs. *J. Vet. Pharmacol. Ther.* 30: 336–344.

Berryhill, E.H., Knych. H., et al. (2019). Pharmacokinetics of single doses of maropitant citrate in adult horses. *J. Vet. Pharmacol. Ther.* 42: 487–491.

Bersenas, A.M., Mathews, K.A., et al. (2005). Effects of ranitidine, famotidine, pantoprazole, and omeprazole on intragastric pH in dogs. *Am. J. Vet. Res.* 66: 425–431.

Boscan, P., Monnet, E, et al. (2011). Effect of maropitant, a neurokinin 1 receptor antagonist, on anesthetic requirements during noxious visceral stimulation of the ovary in dogs. *Am. J. Vet. Res.* 72: 1576–1579.

Breuer, H.W., Meschig, R., et al. (1984). Hemodynamic studies on cimetidine and ranitidine in anesthetized dogs. *Res. Exp. Med. (Berl.)* 184: 265–268.

Chi, T.T., and Hay Kraus, B.L. (2020). The effect of intravenous maropitant on blood pressure in healthy awake and anesthetized dogs. *PLoS One* 15: e0229736.

Costa, R.S., Abelson, A.L., et al. (2020). Postoperative regurgitation and respiratory complications in brachycephalic dogs undergoing airway surgery before and after implementation of a standardized perianesthetic protocol. *J. Am. Vet. Med. Assoc.* 256: 899–905.

Desta, Z., Soukhova, N., et al. (2001). Stereoselective metabolism of cisapride and enantiomer-enantiomer interaction in human cytochrome P450 enzymes: major role of CYP3A. *J. Pharmacol. Exp. Ther.* 298: 508–520.

Eddershaw, P.J., Chadwick, A.P., et al. (1996). Absorption and disposition of ranitidine hydrochloride in rat and dog. *Xenobiotica* 26: 947–956.

Favarato, E.S., Souza, M.V., et al. (2012). Evaluation of metoclopramide and ranitidine on the prevention of gastroesophageal reflux episodes in anesthetized dogs. *Res. Vet. Sci.* 93: 466–467.

Figueiredo, J. (2022). Gastrointestinal disease. In: *Canine and Feline Anesthesia and Co-Existing Disease*, 2e (ed. R.A. Johnson), 155–201. Hoboken NJ: Wiley Blackwell.

Fitzpatrick, R.L., Wittenburg, L.A., et al. (2016). Limited sampling pharmacokinetics of subcutaneous ondansetron in healthy geriatric cats, cats with chronic kidney disease, and cats with liver disease. *J. Vet. Pharmacol. Ther.* 39: 350–355.

Fladung, R., Smith, J.S., et al. (2022). Pharmacokinetics of esomeprazole in goats (*Capra aegagrus hircus*) after intravenous and subcutaneous administration. *Front. Vet. Sci.* 9: 968–973.

Fukui, S., Ooyama, N., et al. (2017). Interaction between maropitant and carprofen on sparing of the minimum alveolar concentration for blunting adrenergic response (MAC-BAR) of sevoflurane in dogs. *J. Vet. Med. Sci.* 79: 502–508.

Garcia, R.S., Belafsky, P.C., et al. (2017). Prevalence of gastroesophageal reflux in cats during anesthesia and effect of omeprazole on gastric pH. *J. Vet. Intern. Med.* 31: 734–742.

Grubb, T., Sager, J., at al. (2020). 2020 AAHA anesthesia and monitoring guidelines for dogs and cats. *J. Am. Anim. Hosp. Assoc.* 56: 59–82.

Hay Kraus, B.L. (2013). Efficacy of maropitant in preventing vomiting in dogs premedicated with hydromorphone. *Vet. Anesth. Analg.* 40: 28–34.

Hay Kraus, B.L. (2014). Effect of dosing interval on efficacy of maropitant for prevention of hydromorphone-induced vomiting and signs of nausea in dogs. *J. Am. Vet. Med. Assoc.* 245: 1015–1020.

Hay Kraus, B.L. (2017). Spotlight on the perioperative use of maropitant citrate. *Vet. Med. (Auckl.)* 8: 41–51.

Henze, L., Foth, S., et al. (2022). Ondansetron in dogs with nausea associated with vestibular disease: a double-blinded, randomized placebo-controlled crossover study. *J. Vet. Intern. Med.* 36: 1726–1732.

Hickman, M.A., Cox, S.R., et al. (2008). Saftey, pharmacokinetics and use of the novel NK-1 receptor antagonist maropitant (Cerenia) for the prevention of emesis and motion sickness in cats. *J. Vet. Pharmacol. Ther.* 31: 220–229.

Hoffmann, K.J., Renberg, L., and Olovson, S.G. (1986). Comparative metabolic disposition of oral doses of omeprazole in the dog, rat, and mouse. *Drug Metab. Dispos.* 14: 336–340.

Hultman, I., Stenhoff, H., and Liljeblad, M. (2007). Determination of esomeprazole and its two main metabolites in human, rat and dog plasma by liquid chromatography with tandem mass spectrometry. *J. Chromatogr. B. Analyt. Technol. Biomed. Life. Sci.* 848: 317–322.

Johnson, R. (2014). Maropitant prevented vomiting but not gastroesophageal reflux in anesthetized dogs premedicated with acepromazine-hydromorphone. *Vet. Anesth. Analg.* 41: 406–410.

Jones, C.T. and Fransson, B.A. (2019). Evaluation of the effectiveness of preoperative administration of maropitant citrate and metoclopramide hydrochloride in preventing postoperative clinical gastroesophageal reflux in dogs. *J. Am. Vet. Med. Assoc.* 255: 437–445.

Jones, S.M., Gaier, A., et al. (2020). The effect of combined carprofen and omeprazole administration on gastrointestinal permeability and inflammation in dogs. *J. Vet. Intern. Med.* 34: 1886–1893.

Kenward, H., Elliott, J., et al. (2017). Anti-nausea effects and pharmacokinetics of ondansetron, maropitant and metoclopramide in a low-dose cisplatin model of nausea and vomiting in the dog: a blinded crossover study. *BMC Vet. Res.* 13: 244.

Lorenzutti, A.M., Martín-Flores, M., et al. (2017). A comparison between maropitant and metoclopramide for the prevention of morphine-induced nausea and vomiting in dogs. *Can. Vet. J.* 58: 35–38.

Lotti, F., Twedt, D., et al. (2021). Effect of two different pre-anaesthetic omeprazole protocols on gastroesophageal reflux incidence and pH in dogs. *J. Small Anim. Pract.* 62: 677–682.

Marks, S.L., Kook, P.H., et al. (2018). ACVIM consensus statement: support for rational administration of gastrointestinal protectants to dogs and cats. *J. Vet. Intern. Med.* 32: 1823–1840.

Marquez, M., Boscan, P., et al. (2015). Comparison of NK-1 receptor antagonist (maropitant) to morphine as a pre-anaesthetic agent for canine ovariohysterectomy. *PLoS One* 10: e0140734.

Martin-Flores, M., Sakai, D.M., et al. (2016). Effects of maropitant in cats receiving dexmedetomidine and morphine. *J. Am. Vet. Med. Assoc.* 248: 1257–1261.

Michiels, M., Monbaliu, J., et al. (1987). Pharmacokinetics and tissue distribution of the new gastrokinetic agent cisapride in rat, rabbit and dog. *Arzneimittelforschung* 37: 1159–1167.

Miyata, K., Kamato, T., et al. (1990). Cardiovascular and bronchial actions of famotidine in anesthetized dogs. *Arzneimittelforschung* 40: 1234–1238.

Narishetty, S.T., Galvan, B., et al. (2009). Effect of refrigeration of the antiemetic Cerenia (maropitant) on pain on injection. *Vet. Ther.* 10: 93–102.

Niyom, S., Boscan, P., et al. (2013). Effect of maropitant, a neurokinin-1 receptor antagonist, on the minimum alveolar concentration of sevoflurane during stimulation of the ovarian ligament in cats. *Vet. Anaesth. Anlag.* 40: 425–431.

Odunayo, A., Galyon, G., et al. (2022). Evaluation of a long-acting injectable formulation of omeprazole in healthy dogs. *J. Vet. Intern. Med.* 36: 1416–1421.

Olivarez, J.D., Kreuder, A.J., et al. (2020). Pharmacokinetics and tissue levels of pantoprazole in neonatal calves after intravenous administration. *Front. Vet. Sci.* 7: https://doi.org/10.3389/fvets.2020.580735.

Ollerstam, A., Persson, A.H., et al. (2007). A novel approach to data processing of the QT interval response in the conscious telemetered beagle dog. *J. Pharmacol. Toxicol. Methods* 55: 35–48.

Oosterhuis, B. and Jonkman, J.H. (1989). Omeprazole: pharmacology, pharmacokinetics and interactions. *Digestion* 44 S: 9–17.

Panti, A., Bennett, R.C., et al. (2009). The effect of omeprazole on oesophageal pH in dogs during anaesthesia. *J. Small Anim. Pract.* 50: 540–544.

Perry, M.J. and Lawson, S.N. (1998). Differences in expression of oligosaccharides, neuropeptides, carbonic anhydrase and neurofilament in rat primary afferent neurons retrogradely labelled via skin, muscle or visceral nerves. *Neuroscience* 85: 293–310.

Piana, F. and Minghella, E. (2021). Extrapyramidal signs following a single intravenous dose of metoclopramide in an English Bulldog. *Vet. Anaesth. Analg.* 48: 977–978.

Quimby, J.M., Lake, R.C., et al. (2014). Oral, subcutaneous, and intravenous pharmacokinetics of ondansetron in healthy cats. *J. Vet. Pharmacol. Ther.* 37: 348–353.

Ramsey, D., Fleck, T., et al. (2014). Cerenia prevents perioperative nausea and vomiting and improves recovery in dogs undergoing routine surgery. *Intern. J. Appl. Res. Vet. Med.* 12: 228–237.

Regårdh, C.G., Gabrielsson, M., et al. (1985). Pharmacokinetics and metabolism of omeprazole in animals and man--an overview. *Scand. J. Gastroenterol. Suppl.* 108: 79–94.

Ryan, C.A., Sanchez, L.C., et al. (2005). Pharmacokinetics and pharmacodynamics of pantoprazole in clinically normal neonatal foals. *Equine Vet. J.* 37: 336–341.

Santos, L.C. (2011). A randomized, blinded, controlled trial of the antiemetic effect of ondansetron on dexmedetomidine-induced emesis in cats. *Vet. Anaesth. Analg.* 38: 320–327.

Saynor, D.A. and Dixon, C.M. (1989). The metabolism of ondansetron. *Eur. J. Cancer Clin. Oncol.* 1: S75–S77.

Seo, D.-H., Lee, J.-B., Song G-H., et al. (2019). Pharmacokinetics and pharmacodynamics of intravenous esomeprazole at 2 different dosages in dogs. *J. Vet. Intern. Med.* 33: 531–535.

Smith, G.W., Davis, J.L., et al. (2010). Efficacy and pharmacokinetics of pantoprazole in alpacas. *J. Vet. Intern. Med.* 24: 949–955.

Smith, J.S., Gebert, J., et al. (2023). The pharmacokinetics and pharmacodynamics of esomeprazole in sheep after intravenous dosing. *Front. Vet. Sci.* 10: https://doi.org/10.3389/fvets.2023.1172023.

Sugiyama, A. and Hashimoto, K. (1998). Effects of gastrointestinal prokinetic agents, TKS159 and cisapride, on the in situ canine heart assessed by cardiohemodynamic and electrophysiological monitoring. *Toxicol. Appl. Pharmacol.* 152: 261–269.

Sykes, B.W., Kathawala, K., et al. (2017). Preliminary investigations into a novel, long-acting, injectable, intramuscular formulation of omeprazole in the horse. *Equine Vet. J.* 49: 795–801.

Trepanier, L. (2010). Acute vomiting in cats: rational treatment selection. *J. Feline Med. Surg.* 12: 225–230.

Uno, Y., Morikuni, S., et al. (2023). Novel cytochrome P450 2C94 functionally metabolizes diclofenac and omeprazole in dogs. *Drug Metab. Dispos.* 51: 637–644.

Wallmark, B. (1989). Omeprazole: mode of action and effect on acid secretion in animals. *Scand. J. Gastroenterol. Suppl.* 166: 12–18.

Wilson, D.V., Evans, A.T., and Mauer, W.A. (2006). Influence of metoclopramide on gastroesophageal reflux in anesthetized dogs. *Am. J. Vet. Res.* 67: 26–31.

Wynn, R.L. (1993). The effects of different antiemetic agents on morphine-induced emesis in ferrets. *Eur. J. Pharmacol.* 241: 47–54.

Zacuto, A.C., Marks, S.L., et al. (2012). The influence of esomeprazole and cisapride on gastroesophageal reflux during anesthesia in dogs. *J. Vet. Intern. Med.* 26: 518–525.

28

Insulin

Phillip Lerche

Introduction

Diabetes mellitus is a common endocrinopathy in cats and dogs (McCann and Simpson 2007), while being rarely encountered in horses, ruminants and pigs (Durham 2017; Mostaghni and Ivoghli 1977; Gerstein and Waltman 2006), and results from low serum insulin concentrations or decreased response to insulin at the tissue level. It is associated with the clinical signs of polyuria, polydipsia, and weight loss. Severe hyperglycemia associated with uncontrolled diabetes mellitus can lead to life-threatening diabetic ketoacidosis or non-ketotic diabetic coma. Management of the diabetic patient is achieved by administration of exogenous insulin, typically timed to coincide with meals. Goals of insulin therapy in dogs are to maintain blood glucose in a mildly hyperglycemic range (90–250 mg/dl), and to reduce or eliminate polyuria (Fracassi 2017). Tighter control of glucose in diabetic cats is recommended (72–180 mg/dl), particularly in the early stages of this disease, as this has been shown to improve the chance of remission (Roomp and Rand 2009).

When diabetic patients present for anesthesia, several factors disrupt the animal's routine, including fasting and stress associated with transport to the unfamiliar environment of the veterinary hospital, all of which can lead to a decrease in stability of blood glucose concentrations.

Detailed management of the diabetic patient for anesthesia is outside the scope of this chapter, and the reader is referred elsewhere (Fischer 2022). Briefly, blood glucose is checked prior to, and at approximately 30-minute intervals during, anesthesia. Insulin and/or dextrose are then used to maintain blood glucose in an acceptable range for the diabetic patient. Insulin can be administered in either a "loose" protocol (insulin given by repeated injections as needed), or a "tight" protocol (insulin given by infusion and adjusted throughout the procedure). Insulin given

prior to anesthesia is typically the type of insulin given at home. During anesthesia, short-acting regular insulin is preferred due to its shorter duration of action, allowing for easier control of blood glucose. Several groups of anesthetic and other drugs can impact insulin and/or blood glucose levels and are discussed below.

Additionally, animals may not resume eating normally after anesthesia, which can delay return to normal diabetic management.

Pharmacology

Chemical Structure

Endogenous Insulin

The peptide hormone insulin consists of two chains of polypeptides, an A chain containing 21 amino acids, and a B chain containing 30 amino acids. The structure is not identical across all species due to small variations in amino-acid sequencing. Insulin preparations have been sourced from cattle (bovine insulin), pigs (porcine insulin) and people (recombinant human insulin). Porcine insulin differs by one amino acid from human insulin and is identical to canine insulin. Similarly, bovine insulin differs from feline insulin by one amino acid (Greco and Broussard 1995). Endogenous insulin has a short elimination half time of five-to-ten minutes in people, however, since it binds tightly to tissue insulin receptors, the duration of action is up to one hour. In non-diabetic patients, insulin secretion is stimulated by eating, beta-adrenergic and parasympathetic activity, and is decreased by alpha-adrenergic activity.

Exogenous Insulin Preparations

Various insulin preparations are available for use in cats and dogs. They are classified based on their onset time, time-to-peak effect, and duration of action, which can be

Table 28.1 Classification of insulin products.

Insulin type	Origin	Onset	Duration (h)
Short-acting			
Regular	Recombinant human	30–60 min	2–4
Intermediate-acting			
Lente	Porcine	1–2 h	8–14 (dogs)
			8–10 (cats)
Neutral protein Hagedorn	Recombinant human	1–2 h	4–10 (dogs)
Protamine zinc	Recombinant human	30–60 min	10–16 (dogs)
			9 to >24 (cats)
Long acting			
Glargine	Recombinant human	1–2 h	8–16 (dogs)
			12 to >24 (cats)
Detemir	Recombinant human	1–2 h	8–16 (dogs)
			11–16 (cats)

short-, intermediate-, or long-acting (Table 28.1). Most insulin formulations originate from human recombinant insulin, although lente insulin is a porcine product.

Synthetic insulin analogs are also available. Insulin glargine has two arginine molecules added to the B chain, resulting in slow absorption, delayed onset, and a long duration of action that provides a constant supply of insulin with no obvious peak. (Heinemann and Linkeschova 2000) Substitution of the fatty acid myristic acid for the amino acid lysin at position 29 in the B chain, along with removal of the amino acid threonine at position 30, yields insulin detemir. These structural changes result in a molecule that can reversibly bind to albumin, resulting in slow absorption and a longer duration. (Chapman and Perry 2004) Ultra-short acting injectable insulin is available in people but has minimal clinical application in veterinary patients. In high concentrations, and in the presence of zinc, insulin forms hexameric complexes which delay absorption, allowing for a longer duration of action.

Mechanism of Action

Insulin release from beta cells in the pancreatic islets is stimulated under normal circumstances by the increase in blood glucose that occurs after eating. Insulin binds to insulin receptors on cell membranes, with the main target organs being the liver, skeletal muscles, and adipose tissue. This results in tyrosine phosphorylation and subsequent phosphorylation of insulin receptor substrates, which then activates phosphoinositide-3-kinase, which phosphorylates protein kinase B, and

ultimately activation of molecular pathways within the cell to allow for glucose storage as glycogen (liver, muscle) and triglycerides and fatty acids (adipose) (Beaupere and Liboz 2021).

Metabolism

Insulin degradation occurs in the liver and kidney via a relatively complex process. Insulin undergoes cellular uptake and, once inside the cell, undergoes degradation. Intracellular insulin-degrading enzyme (IDE) is responsible for most of the degradation of insulin, however, other mechanisms have been shown to be involved (e.g. extracellular IDE activity, glutathione insulin transhydrogenase [or protein disulfide isomerase], carboxypeptidases, and lysosomal activity) (Beaupere and Liboz 2021; Duckworth and Bennett 1998).

Impact of Anesthetic and Other Drugs on Insulin

Inhalant Anesthetics

Isoflurane and sevoflurane have been shown to decrease insulin secretion and glucose utilization in a dose-dependent manner in people (Tanaka and Nabatame 2005). Isoflurane also impairs insulin secretion in rabbits (Tanaka and Kawano 2009). Insulin resistance during isoflurane and sevoflurane has been demonstrated experimentally in dogs (Kim and Broussard 2016). To the author's knowledge, no studies have been performed on the impact of inhalants alone on insulin in cats. One study showed that insulin tended to decrease during anesthesia in cats premedicated with medetomidine, midazolam, ketamine, or combinations of the three, and maintained with isoflurane (Kamohara and Kamohara 2021).

The mechanism of action by which inhalants reduce insulin secretion is via reversal of glucose-induced inhibition of pancreatic adenosine triphosphate-sensitive potassium channel activity (Tanaka and Kawano 2011).

Injectable Anesthetics

It has been demonstrated that propofol does not impact insulin secretion in rats (Tanaka and Kawano 2011), however, in diabetic people total intravenous (IV) anesthesia with propofol resulted in similar levels of hyperglycemia intra-operatively (Kim and Han 2018).

When thiopental was used as the sole anesthetic agent in dogs, moderate insulin resistance was observed compared to when the dogs were awake (Toso and Rodriguez 1993). Blood glucose was elevated in dogs anesthetized with either propofol or isoflurane, however, insulin was only decreased in the isoflurane group (Maeda and Iwasaki 2018). The reason for the elevated blood glucose during propofol anesthesia is unclear but may be due to the increase in free fatty acids in the plasma seen in the dogs given propofol, which may have indirectly impacted glucose uptake. No studies have been conducted with ketamine or alfaxalone as the sole anesthetic agent in dogs. Alfaxalone, given as an induction agent alone, or with ketamine or midazolam prior to isoflurane anesthesia was not associated with a decrease in serum glucose, while insulin concentrations decreased over time and remained in a clinically normal range (Munoz and Robertson 2017). Xylazine and ketamine administered together intramuscularly (IM) decreased insulin concentrations in dogs (Changman and Jianguo 2010).

Insulin was reduced in cats given ketamine prior to isoflurane anesthesia (Kamohara and Kamohara 2021). The impact on insulin of other injectable agents given as the sole anesthetic has not been studied in cats.

Alpha₂ Adrenoceptor Agonists

Xylazine, medetomidine and dexmedetomidine (Kamohara and Kamohara 2021; Guedes and Rude 2013; Kallio-Kujala and Bennett 2018) have all been shown to decrease insulin release in dogs.

In cats, medetomidine given prior to isoflurane anesthesia has been shown to decrease insulin during anesthesia

and in the early recovery period after termination of isoflurane delivery (Kamohara and Kamohara 2021).

Alpha₂ Adrenoceptor Antagonists

Yohimbine and atipamezole both increased insulin levels when given to reverse medetomidine (Ambrisko and Hikasa 2003). The peripheral alpha₂ adrenoceptor antagonist vatinoxan has been shown to stimulate insulin release in dogs (Kallio-Kujala and Bennett 2018).

Sympathomimetics

Epinephrine has been shown to decrease glucose uptake by cells via direct antagonism of insulin in people and dogs (Capaldo and Napoli 1992; Sacca and Eigler 1979). Norepinephrine decreased insulin secretion in non-insulin dependent diabetic people, but not in non-diabetics (Walters and Ward 1997). Dopamine has been shown to decrease insulin secretion from isolated mouse and human pancreatic islets, although compared to norepinephrine, the effect was seven times less (Aslanoglou and Bertera 2021). Dobutamine has been shown to have lesser effects on glucose and insulin in rates compared to epinephrine (Rosseau-Migneron and Nadeau 1985).

Parasympatholytics and Mimetics

In a rat model, neostigmine reversed the relative insulin resistance that occurs during partial fasting and following atropine administration (Schafer and Legare 2010).

Corticosteroids

The interaction between corticosteroids and insulin secretion is complex and has been recently reviewed (Beaupere and Liboz 2021). In general, a single corticosteroid dose will not impact insulin, however, after a few days of treatment and long term, corticosteroid therapy leads to insulin resistance, and a high percentage of people with hyperadrenocorticism will develop diabetes. The response of pancreatic islets to corticosteroids *in vivo* differs from that seen *in vitro*, and can include adaptive mechanisms, e.g. neogenesis of pancreatic beta cells and increased production if insulin.

Antibiotics

In people, tetracycline antibiotics have been shown to induce hypoglycemia, although it is not a consistent effect (Tan and Shelley 2016).

References

Ambrisko, T.D. and Hikasa, Y. (2003). The antagonistic effects of atipamezole and yohimbine on stress-related neurohormonal and metabolic responses induced by medetomidine in dogs. *Can. J. Vet. Res.* 67: 64–67.

Aslanoglou, D. and Bertera, S. (2021). Dopamine regulates pancreatic glucagon and insulin secretion via adrenergic and dopaminergic receptors. *Transl. Psychiatry* 16: 59.

Beaupere, C. and Liboz, A. (2021). Molecular mechanisms of glucocorticoid-induced insulin resistance. *Int. J. Mol. Sci.* 22: 623.

Capaldo, B. and Napoli, R. (1992). Epinephrine directly antagonizes insulin-mediated activation of glucose uptake and inhibition of free fatty acid release in forearm tissues. *Metabolism* 41: 1146–1149.

Changman, H. and Jianguo, C. (2010). Effects of xylazole alone and in combination with ketamine on the metabolic and neurohumoral responses in healthy dogs. *Vet. Anaesth. Anlag.* 37: 322–328.

Chapman, M. and Perry, C. (2004). A review of its use in the management of type-1 and type-2 diabetes mellitus. *Drugs* 64: 2577–2595.

Duckworth, W.C. and Bennett, R. (1998). Insulin degradation: progress and potential. *Endocr. Rev.* 19: 608–624.

Durham, A.E. (2017). Therapeutics for equine endocrine disorders. *Vet. Clin. Equine* 33: 127–139.

Fischer, B.L. (2022). Endocrine disease. In: *Canine and Feline Anesthesia and Co-Exisiting Disease* (ed. L. Snyder and R.A. Johnson), 324–329. Hoboken, NJ, USA: Wiley.

Fracassi, F. (2017). Canine diabetes mellitus. In: *Textbook of Veterinary Medicine*, 8e (ed. S.J. Ettinger and E.C. Feldman), 1767–1781. St. Louis MO: Elsevier.

Gerstein, H.C. and Waltman, L. (2006). Why don't pigs get diabetes? Explanations for variations in diabetes susceptibility in human populations living in a diabetogenic environment. *CMAJ* 174 (1): 25–26.

Greco, D.S. and Broussard, J. (1995). Insulin therapy. *Vet. Clin. N. Am.* 25 (3): 677–689.

Guedes, A.G.P. and Rude, E. (2013). Effects of pre-operative administration of medetomidine on plasma insulin and glucose concentrations in healthy dogs and dogs with insulinoma. *Vet. Anaesth. Analg.* 40: 472–481.

Heinemann, L. and Linkeschova, R. (2000). Time action profile of the long-acting insulin analog glargine in comparison with those of NPH insulin and placebo. *Diab. Care* 23: 644–649.

Kallio-Kujala, I.J. and Bennett, R. (2018). Effects of dexmedetomidine and MK-467 on plasma glucose, insulin and glucagon in a glibenclamide-induced canine hypoglycaemia model. *Vet. Dermatol.* J (242): 33–38.

Kamohara, H. and Kamohara, T. (2021). Effects of pretreatment with medetomidine, midazolam, ketamine, and their combinations on stress-related hormonal and metabolic responses in isoflurane-anesthetized cats undergoing surgery. *J. Adv. Anim. Res.* 563–575.

Kim, S.P. and Broussard, J. (2016). Isoflurane and sevoflurane induce severe hepatic insulin resistance in a canine model. *PLOS One* 11: e0163275.

Kim, H. and Han, J. (2018). Comparison of sevoflurane and propofol anesthesia on the incidence of hyperglycemia in patients with type 2 diabetes undergoing lung surgery. *Yeungnam Univ. J. Med.* 35: 54–62.

Maeda, K. and Iwasaki, M. (2018). Effect of propofol continuous-rate infusion on intravenous glucose tolerance test in dogs. *Vet. Sci.* 5: 43.

McCann, T.M. and Simpson, K. (2007). Feline diabetes mellitus in the UK: the prevalence within an insured cat population and a questionnaire-based putative risk factor analysis. *J. Feline Med. Surg.* 9: 289–299.

Mostaghni, K. and Ivoghli, B. (1977). Bovine diabetes mellitus. *Cornell Vet.* 67 (1): 24–28.

Munoz, K.A. and Robertson, S. (2017). Alfaxalone alone or combined with midazolam or ketamine in dogs: intubation dose and select physiologic effects. *Vet. Anesth. Analg.* 44: 766–774.

Roomp, K. and Rand, J. (2009). Intensive blood glucose control is safe and effective in diabetic cats using home monitoring and treatment with glargine. *J. Feline Med. Surg.* 11: 668–682.

Rosseau-Migneron, S. and Nadeau, S. (1985). Hyperglycemic effect of high doses of dobutamine in the rat: studies of insulin and glucagon secretion. *Can. J. Physiol. Pharmacol.* 63: 1308–1311.

Sacca, L. and Eigler, N. (1979). Insulin antagonstic effects of epinephrine and glucagon in the dog. *Am. J. Physiol.* 237: E487–E492.

Schafer, J.S. and Legare, D. (2010). Acetylcholinesterase antagonist potentiated insulin action in fed but not fasted state. *J. Pharmacol. Exp. Ther.* 333: 621–628.

Tan, C.H. and Shelley, C. (2016). Doxycycline-induced hypoglycaemia. *Clin. Exp. Dermatol.* 41: 43–44.

Tanaka, K. and Kawano, T. (2009). Mechanisms of impaired glucose tolerance and insulin secretion during isoflurane anesthesia. *Anesthesiology* 111: 1044–1051.

Tanaka, K. and Kawano, T. (2011). Differential effects of propofol and isoflurane on glucose utilization and insulin secretion. *Life Sci.* 88: 96–103.

Tanaka, T. and Nabatame, H. (2005). Insulin secretion and glucose utilization are impaired under general anesthesia with sevoflurane as well as isoflurane in a concentration-independent manner. *J. Anesth.* 277–281.

Toso, C.F. and Rodriguez, R. (1993). Adrenocorticotrophic hormone, cortisol and catecholamine concentrations during insulin hypoglycaemia in dogs anaesthetized with thiopentone. *Can. J. Anesth.* 40: 1084–1091.

Walters, J.M. and Ward, G. (1997). The effect of norepinephrine on insulin secretion and glucose effectiveness in non-insulin-dependent diabetes. *Metabolism* 46: 1448–1453.

29

Electrolytes

Teresa A. Burns

Introduction

Diseases and disorders associated with electrolyte abnormalities are encountered frequently in veterinary patients of all species and breeds, and most veterinary clinicians have some degree of comfort and familiarity in dealing with these problems in their patients. When an animal with an electrolyte abnormality also requires general anesthesia, it is frequently recommended that the patient's biochemical problem be addressed prior to anesthesia; given the importance of maintenance of serum electrolyte concentrations within narrow physiologic ranges for optimal functioning of electrically excitable tissues, this recommendation is theoretically sound and likely ensures that the risk of anesthetic complication (hypotension, arrhythmia, myopathy, etc.) is minimized. The content of this chapter is meant to describe common scenarios presented to the veterinary anesthetist in which an electrolyte abnormality might be expected and to recommend strategies to treat the problem and minimize risk of complications during and following general anesthesia. Situations in which serum electrolyte concentrations might be manipulated to treat an anesthetic complication (tissue edema, arrhythmia, etc.) are also described where appropriate.

Sodium

Sodium is the primary cation in extracellular fluid; it is responsible for the generation and maintenance of the "osmotic skeleton" of the body, as it is the primary determinant of the distribution of total body water within intra- and extracellular fluid compartments (Marino 2007b). Further, it is critically important in the generation of action potentials in electrically excitable tissues (skeletal muscle,

cardiac muscle, smooth muscle, nervous tissue), and disorders of sodium can pose a challenge for the anesthetist. In human medicine, it has been suggested that as many as 40% of critically ill patients have a pathologic change in serum sodium concentration (hyper- or hyponatremia; [Pokaharel and Block 2011]); given the number of diseases associated with these abnormalities in veterinary patients, the likelihood is high that clinicians will encounter a patient with an abnormal serum sodium concentration that requires anesthetic management.

Additionally, medications and fluids administered during anesthesia can contribute to derangements in serum sodium concentration. For example, α-2 agonists such as xylazine have been shown to increase the urinary clearance of sodium in veterinary species and may enhance hyponatremia if given to an otherwise untreated patient with this disorder (Trim and Hanson 1986). Both hyper- and hyponatremia are associated with pathologic changes in cell volume associated with fluid shifts, particularly if the change in sodium concentration is acute; this is most notable within the central nervous system (CNS). Severe hyponatremia is associated with risk of cerebral edema, but correction of hyponatremia that is performed too rapidly has been associated with osmotic demyelination syndrome in several species (Mascarenhas and Jude 2014; Snell and Bartley 2008). Conversely, rapid correction of chronic hypernatremia is also associated with cerebral edema, reportedly secondary to neuronal generation of so-called "idiogenic osmoles" that draw free water from the extracellular fluid as it becomes more hypotonic following initiation of fluid therapy. Post-anesthetic decreases in colloid oncotic pressure (COP) and serum sodium concentration appear to be common and have been reported in multiple species (Wendt-Hornickle et al. 2011; Raftery et al. 2015; Wright and Hopkins 2008) for the most part, these appear to be self-limiting and associated with

Pharmacology in Veterinary Anesthesia and Analgesia, First Edition. Edited by Turi Aarnes and Phillip Lerche.
© 2024 John Wiley & Sons, Inc. Published 2024 by John Wiley & Sons, Inc.

little long-term morbidity. However, when this expected change in serum sodium concentration is superimposed on a pre-existing sodium disorder (esp. hyponatremia), management changes may be necessary. In general, unless the sodium imbalance has occurred acutely, it is recommended that changes in plasma sodium concentration (increase or decrease) occur at a rate of no more than 0.5–1.0 mEq/l/h to minimize the risk of cerebral edema or iatrogenic central pontine myelinolysis (Guillaumin and DiBartola 2017).

Sodium-based crystalloid fluids administered intravenously (IV) form the basis for support of blood volume and blood pressure in the anesthetized patient; however, few studies describe the effects of hyper- or hyponatremia on the anesthetized patient. Previous work has demonstrated an effect of plasma and CSF sodium concentration on halothane requirement (MAC) in dogs; in one study, hypernatremia increased halothane MAC by 43%, an effect which was not observed with hyperglycemia or hyperkalemia (Tanifuji and Eger 1978). Preliminary evidence suggests that chronic hypernatremia delays recovery from general anesthesia induced with ketamine in rodents, and the authors of that study suggest that ketamine doses should be reduced in the setting of hypernatremia (Heydarpour et al. 2007); further study is warranted to refine this recommendation, however. Finally, while sodium disorders may affect hemodynamic variables in anesthetized patients (Kozeny et al. 1985), hyper- and hyponatremia do not typically induce characteristic ECG changes that might be useful for monitoring response to fluid therapy under anesthesia.

Infusions of sodium-based crystalloid fluid can also be exploited therapeutically for inducing fluid shifts in the anesthetized patient; perhaps the situation in which this becomes most useful is in anesthesia of the patient with brain disease (head trauma, malignancy, encephalitis, etc.) and consequently at risk for cerebral edema. Animal and human studies have demonstrated that hypertonic saline has clinically desirable physiologic effects on cerebral blood flow, intracranial pressure (ICP), and inflammatory changes within the neuropil in the setting of neurotrauma. Administration of hypertonic sodium chloride solutions (3–23.4%) for the treatment and prevention of elevated ICP has been shown in several human and animal studies to be effective and may be useful in the treatment of intracranial hypertension and cerebral edema if suspected under general anesthesia (Harutjunyan et al. 2005; Taylor et al. 1996; Peterson et al. 2000), such as for animals that have sustained a traumatic brain injury (TBI) and require general anesthesia for brain imaging. When administering hypertonic saline solutions therapeutically, one should use caution in patients with underlying cardiac or renal disease.

Potassium

Potassium is the major intracellular cation, with a relatively small amount of the total body potassium content represented in the extracellular fluid; plasma potassium concentrations typically range between 3.5 and 5.5 mEq/l in health (Marino 2007c). Due to its important role as the primary determinant of resting membrane potential and therefore proper function of excitable tissues (including cardiac muscle, skeletal muscle, and nervous tissue), plasma potassium concentration is tightly regulated by several mechanisms, including dietary intake, acid–base balance, hormonal influences (esp. aldosterone and insulin), and renal tubular function.

Hyperkalemia

Elevation in plasma potassium concentration is a frequently encountered problem in veterinary species, although the most common underlying etiologies vary among species. Most cases of hyperkalemia, particularly if it develops acutely, are related to decreased urinary excretion of potassium; common causes include urethral obstruction in cats and small ruminants, ruptured urinary bladder in foals, and acute renal failure in multiple species. Hypoadrenocorticism, administration of potassium-containing drugs (such as KCl) or potassium-sparing diuretics (such as spironolactone or triamterene), administration of suxamethonium, and conditions resulting in acute translocation of potassium from ICF to ECF (such as vigorous exercise, capture myopathy, acute tumor lysis syndrome, hemolysis, hyperkalemic periodic paralysis [HYPP], and acute mineral acidosis) are also reported to result in clinically significant hyperkalemia. Hyperkalemia has also been documented in response to transfusion of senescent packed red cells in a dog under general anesthesia (Nickell and Shih 2011). Importantly, if hyperkalemia is detected unexpectedly in an otherwise healthy patient, sample handling artifact should be investigated. The plasma [K$^+$] should be measured again and confirmed prior to any therapeutic action, as even minor *in vitro* hemolysis can cause spurious elevation of [K$^+$] outside of reference ranges (pseudohyperkalemia); this can also be observed in samples containing significantly elevated platelet and white blood cell counts and in samples collected from blood vessels occluded by prolonged tourniquet application, and these details should be accounted for in interpretation of results (Asirvatham et al. 2013; Colussi and Cipriani 1995; Stankovic and Smith 2004). Finally, malignant hyperthermia should be considered as an important differential diagnosis for a patient that develops hyperkalemia during general anesthesia (particularly if halothane is used); other clinical findings (such as muscle rigidity, hypercarbia, lactic acidemia, elevated serum creatine kinase [CK] concentration, and hyperthermia) support this diagnosis. Genetic predispositions to this condition have been documented in swine, horses, and dogs (Brunson and Hogan 2004).

Clinical signs of hyperkalemia are not usually apparent until the plasma [K$^+$] exceeds 7.5 mEq/l and are related to the resultant increase in membrane excitability; the cardiovascular effects of hyperkalemia, notably bradycardia, atrial standstill, diastolic arrest, and vasoconstriction, are of greatest concern to the anesthetist and warrant at least partial correction of hyperkalemia prior to induction of general anesthesia. In fact, in a retrospective study of the perioperative management of ureteral obstruction in cats, preoperative hyperkalemia was significantly associated with mortality (Garcia de Carellan Mateo et al. 2015). While electrocardiographic (ECG) monitoring is the standard of anesthetic practice for most patients, it is particularly important for patients with derangements of potassium, as both hyper- and hypokalemia are predisposing factors for arrhythmogenesis. ECG changes classically associated with hyperkalemia include decreased amplitude to absent P waves; tall, tented T waves; widening of the QRS complex; extrasystoles; ventricular asystole; and ventricular fibrillation.

Treatment of hyperkalemia should begin prior to the induction of general anesthesia and is most effective when multimodal in nature. In theory, patients should be given IV fluids free of potassium at a diuretic rate (1.5–2.0× maintenance, as long as urinary obstruction can be functionally relieved if present) to promote kaliuresis. However, administration of K$^+$-containing fluids to hyperkalemic patients might not be contraindicated. For example, administration of K$^+$-containing balanced electrolyte solutions (Normosol-R™ or lactated Ringer's solution) to cats with urethral obstruction was reported to be *as effective* as administration of K$^+$-free solutions (0.9% NaCl) in decreasing plasma [K$^+$], and fluid type did not appear to affect patient survival or length of hospitalization (Cunha et al. 2010; Drobatz and Cole 2008). That said, isotonic saline (0.9% NaCl) or 5% dextrose in water are frequently selected for use in management of hyperkalemia; 5% dextrose in water has the added benefit of inducing endogenous release of insulin, which also promotes the intracellular translocation of potassium and further reduces plasma [K$^+$]. If necessary, this effect can be augmented through the administration of regular insulin (0.1 IU/kg IV or SQ with careful monitoring of plasma [glucose]); however, this is rarely necessary. Severe and/or refractory cases may also respond to administration of an alkalinizing agent such as sodium bicarbonate (1–2 mEq/kg HCO$_3^-$ or 0.25–0.3 of a calculated base deficit given slowly over 15 minutes) or a β$_2$-agonist like terbutaline (0.01 mg/kg IV) (Beer and Waddell 2015). Calcium gluconate should also be administered IV due to calcium's antagonism of hyperkalemia-induced depolarization and decreased arrhythmogenesis (Baetge 2007; Bailey et al. 1996; Pang et al. 2011).

Hypokalemia

Hypokalemia is most frequently associated with an acute shift of potassium intracellularly, a total body potassium deficit, or a combination of these two mechanisms. Intracellular shifting of potassium (exploited therapeutically in the management of hyperkalemia, described above) is associated with insulin (endogenous or exogenous), β-adrenoreceptor agonists (endogenous catecholamines or exogenous drugs, such as terbutaline or salbutamol), theophylline intoxication, and alkalosis. Total body potassium depletion may result from decreased dietary potassium intake, increased renal and extrarenal losses, or a combination of both mechanisms. For example, a dog or cat with diabetes mellitus may be hypokalemic due to persistent glucosuria and ketonuria that result in osmotic diuresis and excessive kaliuresis; administration of exogenous insulin may exacerbate hypokalemia in these patients if not carefully associated with dietary intake (Kogika and de Morais 2017). Since intracellular potassium content (and therefore total body potassium content) correlates poorly with plasma [K$^+$], suspicion of total body K$^+$ depletion should be based on a carefully collected clinical history of the patient and knowledge of the disease process(es) present and not assumed to be normal based on eukalemia alone.

Clinically, the hypokalemic patient is usually asymptomatic when their plasma [K$^+$] remains above 3.0 mEq/l. When the plasma [K$^+$] decreases below this level, neuromuscular weakness can be observed (becoming very likely when [K$^+$] is below 2.5 mEq/l); this can be of significant importance when dealing with a large animal patient under general anesthesia, as hypokalemia can contribute to anesthetic myopathy and difficulty in standing in the post-anesthetic recovery period. Further, hypokalemia is a predisposing risk factor for ventricular and supraventricular ectopic rhythms (particularly in patients receiving digoxin) and, while a threshold of tolerance for hypokalemia has not been established with rigor in the anesthetized veterinary patient, a prudent rule of thumb would be that care should be taken to ensure that plasma [K$^+$] remains above 3.0 mEq/l during general anesthesia. Additionally, pro-arrhythmogenic drugs (such as α-2 agonists frequently used as premedicants in small and large animal species) should either be avoided or used at decreased dosages in patients with electrolyte dyscrasias that might increase their risk of cardiac arrhythmias. Correction of hypokalemia can be efficiently accomplished by supplementation of crystalloid IV fluids with KCl; regarding safe administration of parenteral potassium, the rate may be more critical than the total amount administered. The rate of K^+ administration should not routinely exceed 0.5 mEq/kg/h, although that rate may be increased up to 1.5 mEq/kg/h with continuous ECG monitoring (Schaer 2008).

Effects of Drugs on Plasma Potassium Concentrations

Changes in pH commonly affect the distribution of potassium between the intra- and extracellular fluid. In the setting of acidemia, potassium moves out of the ICF in exchange for hydrogen ion, which moves intracellularly. Conversely, with alkalemia, potassium moves into the ICF. In general, for every 0.1 unit decrease in pH, the plasma potassium concentration can be expected to rise by 0.6 mEq/l (or the converse). The magnitude of this change, however, may vary with the etiology of the acid–base disturbance (e.g. mineral vs. organic acidosis; [DiBartola 2001, Parker et al. 1980]).

Insulin, bicarbonate ion, catecholamines, and exogenously administered β-adrenergic agonists decrease plasma potassium concentrations by promotion of cellular potassium uptake. General anesthesia itself can have a direct effect on plasma potassium concentrations, primarily thought to be related to acid–base alterations and endogenous catecholamine release. Drugs that induce transcellular K^+ shifts can be used to improve hyperkalemia prior to and following induction of general anesthesia in clinical patients, such as in the case of urinary obstruction (commonly seen in goats and tomcats with urethral obstruction, neonatal foals with ruptured urinary bladder, and animals of multiple species with renal failure); however, effects on plasma $[K^+]$ should be anticipated if they are being administered for another reason (for example, β-adrenergic agonists for bronchodilation or $NaHCO_3$ for metabolic acidosis). Supplementation of IV fluids with KCl (20 mEq/l) should be provided in these circumstances, particularly if the patient is already mildly hypokalemic. However, care should be taken (particularly in anesthetized patients) to prevent inadvertent high-volume administration of potassium-supplemented fluids.

HYPP, an important genetic myopathy of stock breed horses (American Quarter Horse, American Paint Horse, Appaloosa, and crosses), is associated with episodes of weakness and muscle fasciculation during which horses are observed to also have elevated plasma potassium concentrations. In affected horses, general anesthesia and recovery have been associated with precipitation of episodes (Bailey et al. 1996), and plasma potassium concentration should be monitored frequently in horses with this disease while under anesthesia. Calcium salts should be administered to patients experiencing episodes under general anesthesia

(100–500 ml of 23% Ca gluconate in every 5 l bag of 0.9% NaCl), as Ca^{2+} can counteract the adverse effects of hyperkalemia on cardiovascular performance in these patients (Pang et al. 2011).

Calcium

Calcium is a divalent cation involved in diverse biological processes; however, its roles in controlling neuromuscular function, smooth muscle contraction, and coagulation are perhaps most relevant to the anesthetist. Excitation-contraction coupling in both somatic and cardiac muscle are Ca-dependent processes, and derangements in plasma [Ca] are most frequently manifested clinically through dysfunction of these tissues. Hypocalcemia often results in increased cardiac and neuromuscular excitability, negative inotropy, and decreased smooth muscle tone; clinically, an affected patient may display cardiac arrhythmias (particularly ventricular ectopy); somatic muscle weakness and spasticity (which may affect quality of anesthetic recovery in large animals); poor cardiac output, blood pressure, and perfusion under anesthesia; and post-operative ileus. Hypercalcemia is observed less frequently and results in relatively non-specific clinical signs, such as vomiting, polyuria, ectopic mineralization of soft tissues, and altered mentation; ECG changes may include prolongation of QRS duration and bradycardia. Calcium derangements are often noted in the setting of renal disease and malignancy in small animals, periparturient transitional physiology in ruminants, and gastrointestinal (GI) disease in horses; awareness of the pathophysiology of the patient's primary disease may allow the anesthetist to predict Ca abnormalities and pre-emptively treat them before and during an anesthetic episode, thereby minimizing risk of adverse anesthetic events. Additionally, it is important to be aware of the effects that general anesthesia itself may have on blood [Ca], as this may exacerbate a pre-existing abnormality. Brainard and colleagues recently showed that plasma $[Ca^{2+}]$ decreased in healthy dogs and cats in response to anesthesia and surgery; while animals were not observed to become hypocalcemic during this study, Ca disorders were not noted in these patients prior to anesthesia (Brainard et al. 2007). The effects of general anesthesia on Ca homeostasis should be taken into account when assessing the necessity of supplementation during an anesthetic episode.

Calcium exists in plasma in three forms: ionized (free), complexed to plasma anions, and bound to albumin. The assay used by most clinical laboratories to measure calcium measures all three fractions (total Ca); however, abnormalities in total calcium may not be the most relevant monitoring parameter during anesthesia, since neuromuscular and cardiovascular function depend on the plasma concentration of *ionized* Ca^{2+}. Ionized Ca^{2+} concentration in both the intra- and extracellular fluid spaces is tightly regulated, as this is the biologically active form of calcium and the fraction whose derangement is most likely to result in clinical signs of hypo- or hypercalcemia; monitoring of patients under anesthesia should involve assessment and normalization of ionized Ca^{2+} (Marino 2007a).

Assessment of plasma Ca content can be significantly affected by protein concentration (specifically albumin), with hypoalbuminemic patients displaying low total Ca but often normal Ca^{2+} (only the protein-bound fraction of Ca is significantly affected by changes in albumin concentration). Acid–base disturbances can also affect measured Ca concentrations, but unlike albumin changes, pH changes typically affect ionized $[Ca^{2+}]$: acidemia decreases Ca^{2+} binding of albumin and increases plasma Ca^{2+}, whereas alkalemia increases Ca^{2+} binding of albumin. This phenomenon could be exploited therapeutically to manage Ca disorders in anesthetized patients (for example, infusion of $NaHCO_3$ to acutely lower Ca^{2+} in a hypercalcemic patient) but, more often, this is a side-effect that needs to be borne in mind when manipulating acid–base status in patients (i.e. infusion of $NaHCO_3$ for treatment of severe metabolic acidosis will also lower plasma Ca^{2+}, possibly necessitating treatment in an already hypocalcemic patient).

Treatment of hypocalcemia in the anesthetized patient is effectively achieved through IV administration of Ca salts (most frequently $CaCl_2$ or Ca gluconate). A solution of $CaCl_2$ contains approximately three times as much elemental Ca as a Ca-gluconate solution of the same concentration (for example, 10% or 23%); its osmolality is also three times that of a solution of Ca gluconate (Marino 2007a). Ca-containing solutions should be administered into a large central vein, if possible, due to their hypertonicity; if using a peripheral vein, Ca gluconate should be administered and diluted in a balanced electrolyte solution (Marino 2007a). If using a 10% calcium gluconate solution, rates of 1.0–1.5 ml/kg given slowly IV over 20–30 minutes (with frequent assessment of heart rate) are well-tolerated; if bradycardia occurs during infusion, administration should slow or stop until normal rate and rhythm return (Schaer 2008). Hypocalcemia that is refractory to Ca supplementation would suggest the presence of hypomagnesemia; this possibility should be investigated through measurement of $[Mg^{2+}]$ and treated with Mg supplementation if noted (Hardy 2009). Calcium salts can also be useful for mitigating the risk of adverse cardiovascular effects of hyperkalemia in patients undergoing general anesthesia (see above under "Hyperkalemia"); while they have been reported to be useful adjunctive positive inotropic agents to improve cardiovascular performance in horses under general anesthesia, other agents are more effective; calcium salts are primarily useful for this purpose in hypocalcemic patients (Schauvliege and Gasthuys 2013).

Magnesium

Magnesium is the second most abundant intracellular cation, and its broad functions as a cofactor in enzymatic reactions of intermediary metabolism are incredibly diverse. Magnesium is vital for the regulation of cellular energy production and ion concentrations, playing roles in mitochondrial oxidative phosphorylation, anaerobic glycolysis, and facilitation of intracellular ion pumping activity (acting as a cofactor with ATP); Mg^{2+} has been referred to as an endogenous Ca^{2+} antagonist, since its modulation of slow Ca^{2+} channels maintains normal vascular tone and prevents tissue Ca^{2+} toxicity in health (Svensen 2013). Magnesium is additionally involved in the synthesis and degradation of DNA, initiation of ribosomal translation, and synthesis of several important intracellular second messengers (Bateman 2006). While much of the total body Mg stores are within bone mineral, this depot is not readily mobilized during times of Mg depletion; as such, maintenance of normal plasma Mg concentration is highly dependent on regular dietary Mg absorption (Goff 2015).

Plasma magnesium concentration can have profound effects on the regulation of the extracellular concentrations of other electrolytes, most notably K^+ and Ca^{2+}. Mg^{2+} regulates parathyroid hormone (PTH) secretion and end-organ sensitivity to PTH and vitamin D, and it regulates the Na^+/K^+ ATPase and renal tubular resorption of K^+ (Svensen 2013); the clinician should be alerted to the possibility of disorders of K^+ and Ca^{2+} balance when an abnormality of Mg^{2+} is present (especially hypomagnesemia). Conversely, if K^+ or Ca^{2+} disorders are present, therapy to correct them may be ineffective without also accounting for the patient's Mg^{2+} status (this may be particularly true for hypokalemia – Mg supplementation is often helpful in normalizing plasma K^+ concentrations in patients previously refractory to K^+ supplementation [Marino 2014]).

For the purposes of clinical anesthesia, the concentration of Mg in the extracellular fluid may be more immediately important than intracellular $[Mg^{2+}]$ or total body Mg^{2+} stores due to its profound effects on excitable tissue. Mg^{2+} stabilizes axonal membranes and competitively inhibits Ca^{2+} entry at pre-synaptic nerve terminals (required for acetylcholine release); functionally, Mg^{2+}

depletion and hypomagnesemia leads to decreased neuronal stimulation threshold, increased nerve conduction velocity, and increased activity in neuromuscular tissue (with hyperexcitability, tetany, seizure, supraventricular and ventricular tachyarrhythmia, and spontaneous death occurring in affected small (Bateman 2006) and large animal patients (Goff 2015)). Symptomatic hypomagnesemia should be treated with IV infusion of magnesium (sulfate or chloride, diluted to a concentration below 20%); rates below 0.2–0.3 mEq/kg are reportedly well-tolerated (Humphrey et al. 2015).

The opposite, namely, decreased neuromuscular excitability, occurs in the setting of Mg^{2+} excess; in fact, this property has been exploited historically for the purposes of clinical veterinary anesthesia when $MgSO_4$ has been used as a neuromuscular blocking agent in combination with chloral hydrate (Bowen and McMullan 1975; Singh et al. 1971; Kumar et al. 1971; Sharma et al. 1984; Costa et al. 1986). Doses of 0.12–0.16 g/kg of $MgSO_4$ have been associated with partial neuromuscular blockade when given IV to anesthetized horses (Bowen and McMullan 1975), and this property might make it useful for enhancing neuromuscular relaxation in anesthetized veterinary patients with normal renal function; however, its utility is likely limited to an adjunct agent due to its lack of direct anesthetic effect (Posner and Burns 2009). Hypermagnesemia may be associated with atrioventricular and intraventricular conduction disturbances if severe; ECG evaluation in these cases may reveal third-degree AV block or asystole.

Recent studies have evaluated the effect of pre- and intraoperative $MgSO_4$ infusion on the amount of induction drug and maintenance inhalant anesthetic required to anesthetize healthy animals. Anagnostou and colleagues showed a dose-sparing effect of $MgSO_4$ when used as an IV infusion (50 mg/kg before induction, then 12 mg/kg/hour during surgery) on the amount of thiopental required for induction and end-tidal halothane

concentration during maintenance of anesthesia in healthy dogs undergoing ovariohysterectomy (OHE) (Anagnostou et al. 2008). This effect was not detected in two other studies, however, where $MgSO_4$ infusion failed to decrease isoflurane requirements in healthy dogs undergoing OHE (Rioja et al. 2012) or healthy adult goats (Queiroz-Castro et al. 2006). Nausea and vomiting were notable side effects of $MgSO_4$ infusion in conscious dogs (Anagnostou et al. 2008), and patients should be monitored accordingly for this complication.

Magnesium is an N-methyl-D-aspartate (NMDA) receptor antagonist and consequently also has analgesic properties (Coetzee 2013). Because of this effect, recent studies have investigated the utility of magnesium salts in enhancing the effectiveness of local/regional anesthetic techniques. Numerous human studies have documented the effectiveness of magnesium as an adjuvant to local and regional nerve blocks performed with lidocaine or bupivacaine to facilitate surgical and dental procedures (Ammar and Mahmoud 2014; Kim et al. 2014; Shetty et al. 2015); in these studies, Mg^{2+} has been shown to improve both quality of analgesia and return to function following these regional anesthetic techniques. Relatively little work has been done to evaluate the efficacy of Mg^{2+} for this use in veterinary medicine, but a recent study in cattle suggests that the addition of 1 ml of 10% $MgSO_4$ solution to an epidural infusate of 2% lidocaine (0.22 mg/kg) delays the onset of analgesia but prolongs its duration significantly when compared with lidocaine and distilled water (Dehghani and Bigham 2009). The lidocaine-$MgSO_4$ combination provided effective analgesia for 168 ± 2.6 minutes (compared with 59.8 ± 3.4 minutes for lidocaine-distilled water), and the authors suggest that this combination would be very suitable for long-duration obstetric and surgical procedures in this species, given that readministration of anesthetic might not be necessary.

References

Ammar, A.S. and Mahmoud, K.M. (2014). Does the addition of magnesium to bupivacaine improve postoperative analgesia of ultrasound-guided thoracic paravertebral block in patients undergoing thoracic surgery? *J. Anesth.* 28 (1): 58–63.

Anagnostou, T.L., Savvas, I., Kazakos, G.M. et al. (2008). Thiopental and halothane dose-sparing effects of magnesium sulphate in dogs. *Vet. Anaesth. Analg.* 35 (2): 93–99.

Asirvatham, J.R., Moses, V., and Bjornson, L. (2013). Errors in potassium measurement: a laboratory perspective for the clinician. *N. Am. J. Med. Sci.* 5 (4): 255–259.

Baetge, C.L. (2007). Anesthesia case of the month. Hyperkalemic periodic paralysis. *J. Am. Vet. Med. Assoc.* 230 (1): 33–36.

Bailey, J.E., Pablo, L., and Hubbell, J.A. (1996). Hyperkalemic periodic paralysis episode during halothane anesthesia in a horse. *J. Am. Vet. Med. Assoc.* 208 (11): 1859–1865.

Bateman, S. (2006). Chapter 8 – Disorders of magnesium: magnesium deficit and excess. I: (ed. S. DiBartola), *Fluid, Electrolyte, and Acid–Base Disorders in Small Animal Practice*. 210–226. Elsevier.

Beer, K.S. and Waddell, L.S. (2015). Perioperative acid–base and electrolyte disturbances. *Vet. Clin. N. Am. Small Anim. Pract.* 45 (5): 941–952.

Bowen, J.M. and McMullan, W.C. (1975). Influence of induced hypermagnesemia and hypocalcemia on neuromuscular blocking property of oxytetracycline in the horse. *Am. J. Vet. Res.* 36 (7): 1025–1028.

Brainard, B.M., Campbell, V.L., Drobatz, K.J., and Perkowski, S.Z. (2007). The effects of surgery and anesthesia on blood magnesium and calcium concentrations in canine and feline patients. *Vet. Anaesth. Analg.* 34 (2): 89–98.

Brunson, D.B. and Hogan, K.J. (2004). Malignant hyperthermia: a syndrome not a disease. *Vet. Clin. N. Am. Small Anim. Pract.* 34 (6): 1419–1433.

Coetzee, J.F. (2013). A review of analgesic compounds used in food animals in the United States. *Vet. Clin. N. Am. Food Anim. Pract.* 29 (1): 11–28.

Colussi, G. and Cipriani, D. (1995). Pseudohyperkalemia in extreme leukocytosis. *Am. J. Nephrol.* 15 (5): 450–452.

Costa, A.G., Singh, A.P., Peshin, P.K., and Singh, J. (1986). Evaluation of chloral hydrate and magnesium sulphate sedation in buffalo calves (*Bubalus bubalis*). *Zentralblatt fur Veterinarmedizin Reihe A* 33 (5): 349–352.

Cunha, M.G., Freitas, G.C., Carregaro, A.B. et al. (2010). Renal and cardiorespiratory effects of treatment with lactated Ringer's solution or physiologic saline (0.9% NaCl) solution in cats with experimentally induced urethral obstruction. *Am. J. Vet. Res.* 71 (7): 840–846.

Dehghani, S.N. and Bigham, A.S. (2009). Comparison of caudal epidural anesthesia by use of lidocaine versus a lidocaine-magnesium sulfate combination in cattle. *Am. J. Vet. Res.* 70 (2): 194–197.

DiBartola, S.P. (2001). Management of hypokalaemia and hyperkalaemia. *J. Feline Med. Surg.* 3 (4): 181–183.

Drobatz, K.J. and Cole, S.G. (2008). The influence of crystalloid type on acid–base and electrolyte status of cats with urethral obstruction. *J. Vet. Emerg. Crit. Care* 18 (4): 355–361.

Garcia de Carellan Mateo, A., Brodbelt, D., Kulendra, N., and Alibhai, H. (2015). Retrospective study of the perioperative management and complications of ureteral obstruction in 37 cats. *Vet. Anaesth. Analg.* 42 (6): 570–579.

Goff, J. (2015). Calcium, magnesium, and phosphorus. In Chapter 41: Endocrine and metabolic diseases. In: *Large Animal Internal Medicine* (ed. B. Smith), 1258–1266. Elsevier.

Guillaumin, J. and DiBartola, S.P. (2017). Disorders of sodium and water homeostasis. *Vet. Clin. N. Am. Small Anim. Pract.* 47 (2): 293–312.

Hardy, J. (2009). Venous and arterial catheterization and fluid therapy. In: *Equine Anesthesia: Monitoring and Therapy*, 2e (ed. W.W. Muir and J.A.E. Hubbell), 144.

Harutjunyan, L., Holz, C., Rieger, A. et al. (2005). Efficiency of 7.2% hypertonic saline hydroxyethyl starch 200/0.5 versus mannitol 15% in the treatment of increased intracranial pressure in neurosurgical patients – a randomized clinical trial [ISRCTN62699180]. *Crit. Care (London, England)* 9 (5): R530–R540.

Heydarpour, F., Amini, B., Kalantari, S. et al. (2007). Determination of sensitivity of male Wistar rats to an equal dose of ketamine/xylazine injection at anesthetic dose in a chronic model of hypernatremia in comparison with control group. *Saudi Med. J.* 28 (10): 1485–1488.

Humphrey, S., Kirby, R., and Rudloff, E. (2015). Magnesium physiology and clinical therapy in veterinary critical care. *J. Vet. Emerg. Crit. Care (San Antonio, Tex.; 2001)* **25** (2): 210–225.

Kim, E.M., Kim, M.S., Han, S.J. et al. (2014). Magnesium as an adjuvant for caudal analgesia in children. *Paediatr. Anaesth.* 24 (12): 1231–1238.

Kogika, M.M. and de Morais, H.A. (2017). A quick reference on hypokalemia. *Vet. Clin. N. Am. Small Anim. Pract.* 47 (2): 229–234.

Kozeny, G.A., Murdock, D.K., Euler, D.E. et al. (1985). In vivo effects of acute changes in osmolality and sodium concentration on myocardial contractility. *Am. Heart J.* 109 (2): 290–296.

Kumar, A., Singh, H., and Singh, R. (1971). Clinical studies on chloral-mag anaesthesia in dog. *Indian Vet. J.* 48 (2): 185–189.

Marino, P. (2007a). Calcium and phosphorus. In: *The ICU Book*, 3e (ed. P. Marino, L. Williams and Wilkins), 639–647.

Marino, P. (2007b). Hypertonic and hypotonic conditions. In: *The ICU Book*, 3e (ed. P. Marino, L. Williams and Wilkins), 595–610.

Marino, P. (2007c). Potassium. In: *The ICU Book*, 3e, 611–623.

Marino, P. (2014). Magnesium. I: The ICU Book, (ed. P. Marino, L. Williams and Wilkins), 687–699.

Mascarenhas, J.V. and Jude, E.B. (2014). Central pontine myelinolysis: electrolytes and beyond. *BMJ Case Rep.* 2014: //schemas.Openxmlformats.

Nickell, J.R. and Shih, A. (2011). Anesthesia case of the month. Administration of aged packed RBCs. *J. Am. Vet. Med. Assoc.* 239 (11): 1429–1431.

Pang, D.S., Panizzi, L., and Paterson, J.M. (2011). Successful treatment of hyperkalaemic periodic paralysis in a horse during isoflurane anaesthesia. *Vet. Anaesth. Analg.* 38 (2): 113–120.

Parker, M.S., Oster, J.R., Perez, G.O., and Taylor, A.L. (1980). Chronic hypokalemia and alkalosis: approach to diagnosis. *Arch. Intern. Med.* 140 (10): 1336–1337.

Peterson, B., Khanna, S., Fisher, B., and Marshall, L. (2000). Prolonged hypernatremia controls elevated intracranial pressure in head-injured pediatric patients. *Crit. Care Med.* 28 (4): 1136–1143.

Pokaharel, M. and Block, C.A. (2011). Dysnatremia in the ICU. *Curr. Opin. Crit. Care* 17 (6): 581–593.

Posner, L. and Burns, P. (2009). Injectable anesthetic agents. In: *Veterinary Pharmacology & Therapeutics* (ed. J. Riviere and M. Papich), 265–299. Wiley.

Queiroz-Castro, P., Egger, C., Redua, M.A. et al. (2006). Effects of ketamine and magnesium on the minimum alveolar concentration of isoflurane in goats. *Am. J. Vet. Res.* 67 (12): 1962–1966.

Raftery, A.G., Morgan, R.A., and MacFarlane, P.D. (2015). Perioperative trends in plasma colloid osmotic pressure in horses undergoing surgery. *J. Vet. Emerg. Crit. Care (San Antonio, Tex.: 2001)* 26 (1): 93–100.

Rioja, E., Dzikiti, B.T., Fosgate, G. et al. (2012). Effects of a constant rate infusion of magnesium sulphate in healthy dogs anaesthetized with isoflurane and undergoing ovariohysterectomy. *Vet. Anaesth. Analg.* 39 (6): 599–610.

Schaer, M. (2008). Therapeutic approach to electrolyte emergencies. *Vet. Clin. N. Am. Small Anim. Pract.* 38 (3): 513–533. x.

Schauvliege, S. and Gasthuys, F. (2013). Drugs for cardiovascular support in anesthetized horses. *Vet. Clin. N. Am. Equine Pract.* 29 (1): 19–49.

Sharma, S.K., Singh, J., Singh, A.P., and Peshin, P.K. (1984). Haemodynamics, blood gas and metabolic changes after anaesthesia with chloral hydrate and magnesium sulphate in camels (*Camelus dromedarius*). *Res. Vet. Sci.* 36 (1): 12–15.

Shetty, K.P., Satish, S.V., Kilaru, K.R. et al. (2015). Comparison of anesthetic efficacy between lidocaine with and without magnesium sulfate USP 50% for inferior alveolar nerve blocks in patients with symptomatic irreversible pulpitis. *J. Endodont.* 41 (4): 431–433.

Singh, H., Kumar, A., Bagha, H.S., and Singh, R. (1971). Studies on chloral mag anaesthesia with and without premedication in buffaloes. *Indian Vet. J.* 48 (6): 640–645.

Snell, D.M. and Bartley, C. (2008). Osmotic demyelination syndrome following rapid correction of hyponatraemia. *Anaesthesia* 63 (1): 92–95.

Stankovic, A.K. and Smith, S. (2004). Elevated serum potassium values: the role of preanalytic variables. *Am. J. Clin. Pathol.* 121 (Suppl): S105–S112.

Svensen, C. (2013). Chapter 34 – Electrolytes and diuretics. In: *Pharmacology and Physiology for Anesthesia: Foundations and Clinical Application* (ed. H. Hemmings and T. Egan). Saunders.

Tanifuji, Y. and Eger, E.I. 2nd (1978). Brain sodium, potassium, and osmolality: effects on anesthetic requirement. *Anesth. Analg.* 57 (4): 404–410.

Taylor, G., Myers, S., Kurth, C.D. et al. (1996). Hypertonic saline improves brain resuscitation in a pediatric model of head injury and hemorrhagic shock. *J. Pediatr. Surg.* 31 (1): 65–70. discussion 70–1.

Trim, C.M. and Hanson, R.R. (1986). Effects of xylazine on renal function and plasma glucose in ponies. *Vet. Rec.* 118 (3): 65–67.

Wendt-Hornickle, E.L., Snyder, L.B., Tang, R., and Johnson, R.A. (2011). The effects of lactated Ringer's solution (LRS) or LRS and 6% hetastarch on the colloid osmotic pressure, total protein and osmolality in healthy horses under general anesthesia. *Vet. Anaesth. Analg.* 38 (4): 336–343.

Wright, B.D. and Hopkins, A. (2008). Changes in colloid osmotic pressure as a function of anesthesia and surgery in the presence and absence of isotonic fluid administration in dogs. *Vet. Anaesth. Analg.* 35 (4): 282–288.

30

IV Fluids

Anusha Balakrishnan

IV Fluids

The primary goal of perianesthetic fluid therapy is to maintain and improve tissue perfusion and restore optimal oxygen and nutrient delivery to tissues. In the sick anesthetized patient with shock, secondary to an absolute or relative decrease in the effective circulating intravascular volume, such as in hypovolemic or distributive shock, intravenous (IV) fluid therapy is the cornerstone of management. Secondary goals of perianesthetic fluid therapy include restoring or maintaining acid–base and electrolyte balance, as well as maintaining patency of IV catheters. Various factors should be taken into consideration while administering IV fluid therapy in these patients, including timing, volume and rate of fluid administration, as well as safety, efficacy, and cost-effectiveness of the fluids.

Important considerations for providing effective and safe fluid therapy to patients under general anesthesia include:

- **Overall health of the patient:** Healthy patients undergoing elective procedures such as ovariohysterectomy or dental cleaning have different fluid requirements from sicker patients undergoing emergency surgical procedures, such as an exploratory laparotomy for a patient with septic peritonitis. Special consideration must be given to patients with different co-morbidities, such as cardiac disease or renal disease, while formulating a fluid therapy plan under general anesthesia.
- **Effects of anesthetic drugs used:** Several anesthetic drugs used commonly in veterinary medicine have profound effects on the cardiovascular system causing changes in vascular tone and increase or decrease in heart rate and cardiac contractility. Inhalant anesthetics, in particular, cause significant vasodilation and decreased cardiac contractility, and can result in hypotension in the anesthetized patient.
- **Intra-operative volume loss**: Surgical blood loss can be a significant contributor to intra-operative hypotension

and must be taken into account when calculating fluid volumes to be administered to patients for replacement.
- **Insensible losses:** Ongoing losses caused by exposure of body cavities and evaporative loss can be a significant cause of hypovolemia and hypotension in the anesthetized surgical patient.

Fluid Therapy Endpoints and Monitoring

Fluid therapy for the anesthetized patient is performed under close monitoring and should continue until various resuscitation endpoints have been reached. These endpoints include physical examination parameters such as improvement in heart rate, pulse quality, capillary refill time, and temperature of extremities. Maintenance or normalization of arterial blood pressure is another clinical parameter widely used to guide fluid therapy under anesthesia. Bloodwork parameters such as lactate levels and central venous oxygen saturation, when available, can be serially monitored to ensure improvement with fluid therapy. However, these traditional markers of hemodynamic stability may prove insensitive at the detection of hypovolemia. Studies in dogs show that cardiovascular compensatory mechanisms can delay the onset of hypotension following blood loss until 30–40% of blood volume has been lost (Berkenstadt et al. 2005). Therefore, hypotension should be a considered a late and insensitive indicator of adequate tissue perfusion (Navarro et al. 2015).

Fluid responsiveness has been defined in dogs as a 10–15% increase in stroke volume following a 10–20 ml/kg fluid challenge (Celeita-Rodriguez et al. 2019). The prevalence of fluid responsiveness in anesthetized veterinary patients is not well described, although a single study did report that approximately 83% of dogs undergoing abdominal surgery were fluid responsive (Drozdzynska et al. 2018).

Pharmacology in Veterinary Anesthesia and Analgesia, First Edition. Edited by Turi Aarnes and Phillip Lerche.
© 2024 John Wiley & Sons, Inc. Published 2024 by John Wiley & Sons, Inc.

Dynamic markers of volume responsiveness have been studied extensively in recent years, providing tools to guide interventions with fluid therapy. These markers are most easily assessed in anesthetized patients on mechanical ventilation and rely on the dynamic and cyclic heart-lung interactions that occur during this time. In hypovolemic patients, mechanical ventilation causes a much more significant compromise to venous return, increasing the variability noted through the respiratory cycle. These dynamic markers, including pulse pressure variation (PPV), tend to be less reliable in patients with cardiac arrhythmias or in those that are spontaneously ventilating (Araos et al. 2020).

PPV reflects the ratio of the difference between the maximum and minimum pulse pressure between their mean. Several studies in anesthetized dogs have shown that PPV >7–16% are predictive for fluid responsiveness (Endo et al. 2017; Fantoni et al. 2017; Drozdzynska et al. 2018; Celeita-Rodriguez et al. 2019). Another similar dynamic index, stroke volume variation (SVV), has also been evaluated in anesthetized dogs, with an SVV >11% found to be predictive for fluid responsiveness (Endo et al. 2017). More recently, a study comparing PPV and systolic pressure variation (SPV) obtained from the dorsal pedal artery in anesthetized dogs undergoing elective ovariohysterectomy were both useful predictors of fluid responsiveness (Dalmagro et al. 2021).

Fluid Types

Various types of fluids available for fluid therapy of the anesthetized patient include isotonic and hypertonic crystalloids, and natural (including blood products) and synthetic colloids.

Crystalloids

Crystalloids are solutions of small water-soluble molecules that can pass freely across a semi-permeable membrane such as the capillary endothelium. The tonicity of these solutions reflects their osmolality relative to that of plasma.

Isotonic Crystalloids

Composition

Crystalloids have a tonicity relatively similar to that of plasma. The principal component of isotonic crystalloid fluids is the inorganic salt sodium chloride (NaCl), with 0.9% NaCl being the prototype isotonic crystalloid. Normal strength saline has a significantly lower strong ion difference and a higher chloride level (154 mEq/l) than plasma levels in most veterinary patients. Normal canine plasma chloride levels are between 105 and 110 mEq/l, while normal equine plasma chloride ranges from 90 to 102 mEq/l (Raghunathan et al. 2013). This can have a significant impact on the acid–base status of patients, potentially causing a hyperchloremic metabolic acidosis by decreasing the strong ion difference. The use of saline in human patients has also been shown to increase the risk for renal injury, potentially related to a chloride-related renal vasoconstriction and subsequent renal hypoperfusion. For this reason, several "balanced" isotonic crystalloids have been developed where some of the chloride is replaced by buffer ions such as acetate and gluconate which are bicarbonate precursors.

Pharmacology

The fact that isotonic crystalloids have sodium levels relatively comparable to that of plasma limits the movement of water out of the extracellular fluid compartment into the intracellular fluid compartment and vice versa. Sodium is the most abundant solute in the extracellular fluid, and it is distributed uniformly throughout the extracellular space. Because 75% of the extracellular fluids are located in the extravascular (interstitial) space, a similar proportion of the total body sodium is in the interstitial fluids. Exogenously administered sodium follows the same distribution, so approximately 75% of the volume of sodium-based IV fluids are rapidly redistributed within the interstitium. This means that to increase plasma volume by a given amount, four times the desired volume needs to be administered to take account of the interstitial redistribution.

When administered rapidly as a bolus, isotonic crystalloids can effectively expand plasma volume. A 2005 study showed that a rapid infusion of 80 ml/kg of 0.9% saline to four healthy dogs caused a 76.4% increase in intravascular volume (Silverstein et al. 2005). While rapid redistribution did occur, leaving a net intravascular volume increase of only 35% at 30 minutes and 18% at four hours post-infusion, it is possible that a similar volume of infusion to hypovolemic animals may have resulted in a greater, more prolonged expansion of the vascular volume.

The elimination clearance (Cl) for isotonic crystalloids can vary based on several factors, such as hydration levels, physiologic stressors, ongoing surgical procedures and the influence of general anesthesia. Patients under general anesthesia tend to have a lower intravascular hydrostatic pressure secondary to volatile anesthetic-induced vasodilation. This could potentially play a role in reducing the clearance of infused fluids and increasing volume expansion from a given infusion. The proportion of infused crystalloids retained in the intravascular space may approach 100% in hypotensive patients when the arterial blood pressure decreases by 20–30%, such as during acute hemorrhage or during general anesthesia (Hahn and Lyons 2016).

Dosing

Isotonic crystalloids are inexpensive and readily available and, as such, are typically the first choice for perianesthetic fluid therapy in most cases. Fluid therapy in small animal patients undergoing general anesthesia is variable and often dictated by patient needs. Advantages of providing fluid therapy during general anesthesia include correction of normal, ongoing fluid losses and potential countering of volatile-anesthetic induced hypotension. Current recommendations in small animals advise fluid rates of 3 ml/kg/h in cats and 5 ml/kg/h in dogs should be employed as starting rates, with reassessment and adjustment as necessary (Davis et al. 2013). Preoperative volume loading in euvolemic patients is not recommended. Rates are typically lower in patients with cardiac disease, and higher in patients with renal disease. In azotemic patients, generally 1.5–2 times maintenance crystalloid administration for the 12–24 hours prior to anesthesia is recommended. Fluid rates up to 20–30 ml/kg/h during anesthesia have been recommended in patients with renal dysfunction (Bednarski et al. 2011). Fluid therapy rates in horses under general anesthesia start at 3–10 ml/kg/h of an isotonic crystalloid, with reassessment of the patient as needed. In case of significant hypotension, rates of up to 20–30 ml/kg/h may be used (Hardy 2009). IV fluid therapy in ruminants undergoing surgery typically includes the use of a balanced isotonic solution, particularly if the patient has been fasting for 24 hours or longer prior to anesthesia. Normal maintenance fluid therapy in ruminants under anesthesia is typically between 4 and 8 ml/kg/h, but rates of up to 10–25 ml/kg/h may be used in cardiovascularly unstable patients or if blood loss is anticipated intra-operatively. Ruminants tend to lose large volumes of saliva during anesthesia, but replacement of electrolytes lost in this manner is typically not necessary for most anesthetic procedures. Fluid therapy in camelids must be undertaken cautiously since their fluid tolerance tends to be low and fluid overload and subsequent pulmonary edema may result in these species.

When used for rapid intra-vascular volume restoration in a hypotensive patient under anesthesia, the classic "shock dose" is approximately 60–90 ml/kg in dogs, 45–60 ml/kg in cats, and 60–80 ml/kg in horses, which reflects the approximate blood volumes in each of these species. The actual dose used to treat patients with evidence of hypovolemia under anesthesia (absolute or relative) varies widely and is influenced by the species, individual patient, severity of hypovolemia, and any other co-morbidities (e.g. cardiac disease). A common recommendation is to use an aliquot of the shock dose, typically around 25–30% (bolus of 10–20 ml/kg) administered over 15–30 minutes, reassess the patient after this, and repeat if necessary. The patient should be closely monitored during delivery of the bolus, and it should be slowed or discontinued if any adverse effects are seen or if perfusion parameters improve before the end of the predetermined amount.

The effectiveness of isotonic crystalloids in combating volatile anesthetic-induced hypotension in veterinary patients has been called into question. A 2009 study compared the efficacy of administration of 80 ml of LRS/kg with <40 ml/kg of a synthetic colloid in healthy dogs with isoflurane-induced hypotension (Aarnes et al. 2009). This study found that administration of LRS decreased blood viscosity but did not increase arterial blood pressure in any of the patients. Another study in healthy, normovolemic isoflurane-anesthetized dogs administered isotonic crystalloids at a rapid rate of 1 ml/kg/min showed that these fluids were ineffective at treating isoflurane-induced hypotension (Valverde et al. 2012).

Adverse Effects

Aggressive crystalloid-based fluid therapy can lead to several adverse effects, especially in patients predisposed to volume overload (e.g. patients with severe hypoproteinemia or cardiac disease). Because these fluids redistribute into the interstitium, organ edema can occur and may be life threatening. Pulmonary edema and acute lung injury are among the most commonly seen adverse effects of aggressive crystalloid therapy, particularly in patients with increased vascular permeability secondary to systemic inflammation or sepsis.

Other consequences of aggressive and overzealous crystalloid administration include changes to the gastrointestinal (GI) tract resulting in decreased motility, increased intestinal permeability predisposing the patient to bacterial translocation, and increased risk for abdominal compartment syndrome. Cardiac effects of crystalloid therapy have also been documented and include an increased risk of ventricular arrhythmias and disruption of cardiac contractility. Coagulation disturbances can also occur as a result of dilution of coagulation factors and decreased blood viscosity; however, these effects are significantly less than changes caused by synthetic colloids (Shoemaker and Hauser 1979; Cotton et al. 2006).

In recent years, the endothelial glycocalyx, a gel-like layer covering the luminal surface of vascular endothelial cells, has been a focus of interest for its role in regulating vascular permeability, providing anti-coagulant effects, and protecting endothelial cells from oxidative stress (Uchimido et al. 2019). There is increasing evidence that suggests that rapid fluid therapy with both crystalloids and colloids can induce shedding of the endothelial glycocalyx through hemodilution and osmotic changes (Smart et al. 2018).

Isotonic crystalloids, particularly lactated Ringer's solution, have been associated with causing activation of pro-inflammatory mediators. Many formulations of lactated Ringer's solution contain racemic mixtures of both the L- and D-lactate stereoisomers. The D-lactate isomer has been associated with an increase in neutrophil stimulation and migration to the lungs, apoptosis of cells in the lungs, and increased production of reactive oxygen species, thereby potentiating the pro-inflammatory response, whereas the L-lactate isomer is rapidly metabolized by the liver (Rhee et al. 1998; Alam et al. 2004).

Normal strength saline, in particular, can have significant deleterious effects on acid–base and electrolyte status, as a consequence of its high chloride concentration, and can cause a decrease in blood pH, decrease in bicarbonate and strong ion difference resulting in a hyperchloremic metabolic acidosis. This has been evaluated in several human studies in anesthetized patients (McFarlane and Lee 1994; Waters et al. 2001; Tellan et al. 2008). Clear evidence indicating that balanced fluids may be preferred in veterinary patients does not exist. A large Cochrane review in humans did not find a mortality difference between critically ill patients treated with a buffered solution versus. normal saline (Martin et al. 2019) (See Table 30.1).

There is some concern that administration of lactated Ringer's solution can cause an increase in plasma lactate levels, which was borne out by studies in anesthetized human patients undergoing various surgical procedures (Scheingraber et al. 1999; Hadimioglu et al. 2008; Shin et al. 2011). Another study evaluating the effect of rapid administration of LRS in healthy dogs found that plasma lactate levels increased significantly within 10 minutes of administration but decreased back to baseline within 60 minutes (Boysen and Dorval 2014). While the clinical significance of these findings is unknown, caution should be exercised when interpreting serum lactate values in these patients and using them as a marker to guide further fluid therapy.

Acetate containing solutions, such as PlasmaLyte-148®, are widely used in veterinary medicine. However, theoretical concerns exist about the vasodilatory and cardiovascular depressant effects of acetate-containing infusions (Aizawa et al. 1977; Kirkendol et al. 1980; Olinger et al. 1979; Veech and Gitomore 1988). However, this has not been borne out in animal models or any veterinary clinical studies.

Hypertonic Crystalloids

Composition

Hypertonic saline solutions have an effective osmolarity greater than that of normal plasma. Commonly used concentrations range from 3% to 7.5%. Hypertonic saline is available commercially in concentrations of 7.2% and 23.4%. Hypertonic saline has several beneficial properties that make it an excellent choice for rapid, small-volume resuscitation in hypotensive patients. A 2005 study evaluating the changes in blood volume after a bolus of 4 ml/kg of 7.5% sodium chloride showed that the post-infusion plasma volume change was only about 17% despite a brief increase in blood volume about three times the volume of fluid administered (Silverstein et al. 2005). Its ability to cause intravascular volume expansion in excess of the volume infused is due to the osmotic gradient generated by the sudden, dramatic increase in plasma osmolarity after administration, thus making it a good option for small-volume resuscitation. A meta-analysis published in 2010 of studies evaluating the use of hypertonic saline for perioperative fluid therapy in human surgical patients showed that patients receiving hypertonic saline had a significantly less positive postoperative fluid balance and received significantly less volume of fluids overall. The study also showed that hypertonic saline given intraoperatively caused a significantly higher cardiac index without a concomitant increase in pulmonary capillary wedge pressure in these patients. However, no information on the effects on survival and morbidity could be gleaned from the included studies (McAlister et al. 2010). In another more recent study, the use of 3% hypertonic saline was compared to lactated Ringer's solution in human surgical patients undergoing pancreatic surgery, and the hypertonic saline group received lower fluid volumes perioperatively and had a lower incidence of peri- and postoperative complications (Lavu et al. 2014).

Hypertonic saline also has other beneficial properties which make it an attractive choice as a resuscitative fluid. These properties include immunomodulatory effects, such as decreased neutrophil activation and adherence, stimulation of lymphocyte proliferation, and inhibition of pro-inflammatory cytokine production by macrophages. It also improves the rheologic properties of circulating blood, reduces endothelial cell swelling, and helps reduce intracranial pressure (ICP) in patients with traumatic brain injury (TBI) (Rizoli et al. 2006; Bulger et al. 2008; Balbino et al. 2010; Mortazavi et al. 2012). Experimental evidence suggests that hypertonic saline improves myocardial function and causes coronary vasodilation (Mouren et al. 1995), thereby improving overall cardiac function. However, its effect on cardiac contractility in clinical veterinary settings requires further evaluation.

The veterinary literature regarding the use of hypertonic saline solutions during anesthesia or for shock resuscitation is limited. A study in hypovolemic endurance horses showed that hypertonic saline led to faster restoration of

Table 30.1 Commonly available IV fluids for peri-operative use in veterinary medicine.

Solution	Category	Sodium (mEq/l)	Potassium (mEq/l)	Chloride (mEq/l)	Magnesium (mEq/l)	Buffer (mEq/l)	COP (mmHg)	Average molecular weight (kDa)	Molar substitution	C2:C6 ratio
0.9% NaCl	Isotonic crystalloid	154	–	154	–	–	–	–	–	–
Lactated Ringer's solution	Isotonic crystalloid	130	4	109	–	Lactate (28)	–	–	–	–
Plasma-lyte 148®	Isotonic crystalloid	140	5	98	1.5	Acetate (27) Gluconate (23)	–	–	–	–
7.2% NaCl	Hypertonic crystalloid	1232	–	1232	–	–	–	–	–	–
Hetastarch in 0.9% NaCl (Hespan)	Synthetic colloid	154	–	154	–	–	30	670	0.75	5:1
Hetastarch in lactated electrolyte solution (Hextend)	Synthetic colloid	143	3	124	0.9	Lactate (28)	30	670	0.75	5:1
Tetrastarch in 0.9% NaCl (Voluven, Vetstarch)	Synthetic colloid	154	–	154	–	–	–	130	0.4	9 : 1

intravascular volume deficits than isotonic saline (Fielding and Magdesian 2011). A 2006 study in anesthetized horses with experimentally induced endotoxemia revealed that administration of 7.2% hypertonic saline, combined with a synthetic colloid, failed to improve cardiac output, systemic vascular resistance, mean arterial pressure or arterial lactate levels (Pantaleon et al. 2006). In another equine study evaluating preoperative fluid therapy with 7.2% hypertonic saline in surgical colic cases, no benefit to overall long-term survival was noted in the hypertonic saline group (Miller et al. 2013). A more recent study in healthy anesthetized horses reported a significant increase in systolic blood pressure 10 minutes following administration of a 4 ml/kg bolus of 7.2% hypertonic saline that lasted for 25 minutes when compared to baseline (Schnuelle et al. 2020). Further studies in veterinary medicine regarding the use of perioperative fluid therapy with hypertonic saline solutions are warranted.

Dosing

Typically, a 3–5 ml/kg dose of 7–7.5% solution is used for small-volume resuscitation. Because hypertonic saline rapidly redistributes into the interstitium within 30 minutes after administration and also causes an osmotic diuresis, its volume expansion effect is short lived (Oliveira et al. 2002). For this reason, it is often combined with a synthetic colloid. This combined solution, sometimes referred to as "turbostarch," is administered at a dose of 3–5 ml/kg and is prepared by mixing a stock solution of 23.4% hypertonic saline with a synthetic colloid in an approximately 1 : 2 ratio to arrive at a total volume of 3–5 ml/kg. For example, a 5 ml/kg dose for a 12-kg dog would be 60 ml. Therefore, one part 23.4% hypertonic saline (20 ml) with two parts (40 ml) 6% hetastarch would create an approximately 7.5% hypertonic saline solution.

Adverse Effects

The primary adverse effect of hypertonic saline is hypernatremia. This is seen immediately after administration but is usually transient (McAlister et al. 2010). There is a risk for hypernatremia-induced osmotic demyelination syndrome in patients with pre-existing chronic hyponatremia. Most critically ill or anesthetized patients have frequent monitoring of electrolytes, and the risk of transient hypernatremia does not usually outweigh the potential benefits hypertonic saline therapy.

Hypertonic saline should be used cautiously in patients with pre-existing cardiac or pulmonary abnormalities because the increase in intravascular volume and hydrostatic pressure may lead to volume overload or pulmonary edema. It can also cause significant interstitial (and intravascular) volume depletion, particularly in patients that are already dehydrated. Therefore, hypertonic fluid administration should be followed by additional fluid therapy as indicated.

Synthetic Colloids

Composition

Colloids are large molecules (>10 000 Da) of varying sizes that do not readily cross diffusion barriers across normal blood vessels as crystalloids do. Commercially available synthetic colloids used in veterinary medicine typically contain large molecules of amylopectin (a synthetic glucose polymer derived from waxy potato or maize starch) suspended in an isotonic crystalloid solution (typically 0.9% NaCl or LRS) (Table 30.1).

Pharmacology

The three most important properties of synthetic colloids that influence their pharmacologic behavior and half-life include the molecular weight, degree of molar substitution and the C2/C6 ratio.

The degree of molar substitution of a starch is determined by the average number of hydroxyethyl residues per 100 available anhydrous glucose units. This varies widely, and most new solutions contain fewer residues per glucose subunit. Highly substituted starches have a terminal half-life that increases with repetitive dosing as well as with longer infusion durations (Treib et al. 1996).

The other major property of starches that can be modified and play a role in their pharmacokinetic properties is the pattern of hydroxyl substitution with hydroxyethyl groups on the molecule. This is also called the C2/C6 ratio and reflects the relative degree of substitution at the second and sixth carbon atoms on the starch molecule. The speed of metabolism of a given starch molecule is inversely proportional to the C2/C6 ratio.

Colloids are metabolized in the body primarily through enzymatic degradation by plasma α-amylases which cleave within the glucose polymer chain resulting in smaller fragments of the starch molecule.

α-amylase-mediated hydrolysis can reduce the molecular weight of these particles to less than 72 kDa. Starches with a higher degree of molar substitution and a higher C2/C6 ratio tend to have longer elimination half-lives and slower rates of α-amylase mediated hydrolysis (Asskali and Förster 1999; Jungheinrich and Neff 2005). The clearance of starch molecules from the intravascular space depends on the rate of their absorption by tissues (liver, spleen, kidney, and heart), uptake by the reticuloendothelial system and clearance through urine and less significantly, bile (Jungheinrich and Neff 2005). There is some degree of transient tissue retention of starch molecules, which appears to be directly proportional to their molecular weight. A 2003 study in rats showed that tetrastarches with an average molecular weight of 130 kDa had lower tissue storage than hetastarches with an average molecular weight of 450 kDa (Leuschner et al. 2003).

Colloids infused into the vascular space therefore tend to remain in the vascular space rather than redistribute to the interstitial space. This, theoretically, leads to a more sustained intravascular expansion effect. These fluids increase the colloid osmotic pressure of serum, creating a force that opposes the hydrostatic pressure in the vasculature and helps retain fluid in the vascular space by preventing extravasation into the interstitial space. This property of colloids makes them useful for volume expansion in anesthetized, hypotensive patients.

Hetastarch

Hetastarch is a synthetic colloid available as a 6% solution suspended in an isotonic-crystalloid solution such as 0.9% saline (Hespan®) or a lactated-electrolyte solution (Hextend®). Hetastarch has a molar substitution of 70 groups out of 100 (0.7), and a molecular weight around 670 kDa. In a study in healthy dogs, infusion of 20 ml/kg of hetastarch solution produced a 27.2% increase in blood volume immediately after infusion, an increase to 36.8% at 30 minutes, and maintenance of 26.6% at four hours post-infusion (Silverstein et al. 2005).

Tetrastarch

Tetrastarch (Voluven® or Vetstarch®) has particles with a slightly lower weight average molecular weight (130 kDa) and a lower substitution with hydroxyethyl groups (40 groups out of 100, or 0.4) than the previously discussed hetastarch. These properties are likely responsible for causing the purported benefit of fewer adverse effects on coagulation than hetastarch solutions. This product has been approved for use in small animals (Vetstarch®). More studies in veterinary medicine evaluating the effects of this particular synthetic colloid are necessary to assess its effectiveness and safety as a volume expander.

Pentastarch

Pentastarch (Pentaspan®) is a low-molecular-weight derivative of hetastarch with an average molecular weight between 200 and 300 kDa, and a molar substitution of 0.4–0.5 (approximately 45 hydroxyethyl groups per 100 glucose subunits), that is available as a 6% or 10% solution in isotonic saline. Although it is not currently approved for clinical use in the US, it has been used in other parts of the world as an effective volume expander. Pentastarch contains smaller but more numerous starch molecules than hetastarch and thus has a higher colloid osmotic pressure.

Dosing

Because colloids are retained in the vascular space longer than crystalloid solutions and can have adverse coagulation effects, the recommended rates and volumes of administration of these fluids are typically much lower than that of crystalloids. When synthetic colloids are used for the treatment of shock, the typical dose is 10–20 ml/kg in the dog and horse and 5–10 ml/kg in the cat (see Table 30.1). This is commonly administered to effect in incremental boluses of 2–5 ml/kg over 10–20 minutes.

A 2009 study showed that <40 ml/kg of a synthetic colloid was effective in improving isoflurane-induced hypotension in anesthetized dogs (Aarnes et al. 2009). Synthetic colloids have been shown to provide more effective volume expansion and improve arterial blood pressure when compared to crystalloids in awake horses (Epstein et al. 2014). They have also been shown to improve colloid osmotic pressure in awake horses and camelids in several studies (Jones et al. 1997, 2001; Carney et al. 2011). However, a 2011 study in horses anesthetized for non-gastrointestinal tract surgery showed that administration of synthetic colloids at a rate of 2.5 ml/kg over one hour along with crystalloids did not prevent the attenuation of colloid osmotic pressure seen with administration of crystalloids alone (Wendt-Hornickle et al. 2011). A more recent study evaluating 10% hydroxyethyl starch in systemically healthy horses undergoing elective surgical procedures found that 6 ml/kg of the starch was effective at maintaining COP during anesthesia (Brunisholz et al. 2015).

Adverse Effects

Acute Kidney Injury

Much emphasis has been placed in recent years on the various potential adverse effects of synthetic colloids, especially in critically ill people. There has been recent evidence in several human trials and meta-analyses that high molecular-weight starches (HES 200/0.6 and >200) may cause acute kidney injury in patients with severe sepsis, although HES 130/0.4 may be less harmful (Myburgh et al. 2012; Zarychanski et al. 2013; Neto et al. 2014). However, a subsequent study did not support this hypothesis and showed that even 6% HES 130/0.4 can cause more impairment of renal function than resuscitation with crystalloids alone in patients with severe sepsis (Perner et al. 2012). Another veterinary study evaluating the use of 10% hydroxyethyl starch 250/0.5 found an increased risk of acute kidney injury and mortality in the dogs receiving synthetic colloids (Hayes et al. 2016). Other veterinary studies have found mixed results, including in cats (Yozova et al. 2016, 2017; Sigrist et al. 2017a, 2017b; Boyd et al. 2019). A recent prospective study (Boyd et al. 2021) compared biomarkers of acute kidney injury between dogs receiving 6% HES 130/0.4 and Hartmann's Solution, and found no differences between the groups of dogs. Larger studies in different veterinary populations are warranted to further evaluate this.

There are several proposed mechanisms by which synthetic colloids can cause renal injury. One of the earlier proposed theories suggested that ischemic injury occurred secondary to hyperviscosity caused by colloid infusions (particularly with hyperoncotic formulations such as 10% hetastarch), resulting in increased urine viscosity and decreased tubular flow (Hüter et al. 2009). An important mechanism for starch-induced kidney injury is osmotic nephrosis after starch molecules enter renal proximal tubular cells via pinocytosis and cause vacuolization and swelling of these cells. This compromises and occludes the tubular lumen and impedes urine flow. Experimental data from isolated porcine renal perfusion models indicates that synthetic colloid infusions caused reduced urine output, higher levels of N-acetyl-B-aminoglucosidase (a biomarker for acute kidney injury), renal interstitial cell proliferation and the presence of osmotic nephrosis-like lesions. This study also showed that higher molecular weight starches with higher molar substitution (200/0.5) caused more pronounced renal tubular damage than lower molecular weight and less substituted starches (130/0.4) (Schortgen et al. 2008).

Despite these studies in critically ill patients with sepsis, the effects on renal tissue caused by shorter durations of exposure to smaller amounts of starches intraoperatively in anesthetized patients are less clear. A meta-analysis published in 2021 evaluated the safety of tetrastarches used in a perioperative setting in humans showed no increase in postoperative mortality or renal injury (Xu et al. 2021). Studies on the renal impact of starches in anesthetized veterinary patients are sparse – a recent retrospective study examined paired plasma creatinine and chloride concentrations in dogs undergoing general anesthesia for various reasons. This study showed no evidence of AKI following a median dose of 6.3 ml/kg of hetastarch under anesthesia (Zersen et al. 2019)

Coagulopathies

All synthetic colloids have the potential to interfere with hemostasis, either through a nonspecific effect correlated to the degree of hemodilution of coagulation factors, or through specific actions of these macromolecules on platelet function, coagulation proteins, and the fibrinolytic system. High molecular-weight starches can cause decreases in the activity of von Willebrand's factor and its associated factor VIII and ristocetin cofactor activities, decreased platelet aggregation through effects on the platelet integrin $\alpha_{IIb}\beta_3$, and impaired factor XIII- fibrin cross linking as well as enhanced fibrinolysis (de Jonge and Levi 2001; Kozek-Langenecker 2005; Westphal et al. 2009).

Several studies in veterinary medicine have documented the effects of synthetic colloids on hemostasis (Falco et al. 2012; Helmbold et al. 2014). A 2015 study evaluating administration of tetrastarch to dogs with LPS-induced endotoxemia found that tetrastarch administration resulted in transiently prolonged partial thromboplastin time, decreased platelet count, decreased speed of clot formation and weaker clot strength, as well as acquired type 1 von Willebrand disease (Gauthier et al. 2015). Another canine study evaluating coagulation parameters in anesthetized healthy dogs undergoing orthopedic surgery found that a bolus of 10 ml/kg of 6% hetastarch (600/0.75) caused an increase in buccal mucosal bleeding time and decrease in platelet count; however, no clinical bleeding was noticed in these dogs (Chohan et al. 2011). A recent canine study evaluating dogs with spontaneous hemoperitoneum that received 6% hydroxyethyl starch 130/0.4 reported impairment of thromboelastometric parameters of clot formation time and maximum clot firmness with no evidence of fibrinolysis (Iannucci et al. 2021). Caution is recommended when using synthetic colloids in hypocoagulable patients undergoing surgical procedures that may have an increased risk of clinical bleeding.

Coagulation abnormalities following colloid administration have also been described in several studies in horses (Schusser et al. 2007; Blong et al. 2013; Viljoen et al. 2014). Starches induce dose-dependent changes in coagulation parameters in horses, beyond causing just hemodilution. However, none of these studies document clinically significant bleeding tendencies that could be reliably attributed to the use of starches.

Conclusion

IV fluid therapy is a cornerstone of management of anesthetized veterinary patients. While similar underlying physiologic principles of fluid needs and responsiveness apply to these patients, there are unique changes induced by general anesthesia that can alter various aspects of patient management. Judicious, goal-directed fluid therapy tailored to the needs of each individual patient is warranted, and care should be taken to consider co-morbidities, the anticipated complications resulting from any surgical procedures as well as the influence of the other anesthetic drugs used when creating a fluid therapy plan. Crystalloids remain the mainstay of intraoperative fluid management of most veterinary patients, but the use of colloids can be considered in certain situations.

References

Aarnes, T.K., Bednarski, R.M., Lerche, P. et al. (2009). Effect of intravenous administration of lactated ringer's solution or hetastarch for the treatment of isoflurane-induced hypotension in dogs. *Am. J. Vet. Res.* 70 (11): 1345–1353.

Aizawa, Y., Ohmori, T., Imai, K. et al. (1977). Depressant action of acetate upon the human cardiovascular system. *Clin. Nephrol.* 8 (5): 477–480.

Alam, H.B., Stanton, K., Koustova, E. et al. (2004). Effect of different resuscitation strategies on neutrophil activation in a swine model of hemorrhagic shock. *Resuscitation* 60 (1): 91–99.

Araos, J., Kenny, J.S., Rousseau-Blass, F., and Pang, D.S.J. (2020). Dynamic prediction of fluid responsiveness during positive pressure ventilation: a review of the physiology underlying heart-lung interactions and a critical interpretation. *Vet. Anesth. Analg.* 47 (1): 3–14.

Asskali, F. and Förster, H. (1999). The accumulation of different substituted hydroxyethyl starches (HES) following repeated infusions in healthy volunteers. *Anasthesiol. Intensivmed. Notfallmed. Schmerzther.* 34 (9): 537–541.

Balbino, M., Capone Neto, A., Prist, R. et al. (2010). Fluid resuscitation with isotonic or hypertonic saline solution avoids Intraneural calcium influx after traumatic brain injury associated with hemorrhagic shock. *J. Trauma* 68 (4): 859–864.

Bednarski, R., Grimm, K., Harvey, R., and Lukasik, V.M. (2011). AAHA anesthesia guidelines for dogs and cats. *J. Am. Anim. Hosp. Assoc.* 47 (6): 377–385.

Berkenstadt, H., Friedman, Z., Preisman, S. et al. (2005). Pulse pressure and stroke volume variations during severe hemorrhage in ventilated dogs. *Br. J. Anesth.* 94: 721–726.

Blong, A.E., Epstein, K.L., and Brainard, B.M. (2013). in vitro effects of three formulations of hydroxyethyl starch solutions on coagulation and platelet function in horses. *Am. J. Vet. Res.* 74 (5): 712–720.

Boyd, C., Claus, M., Sharp, C. et al. (2019). Biomarkers of acute kidney injury in dogs after 6% hydroxyethyl starch 130/0.4 or Hartmann's solution: a randomized blinded clinical trial. *J. Vet. Emerg. Crit. Care* 29: 13056. https://doi.org/10.1111/vec.13056.

Boyd, C.J., Sharp, C.R., Claus, M.A. et al. (2021). Prospective randomized controlled blinded clinical trial evaluating biomarkers of acute kidney injury following 6% hydroxyethyl starch 130/0.4 or Hartmann's solution in dogs. *J. Vet. Emerg. Crit. Care 31* (3): 306–314.

Boysen, S.R. and Dorval, P. (2014). Effects of rapid intravenous 100% L-isomer lactated Ringer's administration on plasma lactate concentrations in healthy dogs. *J. Vet. Emerg. Crit. Care* 24 (5): 571–577.

Brunisholz, H.P., Schwarzwald, C.C., Bettschart-Wolfenberger, R. et al. (2015). Effects of 10% hydroxyethyl starch (HES 200/0.5) solution in intraoperative fluid therapy management of horses undergoing elective surgical procedures. *Vet. J.* 206: 398–403.

Bulger, E.M., Jurkovich, G.J., Nathens, A.B. et al. (2008). Hypertonic resuscitation of hypovolemic shock after blunt trauma: a randomized controlled trial. *Arch. Surg.* 143 (2): 139–148.

Carney, K.R., McKenzie, E.C., Mosley, C.A., and Payton, M.E. (2011). Evaluation of the effect of hetastarch and lactated ringer's solution on plasma colloid osmotic pressure in healthy llamas. *J. Am. Vet. Med. Assoc.* 238 (6): 768–772.

Celeita-Rodriguez, N., Teixeira-Neto, F.J., Garofalo, N.A. et al. (2019). Comparison of the diagnostic accuracy of dynamic and static preload indices to predict fluid responsiveness in mechanically ventilated, isoflurane anesthetized dogs. *Vet. Anesth. Analg.* 46: 276–288.

Chohan, A.S., Greene, S.A., Grubb, T.L. et al. (2011). Effects of 6% hetastarch (600/0.75) or lactated ringer's solution on hemostatic variables and clinical bleeding in healthy dogs anesthetized for orthopedic surgery. *Vet. Anaesth. Analg.* 38 (2): 94–105.

Cotton, B.A., Guy, J.S., Morris, J.A., and Abumrad, N.N. (2006). The cellular, metabolic and systemic consequences of aggressive fluid resuscitation strategies. *Shock* 26 (2): 115–121.

Dalmagro, T.L., Teixeira-Neto, F.J., Celeita-Rodrígues, N. et al. (2021). Comparison between pulse pressure variation and systolic pressure variation measured from a peripheral artery for accurately predictiing fluid responsiveness in mechanically ventilated dogs. *Vet. Anaesth. Analg.* 48 (4): 501–508.

Davis, H., Jensen, T., Johnson, A., and Knowles, P. (2013). 2013 AAHA/AAFP fluid therapy guidelines for dogs and cats. *J. Am. Anim. Hosp. Assoc.* 49 (3): 149–159.

Drozdzynska, M.J., Chang, Y.M., Stanzani, G., and Pelligand, L. (2018). Evaluation of the dynamic predictors of fluid responsiveness in dogs receiving goal-directed fluid therapy. *Vet. Anesth. Analg.* 45: 22–30.

Endo, Y., Tamura, T., Ishizuka, T. et al. (2017). Stroke volume variation (SVV) and pulse pressure variation (PPV) as indicators of fluid responsiveness in sevoflurane anesthetized mechanically ventilated euvolemic dogs. *J. Vet. Sci.* 79: 1437–1445.

Epstein, K.L., Bergren, A., Giguère, S., and Brainard, B.M. (2014). Cardiovascular, colloid osmotic pressure, and hemostatic effects of 2 formulations of hydroxyethyl starch in healthy horses. *J. Vet. Intern. Med.* 28: 223–233.

Falco, S., Bruno, B., Maurella, C. et al. (2012). in vitro evaluation of canine hemostasis following dilution with hydroxyethyl starch (130/0.4) via thromboelastometry. *J. Vet. Emerg. Crit. Care* 22 (6): 640–645.

Fantoni, D.T., Ida, K.K., Gimenes, A.M. et al. (2017). Pulse pressure variation as a guide for volume expansion in dogs undergoing orthopedic surgery. *Vet. Anesth. Analg.* 44: 710–718.

Fielding, C.L. and Magdesian, K.G. (2011). A comparison of hypertonic (7.2%) and isotonic (0.9%) saline for fluid resuscitation in horses: a randomized, double-blinded, clinical trial. *J. Vet. Intern. Med.* 25 (5): 1138–1143.

Gauthier, V., Holowaychuk, M.K., Kerr, C.L. et al. (2015). Effect of synthetic colloid administration on coagulation in healthy dogs and dogs with systemic inflammation. *J. Vet. Intern. Med.* 29 (1): 276–285.

Hadimioglu, N., Saadawy, I., Saglam, T. et al. (2008). The effect of different crystalloid solutions on acid-base balance and early kidney function after kidney transplantation. *Anesth. Analg.* 107 (1): 264–269.

Hahn, R.G. and Lyons, G. (2016). The half-life of infusion fluids. *Eur. J. Anesthesiol.* 33 (7): 475–482.

Hardy, J. (2009). Fluid therapy. In: *Equine Anesthesia: Monitoring and Emergency Therapy*, 2e (ed. W.W. Muir and J.A.E. Hubbell). St. Loius, MI: Saunders.

Hayes, G., Benedicenti, L., and Mathews, K. (2016). Retrospective cohort study on the incidence of acute kidney injury and death following hydroxyethyl starch (HES 10% 250/0.5/5:1) administration in dogs (2007–2010). *J. Vet. Emerg. Crit. Care* 26: 35–40.

Helmbold, K.A., Mellema, M.S., Hopper, K., and Epstein, S.E. (2014). The effect of hetastarch 670/0.75 administered in vivo as a constant rate infusion on platelet closure time in the dog. *J. Vet. Emerg. Crit. Care* 24 (4): 381–387.

Hüter, L., Simon, T.-P., Weinmann, L. et al. (2009). Hydroxyethylstarch impairs renal function and induces interstitial proliferation, macrophage infiltration and tubular damage in an isolated renal perfusion model. *Crit. Care* 13 (1): R23.

Iannucci, C., Dirkmann, D., Howard, J., and Adamik, K.N. (2021). A prospective randomized open-label trial on the comparative effects of 6% hydroxyethyl starch 130/0.4 versus polyionic isotonic crystalloids on coagulation parameters in dogs with spontaneous hemoperitoneum. *J. Vet. Emerg. Crit. Care* 31 (1): 32–42.

Jones, P.A., Tomasic, M., and Gentry, P.A. (1997). Oncotic, hemodilutional, and hemostatic effects of isotonic saline and hydroxyethyl starch solutions in clinically normal ponies. *Am. J. Vet. Res.* 58 (5): 541–548.

Jones, P.A., Bain, F.T., Byars, T.D. et al. (2001). Effect of hydroxyethyl starch infusion on colloid oncotic pressure in hypoproteinemic horses. *J. Am. Vet. Med. Assoc.* 218 (7): 1130–1135.

de Jonge, E. and Levi, M. (2001). Effects of different plasma substitutes on blood coagulation: a comparative review. *Crit. Care Med.* 29 (6): 1261–1267.

Jungheinrich, C. and Neff, T.A. (2005). Pharmacokinetics of hydroxyethyl starch. *Clin. Pharmacokinet.* 44 (7): 681–699.

Kirkendol, P.L., Pearson, J.E., and Robie, N.W. (1980). The cardiac and vascular effects of sodium glutamate. *Clin. Exp. Pharmacol. Physiol.* 7 (6): 617–625.

Kozek-Langenecker, S.A. (2005). Effects of hydroxyethyl starch solutions on hemostasis. *Anesthesiology* 103 (3): 654–660.

Lavu, H., Sell, N.M., Carter, T.I. et al. (2014). The HYSLAR trial. *Ann. Surg.* 260 (3): 445–455.

Leuschner, J., Opitz, J., Winkler, A. et al. (2003). Tissue storage of 14 c-labelled hydroxyethyl starch (HES) 130/0.4 and HES 200/0.5 after repeated intravenous administration to rats. *Drugs R D* 4 (6): 331–338.

Martin, A., Mendoza, J., Muriel, A. et al. (2019). Buffered solutions versus 0.9% saline for resuscitation in critically ill adults and children. *Cochrane Database Syst. Rev.* 7: 1–101. https://doi.org/10.1002/14651858.CD012247.pub2.

McAlister, V., Burns, K.E., Znajda, T., and Church, B. (2010). Hypertonic saline for perioperative fluid management. *Anesth. Analg.* 110 (5): 1506.

McFarlane, C. and Lee, A. (1994). A comparison of Plasmalyte 148 and 0.9% saline for intra-operative fluid replacement. *Anaesthesia* 49 (9): 779–781.

Miller, A.J., Barron, K.E., Proudman, C.J., and Dugdale, A.H.A. (2013). A prospective randomised study to compare the effects of preoperative hypertonic saline or pentastarch on haematological variables and long-term survival of surgical colic cases. *Equine Vet. J.* 45: 2–3.

Mortazavi, M.M., Romeo, A.K., Deep, A. et al. (2012). Hypertonic saline for treating raised intracranial pressure: literature review with meta-analysis. *J. Neurosurg.* 116 (1): 210–221.

Mouren, S., Delayance, S., Mion, G. et al. (1995). Mechanisms of increased myocardial contractility with hypertonic saline solutions in isolated blood-perfused rabbit hearts. *Anesth. Analg.* 81 (4): 777–782.

Myburgh, J.A., Finfer, S., Bellomo, R. et al. (2012). Hydroxyethyl starch or saline for fluid resuscitation in intensive care. *N. Engl. J. Med.* 367 (20): 1901–1911.

Navarro, L.H., Bloomstone, J.A., Auler, J.O. et al. (2015). Perioperative fluid therapy: a statement from the international fluid optimization group. *Perioper. Med. (London)* 4: 3.

Neto, A.S., Veelo, D.P., Peireira, V.G.M. et al. (2014). Fluid resuscitation with hydroxyethyl starches in patients with sepsis is associated with an increased incidence of acute kidney injury and use of renal replacement therapy: a systematic review and meta-analysis of the literature. *J. Crit. Care* 29 (1): 185.e1–185.e7.

Olinger, G.N., Werner, P.H., Bonchek, L.I., and Boerboom, L.E. (1979). Vasodilator effects of the sodium acetate in pooled protein fraction. *Ann. Surg.* 190 (3): 305–311.

Oliveira, R.P., Velasco, I., Soriano, F.G., and Friedman, G. (2002). Clinical review: hypertonic saline resuscitation in sepsis. *Crit. Care* 6 (5): 418–423.

Pantaleon, L.G., Furr, M.O., McKenzie, H.C. II, and Donaldson, L. (2006). Cardiovascular and pulmonary effects of hetastarch plus hypertonic saline solutions during experimental endotoxemia in anesthetized horses. *J. Vet. Intern. Med.* 20 (6): 1422–1428.

Perner, A., Haase, N., and Guttormsen, A.B. (2012). Hydroxyethyl starch 130/0.42 versus ringer's acetate in severe sepsis. *N. Engl. J. Med.* 367 (2): 124–134.

Raghunathan, K., Shaw, A.D., and Bagshaw, S.M. (2013). Fluids are drugs. *Curr. Opin. Crit. Care* 19 (4): 290–298.

Rhee, P., Burris, D., Kaufmann, C., and Pikoulis, M. (1998). Lactated ringer's solution resuscitation causes neutrophil activation after hemorrhagic shock. *J. Trauma* 44 (2): 313–319.

Rizoli, S.B., Rhind, S.G., and Shek, P.N. (2006). The immunomodulatory effects of hypertonic saline resuscitation in patients sustaining traumatic hemorrhagic shock. *Ann. Surg.* 243 (1): 47–57.

Scheingraber, S., Rehm, M., Sehmisch, C., and Finsterer, U. (1999). Rapid saline infusion produces hyperchloremic acidosis in patients undergoing gynecologic surgery. *Anesthesiology* 90 (5): 1265–1270.

Schnuelle, M., Hopster, K., and Hurcombe, S. (2020). Effects of intravenous administration of 7.2% hypertonic saline on cardiovascular parameters in healthy, anesthetized horses. *Vet. Anesth. Analg.* 47 (6): 855.

Schortgen, F., Girou, E., Deye, N., and Brochard, L. (2008). The risk associated with hyperoncotic colloids in patients with shock. *Intensive Care Med.* 34 (12): 2157–2168.

Schusser, G.F., Rieckhoff, K., and Ungemach, F.R. (2007). Effect of hydroxyethyl starch solution in normal horses and horses with colic or acute colitis. *J. Vet. Med. Ser. A* 54 (10): 592–598.

Shin, W., Kim, Y., and Bang, J. (2011). Lactate and liver function tests after living donor right hepatectomy: a comparison of solutions with and without lactate. *Acta Anaesth. Scand.* 55 (5): 558–564.

Shoemaker, W.C. and Hauser, C.J. (1979). Critique of crystalloid versus colloid therapy in shock and shock lung. *Crit. Care Med.* 7 (3): 117–124.

Sigrist, N.E., Kalin, N., and Dreyfus, A. (2017a). Changes in serum creatinine concentration and acute kidney injury (AKI) grade in dogs treated with hydroxyethyl starch 130/0.4 from 2013-2015. *J. Vet. Intern. Med.* 31: 434–441.

Sigrist, N.E., Kalin, N., and Dreyfus, A. (2017b). Effects of hydroxyethyl starch 130/0.4 on serum creatinine

concentration and development of acute kidney injury in nonazotemic cats. *J. Vet. Intern. Med.* 31: 1749–1756.

Silverstein, D.C., Aldrich, J., Haskins, S.C., and Drobatz, K.J. (2005). Assessment of changes in blood volume in response to resuscitative fluid administration in dogs. *J. Vet. Emerg. Crit. Care* 15 (3): 185–192.

Smart, L., Boyd, C.J., Claus, M.A. et al. (2018). Large volume crystalloid fluid is associated with increased hyaluronana shedding and inflammation in a canine hemorrhagic shock model. *Inflammation* 41: 1515–1523.

Tellan, G., Antonucci, A., Marandola, M. et al. (2008). Postoperative metabolic acidosis: use of three different fluid therapy models. *Chir. Ital.* 60 (1): 33–40.

Treib, J., Haass, A., and Pindur, G. (1996). All medium starches are not the same: influence of the degree of hydroxyethyl substitution of hydroxyethyl starch on plasma volume, hemorrheologic conditions, and coagulation. *Transfusion* 36 (5): 450–455.

Uchimido, R., Schmidt, E.P., and Shapiro, N.I. (2019). The glycocalyx: a novel diagnostic and therapeutic target in sepsis. *Crit. Care* 23: 16.

Valverde, A., Gianotti, G., Rioja-Garcia, E., and Hathway, A. (2012). Effects of high-volume, rapid-fluid therapy on cardiovascular function and hematological values during isoflurane-induced hypotension in healthy dogs. *Can. J. Vet. Res.* 76 (2): 99–108.

Veech, R.L. and Gitomer, W.L. (1988). The medical and metabolic consequences of administration of sodium acetate. *Adv. Enzyme Regul.* 27: 313–343.

Viljoen, A., Page, P.C., Fosgate, G.T., and Saulez, M.N. (2014). Coagulation, oncotic and haemodilutional effects of a third-generation hydroxyethyl starch (130/0.4) solution in horses. *Equine Vet. J.* 46 (6): 739–744.

Waters, J.H., Gottlieb, A., and Schoenwald, P. (2001). Normal saline versus lactated ringer's solution for intraoperative fluid management in patients undergoing abdominal aortic aneurysm repair: an outcome study. *Anesth. Analg.* 93 (4): 817–822.

Wendt-Hornickle, E.L., Snyder, L.B., Tang, R., and Johnson, R.A. (2011). The effects of lactated ringer's solution (LRS) or LRS and 6% hetastarch on the colloid osmotic pressure, total protein and osmolality in healthy horses under general anesthesia. *Vet. Anaesth. Analg.* 38 (4): 336–343.

Westphal, M., James, M.F.M., and Kozek-Langenecker, S. (2009). Hydroxyethyl starches. *Anesthesiology* 111 (1): 187–202.

Xu, J., Wang, S., He, L. et al. (2021). Hydroxyethyl starch 130/0.4 for volume replacement therapy in surgical patients: a systematic review and meta-analysis of randomized controlled trials. *Perioper. Med.* 10 (16).

Yozova, I.D., Howard, J., and Adamik, K.N. (2016). Retrospective evaluation of the effects of administration of tetrastarch (hydroxyethyl starch 130/0.4) on plasma creatinine concentration in dogs (2010-2013): 201 dogs. *J. Vet. Emerg. Crit. Care* 26: 568–577.

Yozova, I.D., Howard, J., and Adamik, K.N. (2017). Effect of tetrastarch (hydroxyethyl starch 130/0.4) on plasma creatinine concentration in cats: a retrospective analysis (2010-2015). *J. Feline Med. Surg.* 19: 1073–1079.

Zarychanski, R., Abou-Setta, A.M., Turgeon, A.F., and Houston, B.L. (2013). Association of hydroxyethyl starch administration with mortality and acute kidney injury in critically ill patients requiring volume resuscitation. *J. Am. Med. Assoc.* 309 (7): 678.

Zersen, K.M., Mama, K., and Mathis, J.C. (2019). Retrospective evaluation of paired plasma creatinine and chloride concentrations following hetastarch administration in anesthetized dogs (2002–2015): 244 cases. *J. Vet. Emerg. Crit. Care* 29 (3): 309–313.

31

Blood and Blood Products

Julien Guillaumin

Blood transfusion is a common practice in both small and large animals. Individual blood components can be used to improve tissue oxygen delivery (with red blood cells [RBC]); to replace blood proteins (e.g. coagulation factors, albumin) (with plasma); or to replace blood volume in exsanguinating patients (Lynch et al. 2015a, 2015b; Piek et al. 2008).

Blood component therapy is recommended in transfusion medicine. Separating fresh whole blood (FWB) in its various components allows for better individual use, improves storage and results in fewer adverse effects (Table 31.1) (Davidow 2013). In dogs, the most common reason for RBC transfusion is hemorrhage and for plasma transfusion is coagulopathy (Hann et al. 2014; Snow et al. 2010).

In cats, both component therapy and FWB transfusion is common, although it is less documented than in dogs. There is minimal data on horses or ruminants, where FWB is mostly used (Balcomb and Foster 2014; Hurcombe et al. 2007; Mudge 2014; Mudge 2015).

Pre-transfusion testing, especially establishment of the correct blood type and blood cross-matching is important to limit the risks of transfusion reactions (Tocci and Ewing 2009). Reactions can vary from life-threatening hemolysis in cases of incompatible transfusions, especially in cats and horses, to mild febrile reactions (Davidow 2013; Mudge 2014).

Packed Red Blood Cells

Packed RBCs (pRBCs) is the most commonly transfused blood product. pRBC is a refrigerated (2–6 °C) stored product obtained after FWB fractionation. Storage medium usually consists of Acid-Citrate-Dextrose (ACD), which allows for a 21-day shelf-life. Adenine (in CPDA) or other additives (e.g. Optisol*, Adsol*) can be added as a source of energy, increasing the shelf-life to 35 or 42 days, respectively (Davidow 2013).

The main indication for RBC transfusion is to treat anemia and improve oxygen delivery (DO_2). DO_2 is composed by cardiac output and arterial oxygen content (CaO_2). CaO_2 is equal $1.34 \times [Hb] \times SaO_2 + 0.003 \times PaO_2$ g/dl. Using normal values for each of the components, CaO_2 is equal to approximately 20 g/dl, with 19.7 g/dl being the oxygen present at the RBC surface, and only 0.3 g/dl being the dissolved oxygen. Therefore, the RBC is the most important part of oxygen *transportation* in the blood, whereas PaO_2 becomes the most important part of oxygen *diffusion* to the cells, for use in cellular adenosine triphosphate (ATP) formation. Transfusion of RBCs also increases blood volume and can improve DO_2 by increasing stroke volume and cardiac output.

In a retrospective study on more than 3000 canine cases, the most common reason for RBC transfusion was hemorrhage (68%), with neoplasia (36%) the leading reason for hemorrhage before trauma (13%) and surgical blood loss (12%). Hemolysis was the major cause of anemia in those dogs (16%), with immune-mediated hemolytic anemia accounting for 90% of these cases (Hann et al. 2014).

In a retrospective study on blood transfusion in 31 horses, 58% of horses received a blood transfusion secondary to blood loss, 26% due to hemolytic anemia and 16% due to erythropoietic failure (Hurcombe et al. 2007). The majority of the transfusions (91%) were whole blood transfusion (Hurcombe et al. 2007).

The decision of transfusion is based on clinical signs. If the anemia is chronic, compensatory mechanisms develop, aiming to maintain energy production. It includes maintenance of normal blood volume (through the renin–angiotensin–aldosterone and antidiuretic hormone systems), improvement of PaO_2, local vasoconstriction to direct blood flow to the most important organs, decreased activity to lower oxygen consumption, and changes in cellular metabolism toward anaerobic ATP production (i.e. hyperlactatemia).

Pharmacology in Veterinary Anesthesia and Analgesia, First Edition. Edited by Turi Aarnes and Phillip Lerche.
© 2024 John Wiley & Sons, Inc. Published 2024 by John Wiley & Sons, Inc.

Table 31.1 Types of blood products, and their components, available in veterinary medicine.

This blood product...	...contains:
Fresh whole blood (FWB)	Red blood cells (RBC), white blood cells, plasma, platelets
Packed red blood cells (pRBC)	Red blood cells, plasma
Fresh frozen plasma (FFP)	Clotting factors, albumin, immunoglobulins, plasma
Frozen plasma (>1 yr or >6 h)	Clotting factors (except FV and FVIII), immunoglobulins, albumin plasma
Cryoprecipitate	Factors VIII, XIII, von Willebrand factor, fibrinogen (Factor I)
Cryopoor plasma	Factors other than VIII, XIII, I and vWF – including vitamin K dependent factors
Platelet rich plasma (PRP) or platelet concentrate (PC)	Platelets, plasma

Therefore, the author uses ten criteria to determine an individual patient's need for an RBC transfusion:

1) Age and co-morbidity of the patient, as it can be related to the ability to develop compensatory mechanisms or oxygen consumption may be higher.
2) Chronicity of the anemia, which is directly related to the development of compensatory mechanisms.
3) Clinical signs is a challenging criteria, as 100% of anemic patients will have clinical signs, which varies from mild (e.g. lethargy, pale mucous membranes) to more severe (e.g. syncope, severe tachycardia). The author recommends transfusion in more severe cases.
4) Failure to maintain energy production, which is usually represented by hyperlactatemia.
5) Presence of blood loss, compared to the euvolemic anemic hemolytic patient.
6) The presence or absence of regenerative response, as the absence of regenerative response makes the patient at risk for more prolonged periods of anemia.
7) The cause of anemia, for example, the transfused RBCs will likely be destroyed by a hemolytic patient.
8) The risks associated with transfusion, depending especially on the screening availability or history of previous transfusion.
9) The need for an anesthesia, as the associated increase in the oxygen consumption may worsen the balance between oxygen supply and demand.
10) The hemoglobin (or hematocrit) level: in critically ill humans, RBC transfusions are recommended at a

hemoglobin level of 7 g/dl or hematocrit of 21% (decreased for the hemoglobin of 10 g/dl and hematocrit of 30% rule) unless the patient has clinically significant heart disease or sepsis, in which case, a level of 10 g/dl (hematocrit of 30%) is recommended (Dellinger et al. 2013; Hébert et al. 1999).

Studies showed that dogs receiving RBC transfusion have an average hematocrit of 18% (Hann et al. 2014). The usual goal of transfusion is to abate clinical signs, and reach a safer hematocrit, usually between 25% and 30%. Therefore, a hematocrit increase of approximately 10% is usually needed. An easy calculation is that 1 ml/kg of pRBCs will increase the patient's hematocrit by 1%. However, that rule of thumb has been challenged, and a 1.5 ml/kg may be required for the same effect. Clinicians can also use the following formula to predict a volume (ml) equal to "BW (kg) × blood volume (90 ml) × [(desired PCV − recipient PCV)/Donor PCV]" (Short et al. 2012). If using FWB, the first formula volume has to be doubled.

Blood Types and Pretransfusion Testing

Eight dog erythrocyte antigens (DEA) exist, with DEA 1.1, 1.2, and 7 being clinically significant. Recently, it has been shown that the DEA 1 group is a continuum from negative to strongly positive antigen expression, meaning that previously typed DEA 1.2+ and 1.3+ are just DEA 1+ (Acierno et al. 2014). The rule of thumb in canine RBC transfusion is that they do not have naturally occurring antibodies against DEA 1 blood type, but they will develop anti-DEA 1 antibody when in contact (i.e. transfused) with DEA 1 positive RBCs. Those antibodies will cause agglutination and hemolysis if DEA 1 positive blood is transfused again. Put in simple terms, dogs have a "free pass" on the first transfusion of RBCs. However, dogs have naturally occurring antibodies for some DEA types that will result in delayed reaction (e.g. DEA 3, DEA 4, DEA 5, and DEA 7). In 2007, a new common blood type named *Dal* was identified on Dalmatians with a presumed prevalence of 20%. Dalmatians lacking the *Dal* antigen are likely at risk of acute and delayed hemolytic reactions (Blais et al. 2007). A 2017 study showed that a high percentage of Doberman Pinchers and Shih Tzus, along with Dalmatians, lack the *Dal* antigen, making this clinically relevant for those species (Goulet et al. 2017). The prevalence of blood types and naturally occurring antibodies' presence is presented in Table 31.2. It is recommended that the blood type of all donors and recipients be known prior to transfusion (for at least DEA 1) so type-specific blood can be administered.

Table 31.2 Prevalence of blood types and naturally occurring antibodies.

DEA group	Population prevalence	Presence of naturally occurring antibody	Transfusion significance
1[a]	62%	No	Acute hemolytic reaction (<12h)
3	6%	Yes (20%)	Delayed reaction (i.e. decreased RBC survival)
4	98%	No	None
5	23%	Yes	Delayed reaction (i.e. decreased RBC survival)
6	98–99%	No	Unknown
7	45%	Yes (20–50%)	Delayed reaction (i.e. decreased RBC survival)
8	40%	No	None

[a] Previously known as 1.1 and 1.2. The blood group system DEA 1 is a continuum from negative to strongly positive antigen expression, meaning that previously typed DEA 1.2+ and DEA 1.3+ appears to be DEA 1+ (Acierno et al. 2014).
Source: Adapted from Hale (1995).

Cats have three major blood types A, B, and AB. A is the most common blood type (95–99% of cats in the US). Type B is less common in domestic breeds but is seen with more frequency in other breeds (e.g. Devon Rex, British Shorthair) or in other geographic locations (e.g. Turkey). Cats have naturally occurring circulating alloantibodies targeting the blood type they don't carry. Type B cats have more antigenic anti-A antibodies, and transfusion of a type B cat with A blood could result in severe hemolytic transfusion reaction. Type A cats have less antigenic anti-B antibodies so transfusion of B blood to a type A cat may result in a shorter life span of the transfused cells. Another erythrocyte antigen, called *Mik*, has also been described and can result in acute hemolytic reaction due to circulating alloantibodies. Due to the risk of reaction, it is recommended that all cats should be blood typed prior to transfusion. Because no test is available for detecting the *Mik* antigen, a crossmatch is also recommended prior to cat's transfusion, even if the cat has not been previously transfused. Crossmatch is done by mixing the RBC of the donor with the plasma of the recipient (major crossmatch) or the RBC of the recipient with the plasma of the donor (minor crossmatch) and observing for agglutination (Davidow 2013).

Horses have seven major blood systems (i.e. A, C, D, K, P, Q, and U) and 34 blood factors within those systems. Because of this, there is no true "universal" equine blood type. The incidence of Aa and Qa blood types is breed-dependent (Table 31.3). Horses have naturally occurring antibodies, and sensitized mares may also have anti-Aa hemolysins (Mudge 2015). In one study, 20% of Standardbred mares and 10% of Thoroughbred mares had antibodies detectable in hemolytic or saline agglutination tests. Most of the antibodies were specific for the Ca blood-group antigen of horses, but antibodies against Aa, Ab, Aa, Ab, Da, Df, Ka, Ua, or Qa blood-group antigens were also found. Antibodies to the Ca antigens cause weak agglutination and hemolytic crossmatch reactions, but the antibodies to Ca do not appear to produce a significant hemolytic reaction *in vivo* (Bailey 1982).

However, out of all equine blood types, Aa and Qa are the most antigenic and have been associated with neonatal isoerythrolysis, so the most appropriate equine donor is Aa and Qa negative. Other blood groups can occasionally give neonatal isoerythrolysis reactions, including Dc, Ua, Ab, and Pa.

Obviously, knowing the blood type of the recipient would be preferable (in addition to the donor). A point-of-care test for Ca using a monoclonal antibody exists, but if more information is needed, blood must be sent to an equine blood typing laboratory (Mudge 2015; Owens et al. 2008).

Cattle have 11 major blood group systems: A, B, C, F, J, L, M, R, S, T, and Z. The B group has over 60 different antigens, making it difficult to closely match donor and recipient. Some animals are J-negative and can develop antibodies against the J-antigen and develop transfusion reactions if transfused with J-positive blood. Therefore, donor cattle should be negative for factor J. Neonatal isoerythrolysis is not a naturally occurring phenomenon in cattle.

Transfusion Administration

RBC are administered through a 170–210 μm filter, available in commercial blood delivery sets. RBC are usually transfused in four hours in normovolemic patients, but can be transfused

Table 31.3 Percentage of animals in the listed breed that are negative for the listed factor.

System	Thoroughbred (%)	Arabian (%)	Standardbred (%)	Quarterhorse (%)
Aa-	15	18	44	51
Qa-	39	79	100	83

much faster, even as a bolus, in hypovolemic patients, such as those actively bleeding and exsanguinating. In theory, no medications or solutions other than 0.9% sodium chloride injection should be administered simultaneously with blood components through the same tubing. Blood should not be given concurrently with hyper- or hypotonic solutions or solutions containing dextrose alone, as they may cause swelling or lysis of red cells. Calcium-containing solutions (e.g. LRS) should also be avoided, as calcium may bind to citrate and "neutralize" the anticoagulant in the fluid line.

The American Association of Blood Banks Standards allows exceptions to the above restrictions either when the drug or solution has been approved by the Food and Drug Administration (FDA) for use with blood administration or there is documentation available to show that the addition is safe and does not adversely affect the blood or component. Acceptable solutions according to these criteria include plasma, 5% albumin, or plasma protein fraction. Certain solutions are compatible with blood or blood components as noted on the package inserts reviewed by the FDA, including Normosol-R and Plasmalyte-A. The literature reports the safe use of morphine, hydromorphone and meperidine administered as a bolus in the same tubing as red cells (*American Association of Blood Banks* 2016). This is especially important in anesthesia when monitoring for transfusion reactions can be limited.

It has been shown that it is preferable to use gravity instead of a fluid pump to better preserve transfused cells, although this concept has been challenged (McDevitt et al. 2011; Weeks et al. 2021).

Storage Lesions

Storage of RBCs is associated with biochemical, biomechanical and immunologic changes that affect red-cell viability, deformability, oxygen carrying capacity, microcirculatory flow and recipient response, collectively known as "storage lesions" (Obrador et al. 2015). It includes decreased ATP (which affect RBC deformability), decreased 2,3-bisphosphoglycerate (which increases RBC oxygen affinity, directly affecting organ oxygen offload), ammonia accumulation, oxidative damage, microparticles accumulation (which can lead to thrombosis) and RBC adhesion to endothelium. A recent meta-analysis in humans found that the transfusion of older stored RBC (using a cutoff as close to 21 days as possible) was associated with a significantly increased risk of death (Wang et al. 2012). Potential clinical consequences of RBC transfusion following development of storage lesions include risk of organ dysfunction, infections, immunomodulation and death (Obrador et al. 2015). In dogs, longer duration of RBC storage was associated with development of new or progressive coagulation failure and thromboembolic disease. Although there was no association between duration of RBC storage and overall survival, longer storage time was a negative risk for survival in the hemolytic anemia group in one large study (Hann et al. 2014).

Transfusion Reactions

Transfusion reactions are usually divided between acute immune-mediated transfusion reactions and non-immune-mediated transfusion reactions (Table 31.4). Non immune-mediated reactions include hemolysis (e.g. inappropriate collection, storage or administration), bacterial contamination, transfusion-associated circulatory overload (TACO), hypothermia (i.e. in case of rapid transfusion of inappropriately warmed products), citrate toxicity (causing hypocalcemia), transfusion-related immunomodulation (TRIM), or transfusion-associated acute lung injury (TRALI), which has been described in humans (Bux and

Table 31.4 List of transfusion reactions, clinical signs and appropriate therapy.

		Clinical signs	Treatment
Hemolytic reactions	Type II hypersensitivity	Vomiting, hypotension, tachycardia, tachypnea, pyrexia	Stop the transfusion, treat symptomatically, intravenous fluids to promote diuresis
Anaphylactic reactions	Type I hypersensitivity	Urticaria, pruritus, often with plasma products	Stop the transfusion, administer anti-histamines or small dose of steroids
Anaphylactic shock	Type I hypersensitivity	Cardiovascular collapse, dyspnea, seizures	Stop the transfusion, treat symptomatically with intravenous fluids, epinephrine
Leukocytes and platelet sensitivity reactions		Increase in body temperature of at least 1 °C	Stop the transfusion, may be re-started at a lower rate

Sachs 2007). Although TRALI is the leading cause of transfusion-related morbidity and mortality in humans, it is due to antibodies directed against human neutrophil antigens present in the plasma of predominantly multiparous female blood donors (Bux and Sachs 2007). Therefore, it is unclear if other species can develop TRALI.

There are limited data regarding veterinary transfusion reactions. In a retrospective study of more than 300 canine plasma transfusions, the only side effects were fever, pruritis and anxiety, noted in less than 1% of cases (Snow et al. 2010). Acute transfusion reactions to RBCs were documented in 15% of cases in another retrospective study on 136 dogs, with fever and vomiting documented in 53% and 18% of cases, respectively (Bruce et al. 2015).

Please note that neonatal isoerythrolysis is possible in horses and cats, but its presence in dogs necessitates a previously sensitized (i.e. transfused) bitch with an incompatible sire (Polkes et al. 2008; Silvestre-Ferreira and Pastor 2010). The effects of leukoreduction (the removal of white blood cells from pRBC) on inflammation markers or overall transfusion reactions post-transfusion showed contradictory results, with some studies demonstrating a decrease in markers of inflammation, especially in critically ill dogs (McMichael et al. 2010; Stefani et al. 2021), while other studies did not show any differences (Bosch Lozano et al. 2019; Radulescu et al. 2021).

Plasma Products

Fresh Frozen Plasma (FFP) is plasma separated from RBC after FWB donation, and frozen within 6–8 hours of collection or stored for less than 1–2 years at T < −30 °C. Frozen Plasma (FP) is FFP stored for >1–2 years or frozen after 6–8 hours of collection. Frozen Plasma is thought to be depleted of co-factors V and VIII, although this human dogma has been challenged in veterinary medicine (Urban et al. 2013). The maximum storage length is five years for FFP/FP (Davidow 2013).

The major indication for FFP transfusion is coagulopathies (e.g. anticoagulant rodenticide intoxication, hemophilia A or B). It is considered an inappropriate use of FFP to treat prolonged clotting times without evidence of clinical bleeding (including for a minor procedure), or for α-macroglobulins replacement in pancreatitis, or anti-thrombin replacement in disseminated intravascular coagulation (Davidow 2013; Rozanski et al. 2001). A secondary indication is species-specific albumin replacement. However, the volume needed for this indication (between 20 and 50 ml/kg depending on reference and formula used) may predispose some patients to volume overload, and an increased cost of hospitalization. Calculations of volume are presented later under the albumin section.

FFP transfusion may also be administered to exsanguinating patients, where it is recommended to provide a 1 : 1 ratio of RBC to plasma products (Sihler and Napolitano 2009). In that case, the volume transfused may reach a total of approximately 20–40 ml/kg.

Considering that clotting times become increased when 70–80% of clotting factors are missing, and that 10–20 ml/kg of FFP will provide a 10–20% replacement of clotting factors, the rule of thumb is to transfuse 10–20 ml/kg of FFP to patients with clinical bleeding due to a coagulopathy. After thawing in (ideally) a warm water bath at 37 °C (which usually takes around 35–45 minutes), FFP can be administered to patients over four hours in normovolemic patients, or faster is hypovolemia is present.

In horses, plasma has been used for treatment of disseminated intravascular coagulation, coagulopathy, species-specific albumin replacement as well as failure of transfer of passive immunity (FTP) in foals (Mudge 2015). Plasma transfusion is recommended for FTP in neonatal foals over 12 hours of age. Commercially available fresh frozen hyperimmune plasma is mostly commonly used for this indication (Mudge 2015). FFP transfusion can also be used for FTP in camelid crias (Anderson et al. 2008). In a five-year study of 107 horses receiving plasma transfusions, 69 were foals (including 62 neonates) and 38 were horses of more than 30 days of age. The main reason for FFP transfusion in neonatal foals was high risk for sepsis. In almost 80% of those, FTP (IgG < 800 mg/dl) was documented. In adult horses, the most common reason for FFP transfusion was acute gastrointestinal (GI) disease with clinical evidence of systemic inflammatory response syndrome and biochemical confirmation of protein-losing enteropathy. Plasma transfusion for coagulopathy was rare in that study (Hardefeldt et al. 2010).

FFP can be further divided in cryoprecipitate and cryopoor plasma (CPP) because different factors have different freezing points. Cryoprecipitate is made by partially thawing FFP at 4 °C for 24 hours and removing the supernatant, which leaves the semi-solid cryoprecipitate, containing factor VIII, fibrinogen and von Willebrand factor (vWf) (Davidow 2013). The supernatant is CPP, also known as cryosupernatant or cryodepleted plasma. Cryoprecipitate is indicated for bleeding associated with vWf deficiency or hemophilia A, as well as hypofibrinogenemia cases such as the exsanguinating patient, whereas CPP is listed for use in vitamin K antagonist rodenticide toxicities and hypoalbuminemia (Davidow 2013). The dose of cryoprecipitate is 12–20 ml/kg (corresponding usually to 1 unit per 10 kg). The dose for CPP is 10–20 ml/kg.

Albumin

Albumin is one of the most important proteins in the body. Its physiologic functions are numerous, including transport proteins for many elements (e.g. hormones, drugs), free radical scavenging, maintenance of oncotic pressure (albumin is responsible for 70–80% of the oncotic pressure), anti-apoptotic effects, anticoagulant and anti-thrombotic, acid–base buffering and anti-inflammatory properties (Craft and Powell 2012; Rozga et al. 2013).

Albumin is a small molecule (66 kDa), synthetized by the liver. Hepatic onco-receptors regulate its synthesis. The usual quoted volume of distribution is 30% intravascular and 70% extravascular, but the transcapillary rate is very slow, as it can take several days for albumin to move across the endothelial membrane. After albumin infusion to healthy patients, only 90% is still intravascular after 2 hours, and 25% after two days. However, that transcapillary flux can be increased up to 13 times in critical illness (e.g. infection, shock, burns). Moreover, albumin's half-life (8.2 days in dogs) is inversely dependent on its concentration, with hypoalbuminemia increasing its half-life (Boldt 2010).

It is well documented that hypoalbuminemia carries a worse prognosis in critically ill humans. Each 1.0 g/dl decrease in albumin increases odds of mortality by 137% and morbidity by 89% (Vincent 2009). This is also documented in veterinary medicine (Roux et al. 2013).

Although hypoalbuminemia is a risk factor for death and worsening illness, the link between albumin replacement and improved outcome continues to be debated. In humans, there is evidence that albumin replacement does not improve mortality for perioperative patients, in the heterogenous intensive care unit (ICU) population, or in trauma patients (Boldt 2010; Roberts et al. 2011; SAFE Study Investigators et al. 2011). Albumin transfusion is contra-indicated in traumatic brain injury (TBI) patients. Potential indications for albumin transfusion in humans are burns (Rozga et al. 2013) and severe sepsis/septic shock (Caironi et al. 2014; SAFE Study Investigators et al. 2011).

Veterinary sources of albumin are canine-specific albumin (CSA) contained in plasma, or human serum albumin (HSA) (Craft and Powell 2012). There are controversies about both the use of plasma as a source of CSA, and HSA in veterinary medicine. The albumin content of FFP is relatively low, around 2.9 g/dl (corresponding to 2.9% albumin), so a large volume of FFP is required to raise albumin level. Most veterinary references use the following formula (Dose (g) = 10 × desired delta albumin × weight (kg) × 0.3) to calculate the amount (in grams) of albumin to provide to patients. Using a 0.029 g/ml albumin in FFP, one can calculate that 50 ml/kg of FFP is needed to raise the albumin level by 0.5 g/

dl (i.e. 2 ml/kg/h). Therefore, volume and costs are legitimate concerns for the use of FFP for CSA replacement.

The origin of the "veterinary" formula is difficult to track and seems to be related to albumin replacement using total parenteral nutrition in studies from the 1980s (Brown et al. 1987). Human studies investigating albumin use for critically ill patients, especially severe sepsis/septic shock, use a fixed dose of 0.875 g/kg/day, regardless of "desired albumin level", which is more than three times less than the volume required to raise the albumin level by 1 g/dl using the "veterinary" formula (Caironi et al. 2014; SAFE Study Investigators et al. 2011).

The use of HSA (25%, or 250 mg/ml, or 0.25 g/ml) is an attractive solution to replenish albumin using lower volumes, although HSA may be cost prohibitive. However, there is only 80% homology between CSA and HSA (Francis et al. 2007). Therefore, transfusion of HSA to dogs will result in the production of anti-HSA antibodies possibly leading to acute anaphylactic reaction and the death of HSA-transfused dogs re-exposed to HSA (Adamantos et al. 2009). Moreover, approximately 8–10% of dogs have naturally occurring anti-HSA antibodies, so may develop an acute anaphylactic reaction during their first HSA transfusion (Adamantos et al. 2009). There are several reports of clinical use of HSA in dogs but concerns about immunization and acute (type I) and delayed (type III) hypersensitivity reactions limit its use, and using HSA multiple times in a patient is strictly contraindicated (Adamantos et al. 2009; Powell et al. 2013; Trow et al. 2008). Also, it is documented that approximately 7% of critically ill dogs receiving HSA will have serious complications (Trow et al. 2008; Viganó et al. 2010). Therefore, clinicians must carefully weigh risk-benefits in individual patients before use.

Platelets

Platelet transfusion is challenging in veterinary medicine. Platelets are anucleate, discoid-shaped, cytoplasmic fragments essential in primary hemostasis (Guillaumin et al. 2008). Platelets are extremely fragile and their viability is compromised when refrigerated or frozen. Therefore, the gold standard in human medicine is platelet concentrate (PC) harvested from FWB kept at room temperature under constant agitation for up to seven days (Marwaha and Sharma 2009). Such a product is not commercially available in veterinary medicine, so veterinarians mostly rely on FWB, fresh platelet-rich plasma (PRP) or fresh PC (Callan et al. 2009). Any fresh product has to be used within 6–8 hours. Platelets can be harvested following a platelet-rich plasma protocol (i.e. hard and soft spin), the buffy coat technique or apheresis (Hoareau et al. 2014).

Preservation of platelets using cryopreservation or the freeze-dry cycle (i.e. lyophilized) have been investigated. A lyophilized canine platelet product is commercially available but its hemostatic activity is unknown (Davidow et al. 2012). A small clinical trial using lyophilized platelets in dogs showed no adverse effects and suggests some efficacy (Goggs et al. 2020). In humans, it appears that some cryopreserved or lyophilized platelets may preserve some hemostatic activity through microparticles (Slichter et al. 2014). Indications for platelet transfusion are severe, life-threatening bleeding due to thrombocytopenia. Commonly quoted platelet numbers that put the patient at risk for spontaneous bleeding are between 5 and 20 000/μl. Besides the platelet count, presence of active bleeding (e.g. dropping hematocrit, visible bleeding) in life-threatening anatomic locations (e.g. lungs, brain), or invasive procedures, are indications for platelet transfusion (Davidow 2013). It is usually recommended that one unit of platelet product should be provided per 10 kg of patients. Please note that the goal may not be an increase in platelet numbers (which can be modest, especially at 24 hours), but an improvement in clinical bleeding.

The Exsanguinating Patient Requiring Emergency Anesthesia and Surgery

In humans, 10% of trauma victims will receive a blood transfusion and 10% of those will require transfusion for exsanguinating hemorrhage. In patients with acute massive bleeding, compensatory mechanisms usually associated with anemia do not have the time to develop and the dogma *"if your patient is losing blood, resuscitate with blood"* makes physiologic sense. The concept of Damage Control Resuscitation (DCR) is a resuscitation strategy used to control damages associated with both the initial trauma and the resuscitation efforts.

In humans, DCR includes early surgical intervention, which necessitates emergency anesthesia in an unstable patient. Because the goal of the emergency surgery is stabilization of the patient, there is no time to wait for patient stabilization to perform anesthesia. DCR also includes hypotensive resuscitation (i.e. goal for systolic blood pressure during resuscitation of 80–100 mmHg until hemorrhage control is achieved); hemostatic resuscitation strategies including early use of FFP and an FFP : RBC : Platelets ratio of 1:1:1; use of antifibrinolytics and other non-surgical hemostatic agents; and minimizing crystalloid use.

Massive transfusion (MT) is most commonly defined as transfusion of a volume of blood products superior to a blood volume (e.g. 80–90 ml/kg for dogs) over 24 hours. In humans, the most common reason for MT is trauma. In a canine study, hemoabdomen accounted for 60% of MT patients (67% from abdominal neoplasia and 33% from trauma); 20% for trauma (all were hemoabdomen) and 13% for gastric dilatation volvulus (GDV) (Jutkowitz et al. 2002). Early identification of the patient needing MT is extremely important and many clinicians struggle with that concept. Recently, human studies have been focusing on admission criteria and scoring systems to predict massive transfusion. The most common are the Assessment of Blood Consumption Score (ABC score) and the Trauma Associated Severe Hemorrhage Score (TASH). All scoring systems are based on logic and objective criteria such as hypotension, tachycardia, base excess or lactate, hemoglobin level on presentation, presence of hemoperitoneum or complex long bone/pelvic fracture (Sihler and Napolitano 2009). A three-point criteria to assess the need for MT in veterinary patients would be (i) evidence of blood loss: hemoabdomen or external hemorrhage; (ii) severe hypovolemia: based on heart rate, blood pressure, mental state and lactate level; and (iii) anemia at admission: most human data shows that a cutoff of hematocrit of 30% is both specific and sensitive (Hardy et al. 2004; Nunez et al. 2009; Yücel et al. 2006).

The use of blood products in MT includes the use of RBC, FFP, cryoprecipitate and platelet product. The rapid infusion of large amounts of compatible blood to acutely bleeding patients is at the center of MT. Retrospective studies in human combat victims showed that mortality increased with low FFP/RBC : 65% for a 1:8 ratio and 19% for a 1:1.4 ratio. Therefore, an FFP/RBC ratio of 1:1 has been advocated in MT patients. Those concepts are now being applied to both civilian and military trauma and for both blunt and penetrating injuries in human medicine. It is important to note that early FFP use is associated with a reduction of the overall volume used (Saxena et al. 2013). In a veterinary study, the mean volume of RBC and FFP were 66.5 and 22.2 ml/kg respectively (Jutkowitz et al. 2002). Cryoprecipitate is transfused in MT as a source of fibrinogen and is recommended when plasma fibrinogen levels are 100–200 mg/dl depending on the source (Sihler and Napolitano 2009). Platelet transfusion is recommended when the platelet count is below 50 000–100 000/μl, although platelet transfusion is challenging in veterinary medicine.

Blood transfusion is an important part of veterinary medicine and may help with patient's stabilization before anesthesia. Blood products should be considered as drugs, with specific mechanisms of action, pharmacology, indications, contraindications, and side effects.

References

Acierno, M.M., Raj, K., and Giger, U. (2014). DEA 1 expression on dog erythrocytes analyzed by immunochromatographic and flow cytometric techniques. *J. Vet. Intern. Med. Am. Coll. Vet. Intern. Med.* 28: 592–598. https://doi.org/10.1111/jvim.12321.

Adamantos, S., Chan, D.L., Goggs, R., and Humm, K. (2009). Risk of immunologic reactions to human serum albumin solutions. *J. Small Anim. Pract.* 50: 206. https://doi.org/10.1111/j.1748-5827.2009.00752.x.

(2016). *Standards for Blood Banks and Transfusion Services*, 30e. American Association of Blood Banks, AABB.

Anderson, D., Cotton, T., and Whitehead, C. (2008). Neonatal care for camelids: breeding to birthing to weaning. In: *Veterinary Medical Continuing Education*. Manhattan, KS: Kansas State University.

Bailey, E. (1982). Prevalence of anti-red blood cell antibodies in the serum and colostrum of mares and its relationship to neonatal isoerythrolysis. *Am. J. Vet. Res.* 43: 1917–1921.

Balcomb, C. and Foster, D. (2014). Update on the use of blood and blood products in ruminants. *Vet. Clin. N. Am. Food Anim. Pract.* 30: 455–474. vii. https://doi.org/10.1016/j.cvfa.2014.04.001.

Blais, M.-C., Berman, L., Oakley, D.A., and Giger, U. (2007). Canine Dal blood type: a red cell antigen lacking in some Dalmatians. *J. Vet. Intern. Med. Am. Coll. Vet. Intern. Med.* 21: 281–286.

Boldt, J. (2010). Use of albumin: an update. *Br. J. Anaesth.* 104: 276–284. https://doi.org/10.1093/bja/aep393.

Bosch Lozano, L., Blois, S.L., Wood, R.D. et al. (2019). A pilot study evaluating the effects of prestorage leukoreduction on markers of inflammation in critically ill dogs receiving a blood transfusion. *J. Vet. Emerg. Crit. Care (San Antonio)* 29 (4): 385–390. https://doi.org/10.1111/vec.12857.

Brown, R.O., Bradley, J.E., and Luther, R.W. (1987). Response of serum albumin concentrations to albumin supplementation during central total parenteral nutrition. *Clin. Pharm.* 6: 222–226.

Bruce, J.A., Kriese-Anderson, L., Bruce, A.M., and Pittman, J.R. (2015). Effect of premedication and other factors on the occurrence of acute transfusion reactions in dogs. *J. Vet. Emerg. Crit. Care San Antonio Tex 2001* 25: 620–630. https://doi.org/10.1111/vec.12327.

Bux, J. and Sachs, U.J.H. (2007). The pathogenesis of transfusion-related acute lung injury (TRALI). *Br. J. Haematol.* 136: 788–799. https://doi.org/10.1111/j.1365-2141.2007.06492.x.

Caironi, P., Tognoni, G., Masson, S. et al. (2014). Albumin replacement in patients with severe sepsis or septic shock. *N. Engl. J. Med.* 370: 1412–1421. https://doi.org/10.1056/NEJMoa1305727.

Callan, M.B., Appleman, E.H., and Sachais, B.S. (2009). Canine platelet transfusions. *J. Vet. Emerg. Crit. Care San Antonio Tex 2001* 19: 401–415. https://doi.org/10.1111/j.1476-4431.2009.00454.x.

Craft, E.M. and Powell, L.L. (2012). The use of canine-specific albumin in dogs with septic peritonitis. *J. Vet. Emerg. Crit. Care San Antonio Tex 2001* 22: 631–639. https://doi.org/10.1111/j.1476-4431.2012.00819.x.

Davidow, B. (2013). Transfusion medicine in small animals. *Vet. Clin. N. Am. Small Anim. Pract.* 43: 735–756. https://doi.org/10.1016/j.cvsm.2013.03.007.

Davidow, E.B., Brainard, B., Martin, L.G. et al. (2012). Use of fresh platelet concentrate or lyophilized platelets in thrombocytopenic dogs with clinical signs of hemorrhage: a preliminary trial in 37 dogs. *J. Vet. Emerg. Crit. Care San Antonio Tex 2001* 22: 116–125. https://doi.org/10.1111/j.1476-4431.2011.00710.x.

Dellinger, R.P., Levy, M.M., Rhodes, A. et al. (2013). Surviving sepsis campaign: international guidelines for management of severe sepsis and septic shock, 2012. *Intensive Care Med.* 39: 165–228. https://doi.org/10.1007/s00134-012-2769-8.

Francis, A.H., Martin, L.G., Haldorson, G.J. et al. (2007). Adverse reactions suggestive of type III hypersensitivity in six healthy dogs given human albumin. *J. Am. Vet. Med. Assoc.* 230: 873–879. https://doi.org/10.2460/javma.230.6.873.

Goggs, R., Brainard, B.M., LeVine, D.N. et al. (2020). Lyophilized platelets versus cryopreserved platelets for management of bleeding in thrombocytopenic dogs: a multicenter randomized clinical trial. *J. Vet. Intern. Med.* 34 (6): 2384–2397. https://doi.org/10.1111/jvim.15922.

Goulet, S., Giger, U., Arsenault, J. et al. (2017). Prevalence and mode of inheritance of the Dal blood Group in Dogs in North America. *J. Vet. Intern. Med.* 31 (3): 751–758. https://doi.org/10.1111/jvim.14693.

Guillaumin, J., Jandrey, K.E., Norris, J.W., and Tablin, F. (2008). Assessment of a dimethyl sulfoxide-stabilized frozen canine platelet concentrate. *Am. J. Vet. Res.* 69: 1580–1586. https://doi.org/10.2460/ajvr.69.12.1580.

Hale, A.S. (1995). Canine blood groups and their importance in veterinary transfusion medicine. *Vet. Clin. N. Am. Small Anim. Pract.* 25: 1323–1332.

Hann, L., Brown, D.C., King, L.G., and Callan, M.B. (2014). Effect of duration of packed red blood cell storage on morbidity and mortality in dogs after transfusion: 3,095 cases (2001–2010). *J. Vet. Intern. Med. Am. Coll. Vet. Intern. Med.* 28: 1830–1837. https://doi.org/10.1111/jvim.12430.

Hardefeldt, L.Y., Keuler, N., and Peek, S.F. (2010). Incidence of transfusion reactions to commercial equine plasma.

J. Vet. Emerg. Crit. Care San Antonio Tex 2001 20: 421–425. https://doi.org/10.1111/j.1476-4431.2010.00545.x.

Hardy, J.-F., De Moerloose, P., Samama, M., and Groupe d'intérêt en Hémostase Périopératoire (2004). Massive transfusion and coagulopathy: pathophysiology and implications for clinical management. *Can. J. Anaesth. J. Can. Anesth.* 51: 293–310. https://doi.org/10.1007/BF03018233.

Hébert, P.C., Wells, G., Blajchman, M.A. et al. (1999). A multicenter, randomized, controlled clinical trial of transfusion requirements in critical care. Transfusion requirements in critical care investigators, Canadian critical care trials group. *N. Engl. J. Med.* 340: 409–417. https://doi.org/10.1056/NEJM199902113400601.

Hoareau, G.L., Jandrey, K.E., Burges, J. et al. (2014). Comparison of the platelet-rich plasma and buffy coat protocols for preparation of canine platelet concentrates. *Vet. Clin. Pathol. Am. Soc. Vet. Clin. Pathol.* 43: 513–518. https://doi.org/10.1111/vcp.12195.

Hurcombe, S.D., Mudge, M.C., and Hinchcliff, K.W. (2007). Clinical and clinicopathologic variables in adult horses receiving blood transfusions: 31 cases (1999–2005). *J. Am. Vet. Med. Assoc.* 231: 267–274. https://doi.org/10.2460/javma.231.2.267.

Jutkowitz, L.A., Rozanski, E.A., Moreau, J.A., and Rush, J.E. (2002). Massive transfusion in dogs: 15 cases (1997–2001). *J. Am. Vet. Med. Assoc.* 220: 1664–1669.

Lynch, A.M., O'Toole, T.E., and Hamilton, J. (2015a). Transfusion practices for treatment of dogs undergoing splenectomy for splenic masses: 542 cases (2001–2012). *J. Am. Vet. Med. Assoc.* 247: 636–642. https://doi.org/10.2460/javma.247.6.636.

Lynch, A.M., O'Toole, T.E., and Respess, M. (2015b). Transfusion practices for treatment of dogs hospitalized following trauma: 125 cases (2008–2013). *J. Am. Vet. Med. Assoc.* 247: 643–649. https://doi.org/10.2460/javma.247.6.643.

Marwaha, N. and Sharma, R.R. (2009). Consensus and controversies in platelet transfusion. *Transfus. Apher. Sci. Off. J. World Apher. Assoc. Off. J. Eur. Soc. Haemapheresis* 41: 127–133. https://doi.org/10.1016/j.transci.2009.07.004.

McDevitt, R.I., Ruaux, C.G., and Baltzer, W.I. (2011). Influence of transfusion technique on survival of autologous red blood cells in the dog. *J. Vet. Emerg. Crit. Care San Antonio Tex 2001* 21: 209–216. https://doi.org/10.1111/j.1476-4431.2011.00634.x.

McMichael, M.A., Smith, S.A., Galligan, A. et al. (2010). Effect of leukoreduction on transfusion-induced inflammation in dogs. *J. Vet. Intern. Med. Am. Coll. Vet. Intern. Med.* 24: 1131–1137. https://doi.org/10.1111/j.1939-1676.2010.0561.x.

Mudge, M.C. (2014). Acute hemorrhage and blood transfusions in horses. *Vet. Clin. N. Am. Equine Pract.* 30: 427–436. ix. https://doi.org/10.1016/j.cveq.2014.04.004.

Mudge, M.C. (2015). Blood and blood product transfusions in horses. In: *Equine Fluid Therapy*, 301–311. Wiley.

Nunez, T.C., Voskresensky, I.V., Dossett, L.A. et al. (2009). Early prediction of massive transfusion in trauma: simple as ABC (assessment of blood consumption)? *J. Trauma* 66: 346–352. https://doi.org/10.1097/TA.0b013e3181961c35.

Obrador, R., Musulin, S., and Hansen, B. (2015). Red blood cell storage lesion. *J. Vet. Emerg. Crit. Care San Antonio Tex 2001* 25: 187–199. https://doi.org/10.1111/vec.12252.

Owens, S.D., Snipes, J., Magdesian, K.G., and Christopher, M.M. (2008). Evaluation of a rapid agglutination method for detection of equine red cell surface antigens (Ca and Aa) as part of pretransfusion testing. *Vet. Clin. Pathol.* 37: 49–56. https://doi.org/10.1111/j.1939-165X.2008.00003.x.

Piek, C.J., Junius, G., Dekker, A. et al. (2008). Idiopathic immune-mediated hemolytic anemia: treatment outcome and prognostic factors in 149 dogs. *J. Vet. Intern. Med. Am. Coll. Vet. Intern. Med.* 22: 366–373. https://doi.org/10.1111/j.1939-1676.2008.0060.x.

Polkes, A.C., Giguère, S., Lester, G.D., and Bain, F.T. (2008). Factors associated with outcome in foals with neonatal isoerythrolysis (72 cases, 1988–2003). *J. Vet. Intern. Med. Am. Coll. Vet. Intern. Med.* 22: 1216–1222. https://doi.org/10.1111/j.1939-1676.2008.0171.x.

Powell, C., Thompson, L., and Murtaugh, R.J. (2013). Type III hypersensitivity reaction with immune complex deposition in 2 critically ill dogs administered human serum albumin. *J. Vet. Emerg. Crit. Care San Antonio Tex 2001* 23: 598–604. https://doi.org/10.1111/vec.12085.

Radulescu, S.M., Skulberg, R., McDonald, C. et al. (2021). Randomized double-blinded clinical trial on acute transfusion reactions in dogs receiving leukoreduced versus nonleukoreduced packed red blood cells. *J. Vet. Intern. Med.* 35 (3): 1325–1332. https://doi.org/10.1111/jvim.16138.

Roberts, I., Blackhall, K., Alderson, P. et al. (2011). Human albumin solution for resuscitation and volume expansion in critically ill patients. *Cochrane Database Syst. Rev.* CD001208. https://doi.org/10.1002/14651858.CD001208.pub4.

Roux, F., Deswarte, A., and Deschamps, J. (2013). Prognostic value of preoperative serum albumin level in canine and feline gastro-intestinal surgery: 150 cases (2009–2012). *J. Vet. Emerg. Crit. Care* 23: S17.

Rozanski, E.A., Hughes, D., and Giger, U. (2001). The effect of heparin and fresh frozen plasma on plasma antithrombin III activity, prothrombin time and activated partial thromboplastin time in critically ill dogs. *J. Vet. Emerg. Crit. Care* 11: 15–21.

Rozga, J., Piątek, T., and Małkowski, P. (2013). Human albumin: old, new, and emerging applications. *Ann. Transplant. Q. Pol. Transplant. Soc.* 18: 205–217. https://doi.org/10.12659/AOT.889188.

SAFE Study Investigators, Finfer, S., McEvoy, S. et al. (2011). Impact of albumin compared to saline on organ function and mortality of patients with severe sepsis. *Intensive Care Med.* 37: 86–96. https://doi.org/10.1007/s00134-010-2039-6.

Saxena, A., Chua, T.C., Fransi, S. et al. (2013). Effectiveness of early and aggressive administration of fresh frozen plasma to reduce massive blood transfusion during cytoreductive surgery. *J. Gastrointest. Oncol.* 4: 30–39. https://doi.org/10.3978/j.issn.2078-6891.2012.046.

Short, J.L., Diehl, S., Seshadri, R., and Serrano, S. (2012). Accuracy of formulas used to predict post-transfusion packed cell volume rise in anemic dogs. *J. Vet. Emerg. Crit. Care San Antonio Tex 2001* 22: 428–434. https://doi.org/10.1111/j.1476-4431.2012.00773.x.

Sihler, K.C. and Napolitano, L.M. (2009). Massive transfusion: new insights. *Chest* 136: 1654–1667. https://doi.org/10.1378/chest.09-0251.

Silvestre-Ferreira, A.C. and Pastor, J. (2010). Feline neonatal isoerythrolysis and the importance of feline blood types. *Vet. Med. Int.* 2010: 753726. https://doi.org/10.4061/2010/753726.

Slichter, S.J., Jones, M., Ransom, J. et al. (2014). Review of in vivo studies of dimethyl sulfoxide cryopreserved platelets. *Transfus. Med. Rev.* 28: 212–225. https://doi.org/10.1016/j.tmrv.2014.09.001.

Snow, S.J., Ari Jutkowitz, L., and Brown, A.J. (2010). Trends in plasma transfusion at a veterinary teaching hospital: 308 patients (1996–1998 and 2006–2008). *J. Vet. Emerg. Crit. Care San Antonio Tex 2001* 20: 441–445. https://doi.org/10.1111/j.1476-4431.2010.00557.x.

Stefani, A., Capello, K., Carminato, A. et al. (2021). Effects of leukoreduction on storage lesions in whole blood and blood components of dogs. *J. Vet. Intern. Med.* 35 (2): 936–945. https://doi.org/10.1111/jvim.16039.

Tocci, L.J. and Ewing, P.J. (2009). Increasing patient safety in veterinary transfusion medicine: an overview of pretransfusion testing. *J. Vet. Emerg. Crit. Care San Antonio Tex 2001* 19: 66–73. https://doi.org/10.1111/j.1476-4431.2009.00387.x.

Trow, A.V., Rozanski, E.A., Delaforcade, A.M., and Chan, D.L. (2008). Evaluation of use of human albumin in critically ill dogs: 73 cases (2003–2006). *J. Am. Vet. Med. Assoc.* 233: 607–612. https://doi.org/10.2460/javma.233.4.607.

Urban, R., Guillermo Couto, C., and Iazbik, M.C. (2013). Evaluation of hemostatic activity of canine frozen plasma for transfusion by thromboelastography. *J. Vet. Intern. Med. Am. Coll. Vet. Intern. Med.* 27: 964–969. https://doi.org/10.1111/jvim.12097.

Viganó, F., Perissinotto, L., and Bosco, V.R.F. (2010). Administration of 5% human serum albumin in critically ill small animal patients with hypoalbuminemia: 418 dogs and 170 cats (1994–2008). *J. Vet. Emerg. Crit. Care San Antonio Tex 2001* 20: 237–243. https://doi.org/10.1111/j.1476-4431.2010.00526.x.

Vincent, J.-L. (2009). Relevance of albumin in modern critical care medicine. *Best Pract. Res. Clin. Anaesthesiol.* 23: 183–191.

Wang, D., Sun, J., Solomon, S.B. et al. (2012). Transfusion of older stored blood and risk of death: a meta-analysis. *Transfusion (Paris)* 52: 1184–1195. https://doi.org/10.1111/j.1537-2995.2011.03466.

Weeks, J.M., Motsinger-Reif, A.A., and Reems, M.M. (2021). in vitro iatrogenic hemolysis of canine packed red blood cells during various rapid transfusion techniques. *J. Vet. Emerg. Crit. Care (San Antonio)* 31 (1): 25–31. https://doi.org/10.1111/vec.13020.

Yücel, N., Lefering, R., Maegele, M. et al. (2006). Trauma Associated Severe Hemorrhage (TASH)-Score: probability of mass transfusion as surrogate for life threatening hemorrhage after multiple trauma. *J. Trauma* 60: 1228–1236. discussion 1236–1237. https://doi.org/10.1097/01.ta.0000220386.84012.bf.

Index

Note: Page numbers in "*italics*" represent figures and "**bold**" page number represents tables in text.